Neurodevelopmental Disorders

Developmental Cognitive Neuroscience
Mark Johnson and Bruce Pennington, editors

Neurodevelopmental Disorders, Helen Tager-Flusberg, editor, 1999

Neurodevelopmental Disorders

edited by Helen Tager-Flusberg

A Bradford Book
The MIT Press
Cambridge, Massachusetts
London, England

This book was set in Palatino by Asco Typesetters, Hong Kong and was printed and bound in the United States of America.

Library of Congress Cataloging-in-Publication Data

Neurodevelopmental disorders / edited by Helen Tager-Flusberg.
   p. cm. — (Developmental cognitive neuroscience)
"A Bradford book."
Includes bibliographical references and index.
ISBN 0-262-20116-X (hc : alk. paper)
  1. Developmental disabilities—Etiology. 2. Pediatric neuropsychilogy. 3. Developmental neurobiology. 4. Cognitive neuroscience. I. Tager-Flusberg, Helen. II. Series.
  [DNLM: 1. Mental Retardation—genetics. 2. Child Development Disorders, Pervasive— etiology. 3. Learning Disorders—etiology. 4. Developmental Disabilities—etiology.
WS 107.5.B4N494 1999]
RJ506.D47N48 1999
618.92′8—dc21
DNLM/DLC
for Library of Congress   98-26850
                                                        CIP

Contents

Series Foreword

Mark H. Johnson and Bruce F. Pennington

This volume is the first in a new series on developmental cognitive neuroscience, which is a new discipline concerned with the relation between the developing brain and the emergence of psychological abilities during infancy and childhood. This rapidly expanding field integrates information from both normal and abnormal development in both humans and other species and tackles fundamental issues such as the plasticity and maturation of the developing brain.

One of the strong claims of developmental cognitive neuroscience is that a comprehensive understanding of mature cognition cannot be attained without understanding both the normal and abnormal development of the human brain. In other words, we cannot understand how the mature system works until we understand how it is constructed in development, and we cannot fully understand that process of normal construction without understanding how development may go awry. The current volume provides a state-of-the-science introduction to how development may go awry.

Specifically, the present volume is concerned with abnormal human development and covers a wide range of neurodevelopmental disorders, both those that are currently defined behaviorally, such as autism and dyslexia, and those with known genetic etiologies, such as fragile X syndrome and Williams syndrome. These two kinds of disorders offer complementary strategies for understanding atypical development. In behaviorally defined disorders, one works "backward" from an altered trajectory of cognitive and social development to underlying brain mechanisms and ultimately to genetic and environmental risk factors that cause the perturbation in development. In genetically defined disorders, one works forward from the genotype to identify (1) other etiological factors that modify its expression, (2) underlying brain mechanisms, and (3) the resulting altered trajectory of cognitive and social development. The long-term goal of both strategies is to understand how the interplay of genetic and environmental risk factors alters brain development to produce a distinct profile of behavioral strengths and weaknesses. Both strategies depend on an intimate interaction with studies of typical brain-behavior development.

These two strategies may be contrasted with the study of patients with acquired lesions in both classical neuropsychology and much of current cognitive neuroscience. Such lesion studies usually ignore development, are often focused on localizing functions, and suffer from the methodological weakness that acquired lesions are essentially an irreproducible natural experiment. In contrast, in these two strategies, the altered genotype is a reproducible "lesion" that must be understood developmentally, and can be modeled and manipulated in experiments involving animal models.

Finally, we anticipate that the present volume will leave the reader with a clear impression of both the current achievements, and the future prospects, for a cognitive neuroscience approach to developmental disorders.

Preface

These are exciting times for research on children with neurodevelopmental disorders. Historically, there has always been a strong interest in studying atypical populations because, as "experiments in nature," they offer a window on abnormal development and provide insights into normal developmental processes. Until recently, however, studies into the genetic bases of syndromes, neuroanatomical research, and psychological investigations were carried out quite independently; people working in one field knew little or nothing about research being conducted in other disciplines on the same population. The recent explosion of advances across all disciplines in the cognitive and biological sciences has fundamentally changed the landscape in this field. This book was conceived and developed to present some views of this new landscape.

The human genome project provided a major impetus for discovering the molecular basis of many neurodevelopmental disorders, bringing to fruition decades of work in behavioral and clinical genetics. As we approach the end of the decade of the brain, the technological advances now available in both structural and functional neuroimaging allow us to view living, thinking brains in stunning detail. Concurrently, conceptual and methodological advances in the cognitive sciences have yielded a rich set of sophisticated conceptions about the design and operation of the human mind. The synthesis of ideas and methods across these disciplines has led to the beginning of a new era in the field of neurodevelopmental disorders, in which studies are being designed to yield integrated findings on genetic etiology, neuropathology, and cognitive development. These studies provide fundamentally new ways of looking at the intersection between biology and psychology, as is amply illustrated throughout the chapters in this book.

Part I includes an introductory chapter in which I provide an overview of the history, methods, and developments in the fields that contribute to current research on neurodevelopmental disorders. This introduction also describes the cognitive neuroscience perspective, which guides this new interdisciplinary research program.

Parts II and III contain a series of chapters on genetically based neuro developmental disorders. Case studies are included to provide descriptions of the syndromes and especially to illustrate the variability that is found among children with disorders of the same etiology. Two or more chapters are devoted to every syndrome covered in these sections. In this way, different research perspectives, views, and ways of integrating across disciplines may be considered. Part II (chapters 2–11) focuses on disorders of known etiology, illustrating many different genetic mechanisms, whereas the chapters in Part III (chapters 12–18) focus on complex genetic disorders for which no specific genes have yet been found.

In Part IV, the final section of the book, neurodevelopmental disorders are explored from wider perspectives, including neurobehavioral teratology, sensory disorder, brain damage, and the field of psychiatry. The chapters on teratology (chapters 19 and 20) highlight the common principles that underlie neurodevelopmental disorders that result from either genetic or prenatal exposure to environmental agents, which affect brain development. Chapter 21 discusses the rare and intriguing condition called *synesthesia*, in which cognitive distortions occur at the sensory and perceptual level. This is unlike neurodevelopmental disorders in which only higher-level cognitive domains (such as language, visuospatial, or social cognition) are affected. The next chapter (chapter 22) summarizes research on hydrocephalus, which is defined on the basis of brain dysmorphology rather than by behavioral or physical features. Because it is common in several different neurodevelopmental disorders, hydrocephalus can provide an important model from which to view such disorders. Chapter 23 addresses the development of language in children who have sustained focal lesions in various brain regions. The studies discussed in this chapter challenge the traditional theories of brain and language and provide strong evidence for taking a constrained plasticity view of development. In the final chapter (chapter 24), child psychiatry and clinical genetic perspectives are presented, illustrated by considering two additional genetically based disorders: Tourette syndrome and Marfan syndrome.

One of my primary objectives in editing this book is to cross-fertilize the conceptual models and methods that have been developed in explorations of different disorders or disciplines. By bringing together research that cuts across such a diverse range of syndromes, disorders, and disciplines, I hope that new work in this broad field will be stimulated. The ultimate goal is to understand for each disorder how mutations in genetic material lead to specific alterations in neural development that are realized in unique patterns of cognition and behavior. My aim in this book is to argue that this goal will be achieved by developing and expanding on the cognitive neuroscience perspective that is now beginning to frame research in this field.

Acknowledgments

The idea for this book came from the contributors themselves, whose work on neurodevelopmental disorders has had a profound influence on my own thinking and research program on neurodevelopmental disorders.

Soon after the book was in progress, the National Institute of Child Health and Human Development (NICHD) sponsored a conference that was held at the National Institutes of Health campus in Bethesda, Maryland, in March 1996. The conference, "Cognitive Neuroscience and Neurodevelopmental Disorders: Conceptual and Methodological Challenges," provided an important and invaluable opportunity for many of the contributors to this volume to meet, present, and discuss their research. The conference was made possible by the Mental Retardation and Developmental Disabilities Branch and the Human Learning and Behavior Branch at NICHD. I especially thank Dr. Marie Bristol and Dr. Reid Lyon, who organized the conference, and Dr. Duane Alexander, the Director of NICHD, for his support. This conference was cosponsored by a grant from the March of Dimes Birth Defects Foundation (4 FY 95-1148).

My work on this book has been supported by research grants from the NICHD (RO1 HD -33470) and the National Institute on Deafness and Communication Disorders (RO1 DC 01234; PO1 DC 03610). I am grateful for the support that my work has received over the years from these institutions and for the vision that they have provided to the field of neurodevelopmental disorders.

I am especially grateful to my colleagues at both the University of Massachusetts and the Shriver Center whose advice, knowledge, and friendship have meant so much to me. Jane Adams introduced me to the field of neurobehavioral teratology and taught me everything I know about developmental neuropsychology; Kate Sullivan has been a close friend and collaborator for more than a decade; and Robert Joseph has enriched my clinical perspective on neurodevelopmental disorders.

Finally, I offer my special thanks to Amy Brand at The MIT Press, for her support, faith, encouragement and, especially, her patience!

·

I Introduction

1 An Introduction to Research on Neurodevelopmental Disorders from a Cognitive Neuroscience Perspective

Helen Tager-Flusberg

The last decade has witnessed revolutionary changes in the field of neurodevelopmental disorders. These changes have taken place simultaneously in several different disciplines: molecular biology, behavioral genetics, developmental neurobiology, neuroimaging technology, cognitive science, and developmental psychology. Significant advances in each of these disciplines have radically changed the questions, conceptual frameworks, and research methodologies that have led to dramatic advances in our understanding of genetic causes and the neuropathological underpinnings of cognitive and behavioral deficits across a wide range of neurodevelopmental disorders. These changes have important consequences for individuals with disorders ranging from Down syndrome to dyslexia to autism.

New paradigms of research have provided insights into the role of genes in regulating neural development and organization and into their expression at the cognitive level. Furthermore, the significance of a developmental perspective is becoming increasingly salient as we begin to recognize that genetic factors are integrally linked with environmental variables from the earliest embryological stages to influence the development and organization of dynamic and complex neural systems. This awareness has led to the recognition that the impact of a developmental disorder on the brain, cognition, and behavior must be conceptualized in ways fundamentally different from the measured effects of an acquired lesion to an adult brain.

The chapters in this book bring together some of this new knowledge as a first step in the creation of a new scientific frontier: the integration of molecular genetics with a developmental cognitive neuroscience. The ultimate goal is to understand the basic mechanisms that explain how genes and environmental processes contribute to the development of specific structures and regions of the brain. In turn, we need to elucidate the mechanisms that explain how basic brain structures and function are directly related to specific cognitive processes. That goal also requires us to appreciate both the constraints and the plasticity that are present at neural and behavioral levels and account for particular developmental patterns in the context of neurodevelopmental disorders.

Clearly, we are many decades away from integrating genetics, neurobiology, and developmental cognitive science into a unified view of how the mind develops and functions. Nevertheless, over the last few years, we have begun to take the first steps in this direction. The chapters in this volume provide illustrations of some of these initial achievements from the unique perspective of disorders of development.

In this chapter, we present the historical and methodological background of research on neurodevelopmental disorders from the vantage point of mental retardation and learning disabilities. Then an overview is provided of the exciting conceptual and technological innovations that have been made in genetics, neurobiology, and cognitive science, innovations that allow us to ask new questions about the nature of neurodevelopmental disorders. The concluding section focuses on what interdisciplinary integration across these fields from a developmental approach can offer toward creating new conceptual frameworks within which we can direct future research on neurodevelopmental disorders.

HISTORICAL BACKGROUND

The field of mental retardation has had a rich and lengthy history of research into the psychological characteristics of retarded individuals ranging in age from birth to adulthood. Much of this work has provided important information, particularly of an applied nature, that has significantly improved the lives of retarded people and their families. During this same period, geneticists worked independently to identify the genetic abnormalities that cause mental retardation in significant numbers of cases. To date, more than 1,000 known genetic causes of mental retardation have been found (Moser, 1992), and the rapid rate of identifying new genetic markers for additional retardation syndromes is likely to continue over the next few years, spurred on by the remarkable achievements of the human genome project.

Remarkably, until recently neither of these groups of researchers paid attention to research being conducted in the other discipline (Hodapp & Dykens, 1994). For psychologists and other social scientists working in mental retardation, the only variable of interest was level of global impairment, typically measured by intelligence quotient (IQ). The source of impairment did not arouse interest, nor was much attention paid either to within-child patterns of cognitive strengths and weakness or to defining cognitive phenotypes associated with different disorders. Clinical geneticists, meanwhile, were more concerned with different profiles associated with specific genetic etiologies, however they limited their description of such profiles to physical features, including dysmorphology and malformations, medical complications, salient traits and (perhaps) degree of retardation. Geneticists recognized the significance of classifying different retardation syndromes, though they paid little attention to cognitive features of the syndromes they studied.

Why were psychologists not interested in exploring syndrome-specific aspects of cognition and behavior in mental retardation? One explanation has to do with the theories that dominated psychology. During the early and middle decades of this century, the behaviorist perspective was the primary approach taken by psychological researchers in this field. Within behaviorism, the central focus was directed exclusively toward observable behaviors, response repertoires, and controlling stimuli (rewards and punishments). The nature and age of the organism and underlying brain and cognitive processes were not considered relevant or appropriate for study. Thus, for behaviorists, different psychological characteristics that might be associated with different genetic syndromes comprised a topic outside their conceptual framework.

By the 1970s, the cognitive revolution in psychology had taken hold, and research on mental retardation began to explore aspects of cognitive functioning. At this point, research started from a Piagetian perspective, which incorporated a strong developmental focus. Again, however, the universalist bias within Piaget's developmental theory and its emphasis on *general* cognitive structures and processes led most researchers to neglect the key variables of genetic syndrome and specific cognitive domains. However, exceptions were beginning to emerge at this time as seen in the seminal research by Hermelin and O' Connor (1970) on cognitive deficits in autism and in a focus on psychological functioning in Down syndrome, the most common and easily identifiable genetic syndrome of mental retardation (e.g., Gibson, 1978). These studies paved the way for a new approach to the study of mental retardation that would explore syndrome-specific profiles of cognitive sparing and deficit using established tools and paradigms from psychometrics and cognitive psychology.

Research on learning disabilities followed a history parallel to that of mental retardation. Early on, the construct of "minimal brain dysfunction" was used to cover a wide range of children who showed "soft" neurological signs and learning difficulties but had no clear evidence of frank brain damage. Grouping diverse children under the umbrella of minimal brain dysfunction produced major confusion and questions about the heterogeneity of the children and their particular kinds of problems (Fletcher, 1994). Only when researchers began the task of classifying learning difficulties into discrete subtypes was progress made in understanding specific aspects of the underlying etiology and unique cognitive deficits associated with various learning and attentional disorders. By the 1980s a clear recognition, both in mental retardation and in the related field of learning disabilities, corroborated that progress in understanding the neuropathology associated with a particular disorder depended on paying careful attention to issues of classification (genetic or other), subtypes, and definition.

METHODOLOGICAL ISSUES

The last 20 years has seen great advances in our understanding of the underlying cognitive and behavioral profiles of a number of different syndromes (e.g., Broman & Grafman, 1994). The call for studies on behavioral phenotypes has energized this field by initiating research that explores specific links between genetic abnormalities and psychological profiles (e.g., Dykens, 1995). Yet, a considerable number of conceptual and methodological problems still plague research in this area and significantly limit the rate of progress. Questions remain about the definition of a behavioral phenotype, and studies continue to be conducted that do not meet minimal design standards.

The construct of a behavioral phenotype can be taken to imply that for each identifiable genetic syndrome, a unique, invariant, and specific behavioral pattern is directly linked to the underlying genetic abnormality. Significant problems are associated with such a stringent definition (Flint, 1996). For example, with few exceptions, difficulty arises in finding a behavioral pattern in all and only members of a particular genetic population. This definition ignores the crucial fact of variability. Within any syndrome exists considerable phenotypic variability, some of which may be traced to developmental level or plasticity, some to prenatal, family, or experiential factors, and some to genetic variability. To accommodate such variability, Dykens (1995) suggested that we define a behavioral phenotype in terms of a heightened probability of a behavior or cognitive feature that characterizes a particular syndrome. Such phenotypic characteristics may not be unique or pathognomic because overlap occurs across syndromes.

Some significant limitations arise in measuring the uniqueness of a particular feature of a behavioral phenotype if inadequate assessment tools are used (Flint, 1996). At the cognitive level, for example, relying exclusively on such psychometric measures as IQ tests precludes the investigation of features that are not included in such measures. Examples include a detailed analysis of the language profile that might characterize a disorder such as Down syndrome or the visuospatial deficits that might be associated uniquely with either Williams syndrome or Turner syndrome. IQ tests do not provide this kind of information. Other psychometric measures may also lack the sensitivity needed to identify subtle features associated with a particular linguistic or spatial deficit. Furthermore, no comparable measures of affect or social functioning exist to advance our understanding of either autism or fragile X syndrome, if we remain limited to using existing psychometric tools. We return to these issues of methodological approaches in exploring cognitive profiles associated with specific syndromes in a later section of this chapter on Cognitive Psychology and Neurodevelopmental Disorders.

Other methodological concerns can be found also in the literature on behavioral phenotypes. One serious problem is the absence of appropriate comparison groups in many studies; without them, judging whether one has identified deficits that are unique to a syndrome is not possible. Exactly who to include in a comparison group and how to match subjects across groups are the subjects of significant controversy. Some studies limit themselves to a control group of normally developing individuals who are age-matched to the group of interest. The problem with this approach is that retarded individuals across a broad range of syndromes differ from normals on virtually all measurable characteristics; therefore, it does not allow for a clearer delineation of a particular phenotype.

A more sophisticated solution is to include a comparison group that not only controls for age but for developmental level. Thus, other groups of retarded individuals often are considered for comparison purposes. These groups may include either a different, clearly identifiable syndrome or a group of mentally retarded subjects in whom the disorder's etiology is unknown. Both benefits and limitations are associated with each of these alternatives. Choosing another clearly defined syndrome allows one to compare two different phenotypes. For example, research by Bellugi et al. (e.g., Bellugi et al., 1994) on Williams syndrome typically has included Down syndrome as a comparison group. However, comparing individuals with Williams syndrome to a group of individuals who well may have specific impairments in language, particularly in morphosyntax, does not clarify whether Williams syndrome involves genuine sparing in this domain (because these individuals perform significantly better than do the Down syndrome comparison subjects on measures of morphosyntax) or just relative sparing (i.e., their language is at their overall mental age level but significantly better than their visuospatial skills). This concern is less likely to arise if a group with mental retardation of unknown etiology is included. However, this kind of group is significantly more heterogeneous than is that which includes individuals with a well-defined syndrome, most likely including a "mixed bag" of different genetic syndromes and other types of developmental disorders, thus presenting other limitations by introducing more variance. One compromise that has been advocated by several research groups is to include all three kinds of comparison groups: normals, a group with a contrasting well-defined syndrome, and a group with mental retardation of unknown etiology (Denckla, 1994).

The inclusion of comparison groups raises the issue of how the groups should be matched. Again, studies that focus on defining the phenotype of a particular syndrome often fall short by not matching on all the relevant variables. These include, at a minimum, age and developmental level. Typically, IQ tests are used for matching on developmental level, but one must take care to use a sensitive measure of IQ that covers the full range of intellectual impairment found in the population of interest. Specifically, many tests do not go below an IQ of 40, though it is not unusual to find across a range of neurodevelopmental disorders individuals whose IQ falls below this level. If research on defining the phenotype includes a focus on language or language-related performance, groups should be matched on language ability, again using sensitive standardized measures. Also, as both language and IQ are influenced by family background variables, including socioeconomic level as a matching variable is important.

The majority of studies conducted these days do include comparison groups that are matched on at least some key variables. However, other methodological pitfalls affect studies in this area. To include a sufficiently large sample, studies often include subjects that vary widely in age, thus obscuring the role of developmental and experiential factors. This approach might raise difficulties because possibly behavioral phenotypes may be expressed more clearly only at younger ages; older children and adults might have found ways for compensating areas of deficit using alternative strategies. From this viewpoint, 5-year-old children with autism and Down syndrome, for example, may be significantly more different and show clearer syndrome-specific phenotypic expression than would 25-year-old adults with these disorders. Another concern is the observation in some syndromes of a measurable decline in IQ by adolescence (e.g., fragile X syndrome), which would influence studies that included a wide age range.

One final methodological issue is the inclusion of heterogeneous groups of subjects. As we have noted, all neurodevelopmental disorders are inherently variable, especially at the level of phenotypic expression. Even in well-defined single-gene disorders, such as fragile X syndrome, a wide range is seen in IQ, for example. Heterogeneity is compounded when we look at more complex disorders, such as the spectrum of autistic disorders, in which IQ varies from profoundly retarded to superior, and the phenotypic expression of the core characteristics is similarly disparate. On the one hand, studies focusing on behavioral phenotypes must capture the full range and variability that is found in any disorder. On the other hand, if the goal is to search for the genetic and neurobiological bases of a disorder, including such heterogeneity can be a serious liability because of a greater chance of including false-positives, which will adversely affect chances for success. Research studies designed to address these goals might better include more homogeneous groups that are defined using conservative criteria.

Research on the psychological characteristics of neurodevelopmental disorders has advanced considerably in recent years as a result of increased awareness about how to resolve methodological concerns. At the same time, room still exists for more sophisticated and rigorous procedures that are sensitive to the kinds of questions that studies seek to address. Furthermore, the recent explosion of studies that focus on the neurobiological impairments in different disorders using advances in both structural and functional neuroimaging must consider also all these methodological issues. Thus far, progress in this area has been limited by lack of attention to these concerns (Filipek, 1996). One of the major limitations that all researchers face is the rarity of the populations we seek to study, which creates an impact on the size of the samples that can be included. The future of work in this area lies in advances in statistical analyses that allow one to address sophisticated, theoretically driven questions using small samples (Bates & Appelbaum, 1994; Bakeman & Robinson, 1997).

GENETICS AND NEURODEVELOPMENTAL DISORDERS

The technical and conceptual advances that have taken place in molecular genetics over the last decade have sparked revolutionary changes in our understanding of neurodevelopmental disorders. The advent of recombinant DNA technology led the development of positional cloning: isolating a gene solely on the basis of its location on a particular chromosome. Using these genetic mapping techniques allows one to locate a gene without regard to how it works, so that genes that cause diseases may be discovered without any prior biological clue about its protein products, where it is expressed, and how it functions at the biochemical level.

Initially, an explosion of interest was seen in Mendelian disorders: straightforward, single-gene disorders that follow classic recessive or dominant inheritance patterns. The best-known example of this kind of disorder in the neurodevelopmental literature is phenylketonuria (PKU), a metabolic disorder that leads to mental retardation if left untreated by dietary restrictions. Most cases of PKU are due to the altered function of the enzyme phenylalanine hydroxylase, which has been linked to chromosome 12 (Lidsky et al., 1984). However, research on the molecular basis of PKU has demonstrated that genetics does not provide simple answers, even when dealing with a well-understood single-gene disorder. More than 60 different mutations of the gene associated with PKU have been identified, some of which are associated with variations in phenotypic expression. Now recognized is the existence of variants of classic PKU that reflect mutations in others enzymes and cofactors involved in phenylalanine metabolism (Simonoff et al., 1996).

The lesson to be learned from the PKU example is that the genetic basis of even a well-characterized Mendelian neurodevelopmental disorder is complex and highly variable. We can no longer look at genetics in an unsophisticated way or as a means for providing simple answers to our questions about etiology. The effects of genes on behavioral function are pleiotropic and probabilistic; these effects may provide important clues to the wide range in IQ and to variable cognitive and behavioral expression that we see across all genetically based neurodevelopmental disorders (Simonoff et al., 1996).

The study of the genetic basis of different neurodevelopmental disorders illustrates the variety of mechanisms that are involved in the genetic transmission of disease (see part II, chapters 2–11). The most common causes of neurodevelopmental disorders can be linked to chromosomal anomalies called *aneuploidies*, in which all or part of a complete chromosome may be absent or added, as in trisomies. Chromosomal abnormalities may involve autosomes, as in trisomy 21, better known as *Down syndrome* (see chapters 8 and 9), or sex chromosomes, as in Turner syndrome, in which one of the X chromosomes is missing in girls with this disorder (see chapters 10 and 11). Typically, sex chromosomal anomalies produce less devastating impairments than those in autosomal aneuploidies. Our understanding of the mechanisms by which such chromosomal anomalies cause retardation or learning disabilities is decidedly rudimentary. Perhaps absent genetic material means that the gene product needed for normal morphogenesis is not provided or that additional genetic material leads to the overproduction of gene products that interfere with development (Bregman & Hodapp, 1991).

The most common form of inherited mental retardation is fragile X syndrome, which accounts for perhaps half of all X-linked retardation syndromes (see chapters 2 and 3). It illustrates one of the most intriguing genetic patterns associated with a single-gene disorder that was only recently discovered (Verkerk et al., 1991). This pattern is called the *trinucleotide repeat pattern*, which exhibits interesting generational effects called *anticipation*. Carriers of the fragile X mutation have longer-than-normal DNA nucleotide repeat patterns [cytosine-guanine-guanine (CGG)], but these premutation levels are not sufficient to disrupt the normal functioning of the gene. Female carriers pass on to the next generation even longer repeat sequences, to reach a full mutation leading to the disruption of the pre–messenger RNA transcription process. Since the discovery of the trinucleotide pattern in fragile X syndrome, other disorders also have been found to involve a similar genetic mechanism (e.g., Huntington disease). Interestingly, all the known disorders that fit this genetic pattern involve the central nervous system, and some have speculated that it may be the most important cause of neurally based psychiatric disorders (Ross et al., 1993).

Other genetic causes of mental retardation involve microscopic or submicroscopic deletions that can be found in different regions of particular chromosomes, which almost always arise spontaneously. Such disorders tend to be quite rare, including Williams syndrome and Prader-Willi syndrome. The deleted regions include more than one gene (though the exact number is not yet known for any disorder) and well may be variable. Disorders that involve microdeletions lead to a complex of phenotypic characteristics, including medical, physical, and neuropsychological features. Likely, many new syndromes associated with this kind of genetic basis remain to be identified (Flint et al., 1995).

All cases of Williams syndrome are associated with a microdeletion on the long arm of chromosome 7, and it does not seem to matter on which chromosome 7 the deletion occurs (see chapters 4 and 5). In contast, only some 70% to 75% of individuals with Prader-Willi syndrome show evidence of a microdeletion in the critical region of the long arm of chromosome 15, and it occurs always on the paternally derived chromosome (see chapters 6 and 7). The remaining 25% to 30% of individuals with Prader-Willi syndrome have inherited both copies of chromosome 15 from the mother and, therefore, are missing the paternal genes on the critical region of that chromosome (Butler, 1990; Magenis et al., 1990). This kind of genetic abnormality is known as an *imprinting* disorder, illustrating a new kind of genetic mechanism that had not been previously known in humans.

This brief overview of the range of genetic abnormalities that are associated with syndromes of mental retardation demonstrates the complexity and variability of genetic etiologies that have been discovered thus far by molecular biologists. At the same time, certain other known neurodevelopmental disorders do not fit any of these known patterns; instead, they fall into the category of "complex" disorders (see part III, chapters 12–18). Complex disorders are defined as inherited traits, which do not show classic single-gene Mendelian patterns, covering a large number of both medical and psychological diseases. The next stage in the genetics revolution will be to conquer the challenges posed by complex traits (Lander & Schork, 1994).

The first step in identifying a disorder as involving complex genetic patterns of inheritance is to conduct twin and family studies that establish whether the disorder is indeed of genetic origin. Considerable success has been achieved in these kinds of behavioral genetics studies for a number of neurodevelopmental disorders, including dyslexia (see chapters 12 and 13), specific language impairment (see chapters 14 and 15), and autism (see chapters 16–18). Then, using family data, segregation analyses or pedigree analyses are performed to determine the genetic model that best explains the pattern of inheritance. The final steps in this kind of research involve linkage studies or population-based association analysis and consequent physical mapping of the genes in question.

However, many complications arise in finding the genetic markers for complex disorders; the reason is why so few genes associated with complex neurodevelopmental and other psychiatric disorders have actually been identified (Risch, 1990). The basic assumptions of traditional linkage analysis probably do not hold in these cases (Pauls, 1993). Genetic heterogeneity is possible (i.e., several different mutations in different loci, each causing the disorder). Another possibility is that the disorder is the result of several genes, each causing a small effect in isolation, which cannot be detected easily in linkage studies (Lombroso et al., 1994). Also possible is incomplete penetrance, in which the genotype affects the probability of developing the disorder but does not fully determine the outcome (Lander & Schork, 1994).

Studies into the genetic bases of both simple and complex disorders all focus on identifying genes that explain variation in the phenotype associated with that disorder. In most cases, the relationship between the genes and the resulting phenotypic variation actually is quite indirect. Genes may determine behavior through interactions with a network of other similar genes so that the specific effects result from a disturbance in the balance of the network rather than in a particular gene. Furthermore, genes may participate in a number of different such networks (Flint, 1996). In this view, the relationship between genes and behavior involves a network of interacting factors, each with a degree of redundancy, rather than a linear link between a mutant gene to a specific, yet distant, phenotype. Finally, in some cases, the gene (or genes) associated with a disorder actually may not be a "disease" gene; instead, it may be responsible for normal variation in the behavior associated with it. Now, apparently, this likely is the case for one of the gene linkages that has been identified for dyslexia (see chapters 12 and 13). This more complex and indirect perspective that can be applied to the genetic bass of neurodevelopmental disorders suggests that we must be cautious in the way we describe achievements in finding genes or genetic markers associated with a particular disorders.

NEUROBIOLOGY AND NEURODEVELOPMENTAL DISORDERS

Neurodevelopmental disorders now are recognized to arise from either endogenous (i.e., genetic) or exogenous disturbances in brain development, often beginning in the earliest stages of embryonic development. The last two decades have seen tremendous growth in our knowledge of the developing brain, owing to rapid advances in many fields, particularly in developmental neurobiology and neuroscience.

Brain ontogeny is a product of intrinsic and extrinsic processes taking place both prenatally and postnatally (Todd et al., 1995). Over the course of development, a process of structural organization unfolds, which can be characterized as progressive regional specialization. This specialization is the product of a complex interplay of genetic and environmental variables. For example, Rakic (1988) introduced the concept of a *protomap*, which refers to the underlying genetic determination of different regions of the cortex. At the same time, the developing brain constantly is adapting to changes in the environment and continues fine-tuning neuronal and regional connections. The normal development of the brain unfolds as a series of timed genetic events, the expression of which depends on properly timed and delivered environmental stimuli (Nowakowski, 1987). The degree of malleability of the nervous system, however, varies greatly across cell types and brain regions and over time (Greenough et al., 1987) both prenatally and extending well into postnatal development.

The major stages in the development of the nervous system begin with the initial induction of a primitive neural tube that is derived from the sheet of epithelial cells that line the outer cellular layer (ectoderm) of the embryo. The forebrain region of the neural tube eventually becomes the cerebral cortex (from the telencephalon), thalamus, and hypothalamus (from the diencephalon). The midbrain and hindbrain regions form the other major subcortical structures of the brain. These early regional divisions are followed by rapid cell proliferation, differentiation, and migration. In the human cortex, neurons assemble into a multilayered laminar structure beginning with migration toward the deepest layers of the cortex, with later cells reaching progressively more superficial cortical layers (Rakic, 1972). By 18 weeks' gestational age, virtually all neurons in the cortex have reached their major destinations (Sidman & Rakic, 1973).

The final stages of brain development involve the elaboration of connections, the growth of axons and dendritic trees, and the establishment of synaptic circuits. These events begin in the second trimester of gestation and extend well into childhood (Huttenlocher, 1994). The extremely large number of synaptic connections in the human cortex render likely that only an outline of neural connectivity is genetically determined and that many synapses are formed randomly and in overabundance. Eventually, organized coherent functional circuits become established, with the strengthening of some connections and the elimination of the inactive. This latter phase now is understood to depend crucially on sensory or afferent inputs that produce neuronal activity, as exemplified in the classic work on the development of the visual cortex by Hubel and Wiesel (1970; Hubel et al., 1977). Apparently, in humans differences exist in the time course of synapse elimination in different cortical areas. Synapse elimination in the visual cortex appears to begin at approximately age 1 year and reach completion by the age 10 years, whereas in the frontal cortex, this process occurs between age 7 years and adolescence (Huttenlocher, 1979). Thus, throughout the course of childhood, experience is playing a key role in ongoing brain developments.

Unclear is whether loss of synapses in humans during the postnatal period reflects pruning of synapses or the elimination of entire neurons (Huttenlocher, 1994). In contrast to programmed cell death, elimination of synaptic connections is more closely associated with increasingly complex neural systems, and no real evidence explains neuronal loss in human cortex. The development of complex neural circuits that underlie higher cognitive functions well may require a large number of unspecified synapses that are available during the key developmental phases (Huttenlocher, 1994). Indeed, functional plasticity, an important aspect of development, may critically depend on this early excess of synaptic connections. The notion of plasticity is crucial for understanding brain development, as it serves a primary organizational and adaptive role (Nelson & Bloom, 1997). Perhaps, however, certain brain regions (because of their evolutionary history) have greater or lesser developmental plasticity than do other regions. This differential plasticity has important functional implications and may help to explain the kinds of neuropsychological profiles that are found in developmental disorders (Pennington & Walsh, 1995).

Disruptions in the normal process of brain development can occur at all stages and may affect any aspect of the process outlined here. At the genetic level is found a class of regulatory genes that are critical to the very early stages in the development of the nervous system but are expressed only during a transitory period of embryonic development. Similarly, certain neurons exist briefly to help migrating neurons find their targets (Ciaranello et al., 1995). Certain important implications of these genetic and cellular events are expressed only transiently. In particular, defects in these regulatory genes or neurons may lead to the kind of subtle neuropathology that is involved in some neurodevelopmental disorders but cannot be detected easily. Anomalies in synaptic connections, cell migration, axonal pruning, or dendritic arborization may be the hallmarks of neurological impairment in neurodevelopmental disorders, yet may not be directly observable. These kinds of abnormalities may be due to primary genetic causes or may be secondary to environmental insults to the developing brain. Some genetically based migration disorders result in widespread disruption of normal brain architecture, whereas others may lead to abnormalities that are sporadically distributed or limited to a single brain region (Goodman, 1994). Abnormalities in the selective pruning of synaptic connections can have consequences also at the level of functional deficit. Diffuse overconnection or misconnection might result in a poor signal-to-noise ratio reflected in impairments in attention, learning, or coordination (Goodman, 1994).

The advent of new neuroimaging technologies has provided a direct window on at least some of the abnormalities that characterize the brains of children with various neurodevelopmental disorders. These technologies allow us to go beyond small-scale neuropathological investigations in postmortem studies to studies that include larger numbers of in vivo brains from children at a range of developmental stages. The revolution in neuroimaging began with the development of computed tomography in the early 1970s, followed by positron emission tomography and magnetic resonance imaging, which can provide detailed three-dimensional images of both cortical and subcortical brain structures. Innovations in neuroimaging offer the potential for dramatically advancing our understanding of the pathogenic mechanisms that underlie impairments in neurodevelopmental disorders, opening up many new research possibilities. At this point, magnetic resonance imaging appears to be the preferred modality for studying structural brain abnormalities in children with neurodevelopmental disorders, because it offers a safe, flexible method for obtaining high-resolution three-dimensional images (see Lyon & Rumsey, 1996; Thatcher et al., 1996).

At the same time, we must recognize that when we look at a brain image of a child with a neurodevelopmental disorder obtained through one of these methods, we are simply viewing the *end product* of abnormal brain development (Courchesne et al., 1995). Developmental studies that follow a sample of children longitudinally during the period of important brain growth and change have not yet been conducted. Furthermore, significant limitations still are found in the methods used in these studies. Many controversial issues continue to plague discussions of how to collect brain scans (e.g., thickness of slices), what to measure (e.g., global or regional volumes or areas), how to conduct the measurements, and how to analyze the data using statistical approaches (Courchesne & Plante, 1996; Filipek, 1996).

Thus far, research on structural abnormalities in the brains of children with a range of neurodevelopmental disorders has led to complex, often contradictory findings across different studies. Unlike acquired disorders either in adults or older children, developmental disorders typically are not associated with clear images of focal cortical damage. Many congenital syndromes are associated with overall changes in brain size (e.g., microcephaly in Williams syndrome and Down syndrome, or macrocephaly in at least some cases of autism; see chapters 5, 9, and 16), which affect how one measures more localized structures in the brain. Many studies use measures of *relative* size comparing different regions of the brain, such as focus on the left versus the right hemisphere or on the relative size of frontal to posterior regions. These comparisons have yielded some interesting data but only for some syndromes (for example, chapter 5). By and large, these kinds of approaches have been informative at only a limited level. Interestingly, neurodevelopmental disorders are more often associated with *diffuse* cortical damage, which suggests that the impact of such disorders is more widespread, affecting complex neural systems rather than simple localized areas (for example, see chapters 3 and 13). Furthermore, across a range of developmental syndromes, we find that not only are particular cortical systems affected but often associated atypical subcortical structures are involved as well. For example, in Prader-Willi syndrome, the hypothalamus has been implicated (see chapter 7); in Down syndrome, the hippocampus and associated areas have been implicated (see chapter 9); and in autism, both the cerebellum and limbic system show significant abnormalities (see chapter 16). These findings suggest deviations in brain development that begin early in embryology and cannot be as easily classified and interpreted as later acquired focal lesions. Our theories of structural brain abnormalities in neurodevelopmental disorders will have to incorporate these kinds of developmental complexities rather than relying on more established studies from work with adults.

The greatest challenges and most exciting opportunities have been opened up by neuroimaging advances that provide images of brain *function*. Functional neuroimaging allows scientists to observe and quantify human cognitive activities and to directly measure the localization of cognitive functions to particular brain regions. The initial use of positron emission tomography and single-photon emission computed tomography as functional technologies were of only very limited use to developmental researchers because they depend on radioactive isotopes to measure local pharmacology, chemistry, metabolism, and blood volume and flow as indices of brain function. The risks associated with the use of such isotopes could not be justified for conducting functional neuroimaging research investigations with child populations.

The recent advent of noninvasive technologies, including magnetic resonance spectroscopy and functional magnetic resonance imaging (fMRI), has just begun to open up new possibilities for studying brain function in children with neurodevelopmental disorders. For example fMRI measures cerebral blood flow, which provide images of very high spatial resolution that can be used to detect quite specific cognitive activity. These technologies will add to the more established use of electrophysiological methods, including quantitative electroencephalography and event-related potentials, that yield excellent information about the timing of neural events underlying perceptual and cognitive processing but yield only limited spatial information. Using these various approaches and the new methods that are being developed to combine electroencephalography and fMRI, we have the opportunity to view how the brains of children with neurodevelopmental disorders at different developmental stages process sensory and cognitive stimuli. Functional neuroimaging will provide important clues to the underlying brain mechanisms and impaired neural systems that account for the specific cognitive and behavioral deficits found in particular disorders.

COGNITIVE PSYCHOLOGY AND NEURODEVELOPMENTAL DISORDERS

From the psychological perspective, the key questions about neurodevelopmental disorders center on the behavioral manifestations or "symptoms" of specific disorders. This level is important not only for tracing symptoms to underlying biological causes but for considering therapeutic interventions. Defining the phenotype of a disorder remains pivotal to addressing issues of intervention or remediation because, to date, pharmacological treatments have been of very limited value for most neurodevelopmental disorders, and the hopes for genetic therapies still lie in the next century. Instead, most efforts at intervention are directed toward educational, cognitive, and behavioral change. To be most effective, such approaches must focus on areas of specific deficit. Thus, the more precisely we define the phenotype of a disorder, the more targeted the interventions can be, which are designed to improve the quality of life and achievements of children with neurodevelopmental disorders.

Earlier in this chapter, we discussed some of the history and current concerns that have been raised in connection with the goal of defining phenotypes associated with particular neurodevelopmental disorders. The growing consensus is that, despite these concerns, major advances in our understanding of neurodevelopmental disorders depend on studies designed to provide a clear definition of the phenotype at the psychological level. Such definition includes identifying both core or primary characteristics of a disorder and secondary features, which may be shared by other disorders or may not be universally true of all individuals with a particular syndrome. Instead of being limited to considering phenotypes as a set of observable behaviors or symptoms, the field of neurodevelopmental disorders has become increasingly interested in identifying core features of a phenotype at the more abstract and mediating level of cognition. This development allows one to go from a description of seemingly unrelated behaviors to a conceptually integrated psychological explanation. One example is offered by current theoretical views of autism in which the primary social and language impairments and repetitive behavior symptoms may be explained by interpreting the underlying deficit as involving either deficits in understanding mental states or in executive dysfunction (see chapter 17).

The bulk of research in this area has taken advantage of methodological and conceptual approaches developed in the field of neuropsychology, which investigates the cognitive deficits in neurological patients. The measures used to identify such deficits are typically psychometrically defined and include both intelligence tests and associated batteries of neuropsychological tests, both of which measure functions that putatively map onto particular brain regions. For example, widely used tests of executive functions (such as the Wisconsin Card Sort Test or the Tower of Hanoi) are designed to tap frontal lobe functions. The advantage of using psychometrically based tests is that they have been carefully designed to be used in a standardized way, and performance by individuals can be compared to population norms. Typically, the pattern of performance across tests can be used to identify areas of deficit and sparing across a range of cognitive domains relative to these norms. In turn, this pattern often is used to interpret areas of brain dysfunction. For some disorders, a unique and consistent profile can be quantified across a specific set of tests that may define the phenotype (see chapter 4 for an excellent example of this approach for Williams syndrome).

Limitations restrict relying exclusively on this type of neuropsychological approach, making use only of standardized test batteries. The models of brain function on which these neuropsychological tests have been based are derived from the adult brain lesion literature (Bishop, 1997). Conceptually, then, this approach is not especially sensitive to the very distinct characteristics of neurodevelopmental disorders that involve dynamic alterations to brain organization that are likely to begin very early in embryology. Tests that capture the parameters of a static focal injury to the adult brain may not map onto the same brain and behavior relations in children. Some tests (though not all) have been modified for use with younger children, so the developmental sensitivity of particular tests may be questioned. Thus, for example, the Wisconsin Card Sort Test can be used only with older children and adolescents for whom norms are available. This test does not yield an adequate measure of frontal lobe functioning for younger children, who simply perform at floor levels.

Another concern about many psychometric tests is that they are only indirect and often fairly "impure" measures of the abilities they are assumed to measure. For example, the Wisconsin Card Sort Test taps a number of different aspects associated with frontal lobe functions, including flexibility, working memory, inhibition, and perseveration. Other frontal lobe functions, such as planning, are not measured by this test. Many tests of language often tap both knowledge of linguistic representations (e.g., grammatical or morphological rules) and working memory that is needed for implementing those representations in either production or comprehension. Poor performance on such tests cannot distinguish between deficits in linguistic knowledge from deficits in working memory (see chapter 14). Finally, what should be noted is that certain cognitive domains as yet cannot be tested by standardized available tests. Thus, recent advances in our knowledge of the developmental and neural bases of social cognition, including understanding the mental states of people or "theory of mind," are not incorporated within the established canon of neuropsychological test batteries. This condition has important consequences for a disorder such as autism, which is known to involve deficits in this cognitive domain (see chapter 17).

Because of these limitations in the use of standardized measures, studies of the cognitive characteristics associated with neurodevelopmental disorders (and other types of neuropsychological investigations; Shallice, 1988) have been enriched by adding the conceptual framework and methodologies developed within the cognitive sciences, especially cognitive psychology. The main goal of cognitive science over the last few decades has been to dissect such broad domains as language, memory, visuospatial cognition, or social cognition into their fundamental component units, each of which is assumed to be associated with a unique neural substrate. This computational view of cognitive systems argues that the mind is best viewed as a series of functionally specialized mechanisms that interact to produce the highly complex, flexible, and adaptive human action (Marr, 1976; Pinker, 1997). Cognitive psychology, then, is interested in identifying the key processes and subsystems involved in broader cognitive domains, such as vision, language, reasoning, and social interaction. The methods used in this analysis are usually experimental and derive from the laboratory-based studies of normal individuals. Such methods are tailored to provide relatively purer measures of individual cognitive subprocesses.

This cognitive perspective, which is concerned both with the nature of the representations that underlie different cognitive operations and with the operations or processes themselves, has particular advantages for identifying cognitive aspects of dysfunction in neurodevelopmental disorders. A broader set of cognitive domains is encompassed by this approach, including social cognition, affective processing, and communication, each of which has been implicated in neurodevelopmental disorders ranging from Down syndrome (see chapter 8), Williams syndrome (see chapter 5), and autism (see chapter 17). It is also especially well suited to a developmental approach because of its concern with representational change and processing aspects of cognition. Examples of how computational approaches have enriched research on neurodevelopmental disorders can be found in studies of visuospatial cognitive impairment in both Williams syndrome (chapters 4 and 5), and Turner syndrome (chapter 10); learning and memory deficits in Down syndrome (chapter 9); deficits in social cognition in autism (chapter 17); and language in dyslexia (chapters 12 and 13), specific language impairment (chapter 14), and children with focal lesions (chapter 23).

In each of these cases, illustrated throughout this volume, the complex design of cognitive systems is further illuminated by the study of children whose deficits can be defined with greater precision using this conceptual approach. Thus, we find that the impairments in neurodevelopmental disorders do not occur across broadly defined functional systems; instead, we see fractionation and dissociations *within* major domains. Cognitive deficits in neurodevelopmental disorders map onto narrower, more specialized cognitive mechanisms or subsystems than have been identified from more traditional neuropsychological studies and have thus advanced our understanding of the nature of the core phenotypes associated with such syndromes.

At the same time, defining cognitive deficits in developmental syndromes remains a challenge for research in this area because patterns of impairment and cognitive dissociations might change over time. Cognitive systems are defined by their plasticity in development, which means that some early deficits might be resolved while others remain (see chapter 23). Some aspects of this kind of change may be the result of developmental factors; others might be because of compensation, which might affect how we interpret a child's performance on a particular task or test (Bishop, 1997). These complications highlight the need for more longitudinal studies that can illuminate the nature of changing cognitive profiles in neurodevelopmental disorders and capture changes in underlying cognitive representations.

A COGNITIVE NEUROSCIENCE FRAMEWORK

The ultimate goal for research on neurodevelopmental disorders is to develop a theoretical integration of knowledge across all the levels of analysis discussed in this chapter. This kind of comprehensive approach would provide a complete description and understanding of a syndrome from the level of DNA sequences to the level of observable behavior and symptoms. In this view, the theoretical explanation for how alterations to the genotype are translated into a particular developmental phenotype can be given at both the cognitive and biological systems levels. Indeed, we are beginning to see conceptual models that explicitly discuss the causal connections among genes, brain mechanisms, cognition, and behavior (Morton & Frith, 1995; Pennington & Walsh, 1995; see chapter 13). This emerging integrative perspective on neurodevelopmental disorders is now possible because of the revolutionary changes that have taken place in each of the disciplines that must contribute to this new framework, as described earlier in this chapter.

Thirty years ago, this kind of cross-disciplinary synthesis simply would have been inconceivable. Concepts in the genetics of developmental disorders were in their infancy, although the notion that each syndrome must have its own unique genetic etiology was then recognized by biologists. At that time, however, researchers in the behavioral sciences were pooling individuals with diverse etiologies, and descriptions of behavior were still limited to the observable level of analysis or in terms of general and universal cognitive processes. These conceptions within psychology were fundamentally irreconcilable with a growing view in neurobiology that the brain was made up of a set of functionally specialized regions. Only with the theoretical changes that have taken place within psychology, especially with the advent of a computational view of cognition, has a new integrative model of neurodevelopmental disorders become a possibility.

In recent years, the emergence of the field of cognitive neuroscience has demonstrated the rewards that may be reaped from a synthesis among cognitive psychology, neuroscience, and clinical studies of brain-damaged patients (e.g., Kosslyn, 1994; Gazzaniga, 1995; Schachter, 1996). The goal of this book is to suggest that a similar synthesis is possible for neurodevelopmental disorders, with the added contributions of molecular genetics and a developmental framework. The chapters in this volume vividly illustrate how a cognitive neuroscience perspective enriches the theoretical models and research paradigms that are beginning to be implemented in the study of neurodevelopmental disorders. Consider, for example, current work on Williams syndrome. In chapter 4, Mervis et al. illustrate how one of the genes deleted in Williams syndrome can be directly associated to one component of the cognitive phenotype. Working in isolation, molecular biologists could identify the gene (LIMK1) and fully sequence its DNA. However, without the contribution of cognitive psychology, we would not know how this gene is connected to the phenotype of Williams syndrome, particularly its direct link to the visual-spatial deficits that are a core feature of the disorder. Similarly, in chapter 5, Bellugi et al. are able to draw parallels between the fractionated cognitive profile in Williams syndrome, with its striking peaks and valleys, and some characteristic neuroanatomical and neurophysiological markers of individuals with Williams syndrome.

An integrated cognitive neuroscience framework not only enhances our conception of neurodevelopmental disorders; in turn, the study of neurodevelopmental disorders also expands the definition and scope of cognitive neuroscience. By focusing on disorders that affect how the brain develops early in prenatal life (disorders that may be genetically caused), research on neurodevelopmental disorders adds both genetics and a developmental perspective to the established framework of cognitive neuroscience (cf. Gazzaniga, 1995). Studies of children with neurodevelopmental disorders explore the role and interaction of genetic, biological, and environmental experiences at all points in development, ranging from the earliest embryological stages through the end of puberty (see especially chapters 19 and 20) providing insights into how the biological substrate of behavior changes with age and development. Research on neurodevelopmental disorders may demonstrate where these developmental pathways may be carved at their joints, and can provide a rich picture of basic cognitive architecture as it is constructed over time. In this way, as has been the tradition in psychology for more than 100 years, we can look at neurodevelopmental disorders for insights into normal brain and cognitive development.

Genetic or environmental agents may affect highly localized brain regions and cognitive processes. Alternately, depending of the nature of the agent, they may alter neural connectivity more widely, thus changing the computational properties of neural networks, a process that may explain decrements in intelligence that are commonly found in many neurodevelopmental disorders. Because the brain is a self-organizing system, neurodevelopmental disorders alter the reaction range of brain development, which in turn affects cognitive development and behavior. Unlike the effects of brain damage in adulthood, no static localized lesion exists; development of both neural systems and cognitive pathways occur in ways that are fundamentally similar to what is seen in normal development (Pennington & Walsh, 1995). This similarity provides evidence for the view that supports constraints on development (see chapter 23) at both the neural and cognitive level, and it provides further support for the idea that the study of neurodevelopmental disorders can contribute to an integrated developmental cognitive neuroscience (Johnson, 1997).

Of course, a long way to go remains before we can begin to stitch together the components that make up a cognitive neuroscience of neurodevelopmental disorders in a meaningful and mechanistic way. We are just beginning the work that will take us to a science that truly links neuroscience to cognition in a developmental framework. The task is not easy, and many neurodevelopmental disorders are not yet ready for this kind of analysis. However, the chapters in this book demonstrate that progress has been made in recent years in moving us beyond the limitations of a unidimensional view of neurodevelopmental disorders. Over the next decades, research into particular syndromes will begin to address the four dimensions that make up the cognitive neuroscience of neurodevelopmental disorders: genes, brain systems, cognition, and time or development. The findings of this complex multidimensional research program will begin to provide a detailed portrait and theoretical model of how basic genetic and environmental building blocks build a brain and mind.

ACKNOWLEDGMENT

This chapter was written with grant support from the National Institute on Child Health and Human Development (RO1 HD 33470) and the National Institute on Deafness and Other Communication Disorders (RO1 DC 01234).

REFERENCES

Bakeman, R., & Robinson, B. F. (1997). When Ns do not justify means: Small samples and scientific conclusions. In L. B. Adamson & M. A. Romski (Eds.), *Communication and language acquisition: Discoveries from atypical development* (pp. 49–72). Baltimore: Paul Brookes.

Bates, E., & Appelbaum, M. (1994). Methods of studying small samples: Issues and examples. In S. H. Broman & J. Grafman (Eds.), *Atypical cognitive deficits in developmental disorders: Implications for brain function* (pp. 245–280). Hillsdale, NJ: Lawrence Erlbaum Associates.

Bishop, D. V. M. (1997). *Uncommon understanding: Development and disorders of language comprehension in children*. London: Psychology Press.

Bellugi, U., Wang, P. P., & Jernigan, T. L. (1994) Williams syndrome: An unusual neuropsychological profile. In S. H. Broman & J. Grafman (Eds.), *A typical cognitive deficits in developmental disorders: Implications for brain function* (pp. 23–56). Hillsdale, NJ: Erlbaum

Bregman, J. D., & Hodapp, R. M. (1991). Current developments in the understanding of mental retardation: I. Biological and phenomenological perspectives. *Journal of the American Academy of Child and Adolescent Psychiatry, 30*, 707–719.

Broman, S. H., & Grafman, J. (Eds.). (1994). *Atypical cognitive deficits in developmental disorders: Implications for brain function*. Hillsdale, NJ: Lawrence Erlbaum Associates.

Butler, M. (1990). Prader-Willi syndrome: Current understanding of cause and diagnosis. *American Journal of Medical Genetics, 35*, 319–332.

Ciaranello, R. D., Aimi, J., Dean, R. R., Morilak, D. A., Porteus M. H., & Cicchetti, D. (1995). Fundamentals of molecular neurobiology. In D. Cicchetti & D. J. Cohen (Eds.), *Developmental psychopathology: Vol. 1. Theory and methods* (pp. 109–160). New York: Wiley.

Courchesne, E., & Plante, E. (1996). Measurement and analysis issues in neurodevelopmental magnetic resonance imaging. In R. W. Thatcher, G. R. Lyon, J. Rumsey, & N. Krasnegor (Eds.), *Developmental neuroimaging: Mapping the development of brain and behavior* (pp. 43–65). New York: Academic Press.

Courchesne, E., Townsend, J., & Chase, C. (1995). Neurodevelopmental principles guide research on developmental psychopathologies. In D. Cicchetti & D. J. Cohen (eds.), *Developmental psychopathology Volume 1: Theory and Methods*, (pp. 195–226). New York: Wiley.

Denckla, M. B. (1994). Interpretations of a behavioral neurologist. In S. H. Broman & J. Grafman (Eds.), *Atypical cognitive deficits in developmental disorders: Implications for brain function* (pp. 283–295). Hillsdale, NJ: Lawrence Erlbaum Associates.

Dykens, E. M. (1995). Measuring behavioral phenotypes: Provocations from the "new genetics." *American Journal on Mental Retardation, 99*, 522–532.

Filipek, P. A. (1996). Structural variations in measures in the developmental disorders. In R. W. Thatcher, G. R. Lyon, J. Rumsey, & N. Krasnegor (Eds.), *Developmental neuroimaging: Mapping the development of brain and behavior* (pp. 169–186). New York: Academic Press.

Fletcher, J. (1994). Afterword: Behavior-brain relationships in children. In S. H. Broman & J. Grafman (Eds.), *Atypical cognitive deficits in developmental disorders: Implications for brain function* (pp. 297–325). Hillsdale, NJ: Lawrence Erlbaum Associates.

Flint, J. (1996). Annotation: Behavioral phenotypes. A window onto the biology of behavior. *Journal of Child Psychology and Psychiatry, 37*, 355–367.

Flint, J., Wilkie, A. O. M., Buckle, V. J., Winter, R. M., Holland, A. J., & McDermid, H. E. (1995). The detection of subtelomeric chromosomal rearrangements in idiopathic mental retardation. *Nature Genetics, 9*, 132–139.

Gazzaniga, M. S. (Ed.). (1995). *The cognitive neurosciences*. Cambridge, MA: MIT Press.

Gibson, D. (Ed.). (1978). *Down's syndrome: The psychology of mongolism*. Cambridge, UK: Cambridge University Press.

Goodman, R. (1994). Brain development. In M. Rutter & D. Hay (Eds.), *Development through life: A handbook for clinicians* (pp. 49–78). Oxford: Blackwell Scientific Publications.

Greenough, W., Black, J. E., & Wallace, C. S. (1987). Experience and brain development. *Child Development, 58*, 539–559.

Hermelin, B., & O'Connor, N. (1970). *Psychological experiments with autistic children*. Oxford: Pergamon Press.

Hodapp, R. M., & Dykens, E. M. (1994). Mental retardation's two cultures of behavioral research. *American Journal on Mental Retardation, 98*, 675–687.

Hubel, D. H., & Wiesel, T. N. (1970). The period of susceptibility to the physiological effects of unilateral eye closure in kittens. *Journal of Physiology, 206*, 419–436.

Hubel, D. H., Wiesel, T. N., & LeVay, S. (1977). Plasticity of ocular dominance columns in the monkey striate cortex. *Philosophical Transactions of the Royal Society of London, 278*, 377–409.

Huttenlocher, P. R. (1979). Synaptic density in human frontal cortex: Developmental changes and effects of aging. *Brain Research, 163*, 195–205.

Huttenlocher, P. R. (1994). Synaptogenesis in human cerebral cortex. In G. Dawson & K. W. Fisher (Eds.), *Human behavior and the developing brain* (pp. 137–152). New York: Guilford Press.

Johnson, M. H. (1997). *Developmental cognitive neuroscience*. Oxford: Blackwell.

Kosslyn, S. (1994). *Image and brain*. Cambridge, MA: MIT Press.

Lander, E. S., & Schork, N. J. (1994). Genetic dissection of complex traits. *Science, 265*, 2037–2048.

Lidsky, A. S., Robson, K. J. H., Thirumalachary, C., Baker, P. E., Ruddle, F. H., & Woo, F. H. C. (1984). The PKU locus in man is on chromosome 12. *American Journal of Human Genetics, 36*, 527–535.

Lombroso, P. J., Pauls, D. L., & Leckman, J. F. (1994). Genetic mechanisms in childhood psychiatric disorders. *Journal of the American Academy of Child and Adolescent Psychiatry, 33*, 921–938.

Lyon, G. R., & Rumsey, J. M. (Eds.). (1996). *Neuroimaging: A window to the neurological foundations of learning and behavior in children*. Baltimore: Paul Brookes.

Magenis, R. E., Toth-Fejel, S., Allen, L. J., Black, M., Brown, M. G., Budden, S., et al. (1990). Comparisons of the 15q deletions in Prader-Willi and Angelman syndromes: Specific regions, extent of deletions, parental origin and clinical consequences. *American Journal of Medical Genetics, 35*, 333–349.

Marr, D. (1976). Early processing of visual information. *Philosophical Transactions of the Royal Society of London [B], 275*, 483–524.

Morton, J., & Frith, U. (1995). Causal modeling: S structural approach to developmental psychopathology. In D. Cicchetti & D. J. Cohen (Eds.), *Developmental psychopathology: Vol. 1. Theory and methods* (pp. 357–390). New York: Wiley.

Moser, H. W. (1992). Prevention of mental retardation (genetics). In L. Rowitz, (Ed.), *Mental retardation in the year 2000*. New York: Springer-Verlag.

Nelson, C. A., & Bloom, F. E. (1997). Child development and neuroscience. *Child Development, 68*, 970–987.

Nowakowski, R. S. (1987). Basic concepts of CNS development. *Child Development, 58*, 568–595.

Pauls, D. L. (1993). Behavioral disorders: Lessons in linkage. *Nature Genetics, 3*, 4–5.

Pennington, B. F., & Walsh, M. (1995). Neuropsychology and developmental psychopathology. In D. Cicchetti & D. J. Cohen (Eds.), *Developmental psychopathology: Vol. 1. Theory and methods* (pp. 254–290). New York: Wiley.

Pinker, S. (1997). *How the mind works*. New York: Norton.

Rakic, P. (1972). Mode of cell migration to the superficial layers of fetal monkey neocortex. *Journal of Comparative Neurology, 145,* 61–84.

Rakic, P. (1988). Specification of cerebral cortical areas. *Science, 241,* 170–176.

Risch, N. (1990). Genetic linkage and complex diseases, with special reference to psychiatric disorders. *Genetic Epidemiology, 7,* 3–16.

Ross, C. A., McInnis, M. G., Margolis, R. L., & Li, S. (1993). Genes with triplet repeats: Candidate mediators of neuropsychiatric disorders. *Genetic Epidemiology, 7,* 3–16.

Schachter, D. L. (1996). *Searching for memory.* New York: Basic Books.

Shallice, T. (1988). *From neuropsychology to mental structure.* Cambridge: Cambridge University Press.

Sidman, R. L., & Rakic, P. (1973). Neuronal migration with special reference to developing human brains: A review. *Brain Research, 62,* 1–35.

Simonoff, E., Bolton, P., & Rutter, M. (1996). Mental retardation: Genetic findings, clinical implications, and research agenda. *Journal of Child Psychology and Psychiatry, 37,* 259–280.

Thatcher, R. W., Lyon, G. R., Rumsey, J., & Krasnegor, N. (Eds.). (1996). *Developmental neuroimaging: Mapping the development of brain and behavior.* New York: Academic Press.

Todd, R. D., Swarzenski, B., Rossi P. G., & Visconti, P. (1995). Structural and functional development of the human brain. In D. Cicchetti & D. J. Cohen (Eds.), *Developmental psychopathology: Vol. 1. Theory and methods* (pp. 161–194). New York: Wiley.

Verkerk, A. J., Pieretti, M., Sutcliffe, J., Fu, Y., Kuhl, D. P., & Warren, S. T. (1991). Identification of a gene containing a CGG repeat coincident with a breakpoint cluster region exhibiting length variation in fragile X syndrome. *Cell, 65,* 905–914.

II Neurodevelopmental Disorders: Syndromes with Known Genetic Etiologies

2 Clinical and Molecular Aspects of Fragile X Syndrome

Randi Jenssen Hagerman

The discovery of the fragile X mental retardation 1 gene (*FMR1*) has broadened our understanding of the spectrum of involvement in fragile X syndrome (Verkerk et al., 1991; Hagerman, 1996b). Although fragile X syndrome is the most common known cause of inherited mental retardation, it also can cause learning disabilities and emotional problems. Throughout the 1980s, individuals were diagnosed by cytogenetic testing in folate-deficient tissue culture media, which demonstrates a fragile site at Xq27.3 termed *FRAXA* in individuals affected by fragile X syndrome (Sutherland, 1977, 1979). In 1991, Verkerk et al. detected a trinucleotide $(CGG)_n$ expansion within the 5' untranslated region of *FMR1*, which repeats approximately 6 to 52 times within the normal population (Fu et al., 1991). Individuals who are carriers but are unaffected by fragile X syndrome have approximately 53 to 200 repeats (premutation). Individuals who are affected by fragile X syndrome have a full mutation that is more than 230 repeats and often greater than 1,000 CGG repeats. The full mutation usually is associated with a process of methylation, the addition of CH_3 (methyl) groups along the backbone of the DNA helix. The process of methylation silences transcription, the reading of the DNA message for the production of messenger RNA (mRNA), which subsequently will be translated into protein. In a fully methylated full mutation, no FMR1 protein is produced, and the absence of the FMR1 protein causes fragile X syndrome.

THE GENETICS OF FRAGILE X SYNDROME

Known since the last century is the existence of more retarded male than female individuals (Sherman 1996), but not until publication of the Martin and Bell pedigree (1943) did researchers focus on disorders of the X chromosome as a cause of the male predominance in mental retardation. In the Martin-Bell pedigree were 11 retarded male patients, and the study is recognized as the first published pedigree of X-linked mental retardation. The affected male subjects were noted to have no distinguishing physical features, and the etiology for their mental retardation was not sorted out until the 1980s, when cytogenetic testing revealed the fragile site at Xq27.3 and a diagnosis of fragile X syndrome was made. In retrospect, after the diagnosis was made, all the affected men were noted to have features of fragile X syndrome, including prominent ears and macroorchidism (large testicles).

Presently, fragile X syndrome represents 30% of X-linked metal retardation so it is essential to test for this disorder when there are two or more mentally retarded males in a family. A recent update reports 105 X-linked mental retardation syndromes (Lubs et al., 1996). Two additional disorders cause a fragile site at the Xq27.3 area: *FRAXE*, which is usually associated with a milder version of mental retardation as compared to fragile X syndrome (Brown, 1996), and *FRAXF*, which is not consistently associated with mental retardation. Therefore, all individuals who are given a diagnosis of fragile X syndrome on the basis of cytogenetic testing should have DNA testing to confirm the diagnosis and clarify the mutation status at *FMR1*.

For more than a decade, a process of anticipation (greater involvement in subsequent generations) has been known to be present in the pedigrees with fragile X syndrome. Sherman et al. (1984, 1985) reported the fact that daughters of nonexpressing male carrier were not mentally impaired, whereas female carriers had a 30% risk of having daughters with fragile X syndrome, and the risk of having offspring with fragile X syndrome increased in each succeeding generation. These phenomena were called *Sherman's paradox*, and not until the gene was sequenced in 1991 was the trinucleotide repeat found to be responsible for anticipation.

Women who are carriers of the premutation usually are unaffected cognitively themselves, but the premutation has a high risk of expanding to a full mutation in subsequent generations. Expansion to a full mutation becomes more likely as the CGG repeat number increases, although expansion has occurred with a premutation as low as 55. Expansion to a full mutation occurs only when the premutation is passed on by a woman, although the reason for this is unknown. Male carriers will pass on only a premutation, but it will be passed to all of their daughters and none of their sons. One cause of instability of the premutation is the loss of the AGG anchors usually interspersed within the CGG expansion at approximately every tenth repeat in the normal population. The premutation carriers usually have a pure CGG run of more than 35 repeats, which leads to instability (Imbert & Mandel, 1995).

Men are more severely affected than are women because the former have only one X chromosome. If a male subject has a full mutation that is completely methylated, typically he will be retarded and will not have detectable FMR1 protein levels. Female subjects, on the other hand, have two X chromosomes, although one is routinely inactivated. The percentage or ratio of cells that have the normal X chromosome as the active X chromosome (activation ratio) correlates with less involvement from fragile X syndrome (Rousseau et al., 1991b; Reiss et al., 1995; Sobesky et al., 1996).

The phenomenon of anticipation has been noted in other disorders and, in many cases, has led to the discovery of additional trinucleotide repeat mutations in other genes. Some examples are Huntington disease, myotonic dystrophy, two types of spinocerebellar ataxias, Friedreich's ataxia, a rare form of spinal and bulbar muscular atrophy, dentatorubral-pallidoluysian atrophy, and the previously mentioned *FRAXE* and *FRAXF* mutations (Imbert & Mandel, 1995; Warren & Ashley, 1995; Warren, 1996). Certain types of depression also appear to have anticipation, but specific genes associated with a trinucleotide repeat mutation and depression have yet to be discovered.

PREVALENCE

The prevalence of fragile X syndrome with mental retardation was first estimated by cytogenetic screening studies. Work by Webb et al. (1986; 1991) in County Coventry, England, placed the prevalence at perhaps 1 in 1,040 school children. However, DNA studies on the same population have corrected this figure to 1 in 2,200 because the *FMR1* mutation was not found in everyone who demonstrated the fragile site on cytogenetic testing (Morton et al., 1995). Two separate mutations—*FRAXE* and *FRAXF*—that also have CGG repeat expansions are distal to the *FMR1* mutation but were previously confused with fragile X syndrome.

The largest DNA study regarding the prevalence of the premutation was carried out by Rousseau et al. (1995) in 10,624 Quebec women who donated blood to a blood bank. He found 1 in 259 women with a premutation of 55 repeats or larger. More recent studies by Rousseau et al. (1996) have found the premutation in approximately 1 in 755 male subjects in the general population in Quebec. The frequency of the premutation and full mutation may by fairly variable in different populations because of founder effects. Recent work by Turner in Australia suggested that the frequency of fragile X syndrome with mental retardation is 1 in 4,000 (Turner et al., 1996), whereas in Finland the prevalence is much higher (Sherman, 1996). The increased prevalence in Finland led to the hypothesis that the initial settlers 20 centuries ago included one or more fragile X carriers, causing founder effect leading to a high prevalence (Oudet et al., 1993; Haataja et al., 1994; Imbert & Mandel, 1995).

PHYSICAL PHENOTYPE

The physical features associated with fragile X syndrome include a long face, large prominent ears, high arched palate, hyperextensible finger joints, flat feet, and macroorchidism. Some of these features are related to a connective tissue abnormality associated with fragile X syndrome, which leads to soft, velvetlike skin and ligamentous laxity in several joints (Hagerman et al., 1984; Opitz et al., 1984), whereas other features are related to growth abnormalities, including a long face and a large head circumference. Waldstein et al. (1987) carried out histological studies and found the elastin fibers to be abnormal in fragile X syndrome. The elastin findings require further study and are probably related to a pleiotropic effect of the absence of FMR1 protein. Loesch et al. (1995) carried out detailed growth studies in fragile X syndrome and found enhanced growth in childhood but predominately short stature in adulthood. Hypothalamic dysfunction has been postulated in fragile X syndrome (Fryns et al., 1986), and this dysfunction may lead to growth abnormalities and macroorchidism. Even a Sotos syndrome phenotype has been described in fragile X syndrome, including cerebral gigantism and general overgrowth (deVries et al., 1995).

In female individuals, the typical physical features are most common in those with the greatest cognitive deficits (Fryns, 1986). The most common features are prominent ears, long face, high palate, hyperextensible finger joints, and flat feet (Hagerman, 1996b). Even some women with the premutation may have prominent ears as compared to controls (Riddle et al., 1998).

Medical problems, including recurrent otitis media and sinusitis, associated with the physical abnormalities can be common in young children with fragile X syndrome (Hagerman, 1996a). Mitral valve prolapse is seen in approximately 50% of adult patients with fragile X syndrome (Loehr et al., 1986). Usually, significant arrhythmias are not a problem, and mitral regurgitation is a rare complication. Joint dislocations and hernias are an occasional problem associated with the looseness of the connective tissue. Seizures occur in approximately 20% of patients with fragile X syndrome, and they include generalized, absence, and partial complex seizures (Musumeci et al., 1988; Wisniewski et al., 1991). Sleep disturbances are also common in fragile X syndrome, particularly in young patients (Hagerman, 1996b; Musumeci et al., 1996). Strabismus is seen in approximately 30% to 40% of patients with fragile X syndrome, and it requires early treatment and follow-up to avoid amblyopia (Maino et al., 1991; King et al., 1995).

BEHAVIORAL PHENOTYPE

The behavioral phenotype has remarkable consistency among individuals with fragile X syndrome. It is often more helpful than is the physical phenotype in considering the diagnosis, because most prepubertal patients do not have the macroorchidism or the long face, and some do not even have prominent ears. The typical behavioral features are considered autistic-like and include hand flapping, hand biting, poor eye contact, preservation, and tactile defensiveness. In addition, a short attention span, impulsivity, and hyperactivity are seen in the majority of boys with fragile X syndrome. Many of these features are related to hypersensitivity or overarousal to environmental stimuli (Cohen, 1995). Some patients can hear noises, such as a siren in the distance, before normal individuals can. Patients with fragile X syndrome usually are extrasensitive to touch or the textures of clothing. Children with fragile X syndrome have a greater aversion to direct eye contact, as compared to children with Down syndrome or autism without fragile X syndrome (Cohen et al., 1989b; Cohen, 1995). A characteristic pattern of approach and then avoidance is seen in the social interaction of patients with fragile X syndrome. These patients typically are more interested in social interactions than is a child with autism, but the avoidance appears to be secondary to the hyperarousal or extrasensitivity to the stimuli of social interactions. Perhaps this effect relates to a lack of appropriate inhibitory responses to extraneous or excessive stimuli. In noisy or crowded environments, such as the grocery store, children with fragile X syndrome often become hyperaroused, leading to tantrum behavior (Hagerman, 1996b). Belser and Sudhalter (1995) have shown an enhanced galvanic skin response in patients with fragile X syndrome during eye contact, as compared to controls. The neuroanatomical correlates to the enhanced behavioral and physiological responses in fragile X syndrome may relate to the hypothesized lack of pairing down of neuronal connections, leading to larger brain structures (at least in the hippocampus and caudate) as described in chapter 3.

Many individuals with fragile X syndrome have autistic features but do not meet diagnostic criteria for autism. Approximately 15% of male patients with fragile X syndrome have autism, and approximately 6% of male subjects with autism have fragile X syndrome (Brown et al., 1986; Hagerman et al., 1986; Baumgartner et al., 1995). Therefore, individuals who present with autism or mental retardation of unknown etiology should have DNA *FMR1* testing to rule out the possibility of fragile X syndrome. This recommendation is also true for female patients, because a 12% rate of fragile X syndrome in such individuals with autism has been reported (Cohen et al., 1989a).

Controlled studies have also shown a unique behavioral profile regarding autistic features in fragile X syndrome. Reiss and Freund (1991) used the *Diagnostic and Statistical Manual of Mental Disorders* (revised) (APA, 1987) criteria for autism and demonstrated more stereotypies, unusual nonverbal interactions, and difficulty with peer interactions as opposed to adult interactions in male patients with fragile X syndrome, compared to IQ-matched controls. Maes et al. (1993) and Lachiewicz et al. (1994) also found a unique profile of autism-like features, including unusual vocal and speech habits, verbal perseverations, tactile defensiveness, and social-avoidance reactions in male patients with fragile X syndrome as compared to IQ-matched controls. Maes et al. (1993) attributed these problems to excessive social anxiety. However, the association between fragile X syndrome and autism relates to a variety of neurobehavioral problems in fragile X syndrome that overlap with autism, including social anxiety, sensory aversions, and perseverations. These problems are caused by the lack of FMR1 protein, which leads to neurochemical and neuroanatomical changes (described in chapter 3). Most importantly, the autistic features in fragile X syndrome often improve with time. Baumgardner et al. (1995) found a diagnosis of autism presently or in the past in 38.7% of boys with fragile X syndrome, as compared to 6.7% of controls, which represented a significant difference. However, only 16% of the male subjects with fragile X syndrome had a current diagnosis of autism, demonstrating a significant improvement in time (perhaps related to therapy).

Hyperactivity or attention deficit hyperactivity disorder (ADHD) is seen in the majority of boys and in approximately one-third of girls with the full mutation (Freund et al., 1993; Hagerman, 1996b). Controlled studies have shown hyperactivity to be more common in boys with fragile X syndrome as compared to IQ-matched controls (Borghgraef et al., 1987; Turk, 1994; Baumgardner et al., 1995). ADHD symptoms are more common in girls with the full mutation, compared to their normal female siblings (Hagerman et al., 1992). However, Freund et al. (1993) did not find ADHD to be more common in girls with the full mutation in comparison with IQ-matched controls.

The majority of girls with the full mutation exhibit shyness and social anxiety (Hagerman et al., 1992). The presence of significant ADHD symptoms can counteract the problems of shyness, rendering the individual usually more impulsively outgoing (Sobesky et al., 1995). The shyness in women with the full mutation is associated with social awkwardness and schizotypal features, including odd communication patterns and odd mannerisms (Sobesky et al., 1995). Shyness is also associated with anxiety, and Lachiewicz and Dawson (1994) found that 40% of girls with fragile X syndrome had an anxiety score on the Conners Parent Questionnaire (which included shy and fearful behavior) in the clinical range as compared to none of the controls. Freund et al. (1993) found avoidant disorders in 65% of girls with the full mutation, which was significantly different from IQ-matched controls. In addition, a mood disorder, including depression or dysthymia, was present in 47% of females with fragile X syndrome as compared to 6% of controls, a significant difference.

Overall, shyness, anxiety, and mood problems are common in female patients affected by fragile X syndrome, whereas male patients typically have problems with ADHD and anxiety. The male autistic features are also seen in female patients but are more commonly described as schizotypal features because they are milder, although they interfere with interpersonal communication (Sobesky et al., 1994a). Mood problems or mood instability also are seen commonly in male patients, but they present as outburst behavior, such as tantrums in childhood and episodic aggression in approximately 40% of adolescents and adults (Hagerman, 1996b).

FMR1 PROTEIN

The FMR1 protein appears to regulate translation by binding to the 60s ribosome in the cytoplasm (Khandjian et al., 1996). FMR1 protein also binds to approximately 4% of the messages present in the human fetal brain; therefore, it may be involved with the regulation of translation of these messages (Ashley et al., 1993). In addition, alternative splicing of the *FMR1* genes in a variety of tissues leads to at least 12 isoforms, which suggests functional diversity for FMR1 protein and pleiotropic effects on the phenotype (Warren & Ashley, 1995). The widespread low-level distribution of FMR1 protein in all tissues suggests a general housekeeping function (Bachner et al., 1993).

Devys et al. (1993) found expression of FMR1 protein to be most abundant in neurons and testes with a predominantly cytoplasmic localization. The high levels of FMR1 protein in brain and testes suggest a special function in these tissues. Greenough's laboratory (Witt et al., 1995) has found high concentrations of FMR1 mRNA at the synapse in rat brains, particularly in areas involved with synaptogenesis in the hippocampus, cerebral cortex, and cerebellum. FMR1 protein appears to be stimulated when rats are raised in enriched environments, leading to modification of their synaptic structures (Greenough, personal communication, 1996). This finding is consistent with neuroanatomical studies by Hinton et al. (1991), which demonstrate thin and immature dendritic branches and small synapses in patients with fragile X syndrome as compared to normals. The FMR1 protein appears to be necessary for the maturation of the synapse, particularly in response to environmental stimuli.

Abitbol et al. (1993) found intense staining of FMR1 protein in the hippocampus and thalamus and the nucleus basalis magnocellularis (nbM) in normal human fetuses. The nbM is the major source of cholinergic innervation to the limbic area and cortex, and Abitbol et al. (1993) hypothesize that deficits in the cholinergic system may be related to the hyperarousal, mood lability, and anxiety seen in fragile X syndrome. The neuroanatomical findings in patients with fragile X syndrome, including the large hippocampus and small cerebellar vermis, are described by Mazzocco and Reiss in chapter 3.

Evidence also suggests that the FMR1 protein is important for the normal pruning process of neuronal connections that occurs early in normal development. The larger size of the hippocampus, caudate, and thalamus in patients with fragile X syndrome (described in chapter 3) is consistent with a focal lack of the normal pruning process. In addition, the development of a knockout mouse model for fragile X, wherein the *FMR1* gene is eliminated, has yielded support for this hypothesis. The knockout mouse demonstrates hyperactivity and deficits on the Morris water maze (Bakker et al., 1994; Oostra, 1996). In neuroanatomical studies, the dendritic spines are longer, and the spine density is increased in the knockout mouse as compared to controls, suggesting a deficit in maturation (Comery et al., 1996).

INVOLVEMENT IN INDIVIDUALS WITH THE PREMUTATION

Individuals with the premutation may have some limited features of the phenotypic spectrum of fragile X syndrome, although their cognitive abilities usually are normal (Mazzocco et al., 1993; Reiss et al., 1993). Franke et al. (1996) recently demonstrated an increased incidence of anxiety disorders in women with the premutation compared to controls. Although the majority of women with the premutation experienced an affective disorder, it was not significantly different from controls, which is similar to the data of Sobesky et al. (1994b) and Reiss et al. (1993). Women with the premutation may also have prominent ears or a greater number of physical features associated with fragile X syndrome as compared to controls (Hull & Hagerman, 1993; Riddle et al., 1998). Loesch et al. (1994) found that male subjects with the premutation had bigger ears than did their normal relatives and that female subjects with the premutation had shorter stature and a wider ridge width on their palms than did the normal relatives. Additionally, the twinning rate and the incidence of premature ovarian failure in women with the premutation are higher as compared to controls (Schwartz et al., 1994; Turner et al., 1994). Dorn et al. (1994) found a history of a higher incidence of behavioral problems, including ADHD symptoms, alcoholism, obsessive-compulsive symptoms, and social deficits in fathers who were carriers, as compared to control fathers. Hagerman et al. (1996) recently reported three male patients who had the premutation (between 130 and 210 CGG repeats); mild symptoms of fragile X syndrome, including ADHD symptoms; learning problems without mental retardation; shyness; and prominent ears. All three had a mild deficit of FMR1 protein (70%–90% of normal levels) in blood. Also possible is that an individual with a premutation can be mildly affected because of expansion of the CGG repeat number to the full mutation in other tissues. Likely, a high-end premutation (150–200 CGG repeats) would be more apt to expand to a mosaic pattern (premutation in some cells and full mutation in other cells) or to a full mutation in other tissues. Brown et al. (1995) described a socially reclusive man who had a premutation (125 repeats) in his blood. However, at autopsy, he had a mosaic pattern in his cerebral cortex, which probably explains his social deficits. Further study of occult mosaicism in premutation carriers who appear to be mildly affected is warranted.

MOLECULAR AND CLINICAL CORRELATIONS

The molecular studies have enhanced our understanding of the broad spectrum of involvement in fragile X syndrome. Although the majority of male individuals with fragile X syndrome have mental retardation, approximately 13% have an IQ of 70 or higher, which is associated with variations in the molecular pattern (Hagerman et al., 1994b). Long-term high-functioning (IQ $\geq$ 70) male subjects or those minimally affected usually have a partial or complete lack of methylation of the full mutation expansion of CGG repeats (Loesch et al., 1993a,b; McConkie-Rosell et al., 1993; Merenstein et al., 1994; Milà et al., 1994; Rousseau et al., 1994; Smeets et al., 1995; Steyaert et al.,

1996). Individuals with incomplete methylation have been shown to produce FMR1 protein to a limited extent (10%–35% of normal levels) in peripheral blood samples (Hagerman et al., 1994b; Merenstein et al., 1994). Apparently, a limited degree of FMR1 protein production is protective against the more severe cognitive deficits associated with fragile X syndrome. However, the higher-functioning male patients may often have learning problems or emotional problems, such as social anxiety or schizotypal features, which are common in the female individuals (Merenstein et al., 1994). Although early studies did not show a significant difference in involvement between male patients with the full mutation and those with a mosaic pattern (Rousseau et al., 1991a; deVries et al., 1993), more recent work suggests that a subgroup of mosaic male patients may indeed be higher-functioning. Merenstein et al. (1996) studied 218 male subjects with fragile X syndrome and found that mosaic male patients after puberty had a mean IQ of 60, significantly different from the IQ of those with a fully methylated full mutation (41), although those with less than 50% methylation had the highest IQ (88). Cohen et al. (1996) also found that mosaic male patients had a faster rate of adaptive skills development than did those with full mutation. One could hypothesize that mosaic male subjects who had the largest percentage of cells in the premutation range would be the highest-functioning because these cells should be producing FMR1 protein. Verheij et al. (1993) has demonstrated FMR1 protein production in a mosaic male patient, but further work regarding protein and clinical correlations is necessary.

Female patients provide a broader spectrum of involvement than do males because they have two X chromosomes, and at least some level of FMR1 protein should be produced in the majority of those with the full mutation. Abrams et al. (1994) have shown a correlation between IQ and the activation ratio (the number of normal X chromosomes that are the active X chromosome over the total number of active and inactive X chromosomes). Therefore, the larger the activation ratio, the more FMR1 protein production from the normal X chromosome, because the fully methylated, full-mutation X chromosome should not produce FMR1 protein. Taylor et al. (1994) did not find a significant correlation between IQ and activation ratio and warned against using the activation ratio as a predictive measure in prenatal diagnostic testing. According to a recent article by Sobesky et al. (1996), in nonretarded female patients, the correlation between activation ratio and IQ was close to significance, but the correlation between activation ratio and executive function abilities did achieve significance, suggesting that executive function is more strongly related to the effect of the *FMR1* gene than is IQ alone. DeVries et al. (1996) found in a study of female patients with the full mutation that the performance IQ, but not the verbal IQ, correlated with the activation ratio. This finding was confirmed by Riddle et al. (1998) in a separate group of female subjects with the full mutation. The significant impact of the *FMR1* mutation in the performance areas is discussed further in chapter 3.

FUTURE STUDIES

The molecular age has helped us to understand the broad spectrum of involvement in fragile X syndrome. Although examination of this disorder has resulted in significant advances in mental retardation research, future study must also focus on psychopathology. Deficits in FMR1 protein production have a significant impact on temperament and personality before cognitive functions are affected. With a molecular handle on the genetic component of behavior and cognitive functions in fragile X syndrome, the role of the environment and the rest of the human genome can be assessed. Reiss et al. (1995) have begun to study the influence of the parental IQ in addition to the mutation status in girls with fragile X syndrome, but this study is just the beginning of efforts that will assess all aspects of the phenotype.

Most importantly, studies of treatment to improve the outcome of both children and adults with fragile X syndrome are necessary (Hagerman, 1996a). The molecular advances help us to understand the mechanisms of mutation that ultimately will lead to a molecular cure for fragile X syndrome (Rattazzi & Ioannou, 1996).

REFERENCES

Abitbol, M., Menini, C., Delezoide, A. L., Rhymer, T., Verkemans, M., & Mallet, J. (1993). Nucleus basalis magnocellularis and hippocampus are the major sites of FMR-1 expression in the human fetal brain. *Nature Genetics, 4,* 147–153.

Abrams, M. T., Reiss, A. L., Freund, L. S., Baumgardner, T., Chase, G. A., & Denckla, M. B. (1994). Molecular-neurobehavioral associations in females with the fragile X full mutation. *American Journal of Medical Genetics, 51,* 317–327.

Ashley, Jr., C. T., Wilkinson, K. D., Reines, D., & Warren, S. T. (1993). FMR-1 protein: Conserved RNP family domains and selective RNA binding. *Science, 262,* 563–565.

American Psychiatric Association (1987). *Diagnostic and statistical manual of mental disorders* (3rd ed. rev.) Washington, DC: Author.

Bachner, D., Steinbach, P., Wohrle, D., Just, W., Vogel, W., & Hameister, H. (1993). Enhanced FMR-1 expression in testis [Correspondence]. *Nature Genetics, 4,* 115–116.

Bakker, C. E., Verheij, C., Willemsen, R., Vanderhelm, R., Oerlemans, F., Vermey, M., Bygrave, A., Hoogereen, A. T., Oostra, B. A., Reyniers, E., Deboulle, K., Dhooge, R., Cras, P., Van Velzen, D., Nagels, G., Martin, J. J., Dedeyn, P. P., Darby, J. K., & Willems, P. J. (1994). FMR1 knockout mice: A model to study fragile X mental retardation. *Cell, 78,* 23–33.

Baumgardner, T., Reiss, A. L., Freund, L. S., & Abrams, M. T. (1995). Specifications of the neurobehavioral associations in males with fragile X syndrome. *Pediatrics, 95,* 744–752.

Belser, R. C., & Sudhalter, V. 1995. Arousal difficulties in males with fragile X syndrome: A preliminary report. *Developmental Brain Dysfunction, 8,* 270–279.

Borghgraef, M., Fryns, J. P., Dielkens, A., Dyck, K., & Van den Berghe, H. (1987). Fragile X syndrome: A study of the psychological profile in 23 prepubertal patients. *Clinical Genetics, 32,* 179–186.

Brown, C. A., Brasingont, C. K., & Grass F. S. (1995). Paternal transmission of a full mutation in the *FMR1* gene. Identification of paternal CGG repeat sizes in multiple tissues. *American Journal of Human Genetics, 57* (Suppl. A335), 1947.

Brown, W. T. (1996). The molecular biology of the fragile X mutation. In R. J. Hagerman & A. C. Cronister (Eds.), The fragile X syndrome: Diagnosis, treatment, and research (2nd ed., pp. 88–113). Baltimore: Johns Hopkins University Press.

Brown, W. T., Jenkins, E. C., Cohen, I. L., Fisch, G. S., Wolf-Schein, E. G., Gross, A., Waterhouse, L., Fein, D., Mason-Brothers, A., Ritvo, E., Rittenberg, B. A., Bentley, W., & Castells, V. (1986). Fragile X and autism: A multicenter survey. *American Journal of Medical Genetics, 23,* 341–352.

Cohen, I. L. (1995). A theoretical analysis of the role of hyperarousal in the learning and behavior of fragile X males. *Mental Retardation and Developmental Disabilities Research Review, 1,* 286–291.

Cohen, I. L., Brown, W. T., Jenkins, E. C., French, J. H., Raguthu, S., Wolf-Schein, E. G., Sudhalter, V., Fisch, G., & Wisniewski, K. (1989a). Fragile X syndrome in females with autism [letter to the editor]. *American Journal of Genetics, 34,* 302–303.

Cohen, I. L., Nolin, S. L., Sudhalter, V., Ding, X.-H., Dobkin, C. S., & Brown, W. T. (1996). Mosaicism for the *FMR1* gene influences adaptive skills development in fragile X–affected males. *American Journal of Medical Genetics, 64,* 365–369.

Cohen, I. L., Vietze, P. M., Sudhalter, V., Jenkins, E. C., & Brown, W. T. (1989b). Parent-child dyadic gaze patterns in fragile X males and in non–fragile X males with autistic disorder. *Journal of Child Psychology and Psychiatry and Allied Disciplines, 30,* 845–856.

Comery, T. A., Harris, J. B., Willems, P. J., Oostra, B. A., & Greenough, W. T. (1996). Dendritic spine morphology in the fragile-X knockout mouse: A model of the fragile X syndrome? *Society for Neuroscience Abstracts, 22,* 1132.

deVries, B. B. A., Robinson, H., Stolte-Dijkstra, I., Gi, C. V. T. P., Dijkstra, D. V., vanDoorn, J., Halley, D. J. J., Oostra, B. A., Turner, G., & Niermeijer, M. F. (1995). General overgrowth in the fragile X syndrome: Variability in the phenotype expression of the *FMR1* gene mutation. *Journal of Medical Genetics, 32,* 764–769.

deVries, B. B. A., Wiegers, A. M., deGraaff, E., Verkerk, A. J. M. H., Van Hemel, J. O., Halley, D. T. J., Fryns, J.-P., Curfs, L. M. G., Niermeijer, M. F., & Oostra, P. A. (1993). Mental status and fragile X expression in relation to *FMR1* gene mutation. *European Journal of Human Genetics, 1,* 72–79.

deVries, B. B. A., Wiegers, A. M., Smits, A. P. T., Mohkamsing, S., Duivenvoorden, H. J., Fryns, J.-P., Curfs, L. M. G., Halley, D. J. J., Oostra, B. A., van den Ouweland, A. M. W., Niermeijer, M. F. (1996). Mental status of females with an *FMR1* gene full mutation. *American Journal of Human Genetics, 58,* 1025–1032.

Devys, D., Lutz, Y., Rouyer, N., Bellocq, J. P., & Mandel, J. L. (1993). The FMR-1 protein is cytoplasmic, most abundant in neurons and appears normal in carriers of a fragile X premutation. *Nature Genetics, 4,* 335–340.

Dorn, M., Mazzocco, M., & Hagerman, R. J. (1994). Behavioral and psychiatric disorders in adult fragile X carrier males. *Journal of the American Academy of Child and Adolescent Psychiatry, 33,* 256–264.

Franke, P., Maier, W., Iwers, B., Hautzinger, M., & Froster, U. G. (1996). Fragile X carrier females: Evidence for a distinct psychopathological phenotype?. *American Journal of Medical Genetics, 64,* 334–339.

Freund, L. S., Reiss, A. L., & Abrams, M. (1993). Psychiatric disorders associated with fragile X in the young female. *Pediatrics, 91,* 321–329.

Fryns, J. P., Dereymaeker, A. M., Hoefnagels, M., Volcke, P., & Van den Berghe, H. (1986). Partial fra(X) phenotype with megalotestes in fra(X) negative patients with acquired lesions of the central nervous system. *American Journal of Medical Genetics, 23*, 213–219.

Fu, Y.-H., Kuhl, D. P. A., Pizzuti, A., Pieretti, M., Sutcliffe, J. S., Richards, S., Verkerk, A. J. M. H., Holden, J. J. A., Fenwick, Jr., R. G., Warren, S. T., Oostra, B. A., Nelson, D. L., & Caskey, C. T. (1991). Variation of the CGG repeat at the fragile X site results in genetic instability: Resolution of the Sherman paradox. *Cell, 67*, 1047–1058.

Haataja, R., Väisänen, M. L., Li, M., et al. (1994). The fragile X syndrome in Finland: Demonstration of a founder effect by analysis of microsatellite haplotypes. *Human Genetics, 94*, 479–483.

Hagerman, R. J. (1996a). Medical follow-up and psychopharmacology. In R. J. Hagerman & A. C. Cronister (Eds.), The fragile X syndrome: Diagnosis, treatment, and research (2nd ed., pp. 283–331). Baltimore: Johns Hopkins University Press.

Hagerman, R. J. (1996b). Physical and behavioral phenotype. In R. J. Hagerman & A. C. Cronister (Eds.), The fragile X syndrome: Diagnosis, treatment and research (2nd ed., pp. 3–87). Baltimore: Johns Hopkins University Press.

Hagerman, R. J., Hull, C. E., SaLanda, J. F., Carpenter, I., Staley, L. W., O'Connor, R., Seydel, C., Mazzocco, M. M., Snow, K., Thibodeau, S., Kuhl, D., Nelson, D. L., Caskey, C. T., & Taylor, A. (1994b). High functioning fragile X males: Demonstration of an unmethylated, fully expanded FMR-1 mutation associated with protein expression. *American Journal of Medical Genetics, 51*, 298–308.

Hagerman, R. J., Jackson, A. W., Levitas, A., Rimland, B., & Braden, M. (1986). An analysis of autism in 50 males with the fragile X syndrome. *American Journal of Medical Genetics, 23*, 359–370.

Hagerman, R. J., Jackson, C., Amiri, K., Silverman, A. C., O'Connor, R., & Sobesky, W. E. (1992). Fragile X girls: Physical and neurocognitive status and outcome. *Pediatrics, 89*, 395–400.

Hagerman, R. J., Staley, L. W., O'Conner, R., Lugenbeel, K., Nelson, D., McLean, S., & Taylor, A. (1996). Learning disabled males with a fragile X CGG expansion in the upper premutation size range. *Pediatrics, 97*, 8–12.

Hagerman, R. J., van Housen, K., Smith, A. C. M., & McGavran, L. (1984). Consideration of connective tissue dysfunction in the fragile X syndrome. *American Journal of Medical Genetics, 17*, 123–132.

Hinton, V. J., Brown, W. T., Wisniewski, K., & Rudelli, R. D. (1991). Analysis of neocortex in three males with fragile X syndrome. *American Journal of Medical Genetics, 41*, 289–294.

Hull, C., & Hagerman, R. J. (1993). A study of the physical, behavioral, and medical phenotype, including anthropometric measures of females with fragile X syndrome. *American Journal of Diseases of Children, 147*, 1236–1241.

Imbert, G., & Mandel, J.-L. (1995). The fragile X mutation. *Mental Retardation and Developmental Disabilities Research Review, 1*, 251–262.

Khandjian, E. W., Corbin, E., Woerly, S., & Rousseau, F. (1996). The fragile X mental retardation protein is associated with ribosomes. *Nature Genetics, 12*, 91–93.

King, R. A., Hagerman, R. J., & Houghton, M. (1995). Ocular findings in fragile X syndrome. *Developmental Brain Dysfunction, 8*, 223–229.

Lachiewicz, A. M., & Dawson, D. V. (1994). Behavioral problems of young girls with fragile X syndrome: Factor scores on the Conner's parent questionnaire. *American Journal of Medical Genetics, 15*, 364–369.

Lachiewicz, A. M., Spiridigliozzi, G. A., Gullion, C. M., Ransford, S. N., & Rao, K. (1994). Aberrant behaviors of young boys with fragile X syndrome. *American Journal of Mental Retardation, 98,* 567–579.

Loehr, J. P., Synhorst, D. P., Wolfe, R. R., & Hagerman, R. J. (1986). Aortic root dilatation and mitral valve prolapse in the fragile X syndrome. *American Journal of Medical Genetics, 23,* 189–194.

Loesch, D. Z., Huggins, R. M., & Chin, W. F. (1993a). Effect of fragile X on physical and intellectual traits estimated by pedigree analysis. *American Journal of Medical Genetics, 46,* 415–422.

Loesch, D. Z., Huggins, R. M., Hay, D. A., Gedeon, A. K., Mulley, J. C., & Sutherland, G. R. (1993b). Genotype-phenotype relationships in fragile X syndrome: A family study. *American Journal of Medical Genetics, 53,* 1064–1073.

Loesch, D. Z., Hay, D. A., & Mulley, J. (1994). Transmitting males and carrier females in fragile X—revisited. *American Journal of Medical Genetics, 51,* 392–399.

Loesch, D. Z., Huggins, R. M., & Hoang, N. H. (1995). Growth in stature in fragile X families: A mixed longitudinal study. *American Journal of Medical Genetics, 58,* 249–256.

Lubs, H. A., Chiurazzi, P., Fernando Arena, J., Schwartz, C., Tranebjaerg, L., & Giovanni, N. (1996). XLMR genes: Update 1996. *American Journal of Medical Genetics, 64,* 147–157.

Maes, B., Fryns, J. P., van Walleghem, M., & van den Berghe, H. (1993). Fragile X syndrome and autism: A prevalent association or a misinterpreted connection. *Genetics Counselling, 4,* 245–263.

Maino, D. M., Wesson, M., Schlange, D., Cibis, G., & Maino, J. H. (1991). Optometric findings in the fragile X syndrome. *Optometry and Vision Science, 68,* 634–640.

Martin, J. P., & Bell, J. (1943). A pedigree of mental defect showing sex-linkage. *Journal of Neurology and Psychiatry, 6,* 154–157.

Mazzocco, M. M. M., Pennington, B., & Hagerman, R. J. (1993). The neurocognitive phenotype of female carriers of fragile X: Further evidence for specificity. *Journal of Developmental and Behavioral Pediatrics, 14,* 328–335.

McConkie-Rosell, A., Lachewicz, A., Spiridigliozzi, G. A., Tarleton, J., Scheonwald, S., Phelan, M. C., Goonewardena, P., Ding, X., & Brown, W. T. (1993). Evidence that methylation of the *FMR1* locus is responsible for variable phenotypic expression of the fragile X syndrome. *American Journal of Human Genetics, 53,* 800–809.

Merenstein, S. A., Shyu, V., Sobesky, W. E., Staley, L. W., Taylor, A. K., & Hagerman, R. J. (1994). Fragile X syndrome in a normal IQ male with learning and emotional problems. *Journal of the American Academy of Child and Adolescent Psychiatry, 33,* 1316–1321.

Merenstein, S. A., Sobesky, W. E., Taylor, A. K., Riddle, J. E., Tran, H. X., & Hagerman, R. J. (1996). Molecular-clinical correlations in males with an expanded *FMR1* mutation. *American Journal of Medical Genetics, 64,* 389–394.

Milà, M., Kruyer, H., Glover, G., Sánchez, A., Carbonell, P., Castellví-Bel, S., Volplni, V., Rosell, J., Gabarrón, J., López, I., Villa, M., Ballestra, F., & Estivill, X. (1994). Molecular analysis of the $(CGG)_n$ expansion in the *FMR1* gene in 59 Spanish families. *Human Genetics, 94,* 395–400.

Morton, J. E., Dindl, P. M., & Bullocks, et al. (1995). Fragile X syndrome is less common than previously estimated. *American Journal Medical Genetics, 32,* 144–145.

Musumeci, S. A., Colognola, R. M., Ferri, R., Gigli, G. L., Petrella, M. L., Sanfilippo, S., Bergonzi, P., & Tassinari, C. A. (1988). Fragile-X syndrome: A particular epileptogenic EEG pattern. *Epilepsia, 29,* 41–47.

Musumeci, S. A., Ferri, R., Elia, M., Del Gracco, S., Scuderi, C., & Stefanini, M. (1996). Normal respiratory pattern during sleep in fragile X syndrome patients. *Journal of Sleep Research, 5*, 272.

Oostra, B. A. (1996). FMR1 protein studies and animal model for fragile X syndrome. In R. J. Hagerman & A. C. Cronister (Eds.), *Fragile X syndrome: Diagnosis, treatment, and Research.* (2nd ed., pp. 193–209). Baltimore: Johns Hopkins University Press.

Opitz, J. M., Westphal, J. M., Daniel A. (1984). Discovery of a connective tissue dysplasia in the Martin-Bell syndrome. *American Journal of Medical Genetics, 17*, 101–109.

Oudet, C., VonKeskull, H., Nordstom, A. M., et al. (1993). Striking founder effect for the fragile X syndrome in Finland. *European Journal of Human Genetics, 1*, 181–189.

Rattazzi, M. C., & Ioannou, Y. A. (1996). Molecular approaches to therapy. In R. J. Hagerman & A. C. Cronister (Eds.), *Fragile X syndrome: Diagnosis, treatment, and research* (2nd ed., pp. 412–452). Baltimore: Johns Hopkins University Press.

Reiss, A. L., & Freund, L. (1991). Behavioral phenotype of fragile X syndrome: DSM-III-R autistic behavior in male children. *American Journal of Medical Genetics, 43*, 35–46.

Reiss, A. L., Freund, L., Abrams, M. T., Boehm, C., & Kazazian, H. (1993). Neurobehavioral effects of the fragile X premutation in adult women: A controlled study. *American Journal of Human Genetics, 52*, 884–894.

Reiss, A., Abrams, M., Greenlaw, R., Freund, L., & Denckla, M., (1995). Neuro-developmental effects of the *FMR-1* full mutation in humans. *Nature Medicine, 1*, 159–167.

Riddle, J. E., Cheema, A., Sobesky, W. E., Gardner, S. C., Taylor, A. K., Pennigton, B. F., & Hagerman, R. J. (1998). Phenotypic involvement in females with the FMR1 gene mutation. *American Journal of Mental Retardation, 102*, 590–601.

Rousseau, F., Heitz, D., Biancalana, V., Blumenfeld, S., Kretz, C., Boue, J., Tommerup, N., Van Der Hagen, C., DeLozier-Blanchet, C., Croquette, M.-F., Gilgenkrantz, S., Jalbert, P., Voelckel, M. A., Oberle, I., & Mandel, J.-L. (1991a). Direct diagnosis by DNA analysis of the fragile X syndrome of mental retardation. *New England Journal of Medicine, 325*, 1673–1681.

Rousseau, F., Heitz, D., Oberle, I., & Mandel, J.-L. (1991b). Selection in blood cells from female carriers responsible for variable phenotypic expression of the fragile X syndrome: Inverse correlation between age and proportion of active X-carrying the full mutation. *Journal of American Genetics, 28*, 830–836.

Rousseau, F., Morel, M.-L., Rouillard, P., Khandjian, E. W., & Morgan, K. (1996). Suprisingly low prevalence of *FMR1* premutation among males from the general population. *American Journal of Human Genetics, 59*(suppl. A188), 1069.

Rousseau, F., Robb, L. J., Rouillard, P., & der Kaloustian, V. M. (1994). No mental retardation in a man with 40% abnormal methylation at the *FMR1* locus and transmission of sperm cell mutations as premutations. *Human Molecular Genetics, 6*, 927–930.

Rousseau, F., Rouillard, P., Morel, M.-L., Khandjian, E. W., Morgan, K. (1995). Prevalence of carriers of premutation-sized alleles of the *FMR1* gene—and implications for the population genetics of the fragile X syndrome. *American Journal of Human Genetics, 57*, 1006–1018.

Scharfenaker, S., O'Connor, R., Braden, M., Stackhouse, T., Hickman, L., & Gray, K. (1996). An integrated approach to intervention. In Hagerman R. J., & Cronister A. C. (Eds.), *Fragile X syndrome: Diagnosis, treatment, and research* (2nd ed., pp. 349–411). Baltimore: Johns Hopkins University Press.

Schwartz, C. E., Dean, J., Howard-Peebles, P. N., Bugge, M., Mikkelsin, M., Tommerup, N., Hull, C. E., Hagerman, R. J., Holden, J. J. A., & Stevenson, R. E. (1994). Obstetrical and gynecological complication in fragile X carriers. A multicenter study. *American Journal of Medical Genetics, 51*, 400–402.

Sherman, S. (1996). Epidemiology. In Hagerman R. J., & Cronister A. C., (Eds.), Fragile X syndrome: Diagnosis, treatment, and research (2nd ed. pp. 165–192). Baltimore: Johns Hopkins University Press.

Sherman, S., Maddalena, A., Howard-Peebles, P. N., Brown, W. T., Nolin, S., Jenkins, E., Schwartz, C., Tarrelton, J., Shapiro, L. R., Smits, A. P. T., Van Oost, B. A., Youings, S., Jacobs, P. A., Martinez, A., Barnicoat, A., Hockey, A., Staley, L., Hagerman, R. J., Kennerknecht, I., Steinbach, P., Barbi, G., Filippi, G., Grasso, M., Taylor, S. A. M., Robinson, H., Webb, T., Broome, D., Dixon, J., Ferreira, P., Gustavson, K. H., Meyer, J. L., & Pai, G. S. (1984). Characteristics of the transmission of the *FMR1* gene from carrier females in a prospective sample of conceptuses. *American Journal of Medical Genetics, 51*, 503–506.

Sherman, S. L., Jacobs, P. A., Morton, N. E., Froster-Iskenius, U., Howard-Peebles, P. N., Nielsen, K. B., Partington, M. W., Sutherland, G. R., Turner, G., & Watson, M. (1985). Further segregation analysis of the fragile X syndrome with special reference to transmitting males. *Human Genetics, 69*, 289–299.

Smeets, H., Smits, J., Verheif, A. P., Theelen, C. E., Willemsen, R. J. P., de Burgt, I. Van, Hoogeveen, A. T., Oosterwijk, J. C., & Oostra, B. A. (1995). Normal phenotype in two brothers with a full *FMR1* mutation. *Human Molecular Genetics, 4*, 2103–2108.

Sobesky, W. E. (1996). The treatment of emotional and behavioral problems in fragile X. In Hagerman R. J., & Cronister A. C. (Eds.), Fragile X syndrome: Diagnosis, treatment, and research (2nd ed., pp. 332–348). Baltimore: Johns Hopkins University Press.

Sobesky, W. E., Hull, C. E., & Hagerman, R. J. (1994a). Symptoms of schizotypal personality disorder in fragile X women. *Journal of the American Academy of Child and Adolescent Psychiatry, 2*, 247–255.

Sobesky, W. E., Pennington, B. F., Porter, D., Hull, C. E., & Hagerman, R. J. (1994b). Emotional and neurocognitive deficits in fragile X. *American Journal of Medical Genetics, 51*, 378–385.

Sobesky, W. E., Porter, D., Pennington, B. F., & Hagerman, R. (1995). Dimensions of shyness in fragile X females. *Developmental Brain Dysfunction, 8*, 280–292.

Sobesky, W. E., Taylor, A. K., Pennington, B. F., Riddle, J. E., & Hagerman, R. J. (1996). Molecular/clinical correlations in females with fragile X. *American Journal of Medical Genetics, 64*, 340–345.

Steyaert, J., Borghgraef, M., Teguis, E., & Fryns, J. P. (1996). Molecular-intelligence correlations in young fragile X males with a mild CGG repeat expansion in the *FMR1* gene. *American Journal of Medical Genetics, 64*, 274–277.

Sutherland, G. R. (1977). Fragile sites on human chromosomes: Demonstration of their dependence on the type of tissue culture medium. *Science, 197*, 265–266.

Sutherland, G. R. (1979). Heritable fragile sites on human chromosomes: I. Factors affecting expression in lymphocyte culture. *American Journal of Human Genetics, 31*, 125–135.

Taylor, A., Safanda, J. F., Fall, M. Z., Quince, C., Lang, K. A., Hull, C. E., Carpenter, I., Staley, L. W., & Hagerman, R. J. (1994). Molecular predictors of involvement in fragile X females. *Journal of the American Medical Association, 271*, 507–514.

Turner, G., Robinson, H., Wake, S., & Martin, N. (1994). Dizygous twinning and premature menopause in fragile X syndrome. *Lancet, 344*, 1500.

Turner, G., Webb, T., Wake, S., & Robinson, H. (1996). Prevalence of the fragile X syndrome. *American Journal of Medical Genetics, 64*, 196–197.

Verheij, C., Bakker, C. E., de Graaf, E., Keulemans, J., Willemsen, R., Verkerk, A. J., Galjaard, H., Reuser, A. J., Hoogeveen, A. T., & Oostra, B. A. (1993). Characterization and localization of the *FMR1* gene product associated with fragile X syndrome. *Nature, 363,* 722−724.

Verkerk, A. J., Pieretti, M., Sutcliffe, J. S., Fu, Y.-H., Kuhl, D. P., Pizzuti, A., Reiner, O., Richards, S., Victoria, M. F., Zhang, F., Eussen, B. E., van Ommen, G. J., Blonden, L. A. J., Riggins, G. J., Chastain, J. L., Kunst, C. B., Galjaard, H., Caskey, C. T., Nelson, D. L., Oostra, B. A., & Warren, S. T. (1991). Identification of a gene (*FMR1*) containing a CGG repeat coincident with a breakpoint cluster region exhibiting length variation in fragile X syndrome. *Cell, 65,* 905−914.

Waldstein, G., Mierau, G., Ahmad, R., Thibodeau, S. N., Hagerman, R. J., & Caldwell, S. (1987). Fragile X syndrome: Skin elastin abnormalities. *Birth Defects Original Article Series, 23,* 103−114.

Warren, S. T. (1996). The expanding world of trinucleotide repeats. *Science, 271,* 1374−1375.

Warren, S.T., & Ashley, C. T., (1995). Triplet repeat expansion mutation: The example of fragile X syndrome. *Annual Review of Neuroscience, 18,* 77−99.

Webb, T. P., & Bundey, S. (1991). Prevalence of fragile X syndrome [letter]. *American Journal of Medical Genetics, 28,* 358.

Webb, T. P., Bundey, S., Thake, A., & Todd, J. (1986). The frequency of the fragile X chromosome among school children in Coventry. *Journal of Medical Genetics, 23,* 396−399.

Wisniewski, K. E., Segan, S. M., Miezejeski, C. M., Sersen, E. A., & Rudelli, R. D. (1991). The fra(X) syndrome: Neurological, electrophysiological, and neuropathological abnormalities. *American Journal of Medical Genetics, 38,* 476−480.

Witt, R. M., Kaspar, B. K., Brazelton, A. D., Comery, T. A., Craig, A. M., Weiler, I. J., & Greenough, W. T. (1995). Developmental localization of fragile X mRNA in rat brain. *Society for Neuroscience Abstracts, 21,* 1 # 293.6.

3 A Behavioral Neurogenetics Approach to Understanding the Fragile X Syndrome

Michele M. Mazzocco and Allan L. Reiss

Research findings from molecular genetic, cognitive, psychiatric, and neuro-anatomical studies of the fragile X syndrome provide consistent support for a detailed description of the fragile X phenotype. The contribution across these multiple areas of research exemplifies the interdisciplinary nature of the field of cognitive neuroscience. Illustrated in this chapter is how this collective contribution provides a cohesive—albeit still incomplete—model for understanding the fragile X syndrome. Also illustrated is how the contributions from a behavioral neurogenetics approach extend far beyond enhancing our understanding of this disorder. Recognition of gene-brain-behavior associations that underlie the fragile X phenotype renders possible the development of models of neurodevelopmental variation that lead to mental retardation, learning disability, and psychopathology. Such models provide an important contribution to the field of developmental cognitive neuroscience.

The current state of knowledge concerning the fragile X phenotype is reviewed in this chapter. Also reviewed are ongoing attempts to specify further the phenotype and efforts to identify underlying mechanisms using a behavioral neurogenetics approach. The case reports presented throughout this chapter help to illustrate how research designed to examine molecular genetic, psychiatric, neuroanatomical, and intellectual associations is an important step toward achieving these goals of specifying the phenotype and identifying the mechanisms underlying fragile X syndrome. The case reports also illustrate the distinction between the fragile X premutation and full mutation, which are defined later in this chapter.

CASE REPORT 1: MONOZYGOTIC TWINS DISCORDANT FOR THE FRAGILE X SYNDROME

Twin teenage girls with the fragile X full mutation recently were evaluated in the context of our ongoing research. Although DNA testing confirmed monozygosity, remarkable differences were observed between these identical twins. Like approximately half of female subjects with the fragile X full mutation, twin A has normal intellectual functioning and does not appear to manifest any obvious psychopathology. She received an overall IQ score of 105 on standardized testing and scored within normal limits on measures of academic and neuropsychological functioning. In contrast, twin B has mental retardation, as do approximately half of female patients with the fragile X full mutation. Twin B showed globally deficient performance across academic, neuropsychological, and social domains, although an analysis of her overall profile revealed selective impairment in mathematics and nonverbal areas.

Whereas an initial review of these twins may indicate that only one girl is affected by fragile X, a closer evaluation reveals that each girl has qualitatively similar effects that vary in degree. Both girls demonstrate relative strengths in verbal skills and facial recognition and weaknesses in visual-spatial and executive function skills. Specifically, each girl's standard scores on naming vocabulary (Boston Naming Test and Peabody Picture Vocabulary Test) and rapid automatized naming tasks were at least 11 points higher than her full-scale IQ score. In contrast, each girl's standard scores on the inventory and organization scores of the Rey-Osterreith Complex Figure Drawing task (copy and recall) were low relative to performance in other domains, and relative to her overall, or full-scale, IQ score. Performance on a spatial memory task (dot localization) and a word fluency task was also relatively weak for each girl.

Both girls were rated by their parents as having significant problems with social skills, attention, hyperactivity, conduct, withdrawal, and anxiety, although neither rated herself as having significant anxiety. Despite her average IQ score, twin A's most significant difficulties were primarily psychosocial, not intellectual. Neither twin showed any apparent physical features of the fragile X syndrome. These profiles illustrate the wide range of effects associated with the fragile X full mutation (see Mazzocco et al., 1995; and Reiss et al., 1995a, for a more thorough description of these twins) and the presence of these effects among individuals who lack the physical characteristics of fragile X syndrome (as described by Hagerman in chapter 2). Explanations for the remarkably different levels of psychological function seen across these twins are presented later.

CASE REPORT 2: VARIABILITY IN AGE AT DIAGNOSIS, EVEN AMONG FAMILY MEMBERS

An extended family agreed to participate in our ongoing research primarily to obtain more information about the proband, a 2-year-old boy previously given a diagnosis of fragile X syndrome. This preschool boy and his mother were accompanied by the boy's maternal aunt and her two children, none of whom had ever been tested for the fragile X mutation. DNA testing was offered to all family members present, and the results revealed the absence of any mutation in the proband's male cousin and a full mutation in the proband's female cousin. The DNA results also confirmed that the proband carried the full mutation.

Like the vast majority of preschool boys with fragile X syndrome, the proband had significant language impairment superimposed on mental retardation. At 2 years 7 months, he received a mental development index of "below 50 points" on the Bayley Scales of Infant Development (second edition) and also scored below 50 on the Preschool Language Scale (third edition); these scores represent the lowest possible score on either measure. His language profile included a two-word expressive vocabulary and revealed significant delays in receptive language. Scores obtained by administration of the Vineland Adaptive Scales interview to his mother demonstrated mild to moderate delays in the communication (61), daily living skills (55), socialization (65), and motor skills (58) domains of adaptive behaviors. Although he did not meet criteria for autistic disorder, this boy manifested autism-like behaviors, including stereotypical movements (e.g., hand flapping). He exhibited a clear preference for, and attachment to, his mother and a positive (albeit nonverbal) rapport with his cousins, despite not interacting well with others in general. His play was immature and lacked symbolic functions. His mother described him as very overactive and impulsive.

The proband's female cousin was 10 years old at the time of her evaluation. She presented as a pleasant, well-groomed girl with no apparent features of fragile X syndrome, although her face was somewhat long. Her brother (who had no fragile X mutation) also had a long face, and both were slenderly built. Despite an overall IQ score within the low average range (84), this young girl's cognitive and psychiatric profile was exemplary of the fragile X female phenotype.

This profile included a relatively high verbal comprehension factor score (96) and bordlerine factor scores on the perceptual organization (73) and freedom from distractibility (75) domains. Her reading achievement scores ranged from 84 to 93 and exceeded her below-average math achievement scores of 72 and 74. She scored in the borderline range (73) on the Beery test of visual motor integration. On the basis of maternal ratings and interview, this girl received clinically significant scores on attention problems and borderline scores on ratings of social problems and anxiety. Her mother described her as having developmentally appropriate adaptive skills in the daily living skills domain (87) but borderline adaptive skills in the areas of communication (72) and socialization (71).

The more severe phenotype seen in a male family member relative to his 10-year-old female cousin illustrates the typical variation in full mutation expression across male and female individuals. The presence of cognitive and behavioral features in the 2-year-old boy illustrates that a psychological phenotype is evident in at least a subgroup of boys with fragile X even during the preschool years. The female cousin illustrates the psychosocial deficits that comprise the phenotype of girls with the fragile X full mutation, which frequently is seen despite a full-scale IQ score in the average range. The fact that this girl's condition was diagnosed later in childhood than that of her cousin—and as the result of having an affected male proband in the extended family—is not an uncommon occurrence for girls with fragile X. Equally common is for children with the full mutation to show no apparent physical features of this disorder.

CASE REPORT 3: VARIATION WITHIN AN IMMEDIATE FAMILY

A family of five that participated in ongoing research included the proband, a 4-year-old girl with the full mutation; her 7-year-old brother, who had no fragile X mutation; and her 10-year-old sister, who carried the premutation. Each of the three children (and their parents) had a relatively round face and lacked any apparent physical feature of the fragile X syndrome. The proband had been tested previously (at 7 months of age), at which time she received a mental development index score of 89 on the Bayley Scales of Infant Development and scores at or above 102 across all domains of the Vineland Adaptive Behavior Scales.

As a 4-year-old, she presented as a pleasant, cooperative, outgoing child. During sessions with the psychologist, she initiated conversation and spoke in full sentences, although her articulation was difficult to discern. She scored 93 on the Stanford Binet (fourth edition), a measure of global intellectual functioning. Her strongest performance was on verbal reasoning area subtests (vocabulary, verbal comprehension; area standard score, 108), whereas her weaker performance was on visual and quantitative reasoning tasks (standard scores of 85 and 88, respectively). She received a standard score of 98 on the Beery test of visual motor integration. On measures of adaptive functioning, her standard scores were in the low average to below average ranges for all four domains assessed: daily living (86), communication (85), socialization (80), and motor skills (75).

The proband's brother, who had no fragile X mutation, did not present with any social or intellectual difficulties. On psychological testing, he received an IQ score of 120, with particular strengths in the nonverbal domain. All behavioral, academic achievement, and adaptive scores obtained for this boy were well within or above the average range.

A similar profile was obtained from the proband's sister, a premutation carrier. Her IQ score of 124 was well above average, as were her reading achievement (128), math calculation (129), and visual motor integration (140) scores. Her factor scores on the Wechsler test indicated no particular area of weakness; her verbal comprehension score (118) and perceptual organization score (128) were both above average, as was her score for freedom from distractibility (129). This girl showed no apparent deleterious effects of the premutation she was known to carry.

Several points are illustrated by the data from this family. First, an adult carrier of the fragile X premutation can have offspring with no mutation, the premutation, or the full mutation. Second, offspring with the premutation typically do not appear affected. Third, a diagnosis of the full mutation in a female subject is not necessarily indicative of mental retardation; in this family, the proband scored within the low-average range on many intellectual measures. Fourth, scores obtained on very young children with the full mutation are often within normal limits. Even among male individuals, preschoolers with fragile X do not necessarily test in the mentally retarded range (Freund et al., 1995). Finally, the degree of involvement associated with the fragile X full mutation should be considered within the context of other influences on intellectual development (described later).

Heritable influences on intellectual development can be estimated through the assessment of a proband's unaffected family members. In this family, the proband's level of functioning was significantly lower than what would be predicted on the basis of the well-established evidence for heritability of intelligence (Plomin, 1990; Plomin & Neiderhiser, 1991) and on the basis of her siblings' and mother's IQ scores, which ranged from 120 to 124. Interestingly, the degree to which this proband's IQ differed from those of her siblings and mother is very similar to the discrepancy observed between the IQ score of the 10-year-old girl described in case report 2 (full-scale IQ = 84) and the IQ score from her brother (102) and mother (111). This measure of deviation from parental IQ has proved to be an important variable in our research (Abrams et al., 1994; Reiss et al., 1995a), as described later in this chapter.

THE FRAGILE X MENTAL RETARDATION GENE MUTATION: DIAGNOSIS, DIFFERENTIATION, AND FUNCTION

The phenotypic variation illustrated in these case reports is at least in part a function of molecular genetic features of the fragile X mutation. One primary feature is the degree of expansion seen in the mutation associated most commonly with the fragile X syndrome. This expansion is a cytosine-guanine-guanine (CGG) nucleic acid repeat within the promoter region of the fragile X mental retardation (FMR1) gene. The recent discovery of this expansion (Verkerk et al., 1991) led to the identification of an approximate threshold (approximately 200 CGG repeats) differentiating the full mutation, which is associated with the fragile X syndrome, from the premutation. Carriers of the premutation have a CGG amplification that exceeds the reported high end of the normal (52) number of CGG repeats (Fu et al., 1991) but that falls below the threshold for the full mutation. Individuals with a combination of premutation and full mutation alleles are described as having a mosaic pattern. The distinction between these categories of molecular genetic status (as described in more detail by Hagerman in chapter 2) is particularly dependent on methylation status, which is in turn related to amplification size. The hypermethylation associated with the full mutation leads to a corresponding interruption in production of FMR1 messenger RNA. Without the presence of FMR1 messenger RNA, no protein is produced. The diminished levels or depletion of FMR1 protein in the brain is what leads to the constellation of features that comprise the fragile X syndrome phenotype.

In female patients, an estimate of FMR1 gene activation and, accordingly, FMR1 protein levels can be derived by evaluating cellular X chromosome inactivation patterns. Specifically, a ratio is calculated to represent the proportion of cells that have an active, unaffected X chromosome (i.e., that have a normal FMR1 allele) versus cells with an active, full-mutation X chromosome. This activation ratio, obtained from lymphocyte-derived DNA, approaches 1 as the number of cells with a normal active X chromosome increases, and approaches 0 when the number of cells having an active X chromosome with a full mutation increases. (See Abrams et al., 1994, and Reiss et al., 1995b, for a description of measurement techniques used to calculate activation ratio.)

On the theoretical basis that activation ratio is an indicator of FMR1 protein level, researchers hypothesized that negative correlations would emerge between activation ratio and degree of deficit or abnormality in areas of functioning associated with the fragile X syndrome. Among individuals with the fragile X full mutation, we have reported significant negative correlations between activation ratio and both intellectual dysfunction (Abrams et al., 1994; Reiss et al., 1995b) and degree of neuroanatomical abnormality (Reiss et al., 1995a). Thus, activation ratio and degree of involvement appear to have an important association.

Activation ratio is irrelevant for the study of premutation effects, because typically none of the cells in an individual with a small premutation are hypermethylated. Unclear is whether large premutations are associated with diminished production of the FMR1 protein (Warren et al., 1994). In male subjects with a mosaic pattern of premutation and full mutation cells (as described by Hagerman in chapter 2), activation ratio can be determined. The method used to quantify this ratio is based on a formula different from that derived for female subjects with the full mutation, as described elsewhere (Baumgardner et al., 1995).

Despite the demonstrated link between FMR1 activation and severity of effects, clinical prognoses cannot be based on activation ratio until further questions are addressed. Critically important is the understanding of whether lymphocyte-derived DNA activation ratio reflects activation ratio in brain tissue and whether it accurately reflects the level of FMR1 protein. Evidence from a case report of two patients with the full mutation supports the contention that lymphoctye-derived DNA (i.e., DNA derived from white blood cells) and olfactory epithelial tissue-derived DNA give rise to molecular genetic features (Abrams et al., 1999). On the basis of the biological link between olfactory epithelial and neuronal tissue, this finding provides preliminary support that activation ratio is a good estimate of *FMR1* gene expression in the brain.

Nevertheless, conclusive evidence for this association has not yet been obtained. Also, activation ratio must be considered in conjunction with other factors that influence degree of involvement, such as genetic contributions to intelligence (Reiss et al., 1995b), as illustrated in case report 3, and the family environment (Reiss, 1996). Finally, exceptions to the associations between high activation ratio and high level of functioning must be identified and understood. A notable example is the report that the activation ratios for both monozygotic twins described in case report 1 were high (above 0.80) and virtually identical (Abrams et al., 1994; Mazzocco et al., 1995; Reiss et al., 1995a). Very possibly, the activation ratio for these twins is distorted as a result of their shared placenta during prenatal development. If this is the case, the activation ratio obtained from each girl's blood sample might not reflect activation ratio in either girl's other tissues, and a discrepancy between lymphocyte-derived and olfactory epithelium—derived or brain-derived DNA would be expected for one or both of these girls. Until these questions concerning the accuracy of activation ratio are resolved, activation ratio should *not* be considered a prognostic measure, despite its importance in research on variability and specificity of the fragile X syndrome.

VARIATION IN THE COGNITIVE AND BEHAVIORAL PHENOTYPE

The Fragile X Premutation

Little if any theoretical bases justify hypothesizing a premutation phenotype, because FMR1 protein is present in premutation cells (Pieretti et al., 1991; Sjak & Meyer, 1993) and because of the absence of compelling evidence to date for effects of the normal *FMR1* gene on normal intellectual variation (Daniels et al., 1994; Mazzocco & Reiss, 1997). The older sister described in case report 3 exemplifies reports of normal development in premutation carriers. However, a definitive conclusion regarding potential effects of the premutation must be based on additional empirical research.

Research findings to date generally are inconsistent with respect to evidence for effects of the premutation (Plomin & Neiderhiser, 1991; Mazzocco et al., 1993; Reiss et al., 1993; Dorn et al., 1994; Loesch et al., 1994; Rousseau et al., 1994; Sobesky et al., 1994; Feng et al., 1995). Although the majority of these studies indicate a *lack* of an effect of the premutation on psychopathology or cognitive performance (Mazzocco et al., 1993; Reiss et al., 1993; Feng et al., 1995; Mazzocco & Holden, 1996), some case reports cite the contrary. From the reports suggesting premutation effects, several limitations must be considered. For instance, Dorn et al. (1994) reported a higher frequency of psychopathology among men *presumed* to be carriers of the premutation, relative to men without a fragile X full mutation. However, the data for their study were obtained from daughter informants, and the male participants in their study may have had a mosaic pattern or a full mutation allele. The lack of available genetic data from these male subjects prohibited examination of these possibilities. Case reports of cognitive effects of the premutation (Hagerman et al., 1996; Mazzocco et al., unpublished data) typically are drawn from clinical populations of children seen as being at risk for fragile X syndrome; thus, these reports are subject to ascertainment bias inherent in clinical research. Some researchers view these cases as "coincidence" (Feng et al., 1995). Others suggest that in the few cases in which a positive phenotype is described, the lymphocyte-derived premutation status may reflect inaccurately a mosaic pattern in the brain (Hagerman et al., 1996). The most convincing report to date of a premutation phenotype is based on a mild physical phenotype, including slightly longer face and more prominent ears among female subjects, with the premutation relative to non–fragile X controls with mental retardation (Hull & Hagerman, 1993). Despite case reports to the contrary, to date no compelling evidence corroborates that the premutation has a negative impact on intellectual or psychological function. Controlled studies of individuals drawn from a general population are needed for more satisfactory closure on this issue.

Effects of the Full Mutation in Male Subjects

Unlike studies of the premutation, unquestionably the fragile X full mutation leads to variable and specific effects. As a group, *male* patients with fragile X syndrome represent individuals at one end of the cognitive and behavioral spectrum of the fragile X phenotype. Their adaptive skills generally are consistent with their level of intellectual functioning, although the association between adaptive behavior and measured intelligence in fragile X is not well understood at this time (Dykens, 1995). The male phenotype, as described by Hagerman in chapter 2, includes mental retardation, hyperactivity and hyperarousal, attentional difficulties, language delay, and autistic behaviors. The autistic behaviors appear to be related primarily to stereotypies and communication abnormalities, including echolalia. The social interaction deficits that are reported typically among children with autism, such as not seeking comfort from a caregiver and not recognizing the emotional state of others, are not seen among children with fragile X (Reiss & Freund, 1992). Language in male individuals with fragile X often is perseverative (Sudhalter et al., 1990), but such perseveration appears related to social stimulation and hyperarousal (such as being looked at) versus syntactical ability (Besler & Sudhalter, 1995). Quantitative skills weakness and social withdrawal (Freund et al., 1995) also have been reported. The specific neurobehavioral profile reported for male subjects with fragile X has been observed as early as age 3 (Freund et al., 1995), as illustrated in case report 2. Between early childhood and adolescence, IQ scores appear to decline among male patients with fragile X (Hagerman et al., 1989; Hodapp et al., 1991). These declines represent a widening gap between boys with fragile X and other children their age, rather than a loss of already acquired skills.

The psychological characteristics of fragile X are more consistent across boys with fragile X than is their physical phenotype; moreover, the domains in which deficits are seen in male subjects are similar to the domains in which female subjects manifest deficits. Nevertheless, the behavioral neurogenetic approach to studying fragile X in *male* subjects is limited by the narrow range and greater severity of these effects. Female individuals with fragile X present with a much wider range of activation ratio scores, cognitive deficits, and psychological dysfunction. For this reason, the emphasis on our description of the fragile X phenotype pertains to *female* individuals with the full mutation.

Effects of the Full Mutation in Female Individuals

Descriptions of the cognitive phenotype in *female* subjects with fragile X has been refined recently, owing in part to the genetic advances described. Until

1991, estimates suggested that approximately one-third of female subjects with fragile X were mentally retarded (Sherman et al., 1985), one-third presented with milder cognitive deficits (including learning disability), and one-third were unaffected. These estimates predated the identification of the premutation and full mutation distinctions and, therefore, were based on female individuals across these genetic categories. Associations were reported between degree of cognitive effects and positive cytogenetic fragility (Prouty et al., 1988; Mazzocco et al., 1992a) and maternal inheritance (Reiss et al., 1989; Hinton et al., 1992), factors that now are considered indicators of the full mutation. Among female subjects with the full mutation, more recent data indicate that approximately half (53%) have mental retardation (Rousseau et al., 1994). A subset of female patients who have the full mutation and are *not* mentally retarded nevertheless manifest a cognitive profile that appears consistent in pattern, yet variable in severity, with IQ scores ranging from below to above average. Of girls who have the fragile X full mutation, the majority are affected cognitively or behaviorally to varying degrees.

With respect to the nature of cognitive and behavioral deficits, preliminary studies revealed weaknesses in performance on specific Wechsler subtests, including block design (Loesch et al., 1987), arithmetic and digit span in both girls and women with fragile X, relative to controls (Kemper et al., 1986; Miezejeski et al., 1986; Grigsby et al., 1987; Brainard et al., 1991). Deficits in visual memory for abstract stimuli and numerical skills were indicated by relatively weak performance on the Stanford-Binet (fourth edition) quantitative and bead memory subtests (Freund & Reiss, 1991) and deficits on achievement measures of arithmetic (Miezejeski et al., 1986; Miezejeski & Hinton, 1992). Results from more recent studies also have been consistent with this pattern of findings for depressed performance on mathematics achievement scores in girls (Kover, 1993) and in women (Mazzocco et al., 1993) with fragile X, relative to non–fragile X comparison groups. Findings inconsistent with this profile of specific mathematics skills difficulties were drawn from mostly fragile X negative obligate carriers (Wolf et al., 1988), who most likely were carriers of the premutation.

Initial IQ profiles provided a foundation for later attempts to specify the neuropsychological nature of the phenotype. Evidence for visual-spatial and mathematical deficits and relative strengths in global verbal performance consistently emerged through this later research. On the Woodcock-Johnson Spatial Relations subtest, women (Mazzocco et al., 1993) and girls (Kovar, 1993) with the full mutation have significantly greater difficulty than do female subjects without fragile X. Girls with fragile X demonstrate remarkable difficulty on the Rey-Osterreith Complex Figure drawing, Benton Judgment of Line Orientation, and the Wechsler Block Design. The visual spatial deficits in conjunction with attentional difficulties (Freund et al., 1997), arithmetical weaknesses, and problem-solving deficits (Mazzocco et al., 1992b), are consistent with the nonverbal learning disability profile proposed by

Rourke (e.g., Harnadek & Rourke, 1994). In an attempt to specify the fragile X phenotype, the similarities between the behaviorally and neuro-psychologically defined nonverbal learning disability and the biologically defined fragile X syndrome have been noted.

The notion that fragile X is an etiology of the nonverbal learning disability has been challenged (Miezejeski & Hinton, 1992; Kovar, 1993) on the basis of inconsistencies seen between these disorders, including preserved performance on visual short- and long-term memory (Mazzocco et al., 1993) and intact social cognition skills (Kovar, 1993; Mazzocco et al., 1993) in female patients with fragile X. Research findings pertaining to memory performance in fragile X may appear inconsistent across studies, but a careful examination of the tasks used across studies may clarify this apparent discrepancy. Girls (and boys) with fragile X perform poorly on immediate recall of visually presented beads that vary in shape and color and are presented individually or in groups of two or more beads (Freund & Reiss, 1991). Similarly, Kovar (1993) demonstrated that girls with fragile X had poorer short-term verbal recall of stories, relative to girls with dyslexia; however, the girls with fragile X had scores that were in the average range and were comparable to their IQ scores, and the amount of information they lost between immediate and delayed recall of the stories did not differ from that of the girls with dyslexia. The performance observed across these (and other) studies may indicate memory deficts or difficulty with the attention skills necessary for success on these tasks. Women with fragile X perform above average when immediately reproducing a visually presented design on paper and have average performance on delayed reproduction of these designs (Mazzocco et al., 1993). Thus, memory difficulties do not appear to be a global component of the fragile X phenotype, and intact visual memory performance is inconsistent with the nonverbal learning disability profile.

Although reports of verbal strengths in female individuals with fragile X are consistent with the nonverbal learning disability profile, these strengths may be limited to reading and naming abilities. Evidence for verbal "strengths" is drawn primarily from measures of global verbal expression (such as the verbal IQ score), reading achievement, and reading decoding skills. Higher-order language skills are not necessarily intact. Some have hypothesized that higher-order problem solving skills, referred to as *executive function skills*, underlie the language errors, such as tangential and perseverative speech (Mazzocco et al., 1992a) and difficulty with linguistic inferences (Simon & Keenan, 1996). Thus, not yet clear is whether the fragile X cognitive phenotype in female subjects represents primary deficits in visual perception or executive function skills, or which features are primary or secondary to the disorder.

Despite the lack of understanding for what underlies the cognitive phenotype in female patients with fragile X, what *is* clear is that the pattern of deficits reported across studies is specific. This pattern includes visual spatial, mathematics, attentional, and problem-solving difficulties. An important feature of our own research and of other neuropsychological studies is that the results are based on groups consisting of female individuals who have fragile X and whose full-scale IQ scores > 70, indicating that these deficits are seen even among the less affected female subjects with fragile X and clearly are *not* linked to mental retardation (Mazzocco et al., 1992a,b; Mazzocco et al., 1993; Kovar 1993). Whether the degree of these deficits changes over age has not been addressed definitely to date. Evidence for an age-related decline in IQ has been reported for female subjects with fragile X (Prouty et al., 1988), but that evidence has not been consistent (Brun et al., 1995).

In addition to specific cognitive deficits, behavioral manifestations are key components of the full mutation phenotype in females. Young girls with fragile X are reported to show clinically significant levels of hyperactive behaviors, as measured by the Child Behavior Checklist (Lachiewicz, 1992). Although hyperactivity and attention problems have been considered correlates of low IQ, girls who have fragile X and have average IQs (>85) have significantly greater attention problems than do age-, IQ-, and gender-matched control participants, including girls with Turner syndrome and girls with neither disorder. Attention and hyperactivity appear to be a specific component of the fragile X phenotype. When compared to IQ-matched girls from a non–fragile X comparison group, girls with fragile X also show significantly higher levels of mood disorders and withdrawn behaviors (Freund et al., 1993); problem behaviors, including anxiety, as measured by the Conners Parent Questionnaire (Lachiewicz & Dawson, 1994); and significantly poorer social skills, including low social competence, low social adaptive behavior, increased social withdrawal, and anxiety (Kovar, 1993; Freund et al., 1996a). Interpersonal skills have been shown to be deficient in girls with fragile X, as marked by infrequent use of socially appropriate behaviors and less social involvement with same-age peers. Despite being described as anxious by parents and teachers, girls with fragile X do not themselves report experiencing anxiety (Kovar, 1993; Sarter, 1996). Reports of social dysfunction in women with fragile X, relative to IQ-matched controls (Freund et al., 1992), suggest that the social dysfunction seen in girls with fragile X does not diminish with development. Awareness of subtle aspects of social awareness (such as perspective taking and emotion perception) appear intact among girls and women with fragile X (Kovar, 1993, Mazzocco et al., 1993, respectively), despite reported deficits in their social behavior and competence. Preliminary paired-sibling studies lend support that this social dysfunction is not explained solely by familial factors (Mazzocco et al., 1998).

Additional behavioral features associated with fragile X syndrome are depression and autistic behaviors. Despite early reports of depression in girls with fragile X (Lachiewicz, 1992; Freund et al., 1993), more recent findings fail to support the notion that depression is a general characteristic of the fragile X phenotype (Kovar, 1993). Autistic behaviors reported among girls with fragile X are similar in nature but milder in severity relative to those reported for male subjects (Reiss & Freund, 1990, 1992), and include a higher degree of stereotypies, restricted behaviors, and communication difficulties (Mazzocco et al., 1997a). These autistic behaviors have been shown not to correlate with mental retardation or with overall full-scale IQ scores.

Hypotheses that the social difficulties seen in fragile X are related to social cognition or cognitive deficits have not received empirical support. Women (Mazzocco et al., 1993) and girls (Kovar, 1993) with fragile X do not appear to have difficulty with perspective taking, nor do women with fragile X have trouble in matching photographs depicting simple or complex emotions (Mazzocco et al., 1994). Sobesky et al. (1994) examined cognitive and psychosocial correlates among women affected by fragile X and found no significant association between cognitive performance and each psychiatric measure from the Minnesota Multiphasic Personality Inventory (second edition) or the schedule for affective disorders and schizophrenia-lifetime version, except with a score indicating denial. These findings lend support for the notion that cognitive and psychosocial effects of the full mutation are independent components of the fragile X phenotype.

As was described relative to conclusions regarding effects of the premutation, an important consideration is the potential influence of ascertainment bias on descriptions of the full mutation phenotype. Possibly individuals who come to clinical attention (and who therefore are identified as potential research participants) represent the tip of the iceberg with respect to persons affected by the fragile X syndrome. If this scenario were accurate, individuals with little or no effect of the full mutation would remain without diagnosis and be underrepresented in phenotype descriptions. Prevalence studies play an important role in identifying the discrepancy between the phenotypes of clinically derived and genetic screening–derived samples. Based on our studies of the prevalence of fragile X among non–mentally retarded children with academic difficulty (Mazzocco et al., 1997b), we find no evidence to suggest that this discrepancy is significant. Findings from additional screening studies support this contention (Holden et al., 1995) although further studies of different population groups are needed to validate or disclaim this preliminary conclusion.

Neuroanatomical Findings in Male and Female Subjects

Neuroimaging research is a relatively new contribution to science in general and to the study of fragile X syndrome. Magnetic resonance imaging allows for noninvasive investigation of brain structure in living persons and yields high-resolution, three-dimensional data. The initial neuroanatomical investigation of the fragile X phenotype was designed to assess posterior cerebellar vermis volumes, in view of the abnormalities reported for this region among a subset of individuals with autism (Courchesne et al., 1988). This initial investigation led to the first experimental support for the notion that specific abnormality in brain structure is a component of the fragile X syndrome. Among 14 male and 12 female subjects with fragile X syndrome examined, decreased volume of the posterior cerebellar volume (particularly lobules VI and VII) was reported relative to developmentally delayed and nondelayed comparison subjects (Reiss et al., 1991a,b). No such differences were found for other neuroanatomical regions examined, including the corpus callosum, cerebellar hemispheres, pons, midbrain, and medulla. Later investigations led to findings that individuals with fragile X have increased size of specific brain regions, including the caudate nucleus, hippocampus, and lateral ventricle. Individuals with the full mutation also have age-related increases in hippo-campal and lateral ventricular volumes and age-related decreases in superior temporal gyral volume. None of these age-related differences was found in the comparison groups examined (Reiss 1994).

The neuroanatomical findings across studies lead to an important conclu-sion concerning phenotype variation and specificity in fragile X. Although none of the neuroanatomical abnormalities observed is specific to fragile X syndrome alone, the evidence across male and female individuals with fragile X indicates a clear pattern of incremental degrees of abnormality consistent with a gene dosage model of the *FMR1* full mutation. Girls with fragile X have neuroanatomical abnormalities in the same brain structures and in the same direction as do male subjects with fragile X, yet their volumetric data are intermediate between those reported for male patients with fragile X and female patients without fragile X (Reiss et al., 1995a). This pattern is similar to findings reported for the cognitive and behavioral phenotypes, and lends support for the notion that increased levels of FMR1 protein are associated with diminished effects of the fragile X full mutation.

A second conclusion to be drawn from the neuroanatomical findings is that these data provide evidence for a brain-behavior relation in fragile X syndrome. The neuroanatomical areas for which brain structure abnormality is reported are brain regions associated with functions now known to be deficient among individuals with the fragile X syndrome (as discussed later). The association between neuroanatomical structure and development, with behavior and genetic variables, is the primary focus of the behavioral neuro-genetics approach to understanding the fragile X syndrome.

LINKING GENETIC, PSYCHOLOGICAL, AND NEUROANATOMICAL PROFILES

Although descriptions of the genetic, psychological, and neuroanatomical findings each contribute to describing the fragile X phenotype, the *associa-tions* among these three levels of variables are most relevant to understand-ing the mechanisms that may underlie the overall phenotype. It is, of course, expected that these associations interact with other influences on function and development. For this reason, such influences are considered whenever possible.

For example, in studies of how the *FMR1* mutation influences intellectual function, we have controlled statistically for additional genetic contributions to intellectual development. We derive this estimate by calculating the difference between a child's IQ score and the IQ score of its parent(s); the mean of both parents' score is used when scores for both are available (Abrams et al., 1994; Reiss et al., 1995b). This difference from parental IQ coupled with the impact of the family environment (Reiss, 1996) provides significant contributions to statistical models of the effects of the *FMR1* full mutation.

Also important are consideration of the limits of brain-behavior associations in determining localization of function in general (e.g., see Sarter et al., 1996) and of the fact that strict localization of function is *not* the goal of our gene-brain-behavior investigations. Indeed, the lack of an association between function and a particular brain region does not implicate a corresponding lack of involvement of that region in the function of interest; nor does the presence of a strong association implicate a primary localization of function. Instead, the identification of gene-brain-behavior associations in individuals with fragile X will help to elucidate both the neurodevelopmental pathways leading to the fragile X phenotype and a general model of developmental variation leading to characteristics associated with this disorder that may occur also in its absence.

An initial effort toward identifying *gene-behavior* relations revealed important associations between activation ratio and cognitive functioning (Abrams et al., 1994; Reiss et al., 1995b). In female subjects, activation ratio correlates with intellectual functioning, particularly in areas that best differentiate female subjects with fragile X from female subjects without fragile X. For instance, activation ratio is correlated most strongly with performance on the block design subtest of the Wechsler scale, a task that requires the deliberate construction of an abstract two-dimensional design composed of individual blocks. In contrast, no correlation has been noted between activation ratio and vocabulary or picture completion subtests, the latter of which requires the identification of an item missing from an illustration of a familiar object. This set of findings indicates that among areas of cognitive functioning that appear affected by the fragile X full mutation, activation ratio is a good estimate of the degree to which an individual is affected. The correlations indicate that as activation ratio increases (which is believed to reflect increased levels of FMR1 protein), the degree of dysfunction associated with fragile X appears to decrease. Similarly, among girls with fragile X with full-scale IQ scores above or equal to 70 points, activation ratio has been shown to correlate significantly with ratings for specific autistic behaviors, including restricted behaviors and interests (Mazzocco et al., 1997ab). Higher ratings (indicating a greater severity and more types of behaviors) on these stereotypical-restricted behavior items were associated with *lower* activation ratio. No significant correlations emerged among these girls between autistic-like social interaction, communication or imagination ratings, and activation ratio. In conclusion, this gene-behavior association based on activation ratio, an estimate of FMR1 protein, is strong, in the predicted direction, and specific.

A similar *gene-brain* association emerged from the study of activation ratio and neuroanatomical variation in fragile X syndrome. Activation ratio has been shown to predict the degree to which the caudate and ventricular volumes are increased, relative to non–fragile X comparison subjects. This correlation illustrates that as activation ratio increases (a reflection of higher levels of FMR1 protein), the degree of caudate and ventricular volume abnormality decreases. Finally, examination of *brain-behavior* associations also illustrate support for a specific link between brain structure abnormality and psychological dysfunction. Caudate and lateral ventricular volume is correlated negatively with full-scale IQ scores among individuals with fragile X but not among controls. Posterior cerebellar vermis size is correlated positively with performance on intellectual and visuospatial measures in female subjects with fragile X (Mostofsky et al., 1996). Among school-age girls who had fragile X and had IQ scores > 70, posterior cerebellar vermis area is correlated negatively with the degree of abnormality in communication and stereotypical-ritualistic behavioral abnormalities corresponding to the criteria for autistic disorder described in the *Diagnostic and Statistical Manual of Mental Disorders* (third edition 1980) (Mazzocco et al, 1997a).

Each of these findings illustrates the contributions of a behavioral neurogenetic approach to the study of fragile X syndrome. As activation ratio decreases, degree of abnormality in brain structure and degree of psychological dysfunction increases. Increases in degree of brain structure abnormality are associated with behavioral dysfunction. Considered together, the results already presented are consistent with the hypothesis that a gene-brain-behavior model of fragile X can be based on estimates of *FMR1* gene inactivation.

IMPLICATIONS FOR THE NEUROBIOLOGICAL ORGANIZATION INVOLVED IN FRAGILE X SYNDROME

An exciting aspect of the molecular genetic and neuroanatomical associations previously described is how closely these associations are linked to specific components of the fragile X phenotype. Associations are seen not only among global behavioral or intellectual functions but particularly for behavioral and cognitive measures that differentiate individuals with fragile X from individuals without the mutation. Moreover, neuroanatomical abnormalities described for fragile X are found in brain regions associated with these differentiating measures. For instance, the cerebellar vermis plays a role in mediating sensory stimulation and arousal through its connections to the somatosensory, auditory, and visual cortices (Joseph et al., 1978; Crispino & Bullock, 1984) and the brainstem reticular formation (Tang & Zhang, 1987). These functions are known to be involved in arousal and may influence the hypersensitivity to tactile stimuli reported for children with fragile X (Hagerman, 1991; Baumgardner et al., 1995). Deficits in attention are consistent with impairment in the capacity to shift attention voluntarily and rapidly, a deficit that has been found independently in both autistic patients and patients with acquired cerebellar lesions (Courchesne, et al., 1994) and in individuals with fragile X (Mazzocco et al., 1992a,b). The caudate is believed to influence mood regulation and the control of higher-order processes, such as voluntary eye movement, problem solving, impulse control, and mental flexibility, through its involvement with frontal-subcortical circuits (Cummings, 1993). Lesions to these circuits have been associated with lack of inhibition and poor cognitive organization, both of which are features of the fragile X phenotype. Influences of the hippocampus on attention and the role of the temporal gyrus in language may further explain aspects of the fragile X phenotype related to these functions. Age-related increases in degree of abnormality may be associated with the IQ decline reported for male and female individuals with fragile X (as discussed earlier).

The precise role of the FMR1 protein on brain development and on the corresponding areas of dysfunction remains unclear. Neural cell proliferation, organization, or programmed cell death have been hypothesized as the neurodevelopmental processes affected by the FMR1 protein, hypotheses that have not been examined in the very few postmortem studies available (Reiss et al., 1995a). Animal studies (Willems et al., 1995) using an *FMR1* knockout mouse are ongoing and, it is hoped, will lead to more specific explanations of the role of FMR1 protein on brain development and function.

SUMMARY AND DIRECTIONS OF FUTURE RESEARCH

The neurobehavioral approach to studying the fragile X phenotype involves identifying genetic, psychological, behavioral, and neuroanatomical features of individuals with this disorder and understanding the relation across these areas of development. The psychological and behavioral phenotype varies quite markedly among female subjects and across male and female subjects with fragile X; this notion was illustrated across the three case reports presented earlier in this chapter. The similarities across individuals with fragile X are qualitative rather than quantitative. Cognitive difficulties in visuospatial, arithmetical, attentional, and executive function skills, in addition to autistic behaviors and tangential and perseverative language, are seen in both male and female individuals. Discerning specific areas of strengths and weaknesses is more difficult in male subjects with fragile X, because most with the syndrome have mental retardation and, thus, are globally deficient. In contrast, female subjects often show deficits in the domains described earlier, even when they have average levels of intellectual functioning. Although a psychological phenotype may be evident even in very young preschoolers (as illustrated by the preschool boy in case report 2), some preschool children with fragile X (male and female) have average intellectual functioning. The 4-year-old girl described in case report 3 is such a preschooler. The primary deficits underlying this well-established psychological profile is a topic of ongoing and future research. Regardless of its underlying components, clearly the psychological phenotype may be a more reliable indicator of fragile X than is the physical phenotype. As was illustrated by the case reports, the absence of a physical phenotype clearly is not an indicator of the absence of the fragile X full mutation. Each of the children described in the case reports lacked any apparent physical features of the fragile X phenotype.

The explanation for this variation in phenotypic expression relies on understanding the role of genetics and brain development in cognition and behavior. The results reported to date provide promising evidence of gene-brain-behavior associations believed to be linked by FMR1 protein production. An obvious direction for future research is directly to assess FMR1 protein level, a process in progress. Of interest is whether variation in protein expression among individuals with the full mutation may account for the phenotypic variations illustrated in the foregoing case reports. Validation of the degree to which lymphocyte-derived DNA accurately reflects activation ratio and FMR1 protein levels in the brain is also necessary to understand the associations heretofore described. Longitudinal studies are needed to address the limitations of these associations over time, the degree to which phenotypic variation relates to postnatal brain development, and the prognostic value of molecular genetic or neuroanatomical variables. Functional imaging studies can contribute toward analysis of neurodevelopment and performance across a wide range of domains. Environmental influences on degree of involvement are not to be ignored and, thus, continue to play an increasingly important role in our research. Each of these future directions will contribute toward understanding neurodevelopmental processes that underlie the fragile X syndrome, which will lead in turn to a model of neurodevelopmental variation in specific cognitive and behavioral dysfunction.

REFERENCES

Abrams, M. T., Kaufmann, W. E., Rousseau, F., Oostra, B. A., Wolozin, B. L., Taylor, C. V., Lishaa, N., & Reiss, A. L. (1999). FMR1 gene expression in olfactory neuroblasts from two males with fragile X syndrome. *American Journal of Medical Genetics, 82,* 25–30.

Abrams, M. T., Reiss, A. L., Freund, L. S., Baumgardner, T. L., Chase, G. A., & Denckla, M. B. (1994). Molecular-neurobehavioral associations in females with the fragile X full mutation. *American Journal of Medical Genetics, 51,* 317–327.

American Psychiatric Association (1980). *Diagnostic and statistical manual of mental disorders* (3rd. Ed.) Washington, DC: Author.

Baumgardner, T., Reiss, A. L., Freund, L., & Abrams, M. (1995). Specification of the neurobehavioral phenotype in males with fragile X syndrome. *Pediatrics, 95,* 744–752.

Besler, R., & Sudhalter, V. (1995). Arousal difficulties in males with fragile X syndrome: A preliminary report. *Developmental Brain Dysfunction, 8*(4–6), 270–279.

Brainard, S. S., Schreiner, R. A., & Hagerman, R. J. (1991). Cognitive profiles of the carrier fragile X woman. *American Journal of Medical Genetics, 38,* 505–508.

Brun, C., Obiols, J. E., Cheema, A., O'Connor, R., Riddle, J., DiMaria, M., Wright-Talamante, C., and Hagerman, R. J. (1995). Longitudinal IQ changes in fragile X females. *Developmental Brain Dysfunction, 8,* 230–241.

Courchesne, E., Townsend, J., Akshoomoff, N. A., Saitoh, O., Yeung-Courchesne, R., Lincoln, A. J., James, H. E., Haas, R. H., Schreibman, L., & Lau, L. (1994). Impairment in shifting attention in autistic and cerebellar patients. *Behavioral Neuroscience, 108,* 848–865.

Courchesne, E., Young-Courchesne, R., Press, G. A., Hesselink, J. R., & Jernigan, T. L. (1988). Hypoplasia of cerebellar vermal lobules VI and VII in autism. *New England Journal of Medicine, 318,* 1349–1354.

Crispino, L., & Bullock, T. H. (1984). Cerebellum mediates modality-specific modulation of sensory responses of midbrain and forebrain in rat. *Proceedings of the National Academy of Sciences, 81,* 2917–2920.

Cummings, J. L. (1993). Frontal-subcortical circuits and human behavior. *Archives of Neurology, 50,* 873–880.

Daniels, J., Owen, M., McGuffin, P., Thompson, L., Detterman, D., Chorney, M., Chorney, K., Smith, D., Skuder, P., Vignetti, S., McClearn, G., & Plomin, R. (1994). IQ and variation in the number of fragile X CGG repeats: No association in a normal sample. *Intelligence, 19,* 45–50.

Dorn, M. B., Mazzocco, M. M., & Hagerman, R. J. (1994). Behavioral and psychiatric disorders in adult male carriers of fragile X. *Journal of the American Academy of Child and Adolescent Psychiatry, 33,* 256–264.

Dykens, E. M. (1995). Adaptive behavior in males with fragile X syndrome. *Mental Retardation and Developmental Disabilities, 1,* 281–285.

Feng, Y., Lakkis, L., Devys, D., & Warren, S. T. (1995). Quantitative comparison of *FMR1* gene expression in normal and premutation alleles. *American Journal of Human Genetics, 56,* 106–113.

Freund, L., Baumgardner, T. L., Mazzocco, M., Reiss, A., & Denckla, M. (1997). *Neuropsychological profiles in X chromosome disorders: Fragile X and Turner syndromes.* Poster presented at the Annual Meeting of the International Neuropsychological Society, February 5–8, Orlando, FL.

Freund, L. S., Peebles, C. D., Aylward, E., & Reiss, A. L. (1995). Preliminary report on cognitive and adaptive behaviors of preschool-aged males with fragile X. *Developmental Brain Dysfunction, 8,* 242–251.

Freund, L. S., & Reiss, A. L. (1991). Cognitive profiles associated with the fra(X) syndrome in males and females. *American Journal of Medical Genetics, 38,* 542–547.

Freund, L. S., Reiss, A. L., & Abrams, M. T. (1993). Psychiatric disorders associated with fragile X in the young female. *Pediatrics, 91,* 321–329.

Freund, L. S., Reiss, A. L., Hagerman, R., & Vinogradov, S. (1992). Chromosome fragility and psychopathology in obligate female carriers of the fragile X chromosome. *Archives of General Psychiatry, 49,* 54–60.

Fu, Y. H., Kuhl, D. P., Pizzuti, A., Pieretti, M., Sutcliffe, J. S., Richards, S., Verkerk, A. J., Holden, J. J., Fenwick, R. G., Warren, S. T., Oostra, B. A., Nelson, D. L., Caskey, C. T. (1991). Variation of the CGG repeat at the fragile X site results in genetic instability: Resolution of the Sherman paradox. *Cell, 67,* 1047–1058.

Grigsby, J., Kemper, M., & Hagerman, R. (1987). Developmental Gerstmann syndrome without aphasia in the fra X syndrome. *Neuropsychologia, 25,* 881–891.

Hagerman, R. J. (1991). Physical and behavioral phenotype. In R. J. Hagerman & A. C. Cronister (Eds.), *Fragile X syndrome* (pp. 3–68). Baltimore: Johns Hopkins University Press.

II. Syndromes with Known Genetic Etiologies

Hagerman, R. J., Schreiner, R. A., Kemper, M. B., Wittenberger, M. D., Zahn, B., & Habicht, K. (1989). Longitudinal IQ changes in fragile X males. *American Journal of Medical Genetics, 33,* 513–518.

Hagerman, R., Staley, L., O'Conner, R., Lugenbeel, K., Nelson, D., McLean, S., & Taylor, A. (1996). Learning-disabled males with a fragile X CGG expansion in the upper premutation size range. *Pediatrics, 97*(1), 122–126.

Harnadek, M. C., & Rourke, B. P. (1994). Principal identifying features of the syndrome of non-verbal learning disabilities in children. *Journal of Learning Disabilities, 27,* 144–154.

Hinton, V. J., Dobkin, C. S., Halperin, J. M., Jenkins, E. C., Brown, W. T., Ding, X. H., Cohen, I. L., Rousseau, R., & Miezejeski, C. M. (1992). Mode of inheritance influences behavioral expression and molecular control of cognitive deficts in female carriers of the fragile X syndrome. *American Journal of Medical Genetics, 43,* 87–95.

Hodapp, R. M., Dykens, E. M., Ort, S. I., Zelinsky, D. G., & Leckman, J. F. (1991). Changing patterns of intellectual strengths and weaknesses in males with fragile X syndrome. *Journal of Autism and Developmental Disorders, 21,* 503–516.

Holden, J. J. A., Chalifoux, M., Wing, M., Julien-Inalsingh, C., Lawson, J. S., Higgins, J. V., Sherman, S., & White, B. N. (1995). Distribution and frequency of FMR1 CGG repeat numbers in the general population. *Developmental Brain Dysfunction, 8,* 405–407.

Hull, C., & Hagerman, R. J. (1993). A study of the physical, behavioral, and medical phenotype, including anthropometric measures, of females with fragile X syndrome. *American Journal of Diseases of Children, 147,* 1236–1241.

Joseph, J. W., Shambes, G. M., Gibson, J. M., & Welker, W. (1978). Tactile projections to granule cells in caudal vermis of the rat's cerebellum. *Brain, behavior, and evolution, 15,* 141–149.

Kemper, M. B., Hagerman, R. J., Ahmad, R. S., & Mariner, R. (1986). Cognitive profiles and the spectrum of clinical manifestations in heterozygous fra(X) females. *American Journal of Medical Genetics, 23,* 139–156.

Kovar, C. (1993). *The neurocognitive phenotype of fragile X girls.* Unpublished Master's thesis, University of Denver, Denver, CO.

Lachiewicz, A. M. (1992). Abnormal behaviors of young girls with fragile X syndrome. *American Journal of Medical Genetics, 43,* 72–77.

Lachiewicz, A. M., & Dawson, D. V. (1994). Behavior problems of young girls with fragile X syndrome: Factor scores on the Conners' Parent's Questionnaire. *American Journal of Medical Genetics, 51,* 364–369.

Loesch, D. Z., Hay, D. A., & Mulley, J. (1994). Transmitting males and carrier females in fragile X—revisited. *American Journal of Medical Genetics, 51,* 392–399.

Loesch, D. Z., Hay, D. A., Sutherland, G. R., Halliday, J., Judge, C., & Webb, G. C. (1987). Phenotypic variation in male-transmitted fragile X: Genetic inferences. *American Journal of Medical Genetics, 27,* 401–417.

Mazzocco, M. M. M., Baumgardner, T. L., Freund, L. S., Reiss, A. L. (1998). Social functioning among girls with fragile X or Turner syndrome and their sisters. *Journal of Autism and Developmental Disorders, 28,* 509–517.

Mazzocco, M. M. M., Freund, L. F., Baumgardner, T. L., & Reiss, A. L. (1995). The neurobehavioral and neuroanatomical effects of the *FMR-1* full mutation: Monozygotic twins discordant for the fragile X syndrome. *Neuropsychology, 9,* 470–480.

Mazzocco, M. M. M., Hagerman, R. J., Cronister, S. A., & Pennington, B. F. (1992a). Specific frontal lobe deficits among women with the fragile X gene. *Journal of the American Academy of Child and Adolescent Psychiatry, 31,* 1141–1148.

Mazzocco, M. M. M., Hagerman, R. J., & Pennington, B. F. (1992b). Problem solving limitations among cytogenetically expressing fragile X women. *American Journal of Medical Genetics, 43*, 78–86.

Mazzocco, M. M. M., & Holden, J. J. A. (1996). Neuropsychological profiles of three sisters homozygous for the fragile X premutation. *American Journal of Medical Genetics, 64*, 001–008.

Mazzocco, M. M. M., Kates, W. R., Freund, L. S., Baumgardner, T. L., and Reiss, A. L. (1997ab). Autistic behavior among girls with fragile X syndrome. *Journal of Autism and Developmental Disorders, 27*, 415–435.

Mazzocco, M. M. M., Pennington, B. F., & Hagerman, R. J. (1993). The neurocognitive phenotype of female carriers of fragile X: Additional evidence for specificity. *Journal of Developmental and Behavioral Pediatrics, 14*, 328–335.

Mazzocco, M. M. M., & Reiss, A. L. (1997). Normal variation in size of the FMR1 gene is not associated with variation in intellectual performance. *Intelligence, 24*, 355–366.

Mazzocco, M. M. M., Sonna, N. L., Teisl, J. T., Pinit, A., Shah, N., Shapiro, B. K., & Reiss, A. L. (1997b). The FMR1 and FMR2 mutations are not common etiologies of academic difficulty among school age children. *Developmental and Behavioral Pediatrics 18*, 392–398.

Miezejeski, C. M., & Hinton, V. J. (1992). Fragile X learning disability: Neurobehavioral research, diagnostic models, and treatment options. In R. J., Hagerman, & P. McKenzie (Eds.), *International 1992 Fragile X Conference Proceedings* (PP. 85–98). Dillon, CO: Spectra Publishers.

Miezejeski, C. M., Jenkins, E. C., Hill, A. L., Wisniewski, K., French, J. H., & Brown, W. T. (1986). A profile of cognitive deficit in females from fragile X families. *Neuropsychologia, 24*, 405–409.

Mostofsky, S., Mazzocco, M. M. M., Aakalu, G., Warsofsky, I. S., Denckla, M. B., & Reiss, A. L. (1996). Decreased posterior cerebellar vermis size in fragile X syndrome. *Neurology, 50*, 121–130.

Pieretti, M., Zhang, F. P., Fu, Y. H., Warren, S. T., Oostra, B. A., Caskey, C. T., & Nelson, D. L. (1991). Absence of expression of the *FMR-1* gene in fragile X syndrome. *Cell, 66*, 817–822.

Plomin, R. (1990). The role of inheritance in behavior. *Science, 248*, 183–188.

Plomin, R., & Neiderhiser, J. (1991). Quantitative genetics, molecular genetics, and intelligence. *Intelligence, 15*, 369–387.

Prouty, L. A., Rogers, R. C., Stevenson, R. E., Dean, J. H., Palmer, K. K., Simensen, R. J., Coston, G. N., & Schwartz, C. E. (1988). Fragile X syndrome: Growth, development, and intellectual function. *American Journal of Medical Genetics, 30*, 123–142.

Reiss, A. L. (1996). *Behavioral neurogenetics: Genetic conditions as models for understanding brain development, cognition and behavior in children.* Presented at the Advancing Research on Developmental Plasticity meeting, Chantilly, VA, May 12–15, 1996.

Reiss, A. L., Abrams, M. T., Greenlaw, R., Freund, L., & Denckla, M. B. (1995a). Neurodevelopmental effects of the FMR-1 full mutation in humans. *Nature Medicine, 1*, 159–167.

Reiss, A. L., Aylward, E., Freund, L. S., Joshi, P. K., & Bryan, R. N. (1991a). Neuroanatomy of fragile X syndrome: The posterior fossa. *Annals of Neurology, 29*, 26–32.

Reiss, A. L., & Freund, L. (1990). Fragile X syndrome, DSM-III-R, and autism. *Journal of the American Academy of Child and Adolescent Psychiatry, 29*, 885–891.

Reiss, A. L., & Freund, L. (1992). Behavioral phenotype of fragile X syndrome: DSM-III-R autistic behavior in male children. *American Journal of Medical Genetics, 43*, 35–46.

Reiss, A. L., Freund, L., Abrams, M. T., Boehm, C., & Kazazian, H. (1993). Neurobehavioral effects of the fragile X premutation in adult women: A controlled study. *American Journal of Human Genetics, 52*, 884–894.

II. Syndromes with Known Genetic Etiologies

Reiss, A. L., Freund, L. F., Baumgardner, T. L., Abrams, M. T., & Denckla, M. B. (1995b). Contribution of the FMR1 gene mutation to human intellectual dysfunction. *Nature Genetics, 11,* 331–334.

Reiss, A. L., Freund, L., Tseng, J. E., & Joshi, P. K. (1991b). Neuroanatomy in fragile X females: The posterior fossa. *American Journal of Human Genetics, 49,* 279–288.

Reiss, A. L., Freund, L., Vinogradov, S., Hagerman, R., & Cronister, A. (1989). Parental inheritance and psychological disability in fragile X females. *American Journal of Human Genetics, 45,* 697–705.

Reiss, A. L., Lee, J., & Freund, L. (1994). Neuroanatomy of fragile X syndrome: The temporal lobe. *Neurology, 44,* 1317–1324.

Rousseau, F., Heitz, D., Tarleton, J., MacPherson, J., Malmgren, H., Dahl, N., Barnicoat, A., Mathew, C., Mornet, E., Tejada, I., Maddalena, A., Spiegel, R., Schinzel, A., Marcos, J. A. G., Schwartz, C., & Mandel, J. L. (1994). A multicenter study on genotype-phenotype correlations in the fragile X syndrome, using direct diagnosis with probe StB12.3: The first 2,253 cases. *American Journal of Human Genetics, 55,* 225–237.

Sarter, M., Berntson, G. G., & Cacioppo, J. T. (1996). Brain imaging and cognitive neuroscience. Toward strong inference in attributing function to structure. *American Psychologist, 51*(1), 13–21.

Sherman, S. L., Jacobs, P. A., Morton, N. E., Froster, I. U., Howard-Peebles, P. N., Nielsen, K. B., Partington, M. W., Sutherland, G. R., Turner, G., & Watson, M. (1985). Further segregation analysis of the fragile X syndrome with special reference to transmitting males. *Human Genetics, 69,* 289–299.

Simon, J., & Keenan, J. (1996). *Investigation of discourse processing skills in women with fragile X syndrome.* Presented at the International Fragile X Conference, Portland, OR, August 6–11.

Sjak, S. N., & Meyer, E. M. (1993). Effects of chronic nicotine and pilocarpine administration on neocortical neuronal density and [^{3}H]GABA uptake in nucleus basalis lesioned rats. *Brain Research, 624,* 295–298.

Sobesky, W. E., Pennington, B. F., Porter, D., Hull, C. E., & Hagerman, R. J. (1994). Emotional and neurocognitive deficits in fragile X. *American Journal of Medical Genetics, 51,* 378–385.

Sudhalter, V., Cohen, I. L., Silverman, W., & Wolf, S. E. (1990). Conversational analyses of males with fragile X, Down syndrome, and autism: Comparison of the emergence of deviant language. *American Journal of Mental Retardation, 94,* 431–441.

Tang, Z., & Zhang, S. (1987). The cerebellar projection from the reticular formation of the brain stem in the rabbit. *Anatomical Embryology, 175,* 521–526.

Verkerk, A. J., Pieretti, M., Sutcliffe, J. S., Fu, Y. H., Kuhl, D. P., Pizzuti, A., Reiner, O., Richards, S., Victoria, M. F., Fuping Zhang, M. F. V., Eussen, B. E., van Ommen, G. J. B., Blonden, L. A. J., Riggins, G. J., Chastain, J. L., Kunst, C. B., Galjaard, H., Caskey, C. T., Nelson, D. L., Oostra, B. A., & Warren, S. T. (1991). Identification of a gene (FMR-1) containing a CGG repeat coincident with a breakpoint cluster region exhibiting length variation in fragile X syndrome. *Cell, 65,* 905–914.

Warren, S. T., Zhang, F., Lokey, L. K., Chastain, I. L., Lakas, L., & Feng, Y. (1994). Influence of CGG-repeat length upon FMR1 transcription and translation. *American Journal of Human Genetics, 55(suppl.),* A18.

Willems, P. J., Reyniers, E., & Oostra, B. A. (1995). An animal model for fragile X syndrome. *Mental Retardation and Developmental Disability Research Review, 1,* 298–302.

Wolf, S. E., Jenkins, E. C., Sklower, S., Cohen, I. L., Wisniewski, K. E., & Brown, W. T. (1988). On the association of fragile X with autism [letter]. *Journal of Autism and Developmental Disorders, 18,* 457–458.

4

Williams Syndrome: Findings from an Integrated Program of Research

Carolyn B. Mervis, Colleen A. Morris,
Jacquelyn Bertrand, and Byron F. Robinson

Carl is a delightful $8\frac{1}{2}$-year-old who, according to his mother, has "never met a stranger." Although he can recite the usual rules about not talking to people he doesn't know, Carl violates these injunctions constantly, confidently approaching people he has never seen before and beginning a lively conversation. He speaks in complete sentences, uses a varied vocabulary, responds to indirect hints, and is sensitive to the feelings of the person with whom he is talking. These characteristics, combined with the fact that he is very small for his age, often lead people who do not know Carl well to overestimate his capabilities.

Carl has an IQ of 54. This single number masks a wide range of ability levels. The area of greatest difficulty for Carl is visuospatial constructive cognition (visual-motor integration). He has a great deal of trouble with drawing and with constructing simple patterns out of colored blocks. In contrast, his verbal abilities are relatively good, and his auditory short-term memory (digit span) is excellent, ranking at the sixty-sixth percentile for his age. Carl's adaptive behavior quotient of 74, which is at the low end of the normal range, masks this same pattern of abilities. Carl cannot yet tie his shoelaces or fasten small buttons, has difficulty in cutting with a knife, and is just beginning to use basic handtools. He has difficulty in paying attention for more than short periods. However, Carl can read stories at the first-grade level and can write simple messages. He reliably remembers the birthdays of close relatives and friends. Carl plays T-ball and soccer and is a Cub Scout. He also collects seashells and enjoys listening to country-western music.

Ray, another $8\frac{1}{2}$-year-old, also is very interested in people. Although he knows that he should not approach strangers, he routinely does so, conversing with them as if they were good friends. Ray is sensitive to other people's feelings toward him but often is not aware of their feelings on other topics. His mother describes him as self-centered in the way that a 3- or 4-year-old would be. Ray has attention deficit hyperactivity disorder, is tactilely defensive, and is compulsive. His IQ of 40 and adaptive behavior quotient of 41 mask large discrepancies among his abilities. His verbal abilities are a relative strength. Ray often speaks in complete sentences. He has a small sight-word reading vocabulary and is able to print his first and last names. His greatest strength is in auditory short-term memory; his performance is at the eighteenth percentile, which is well within the normal range. Ray has extreme difficulty with visuospatial constructive cognition; he is able to copy only the simplest two-block patterns. He cannot yet tie his shoelaces, fasten small buttons, or cut with a knife and has not yet begun to use basic handtools. However, Ray is able to dress himself in everyday play clothes. He is beginning to help his parents with food preparation and is very interested in music.

Kevin also is an outgoing $8\frac{1}{2}$-year-old. He is beginning to inhibit his natural tendency to interact with strangers as if they were old friends. He is very social and concerned with other people's feelings. Kevin's IQ of 76 and adaptive behavior quotient of 90 are in the normal range but still mask serious discrepancies in verbal, reasoning, and spatial abilities. Kevin's verbal abilities are at the level that would be expected for his age. He speaks in complete sentences, using complex syntax and age-appropriate vocabulary, and responds to indirect hints. He reads at the second grade level and is able to write short messages and letters. Kevin's reasoning abilities, although not as good as his verbal ability, are still within age expectations. He is able to count change and has saved money to buy books about dinosaurs. Kevin is a dinosaur expert: He knows far more about dinosaurs than most adults do. He plays several board games that require skill and knowledge of relatively complex sets of rules. Kevin's auditory short-term memory (digit span) is at the fifty-fourth percentile for his age. The area in which Kevin has greatest difficulty is visuospatial constructive cognition. His performance in this area is well below what would be expected for his age. Kevin's drawing ability is quite limited, and he is able to copy only simple block patterns. He has difficulty in fastening small buttons. Kevin has mastered several important daily living skills that require visual-motor integration, however, he is able to tie his shoelaces, cut with a knife, and use basic handtools. Kevin plays baseball and soccer, collects baseball cards and small glass animals, and has a best friend.

Carl, Ray, and Kevin have Williams syndrome, a contiguous gene disorder caused by a hemizygous submicroscopical deletion of chromosome 7q11.23, including the *elastin* (*ELN*) gene. Diagnosis may be made on the basis of a fluorescent in situ hybridization (FISH) test for the deletion of *ELN*; deletions are present in at least 98% of individuals with Williams syndrome (Morris et al., 1994; Lowery et al., 1995). Most of the remainder of the deletion has not yet been characterized. The spectrum of abnormalities included in the Williams syndrome phenotype provides clinical markers for gene functions for as-yet-undiscovered genes in the deleted region.

At the phenotypic level, Williams syndrome is characterized by a distinctive set of facial features (figure 4.1), mental retardation or learning difficulties, unique cognitive and personality profiles, and a recognizable pattern of malformations, including connective tissue abnormalities and cardiovascular disease and especially supravalvular aortic stenosis (SVAS). A detailed

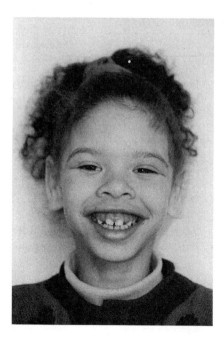

Figure 4.1 Seven-year-old child with Williams syndrome.

description of the Williams syndrome phenotype is presented in table 4.1. This description is based primarily on the reports of Williams et al. (1961), Beuren (1972), and Morris et al. (1988, 1990). In Williams syndrome, as in all syndromes, the expression of particular phenotypic characteristics varies. This variability may result from the actions of other genes or from environmental factors that modulate the phenotype. In contiguous gene syndromes, the variability also may be secondary to differing sizes of deletions, which results in the deletion of different numbers of genes. The incidence of seven key phenotypic features in a cohort of 110 individuals with Williams syndrome is indicated in table 4.2.

In the remainder of the chapter, we summarize the major findings of our research program. These findings are divided into four parts. In the first, we present a proposal for an objective measure of the cognitive profile associated with Williams syndrome and show that this profile accurately differentiates individuals who have Williams syndrome from other individuals with mental retardation or borderline normal intelligence. Evidence that the roots of the profile are apparent even in toddlers is provided. In the four sections that compose the second part, we consider our research relevant to the three major components of the cognitive profile—auditory short-term memory abilities, language abilities, and visuospatial constructive abilities—and to the interrelations among these abilities. In the third part, we describe what is known about the genetics of Williams syndrome. We include both the research that led to the determination of the genetic test for Williams syndrome and also new research with kindreds including members who

Mervis et al.: Williams Syndrome

Table 4.1 Williams syndrome (WS) phenotype

Infancy	Any age	Adulthood
Craniofacial features		
Periorbital fullness	Broad brow	Prematurely gray hair
Strabismus	Stellate iris	Facial asymmetry
Bitemporal narrowing	Full nasal tip	
Low nasal root	Wide mouth	
Flat mala	Full lips	
Long philtrum	Malocclusion	
Full cheeks	Prominent ear lobes	
Small jaw	Long neck	
Cardiovascular features		
Peripheral pulmonic stenosis	Supravalvular aortic stenosis	Other arterial stenoses
Supravalvular pulmonic stenosis	Hypoplasia of aorta	Hypertension
Connective tissue features		
Inguinal hernia	Hoarse voice	Bladder diverticulae
Umbilical hernia	Dental malocclusion	Colon diverticulae
Lax joints	Sloping shoulders	Premature aging of the skin
Rectal prolapse	Kyphosis-lordosis	Joint contractures
Neurobehavioral features		
Developmental delay	WS personality[a]	Anxiety[b]
Irritability-colic	WS cognitive profile[a]	Depression
	Attention deficit disorder	
	Mental retardation or learning difficulties	
Other medical problems		
Born postterm	Hypercalciuria	Stiff gait
Small for gestational age	Nephrocalcinosis	Lower-extremity hyperreflexia
Hypercalcemia	Constipation	Chronic abdominal pain
Failure to thrive		
Chronic otitis media		

[a] Apparent beginning in toddler or preschool period.
[b] May begin in middle childhood.

have small deletions of chromosome 7q11.23 but are not considered to have Williams syndrome. In the fourth part, we provide an integration and conclusion.

WILLIAMS SYNDROME COGNITIVE PROFILE

The results of previous studies of individuals with Williams syndrome suggest a characteristic cognitive profile. Auditory short-term memory is a relative strength; performance on tasks measuring this ability is greater than would be expected for mental age (MA) (Bennett et al., 1978; Udwin & Yule, 1991; Finegan et al., 1995). Language abilities are also relatively good;

Table 4.2 Major clinical features in a cohort of 110 individuals with Williams syndrome[a]

Clinical feature	Number	Percentage
Williams syndrome facial features	110	100
Mental retardation or developmental delay	108	98
Hoarse voice	108	98
Any congenital heart disease[b]	81	74
Supravalvular aortic stenosis	58	53
Inguinal hernia	49	46
Hypercalcemia	17	15

[a]All individuals were examined by Colleen Morris. Fluorescent in situ hybridization studies were completed on 52 individuals; all were positive for *ELN* deletion.
[b]Includes supravalvular aortic stenosis, supravalvular pulmonic stenosis, peripheral pulmonic stenosis, septal defects, and coarctation of the aorta. Degree of congenital heart disease in Williams syndrome is variable, ranging from individuals who die soon after birth as a result of heart failure to individuals with little or no evidence of supravalvular aortic narrowing.

performance on language measures is either greater than (e.g., Bellugi et al., 1992, 1988, 1994) or equivalent to (e.g., Gosch et al., 1994) the level expected for MA. In contrast, visuospatial constructive abilities are a distinct weakness; performance on tasks tapping these abilities is consistently below MA expectations (e.g., Bellugi et al., 1988, 1992, 1994; Milani et al., 1995; Bertrand et al., 1997). Our literature search targeting cognitive profiles associated with other syndromes (e.g., Down, fragile X, Prader-Willi, fetal alcohol) suggested that the Williams syndrome cognitive profile was likely unique.

Assessment of the Williams Syndrome Cognitive Profile in Children and Adults

Demonstration of the consistency and uniqueness of the cognitive profile for Williams syndrome has been hampered, however, by the lack of an explicit quantitative specification of the profile. To address this problem, we recently proposed and tested a systematic method of assessment of the Williams syndrome cognitive profile across a broad age range (Mervis et al., 1996). The profile was operationalized as a specific pattern of performance on particular subtests of the Differential Ability Scales (DAS; Elliott, 1990). The DAS offers two advantages for the study of cognitive profiles. First, it was designed carefully to provide specific information about an individual's strengths and weaknesses across a wide range of intellectual abilities. Second, the very large range of possible standard scores on the DAS provides increased sensitivity to differences in ability across subtests. The upper-preschool and school-age levels of the DAS include six core subtests that contribute to the child's GCA (General Conceptual Ability or IQ) score and also several diagnostic subtests, one of which measures auditory short-term memory. Standard scores (T scores) on each subtest range from 20 to 80, with a standard deviation (SD) of 10. A T score of 50 indicates performance at the fiftieth percentile.

The proposed Williams syndrome cognitive profile takes into account both mean level of overall performance on the core subtests (mean T score) and level of performance on four specific subtests: one measuring auditory short-term memory (digit recall subtest), two measuring verbal abilities (naming and definitions and similarities), and one measuring visuospatial constructive abilities (pattern construction). In determining whether an individual fits this cognitive profile, both absolute levels of performance and level of performance on certain subscales relative to performance on other subscales are considered. An individual was considered to fit the Williams syndrome cognitive profile if all the following criteria were met:

1. Pattern construction standard score (T score) < mean T score (for the core subtests)

2. Pattern construction T score < digit recall T score

3. Pattern construction T score < twentieth percentile

4. T score for either digit recall, naming and definitions, or similarities > first percentile (T ≥ 29).

The first three criteria reflect the expected relative weakness in visuospatial constructive abilities in relation to both overall level of ability and level of auditory short-term memory ability, and they reflect an absolute weakness in visuospatial constructive cognition. The fourth criterion reflects the expected relative strength in either auditory short-term memory or language, even for individuals who are very low-functioning.

For individuals who met all four criteria (and therefore fit the Williams syndrome cognitive profile), we also considered the strength of the match to the profile. Individuals were assigned a score from 1 to 4 on the basis of their fit to the following criteria:

• Digit recall T score > mean T score (2 points)

• Naming-definition T score > pattern construction T score (1 point)

• Similarities T score > pattern construction T score (1 point)

The first criterion provides a stronger test of the expected relative strength in auditory short-term memory. The second and third criteria reflect the expected relative strength in verbal abilities compared to visuospatial constructive abilities.

To determine whether the proposed cognitive profile characterized most individuals with Williams syndrome but did not fit most individuals with other etiologies of mental retardation or learning difficulties, we administered the DAS to 50 individuals who had Williams syndrome and to a contrast group of 40 individuals who did not (mixed-etiology group). The individuals with Williams syndrome ranged in age from 3 years 11 months to 46 years. The individuals in the mixed-etiology group ranged in age from

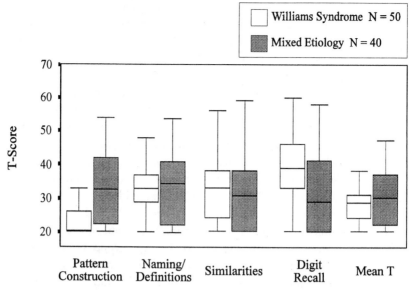

Figure 4.2 Cognitive profile T score distributions of individuals with Williams syndrome and individuals from the mixed-etiology contrast group.

3 years 3 months to 34 years. Included in this group were 20 individuals with a variety of genetic or other congenital disorders (e.g., Down syndrome, fragile X syndrome, Noonan syndrome, fetal alcohol syndrome), 15 individuals with mental retardation or learning difficulties of unknown etiology, and 5 individuals who had borderline normal intelligence. The DAS can be used to determine IQs for individuals between the ages of $2\frac{1}{2}$ and 18 years. Mean IQ for the 38 individuals with Williams syndrome in this age range was 59.32 (SD = 10.74), with a range from 38 to 84. For the 31 individuals in the mixed-etiology group in this age range, mean IQ was 66.03 (SD = 15.71), with a range from 31 to 95.

Box-and-whiskers plots describing the distribution of T scores for the pattern construction, naming and definitions, similarities, and digit recall subtests scores for overall performance on the core subtests are shown in figure 4.2. The fiftieth percentile is represented by the internal bar in each box; the bottom and top of each box correspond to the twenty-fifth and seventy-fifth percentiles, respectively. The end of the bottom whisker corresponds to the minimum score obtained. The end of the top whisker corresponds to the maximum score obtained (excluding outliers). The data presented in figure 4.2 are consistent with the overall pattern found in previous studies of individuals with Williams syndrome: definite weakness in visuospatial constructive abilities, relative strength in language abilities, and definite strength in auditory short-term memory. Performance of the mixed-etiology group appears relatively flat and is more variable than is performance of the Williams syndrome group; this is at least partially due to the averaging together of individuals who show different patterns of strengths and weaknesses.

To determine whether individual participants fit the Williams syndrome cognitive profile, the four profile rules already described were applied to the T scores the individual earned on the various subtests of the DAS. Results indicated that 47 of the 50 individuals with Williams syndrome fit the Williams syndrome cognitive profile. Two of the individuals who did not fit the profile were excluded because none of their subtest T scores was above the first percentile. The third individual was excluded because his pattern construction T score and his mean T score were greater than his digits T score. Of the 47 individuals who had Williams syndrome and fit the cognitive profile, 42 received a score of four points, indicating an excellent fit to the profile. Three received three points, and two received two points. Overall, the proposed cognitive profile fit the individuals with Williams syndrome very well; the sensitivity of the profile was 0.94, and most individuals who fit the profile received the maximum possible points for strength of match.

The results for the mixed-etiology group were very different. Of the 40 individuals in that group, 37 did not fit the Williams syndrome cognitive profile. The three individuals who did fit the profile included one very high-functioning girl who has Down syndrome and two relatively high-functioning male subjects of unknown etiology. The specificity of the Williams syndrome profile was 0.93. The high sensitivity and specificity values indicate that individuals with Williams syndrome have a consistent and relatively unique cognitive profile.

Assessment of the Williams Syndrome Cognitive Profile in Toddlers and Young Preschoolers

Assessment of the Williams syndrome cognitive profile on the basis of the DAS criteria previously described is feasible beginning at approximately age 4 years. No standardized measures are available to assess the complete profile in younger children. However, the mental scale of the Bayley Scales of Infant Development (BSID; Bayley, 1969) may be used to assess a major component of the cognitive profile: language abilities more advanced than nonlinguistic cognitive abilities. To determine whether this component of the Williams syndrome cognitive profile is evident in toddlers and young preschoolers with Williams syndrome, we considered the performance of six children who were participating in a longitudinal study of the early development of children with Williams syndrome. The performance of a contrast group of six children with Down syndrome, followed longitudinally, also was considered. The children with Williams syndrome were assessed three to five times (mean, 4.17 times) on the BSID; the children with Down syndrome were assessed four to five times (mean, 4.67). Assessments were conducted at intervals of approximately 6 months. MA ranges during the period of study were similar for the two groups of children: 6.25 months to 30+ months (the maximum possible) for the children with Williams syndrome and 8.10 months to 30+ months for the children with Down syndrome.

We began our analysis of relative strength of language and nonlanguage abilities by dividing the items on the mental scale of the BSID into two types. Language items were those that involved syllable production, linguistic imitation, language comprehension, or language production; the remaining items were considered nonlanguage. These included measures of nonverbal reasoning (object permanence, means-ends), visual-motor integration (pegboards, form boards, block construction, drawing), and gestural imitation. The majority of the nonlanguage items assessed visual-motor integration; a large proportion of these items measured visuospatial constructive abilities.

To compare the performance of individual children on the language and nonlanguage items, we considered all the items from the child's basal (10 items prior to the first item failed) through the last item the child passed. Determination of which items to include was made separately for each time the BSID was administered. To compare general level of language abilities to general level of nonlanguage cognitive abilities, we determined the proportion of language items passed out of language items attempted and the proportion of nonlanguage items passed out of nonlanguage items attempted, separately for each assessment. We then calculated the mean proportions across assessments for each child.

The mean proportions of language and nonlanguage items passed by the children with Williams syndrome and the children with Down syndrome are presented in figure 4.3. As is clear from the figure, the children with Williams syndrome showed the expected pattern: The mean proportion of language

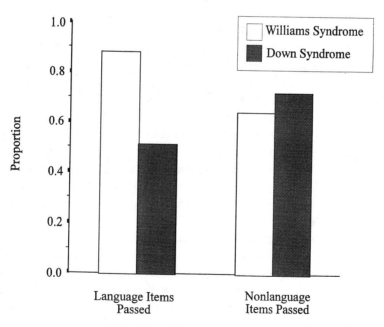

Figure 4.3 Mean proportions of language and nonlanguage items passed by the children with Williams syndrome and the children with Down syndrome.

items passed was significantly greater than the mean proportion of non-linguistic cognitive items passed ($P < .001$). The children with Down syndrome showed the opposite pattern; these children passed a significantly greater proportion of nonlanguage items than language items ($P < .05$). We also calculated the difference between the proportion of language items passed and the proportion of nonlanguage items passed, separately for each child. There was no overlap between the children with Williams syndrome and the children with Down syndrome in the distribution of these difference scores. Difference scores were positive for all the children with Williams syndrome. This pattern of findings indicates that a major component of the Williams syndrome profile—a higher level of language abilities than of non-linguistic cognitive abilities (especially visual-motor integration and visuo-spatial constructive cognition)—is apparent even in toddlers with Williams syndrome.

AUDITORY SHORT-TERM MEMORY

In the next four sections of the chapter, we briefly review our work on the three major aspects of cognition included in the Williams syndrome cognitive profile (auditory short-term memory, visuospatial constructive cognition, and language) and then consider the interrelations among the three types of abilities. In each of the first three sections, we begin by considering the performance of a large sample of children and adults with Williams syndrome on one or more standardized measures. For these analyses, individuals who were 17 years or younger were considered children; individuals who were 18 years or older were considered adults. Performance on these measures supports the general pattern of strengths and weaknesses represented in the Williams syndrome cognitive profile. Although this pattern is maintained across individuals, there is a great deal of variability in absolute levels of performance, not only across individuals of different ages but among individuals of the same age. To provide a visual representation of central tendencies and variability in performance on these measures, we present both scatterplots of raw scores as a function of age and histograms of standard scores. We also report correlations of raw scores and standard scores with chronological age (CA). In the remainder of each section, we describe some of the research we have conducted using measures for which norms are not available.

We begin this section on auditory short-term memory with a consideration of the performance of individuals with Williams syndrome on the DAS digit recall subtest. The digit presentation rate for the DAS is faster than the more commonly used measures of digit span. We also have administered other digit recall tasks that use the standard presentation rate of one item per second. After describing the results for the DAS measure, we present our findings on foward and backward digit spans based on this slower rate of presentation.

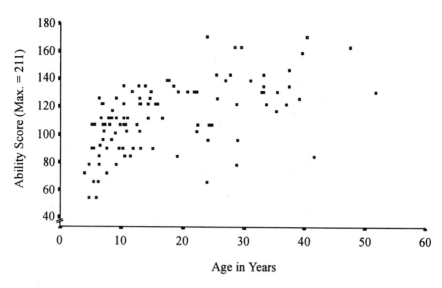

Figure 4.4 DAS recall of digits subtest ability score as a function of age (N = 104).

DAS Digit Recall

The DAS digit recall subtest provides a measure of auditory rote memory. Digit strings to be recalled range in length from two items to nine items. Participants are asked to repeat the digits in the same order as that produced by the researcher. Digits are presented to the participant at a rate of one every half-second. (This presentation rate is twice as fast as that used on the Wechsler IQ tests.) As on all the DAS subtests, raw scores of number of items correct within a designated item set are converted to ability scores. Ability scores then are converted to standard scores based on the participant's CA. (The norms for the oldest age group included in the standardization sample—17 years 6 months to 17 years 11 months—were used for adult participants. This procedure is consistent with subtest standard score determination for the Wechsler Adult Intelligence Scale–Revised (WAIS-R) (Wechsler, 1981).

A scatterplot of the ability scores of the 104 individuals between the ages of 4 and 52 years whom we have assessed on the DAS digit recall subtest is presented in figure 4.4. The pattern of performance suggests consistent growth in digit recall abilities during childhood and maintenance of performance during adulthood. The correlations with age reflect this trend. For the 65 children (ages 4–17 years), the correlation between digit recall ability score and CA was +0.58 (P < .001). The correlation for the 39 adults was +0.29 [nonsignificant (NS)].

A histogram of the T (standard) scores earned by the 104 individuals with Williams syndrome is presented in figure 4.5. The mean T score was 35.38 (SD = 9.99). This T score is at the seventh percentile, which is in the normal range. T scores were consistent across CA (r = +0.12, NS). The data

Mervis et al.: Williams Syndrome

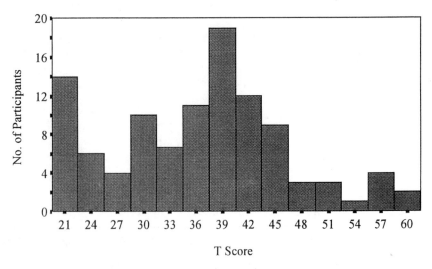

Figure 4.5 DAS recall of digits subtest T score distribution (N = 104).

presented in figure 4.5 indicate a great deal of variability. The percentiles associated with the T scores ranged from the bottom of the first (T = 20) to the eighty-fourth (T = 60). The scores of most of the subjects are distributed normally, with a mode centering around the fourteenth percentile (T = 39). However, a group of individuals also was clustered at the bottom of the distribution at the first percentile (T = 20). Even though most of the individuals tested have full-scale IQs in the mentally retarded range, 73% scored in the normal range for auditory short-term memory, with 9% scoring at or above the fiftieth percentile. Overall, the pattern of findings for the DAS digit recall subtest indicates that auditory short-term memory is a definite strength for individuals with Williams syndrome, beginning by age 4 years and continuing at least through middle adulthood.

One-Item-per-Second Forward Digit Span

We also have assessed the forward digit recall abilities of 86 individuals with Williams syndrome using the more typical presentation rate of one item per second. Participants ranged in age from 4 to 47 years. The digit strings used were taken from the McCarthy Scales of Children's Abilities (MSCA; McCarthy, 1970), the WAIS-R (Wechsler, 1981), the Wechsler Intelligence Scale for Children-III (WISC-III; Wechsler, 1991), or the Test of Auditory Perceptual Skills (Gardner, 1985). In the results reported in this section, data from all four tests were combined.

A scatterplot of the forward digit span (longest string of digits recalled in the correct sequence) for the 86 individuals is provided in figure 4.6. The pattern of performance suggests growth throughout childhood and continuing into adulthood. For the 50 children, the correlation between forward

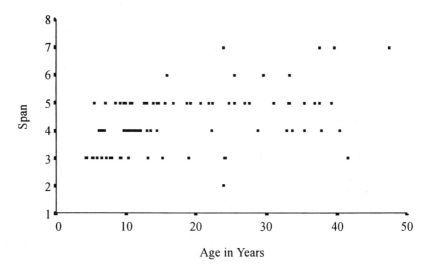

Figure 4.6 One-second digit span (forward) as a function of age (N = 86).

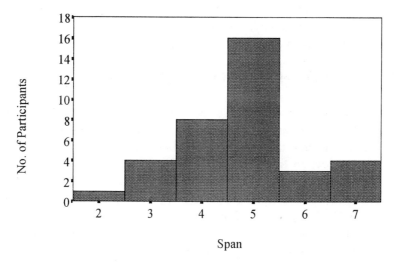

Figure 4.7 One-second digit span (forward) distribution of adult scores (N = 36).

digit span and CA was +0.45 ($P = .001$). The corresponding correlation for the 36 adults was +0.26 (NS). A histogram of the forward digit span lengths of the adults is provided in figure 4.7. Span lengths were normally distributed. Mean span length was 4.40 digits (SD = 1.05). This span length is very similar to the 4.56 digits reported by Wang and Bellugi (1994) for a sample of nine adolescents with Williams syndrome.

Standard scores on the digit recall subtest of the WAIS-R are based on the sum of the raw scores for forward and backward digit recall; separate standard scores for forward recall and backward recall are not provided. Thus, we were unable to compare our sample's adult performance on the forward digit recall task to the performance of the standardization sample. Instead, we compared the performance of the adults with Williams syndrome to the performance reported by Banken (1985) of a sample of 50 adults with low average intelligence (mean WAIS-R IQ = 90.86). Mean CA of the two samples was equivalent: 29.9 years for the individuals with Williams syndrome and 29.4 years for Banken's sample. Banken reported his findings in terms of number of trials correct. To compare the scores of the two groups, we determined the number of trials correct for the individuals with Williams syndrome, beginning with the three-digit trials, even if the test we administered included two-digit trials. (The WAIS-R forward digit span test begins with sequences of three digits.) The adults with Williams syndrome recalled the digit sequences correctly on a mean of 4.89 trials (SD = 2.04). In contrast, the adults in Banken's sample were correct on a mean of 7.32 trials (SD = 1.81). Thus, the mean number of correct trials for the individuals with Williams syndrome was 1.34 SD below the mean for Banken's sample. More than three-fourths of the individuals with Williams syndrome (76%) scored in the normal range as determined by the Banken sample. This level of performance relative to the normal population is comparable to the mean level of performance of the individuals with Williams syndrome on the DAS digit recall task relative to the normal population (1.46 SD below the standardization sample mean; 73% of scores in the normal range).

One-Item-per-Second Backward Digit Span

On backward digit span tests, individuals are presented with a string of digits and then are asked to repeat them in reverse order. Success at this task requires that the participant be able to manipulate a series of items held in memory, so that they can be reported in the order opposite from that in which they were presented. Because of this additional processing component, backward digit span is related more closely to working memory (Baddeley, 1992) than to forward digit span (Wang & Bellugi, 1994). Because working memory appears to play an important role in comprehension and production of complex syntax (e.g., Kemper et al., 1989; Norman et al., 1991) and many individuals with Williams syndrome routinely use complex syntactic constructions, we were especially interested in assessing the backward digit spans of individuals who had Williams syndrome.

Backward digit span was assessed for the same 86 individuals assessed for forward digit span. The sequences of digits presented were taken from the same four standardized tests that were used to measure forward digit span. Rate of presentation of digits is one item per second on all four tests. Data were collapsed across the four tests.

A scatterplot of the backward digit span (longest string of digits correctly recalled in reverse order) for the 86 individuals with Williams syndrome is shown in figure 4.8. The pattern of performance suggests consistent growth throughout childhood and maintenance in adulthood. The correlation between backward digit span and CA was +0.32 ($P < .05$) for the 50 children

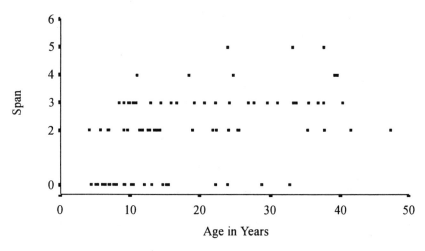

Figure 4.8 One-second digit span (backward) as a function of age (N = 86).

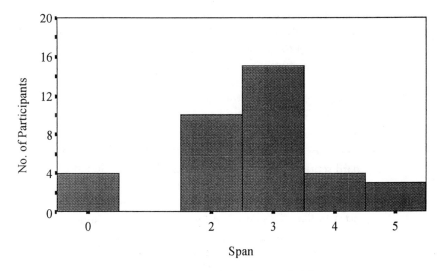

Figure 4.9 One-second digit span (backward) distribution of adult scores (N = 36).

and +0.14 (NS) for the 36 adults. A histogram of the backward digit span lengths of the adults is provided in figure 4.9. Once again, span lengths were distributed normally, with a mode of three digits. Note, however, that four (11%) of the adults were unable to repeat even two-digit sequences in reverse order. Mean span length was 2.67 digits (SD = 1.29). This span length is similar to the 2.67 digits reported by Wang and Bellugi (1994).

The performance of the 36 adults with Williams syndrome again was compared to that of the 50 low-average adults included in Banken's (1985) study. Number of correct trials was determined for each of the individuals with Williams syndrome, beginning with the two-digit trials. (The WAIS-R includes two-digit sequences in the backward digit span test.) The adults

Mervis et al.: Williams Syndrome

with Williams syndrome correctly repeated the digit sequences in reverse order on a mean of 2.97 trials (SD = 1.70). In contrast, the adults in Banken's sample were correct on a mean of 5.70 trials (SD = 2.36). Thus, the mean number of correct trials for the individuals with Williams syndrome was 1.16 SD below the mean for Banken's sample. Most of the individuals with Williams syndrome (89%) scored within the normal range as determined by the Banken sample.

LANGUAGE

In our research on the language abilities of individuals with Williams syndrome, we have considered both the lexicon (vocabulary) and grammar. Our findings for these two aspects of language are presented separately.

Lexicon

Peabody Picture Vocabulary Test–Revised The Peabody Picture Vocabulary Test–Revised (PPVT-R; Dunn & Dunn, 1981) is the test most commonly used to measure receptive vocabulary development, both for research and clinical purposes. Participants are asked to choose from a set of four pictures the one that best matches the word that the researcher says. Words tested include names for objects, actions, descriptors, and abstractions. Raw scores of number of items correct are converted into standard scores, taking into account the participant's CA. To determine standard scores for individuals whose raw scores were less than the raw score corresponding to a standard score of 40 (the lowest standard score included in the PPVT-R manual), we used the supplementary norms provided by the publisher (American Guidance Service, 1981). These norms cover the standard score range of 20–39. We have administered Form L of this measure to 127 individuals who had Williams syndrome and are between the ages of 4 and 52 years.

A scatterplot of the raw scores of the 127 individuals with Williams syndrome is presented in figure 4.10. The pattern of performance suggests consistent growth in vocabulary size during childhood and continuing into adulthood. The correlation between PPVT-R raw score and CA for the 85 children was +0.78 ($P < .001$). The corresponding correlation for the 42 adults was +0.35 ($P < .05$). A histogram of the standard scores earned by the 127 individuals is shown in figure 4.11. The mean standard score was 66.50 (SD = 18.23). Standard scores were consistent across the age range sampled ($r = -0.051$; NS). The distribution of standard scores was normal. However, the SD for this sample was very large, indicating a great deal of variability. The percentiles associated with the standard scores ranged from the very bottom of the first percentile (standard score of 19) to the seventy-fifth percentile (standard score of 110). Although most of the individuals tested have full-scale IQs in the mentally retarded range, 42% scored in the normal range (standard score ≥ 70) on the PPVT-R, with 4% scoring at or

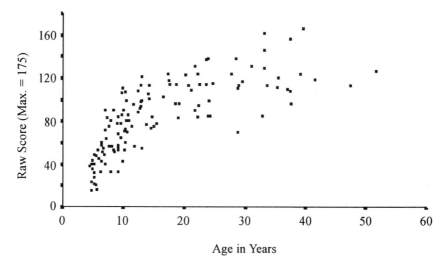

Figure 4.10 PPVT-R raw score as a function of age (N = 127).

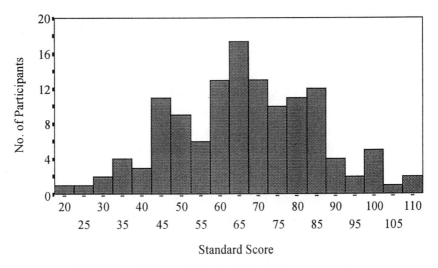

Figure 4.11 PPVT-R standard score distribution (N = 127).

above the fiftieth percentile. Overall, the pattern of findings for the PPVT-R indicates that vocabulary is a strength for individuals who have Williams syndrome.

Semantic Organization During Middle Childhood The semantic organization of a category refers to how an individual cognitively relates the members of the category. This type of organization often is measured by word fluency tests, which involve asking individuals to list all the items that they can bring to mind that are members of a given category (e.g., animal, clothing, food). Bellugi et al. (1992, 1994) used a word fluency task to consider the semantic organization of the *animal* category for adolescents with

Williams syndrome. The lists generated by the six adolescents with Williams syndrome were compared to the lists produced by six IQ- and CA-matched adolescents with Down syndrome and by a group of normally developing second-graders. Based on the findings from this study, Bellugi et al. (1992, 1994) argued that the semantic organization of adolescents with Williams syndrome is deviant. In particular, Bellugi et al. (1992, 1994) found that when asked to list all the animals that they could, adolescents with Williams syndrome were much more likely than either of the other two groups to list unusual (defined as low word frequency) animals, such as yak, weasel, or salamander. This increase in production of low-frequency names was true both for the absolute number of names produced and also for the proportion of low-frequency names out of the total number of names produced. The individuals with Williams syndrome also produced more animal names than did the individuals with Down syndrome.

Our experience with individuals with Williams syndrome suggested that although these individuals occasionally used low-frequency words, the incidence of these words was not substantially greater than would be expected for a normally developing child of the same MA. Because we were surprised by the findings of Bellugi et al. (1992, 1994), we performed an additional study, using a larger sample (Scott et al., 1995). Participants in this study were twelve 9- and 10-year-olds with Williams syndrome, 12 children with Down syndrome individually matched to the children with Williams syndrome for both CA and MA on the MSCA (McCarthy, 1970), 12 normally developing children individually matched to the children with Williams syndrome or Down syndrome for MA, and 12 normally developing children individually matched to the children with Williams syndrome or Down syndrome for CA. Children were asked to tell the researcher the names of all the animals they could think of. The researcher provided two examples: cat, bear. Although children were given unlimited time, they rarely took more than 60 seconds (the time limit in the study by Bellugi et al. 1992, 1994 study) to generate their lists.

We compared the lists of animals generated by the four groups of children on four types of measures: fluency, representativeness, word frequency, and category composition. Fluency was measured by the number of animal names a child produced. Representativeness of the items produced as members of the *animal* category was determined by goodness of example (GOE) ratings obtained using a procedure similar to Rosch (1973, 1975). College students were asked to rate the animal names generated by the children for how well each animal fit the student's idea or image of *animal*. Scores on a scale of 1 (fits idea or image of *animal* very well) to 7 (fits idea or image of *animal* very poorly) were used. We compared the lists generated by the four groups of children on three measures of GOE: mean GOE rating for the animal names produced by a child, GOE rating for the most representative (typical) animal name produced by the child, and mean GOE rating for the least representative (typical) animal name produced by the child. Word frequency was measured in two ways: mean frequency of the animal names the child listed in children's texts [standard frequency index (SFI; Carroll et al., 1971)] and proportion of items with an SFI < 50. The latter measure was the criterion of Bellugi et al. (1992, 1994) for classification of a word as low-frequency (P. P. Wang, personal communication, 1994). Two measures of category composition were used: percentage of animal names produced at the basic level (e.g., dog) and percentage of animal names produced at the subordinate level (e.g., collie).

On all but one of these measures, the children in the three MA-matched groups (Williams syndrome, Down syndrome, MA-match) performed similarly. Performance was equivalent on number of animal names produced, mean GOE rating, GOE rating for the most typical exemplar produced, mean SFI, proportion of items with SFI of less than 50, proportion of items generated at the basic level, and proportion of items generated at the subordinate level. The performance of the three groups differed for one measure: GOE rating for the least typical exemplar named. For this measure, the performance of the children with Williams syndrome and the children with Down syndrome was equivalent to the performance of the CA-match group and differed significantly from that for the MA-match group. The least typical exemplar named by the older groups of children was significantly less representative of the *animal* category than was the least typical exemplar named by the MA-match group.

Performance of the Williams syndrome group was equivalent also to performance of the CA-match group on two other measures: mean SFI value and proportion of animal names that were at the basic level. Performance of the two groups differed on the three remaining measures. The CA-match group demonstrated fluency (mean of 24 animals listed) significantly greater than that of the Williams syndrome group (mean of 9 animals listed). Mean GOE rating was higher for the CA-match group than for the Williams syndrome group, indicating that the exemplars produced by the Williams syndrome group were on average more representative of the *animal* category than were the exemplars listed by the CA-match group. Finally, the lists generated by the CA-match group contained a proportion of subordinate-level animal names significantly greater than that of the lists generated by the children with Williams syndrome.

The pattern of findings we obtained indicated that in some ways, the semantic organization of the *animal* category is similar for all four groups of children. The proportion of items that were basic-level names, the mean SFI value, and the proportion of items for which SFI < 50 were equivalent for all four groups. The latter finding contrasts with that of Bellugi et al., (1992, 1994) who found that adolescents with Williams syndrome produced proportion of low-frequency animal names greater than that of either of the other groups tested. We did find one difference between the children with Williams syndrome and the MA-match group that may be consistent with Bellugi's suggestion that individuals with Williams syndrome produce more unusual animal names than do younger, normally developing children. Although Bellugi et al. (1992, 1994) defined "unusual" animal names in terms of SFI, another possible definition would be "names of atypical exemplars of the *animal* category." In our study, the least typical exemplar produced by the children with Williams syndrome, the children with Down syndrome, and the children in the CA-match group was reliably less representative of the *animal* category than was the least typical exemplar produced by the children in the MA-match group. In this case, amount of experience with animals (as measured by CA), was more important than MA in determining a particular component of semantic organization. On all the other measures of semantic organization, however, the performance of the children with Williams syndrome was consistent with that of the two groups matched to them for MA (Down syndrome and MA-match). Thus, performance was appropriate for MA, suggesting that the development of semantic organization in Williams syndrome is delayed, rather than deviant.

Grammar

Test for Reception of Grammar   The Test for Reception of Grammar (TROG, Bishop, 1989) is a standardized measure of grammatical comprehension. The format of this test is similar to that of the PPVT-R: The participant is shown four pictures and is asked to choose the one that matches the word, phrase, or sentence produced by the researcher. The TROG is composed of 20 blocks of four items. Each block tests a different grammatical construction, ranging from bare nouns to embedded sentences. Most of the blocks assess relatively simple grammatical constructions. Raw scores on the TROG correspond to the number of blocks for which the participant answered all four items correctly and are converted to standard scores based on CA. Standard scores for individuals 13 years or older were assigned according to the instructions in Appendix 11 of the TROG manual.

We have assessed 77 individuals with Williams syndrome between ages 5 and 52 years on the TROG. A scatterplot of their raw scores is shown in figure 4.12. The pattern of raw scores suggests consistent growth in childhood, with performance maintained during adulthood. For the 54 children, the correlation between number of blocks correct and CA was $+0.55$ ($P < .001$). The correlation for the 23 adults was $+0.28$ (NS). A histogram of the standard scores is provided in figure 4.13. The mean standard score was 73.12, with an SD of 13.11. Standard scores increased slightly with increasing CA ($r = +0.24$; $P < .05$). Most of the standard scores (86%) were distributed between 55 and 85. The percentiles associated with the standard scores ranged from the first to the seventy-third. The mean standard score was at the fourth percentile, and 56% of the participants scored in the normal range (standard score ≥ 70). Overall, the pattern of findings for the TROG indicates that grammatical comprehension is a relative strength for individuals with Williams syndrome. It should be noted, however, that performance

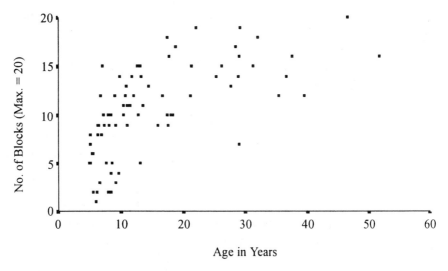

Figure 4.12 TROG raw score as a function of age (N = 77).

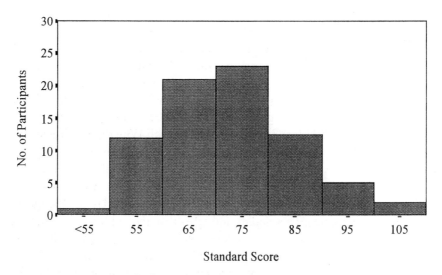

Figure 4.13 TROG standard score distribution (N = 77).

on the most complex constructions was poor. For example, only 18% of the participants (22% of the adults) passed the block assessing relative clauses (right branching), and only 5% (9% of the adults) passed the block assessing embedded sentences (left branching).

Grammatical Development of Preschoolers and Young School-Age Children Most adults with Williams syndrome have good syntactical abilities. However, little research has been concerned with the development of these abilities during childhood. Furthermore, the relation between overall level of syntactical abilities and level of such other intellectual abilities as

Mervis et al.: Williams Syndrome

vocabulary, auditory short-term memory, or spatial cognition has not been considered systematically. To begin to address these questions, members of our laboratory have conducted a cross-sectional study of the syntactical abilities of 39 children with Williams syndrome (Klein, 1995; Klein et al., 1996). Syntactical abilities were assessed on the basis of the Index of Productive Syntax (IPSyn; Scarborough, 1990), a measure of the emergence of syntactical abilities ranging from single word usage to embedded clauses.

The children who participated in the study ranged in age from 2 years 6 months to 12, with a mean age of 7. The children's GCA (IQ as measured by the DAS) ranged from 40 to 88, with a mean of 61.44. Each child participated in a 30-minute play session with a researcher, using a standard set of toys selected to facilitate symbolic and imaginary play. Play sessions were videotaped; videotapes were later transcribed and then coded according to Scarborough's (1990) criteria. Children also completed a series of standardized measures, including the DAS, the PPVT-R, and the TROG.

Results indicated that the syntactical abilities of children with Williams syndrome are considerably delayed. Mean length of utterance (MLU) ranged from 1.52 to 4.82, with a mean of 3.18 (SD = 0.73). IPSyn scores ranged from 20 to 98 (of 112 possible), with a mean of 71.77. This mean is lower than the mean score Scarborough (1990) reported for normally developing children aged 3 years, 6 months. Despite this delay, however, the language of the children with Williams syndrome showed the same relation between MLU and IPSyn as that of children who are developing normally, across the entire MLU range studied. The quadratic curves relating MLU and IPSyn are virtually identical for the children with Williams syndrome and the normally developing preschoolers who participated in Scarborough's study. These curves are illustrated in figure 4.14. (A logarithmic curve would have been more appropriate for measuring the relation between MLU and IPSyn. However, Scarborough only reported the parameters for the quadratic curve for her data.) This finding indicates that the syntactical complexity of the language produced by children with Williams syndrome is appropriate for the length of their utterances. This result contrasts with that previously reported for other groups of children with mental retardation (Scarborough et al., 1991). The language of children with Down syndrome, fragile X syndrome, or autism showed the same relation between utterance length and syntactical complexity as did the language of the normally developing preschoolers until MLU reached 3.00. However, at MLU levels greater than 3.00, syntactical complexity was less than would have been expected on the basis of MLU. Thus, Williams syndrome is the first syndrome for which a normal relation between utterance length and syntactical complexity has been demonstrated.

We also were interested in the relation between the children's level of syntactical ability and their levels of ability for other language and non-linguistic cognitive skills. To address this issue, we compared children's age equivalents on the IPSyn to their age equivalents on five additional measures: receptive vocabulary (PPVT-R age equivalent), verbal ability

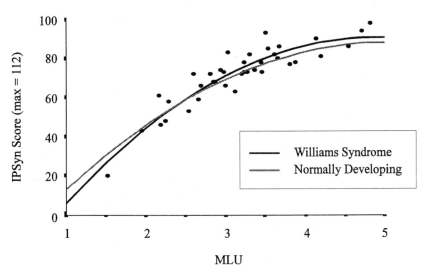

Figure 4.14 IPSyn scores as a function of MLU for children with Williams syndrome and the normally developing preschoolers who participated in Scarborough's (1990) study.

(DAS verbal cluster age equivalent), visuospatial constructive cognitive ability (DAS pattern construction age equivalent), auditory short-term memory (DAS digit recall age equivalent), and composite mental abilities (mean of DAS verbal cluster and pattern construction age equivalents). The standardized test scores of the normally developing preschoolers who had particated in Scarborough's study indicated that the MAs of these children were, on average, 6 months greater than their CAs. Therefore, we adjusted the expected age equivalents on the IPSyn by 6 months, to take into account the above average abilities of these preschoolers.

To determine childrens' relative level of ability on each of these measures, we compared their actual IPSyn scores to the IPSyn scores that would have been expected on the basis of their age equivalent for each of the other five measures. Relative levels of ability were divided into four categories. Observed IPSyn scores were considered very high if they were more than 1 SD above the mean IPSyn score expected for the child's age equivalent on the other relevant measure. Observed IPSyn scores that were above, but within 1 SD of, the expected score, were considered high. Similarly, observed IPSyn scores that were below, but within 1 SD of, the expected score were considered low. Observed IPSyn scores that were more than 1 SD below the expected score were considered very low.

Results of Kolmogorov-Smirnov analyses indicated that the observed distribution of scores in the four possible categories (very high, high, low, very low) differed significantly from the expected (normal) distribution for four of the five comparisons. The observed IPSyn scores were significantly higher than would have been expected on the basis of spatial constructive ability but significantly lower than would have been expected on the basis of receptive vocabulary ability, verbal ability, or auditory short-term memory

Mervis et al.: Williams Syndrome

ability (all $P < .01$). In contrast, observed IPSyn scores were consistent with expected IPSyn scores on the basis of composite mental abilities ($P > .20$). This pattern of findings indicates that the grammatical abilities of children with Williams syndrome are more advanced than would be expected on the basis of their spatial abilites but less advanced than would be expected on the basis of their lexical, semantic, or auditory short-term memory abilities. The finding that level of grammatical ability is consistent with level of composite mental abilities fits with the results of previous studies (Udwin & Yule, 1991; Gosch et al. 1994) in which use of specific grammatical constructions by children with Williams syndrome and matched children with other types of mental retardation were compared.

Summary

The language abilities of most individuals with Williams syndrome are significantly delayed relative to CA expectations. This delay was evidenced by performance on standardized tests of receptive vocabulary (PPVT-R) and receptive grammar (TROG). The delay also was apparent on a measure of semantic fluency (elicited production of animal names) and on grammatical measures (MLU, IPSyn) derived from language samples obtained from free play sessions. Despite these delays, however, the language abilities of individuals with Williams syndrome parallel those of individuals who are developing normally in three important ways. First, the composition of the *animal* category of school-age children with Williams syndrome is very similar to that of MA-matched children who are developing normally, with regard to the number of animal names produced, the average representativeness of the animals as members of the *animal* category, and the proportion of animal names produced that were at the basic level of categorization. Second, syntactical abilities are at the level expected for composite mental abilities. Third, syntactical complexity is at the level expected for mean utterance length.

VISUOSPATIAL CONSTRUCTIVE COGNITION

In the two previous sections, we focused on domains in which individuals with Williams syndrome perform relatively well. In the present section, we turn to the domain in which individuals with Williams syndrome have the most difficulty: visuospatial constructive cognition. We begin by describing performance on the DAS pattern construction subtest. As expected, our findings replicate those of previous researchers, providing still another demonstration that visuospatial constructive cognition represents the area of greatest difficulty for individuals with Williams syndrome. In the remainder of the section, we describe two studies that we have conducted to try to understand the specific difficulties that individuals with Williams syndrome have with visuospatial construction.

DAS Pattern Construction Subtest

The DAS pattern construction subtest is a very sensitive measure of visuo-spatial constructive cognition. The participant is shown a colored picture of a block pattern and is asked to construct the same pattern, using colored cubes. Each cube has one solid yellow side, one solid black side, two sides divided diagonally into yellow and black, and two sides divided horizontally into yellow and black. (The youngest children are asked to copy a different set of patterns, using crepe rubber squares composed of one solid yellow side and one solid black side.) The initial designs are composed of two cubes; if individuals are able to complete some of the two-cube designs, they are asked to complete four-cube designs. (The test also includes nine-cube patterns, but these are used only for individuals who are particularly good at pattern construction.) Points are awarded both for completing the pattern correctly and for speed of completion of correct patterns. As was the case for the DAS digit recall subtest, raw scores consist of ability scores, which are converted to T (standard) scores based on the participant's CA.

The inclusion of two-block patterns provides the DAS pattern construction subtest with an important advantage over the Wechsler IQ block design subtests, which include only four- and nine-block patterns. Bellugi et al. (1992, 1994) have reported that most of the adolescents and young adults with Williams syndrome in their samples have been unable to construct even a four-block checkerboard pattern (the simplest pattern on the Wechsler IQ tests). Thus, detection of any developmental trends in constructing block patterns is likely to require the use of two-block patterns of varying difficulty.

A scatterplot of the ability scores of the 80 individuals between ages 4 and 47 years to whom we have administered the DAS pattern construction subtest is shown in figure 4.15. The data indicate that individuals with Williams syndrome show improvement in visuoconstructive spatial abilities during childhood and maintain this ability in adulthood. The correlation between ability score and CA was $+0.59$ ($P < .001$) for the 47 children and -0.093 (NS) for the 33 adults.

Despite substantive developmental gains in visuospatial constructive abilities, however, the 80 individuals with Williams syndrome had standard scores that were consistently low across the entire age range sampled ($r = -0.12$; NS). A histogram of the T scores is presented in figure 4.16. The mean T score was 22.99 (SD = 4.30). The mean clearly is not representative of the sample distribution, which is highly positively skewed. The modal T score (obtained by 58% of the sample) was 20, the lowest score possible. The T scores of 88% of the participants were at the first percentile. Nevertheless, 10% of the participants scored in the normal range. The highest T score corresponded to the eighth percentile.

These figures are very similar to those reported by Bellugi et al. (1994) for six adolescents with Williams syndrome, tested on either the WISC-R or the WAIS-R block design subtest. Four of these individuals (67%) earned the lowest possible scaled score (1, on a scale from 1 to 19); five (83%) scored at

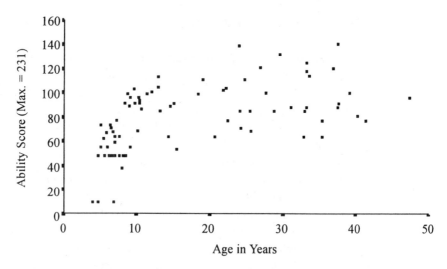

Figure 4.15 DAS pattern construction subtest ability score as a function of age (N = 80).

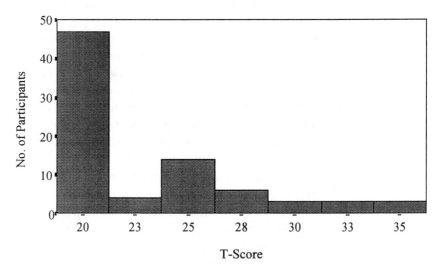

Figure 4.16 DAS pattern construction subtest T-score distribution (N = 80).

the first percentile, and only one individual (17%) scored in the normal range (scaled score of 4). Similar findings also were reported by Udwin and Yule (1991). Thus, our pattern of results for the DAS pattern construction subtest replicates once again the finding of previous researchers that, for individuals with Williams syndrome, visuospatial constructive cognition is an area of pronounced weakness.

Low-Level Spatial Organization

The normal processing of spatial organization involves two levels: global and local. Global processing involves attention to the overall arrangement of the elements of the spatial display. Local processing involves attention to the individual elements of the display. For example, consider a triangle made of small circles. At the global level, a person would focus on the fact that this stimulus is a triangle; the specific elements that compose the triangle would be ignored. At the local level, the person would focus on the fact that the stimulus includes a number of small circles; the overall arrangement of the circles into a triangle would be ignored. Although individuals with normal intelligence attend to both global and local aspects of spatial displays, priority is given to the global aspect (Navon, 1977).

Bellugi et al., (1988, 1992, 1994) have argued, on the basis of findings from a small-sample study of adolescents and young adults with Williams syndrome, that individuals with this syndrome do not follow this normal pattern of spatial processing. Instead, individuals with Williams syndrome focus on the local elements, often to the exclusion of the global organization. For example, Bihrle et al., (1989) found that when asked to draw from memory a large uppercase A composed of small uppercase Ms, participants with Williams syndrome produced a series of small Ms, but did not arrange the Ms into an A. Bihrle et al. (1989) also considered performance on the block design subtest of the WISC-R (Wechsler, 1974), and found that when asked to copy a four-block checkerboard pattern, most of the participants with Williams syndrome not only were unable to produce the correct design but failed to maintain the overall arrangement of the blocks (two rows of two blocks each). Bellugi et. al. (1992, 1994) suggested that the spatial construction problems of individuals with Williams syndrome are due to attention to the local elements of a display, at the expense of the global elements.

It is possible, however, that the spatial construction problems exhibited by individuals with Williams syndrome have a different source. If so, the low-level spatial organization of individuals with Williams syndrome may be normal (i.e., involve global processing). To test this hypothesis, we administered the Banks and Prinzmetal (1976) visual search task to adults with Williams syndrome. In this task, participants are shown a stimulus composed primarily of small elements (distractors) that are halfway between a *T* and an *F*. The stimulus also includes one true *T* or *F* (the target). The participant's task is to indicate, as rapidly as possible, which letter (*T* or *F*) is included in the display. Examples of the stimuli used in this task are presented in figure 4.17. Banks and Prinzmetal (1976) found that performance of normal adults was influenced strongly by Gestalt grouping. In some of the stimulus configurations (e.g., see 2 in figure 4.17), the targets were isolated because the distractors were grouped by proximity. Search times were shortest for this type of stimulus, even though it contained more elements than did stimulus configuration type 1 (in figure 4.17). In contrast, when the target was grouped with the distractors (e.g., configurations 1 and 5 in figure 4.17), search time was significantly longer. Search time was longest for configuration type 5 because for these stimuli, not only was the target grouped with the distractors but more distractors were included than in configuration type 1 (in

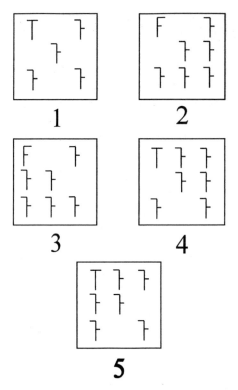

Figure 4.17 Examples of the Gestalt grouping task stimulus configuration types.

figure 4.17). If individuals with Williams syndrome have normal low-level spatial organization, they should show this same pattern of response times. In contrast, if the low-level spatial organization of these individuals stresses local organization, response times should be fastest for such stimuli as 1, because these stimuli have the fewest local elements (five versus seven in the other types of stimuli).

Thirteen adults with Williams syndrome (mean age, 35 years; range, 18–47 years) participated in this study. Mean IQ on the Kaufman Brief Intelligence Test (K-BIT; Kaufman & Kaufman, 1990) was 66 (range, 41–95). (Because the K-BIT does not include any measures of visuospatial construction, the IQs earned by individuals with Williams syndrome on this test are usually higher than those earned on full-scale IQ tests.) The Banks and Prinzmetal (1976) task was presented by computer. Individuals were told that they were to determine whether the target letter in the stimulus configuration was a *T* or an *F*, and then to push the touchpad button labeled with the correct letter. Participants were told that they should respond as quickly as possible without making errors. A series of practice trials was administered prior to the experimental trials.

Results indicated that the responses of the individuals with Williams syndrome were almost always correct (96%). Error rates did not differ as a function of type of stimulus configuration. The response times fit the predicted pattern for normal low-level spatial processing. Participants responded significantly faster to configuration type 2 (see figure 4.17) than to any of the other configurations, even though configuration type 1 contained fewer elements. Response times were significantly slower to configuration type 5 than to any of the other configurations. Response times to configuration types 1, 3, and 4 were intermediate. This pattern indicates that the performance of adults with Williams syndrome was affected strongly by the global characteristics of the stimulus configurations.

Impact of Segmented ("Cued") Designs on Performance on Pattern Construction Tasks

The results of our study of low-level spatial processing by adults with Williams syndrome indicated that these individuals, as did persons with normal intelligence, focused on global information. This finding suggests that the visuospatial construction problems experienced by individuals having Williams syndrome are not caused simply by attention to the individual elements of a design at the expense of the whole.

In fact, the pattern construction problem that individuals with Williams syndrome have may involve difficulty in dividing the whole (global pattern) into its component (local) parts. If so, performance should improve if the parts are made explicit. For example, pattern construction tasks could be modified by placing a grid over the picture of the block pattern to be copied or by separating the blocks in the pictured pattern slightly. These types of modifications have resulted in improved performance by individuals with normal intelligence or mild mental retardation. Royer (1977) and Royer and Weitzel (1977) found that when a grid was present, adults of normal intelligence were able to copy block designs signficantly faster than when the grid was not present. Accuracy was excellent in both conditions. Akshoomoff and Stiles (1996) found that normally developing children ages 4 to 7 years copied block designs more accurately when a grid was superimposed over the pattern to be copied. Shah and Frith (1993) found that normally developing primary-school children and adolescents copied block designs significantly faster when a small space was placed between the blocks in the to-be-copied pattern than when no space was left between the pictured blocks. Accuracy was very high in both conditions. Adolescents with borderline normal intelligence or mild mental retardation (mean IQ, 73) copied the designs more accurately when the blocks in the to-be-copied pattern were separated slightly. In contrast, autistic individuals who excel on tasks requiring a local processing strategy and have difficulty with tasks requiring a global strategy performed highly accurately and equally fast in both conditions in the Shah and Frith study. In the no-separation condition, both high-functioning adolescents (mean performance IQ, 96.7) and lower-functioning adolescents

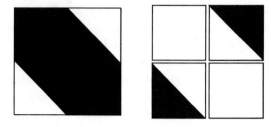

Figure 4.18 Examples of unsegmented and segmented block patterns.

(mean performance IQ, 71.0) with autism copied the designs significantly more rapidly than did controls matched for performance IQ. The copies made by the lower-IQ adolescents with autism were significantly more likely to be correct than were those made by the matched controls.

To test the hypothesis that the very poor performance of individuals with Williams syndrome on pattern construction tasks is due in part to extreme difficulty in correctly segmenting pictured patterns into individual blocks, we compared the performance of 21 adults with Williams syndrome (mean age, 29.5 years; mean K-BIT IQ, 59.1) in two conditions. A within-group design was used. In the first condition, the pictures of the patterns to be copied were presented in the usual manner (as on the DAS or the Wechsler IQ tests). In the second condition, the pictures of the patterns to be copied were presented with a small space separating the blocks. The same designs were used in the two conditions, with the colors reversed. Examples of the stimuli used are shown in figure 4.18.

Each participant copied a total of 16 patterns: 8 in the unseparated condition and 8 in the separated condition. Each set of eight patterns included 4 two-block patterns and 4 four-block patterns. Performance was considerably more accurate in the separated condition ($P < .01$). Nineteen of the 21 participants completed all 4 two-block patterns correctly in that condition (mean correct, 3.86 of possible 4); only 10 participants completed all 4 two-block patterns correctly in the unseparated condition (mean correct, 2.67 of 4). Ten individuals also completed all 4 four-block patterns correctly in the separated condition (mean correct, 2.43); in contrast, only five individuals completed all 4 four-block patterns correctly in the unseparated condition (mean correct, 1.61).

Across the 21 participants, 55 pairs of two-block patterns were completed correctly in both conditions. For 48 of these pairs, response times were shorter in the separated condition ($P < .001$). Of the 33 pairs of four-block patterns completed correctly in both conditions, response times were shorter in the separated condition for 25 of these pairs ($P = .002$). This pattern of findings suggests that when the parts of a whole are not delineated clearly, individuals with Williams syndrome have difficulty in segmenting the whole into its component parts. This difficulty contributes to the extreme problem that individuals with Williams syndrome have in visuospatial construction.

For the four-block patterns, it was possible to determine whether the participants preserved the overall shape of the pattern (a square composed of two rows of two blocks each) even when the design was not copied correctly. In the separated condition, the correct overall shape was maintained on 91% of the four-block patterns that were copied incorrectly. The correct overall shape also was maintained on 76% of the four-block patterns that were copied incorrectly in the unseparated condition. Two individuals produced more than half of the total number of broken configurations (incorrect overall shapes) in this condition. The remaining individuals maintained the correct overall shape on 88% of the patterns that were copied incorrectly. These rates of maintaining the correct global configuration are consistent with those reported by Akshoomoff and Stiles (in press) for normally developing children ages 6 to 8 years.

Summary

The findings from our research converge with those of previous researchers: Individuals with Williams syndrome perform extremely poorly on pattern construction tasks. On the standardized test of pattern construction (DAS), more than half of the participants earned the lowest possible scaled score. At the same time, our results indicate improvement in absolute level of performance as individuals with Williams syndrome get older. Furthermore, despite the extreme difficulty most individuals with Williams syndrome have with pattern construction, we found several important parallels between the spatial abilities of individuals with Williams syndrome and individuals with normal intelligence or mild mental retardation. The low-level spatial organization of adults with Williams syndrome was normal; global processing was given precedence over local processing. The performance of adults with Williams syndrome on pattern construction tasks improved when the delineation of the pattern into individual blocks was made explicit by separating slightly the blocks in the to-be-copied pattern. Better performance was demonstrated both in the number of patterns copied correctly and in the speed of copying patterns correctly. These improvements are consistent with those shown by individuals with mild mental retardation in the Shah and Frith (1993) study; the improvement in speed of correct copying also was shown by individuals with normal intelligence. The improvement in performance in the separated block condition suggests that part of the pattern construction task problem experienced by individuals with Williams syndrome results from difficulty in accurately segmenting into its local components the global pattern to be copied. Finally, like the normally developing 6- to 8-year-olds in the Akshoomoff and Stiles study (1996), adults with Williams syndrome usually maintained the correct overall configuration (a square composed of two rows of two blocks) even when the patterns were copied incorrectly.

INTERRELATIONS AMONG AUDITORY SHORT-TERM MEMORY, LANGUAGE, AND VISUOSPATIAL CONSTRUCTIVE COGNITION

Relative performance on the standardized measures of auditory short-term memory, language, and visuospatial constructive cognition replicated previous findings regarding the strengths and weaknesses of individuals with Williams syndrome in different cognitive domains. Participants performed very well on all the auditory short-term memory measures. Most individuals (73%) scored in the normal range on the two-items-per-second digit recall measure (DAS); 9% scored at or above the fiftieth percentile. Performance on the one-item-per-second digit recall measures was at the same level, with 75% of the individuals with Williams syndrome scoring in the normal range for forward digit span and 89% for backward digit span.

Performance also was good on the language measures. For receptive vocabulary (PPVT-R), 42% of the participants scored in the normal range. Note, however, that level of performance on the DAS digits subtest was substantially higher. The standard scores earned on the DAS digit recall were significantly greater than those on the PPVT-R [paired $t(96) = 6.79$; $P < .001$]. The very good auditory rote memory abilities of individuals with Williams syndrome are probably a major reason why the vocabularies of these individuals are relatively good. The discrepancy between rote memory abilities and vocabulary abilities, even though both are relative strengths for individuals with Williams syndrome, renders it clear that vocabulary development also depends on other abilities (e.g., abstract thought), components that are relatively weak in Williams syndrome.

On the measure of receptive grammar (TROG), 56% of the individuals with Williams syndrome scored in the normal range. Once again, however, auditory short-term memory performance was substantially higher. The DAS digit recall standard scores were significantly higher than were those corresponding to the TROG standard scores [paired $t(70) = 4.62$; $P < .001$]. The strong auditory rote memory skills of individuals with Williams syndrome likely play an important role in grammatical development.

As expected, performance on the measure of visuospatial constructive cognition (DAS pattern construction) was extremely poor. More than half of the individuals with Williams syndrome (57%) received the lowest possible standard score (T = 20). Nevertheless, older individuals with Williams syndrome correctly copied more patterns than did younger individuals, indicating definite improvement with CA. A small proportion of individuals with Williams syndrome (10%) scored in the normal range (third to eighth percentiles).

Despite the large discrepancies in relative level of ability for auditory short-term memory, language, and visuospatial constructive cognition, substantial correlations still may exist in ability across these domains. To address this possibility, we began by computing the simple correlations between

Table 4.3 Simple correlations among DAS digit span, 1-second digit span (forward), 1-second digit span (backward), PPVT-R raw score, TROG raw score, and pattern construction ability score[*]

		DAS Span	Span F	Span B	PPVT	TROG
Span F	r	0.77				
	P	< .001				
Span B	r	0.65	0.61			
	P	< .001	< .001			
PPVT	r	0.70	0.67	0.80		
	P	< .001	< .001	< .001		
TROG	r	0.70	0.72	0.65	0.79	
	P	< .001	< .001	< .001	< .001	
Pattern	r	0.52	0.50	0.62	0.65	0.63
	P	< .001	< .001	< .001	< .001	< .001

DAS, differential ability scales; PPVT-R, Peabody Picture Vocabulary Test–Revised; TROG, test for reception of grammar.
[*]N = 55.

DAS digit recall span length (longest string of digits repeated in the correct order), 1-second forward digit span length, 1-second backward digit span length, PPVT-R raw score, TROG raw score, and DAS pattern construction ability score. We have obtained data for all six of these measures from 55 individuals with Williams syndrome, ranging in age from 5 to 47 years; the correlations reported in table 4.3 are based on these data. All the correlations are positive, highly significant ($P < .001$), and substantial.

These impressive correlations may be an artifact of the wide CA range of the participants, however. To determine whether the relations between domains held even if CA were controlled statistically, we calculated the first-order correlations between the six measures, with CA partialled out. These correlations are presented in table 4.4. All the correlations are significant ($P < .01$); 13 of the 15 are significant at the $P < .001$ level. The large positive correlations between backward digit span and the two language measures (PPVT-R and TROG)—even with CA partialled out—suggest that working memory is related strongly to language level for individuals with Williams syndrome. This relation between working memory and language ability is consistent with previous findings for both individuals with normal intelligence (Kemper et al., 1989; Norman et al., 1991) and individuals with Down syndrome (Chapman, 1995; Rondal, 1995).

We were able to make a direct comparison of the obtained correlations for individuals with Williams syndrome to correlations for individuals who were developing normally for only one of our comparisons. Bishop (1989) reported the partial correlation between raw scores of the British Picture Vocabulary Test (BPVT, the British version of the PPVT-R) and TROG raw scores for the TROG standardization sample. This correlation was +0.44;

Table 4.4 Partial correlations (controlling for CA) among DAS digit span, 1-second digit span (forward), 1-second digit span (backward), PPVT-R raw score, TROG raw score, and pattern construction ability score*

		DAS span	Span F	Span B	PPVT	TROG
Span F	r	0.70				
	P	< .001				
Span B	r	0.51	0.46			
	P	< .001	< .001			
PPVT	r	0.57	0.50	0.69		
	P	< .001	< .001	< .001		
TROG	r	0.58	0.60	0.47	0.64	
	P	< .001	< .001	< .001	< .001	
Pattern	r	0.38	0.35	0.50	0.52	0.50
	P	< .005	< .01	< .001	< .001	< .001

CA, chronological age; DAS, differential ability scales; PPVT-R, Peabody Picture Vocabulary Test–Revised; TROG, test for reception of grammar.
*N = 55.

which is significantly less than the +0.63 obtained for our Williams syndrome sample ($z = 2.03$; $P = .02$).

The most striking result portrayed in table 4.4 is the measure of visuospatial constructive cognition, which is correlated significantly with all the memory measures and both the language measures. This is true even though absolute levels of ability in the three domains differ dramatically for individuals with Williams syndrome. The consistently high correlations among auditory short-term memory, language, and visuospatial constructive cognition obtained for individuals with Williams syndrome are consistent with the Detterman and Daniel (1989) finding that correlations among the subtests of the WISC-R and WAIS-R are highest for individuals with low IQs (in their study, IQ < 78) and lowest for individuals with high IQs. Detterman (1987) and Detterman and Daniel (1989) argued that individuals with mental retardation have deficits in central processes, which limit the efficiency of all the other processes in the system. These limitations reduce the variability in level of ability for other processes, so that all processes tend to operate at the same low level. The result is high correlations among disparate abilities for individuals with mental retardation. In Williams syndrome, other processes have not all been reduced to the same low level; individuals with Williams syndrome have clear and consistent strengths in certain domains and extreme weakness in others. Nevertheless, the correlations among ability levels in these domains are very high, suggesting a powerful role for general intelligence (or *g*; Spearman, 1904) in Williams syndrome, as Detterman (1987) and Detterman and Daniel (1989) suggested is the case for other forms of mental retardation.

GENETICS OF WILLIAMS SYNDROME

The first descriptions of Williams syndrome occurred in Great Britain during a post–World War II epidemic of infantile hypercalcemia, which occurred as a result of overfortification of infant foods with vitamin D (Stapleton et al., 1957). After vitamin D supplementation decreased, the incidence of infantile hypercalcemia dramatically declined, but the result was a subset of children who had hypercalcemia and developmental delay and unusual facies. These children were described as having "idiopathic hypercalcemia of infancy" (Bongiovanni et al., 1957; Joseph & Parrott, 1958).

Garcia et al., (1964) were the first to document a connection between idiopathic infantile hypercalcemia and SVAS. SVAS long had been recognized as an abnormality of great vessels, which either could be inherited in an autosomal dominant fashion or could occur sporadically in association with developmental delay (Merritt et al., 1963; Eisenberg et al., 1964). The sporadic form of the syndrome as described by Williams et al., (1961) and Beuren et al., (1964) became known as *Williams syndrome*.

Genetic Relations between SVAS and Williams Syndrome

Early articles describing families with SVAS and individuals with Williams syndrome debated the possible genetic relations between the two conditions. Proposed mechanisms included the following: Williams syndrome as a variable severe manifestation of the autosomal dominant SVAS; Williams syndrome and SVAS as allelic disorders; Williams syndrome as a nongenetic phenocopy of SVAS; or Williams syndrome and SVAS as contiguous gene disorders (Friedman & Roberts, 1966; Grimm & Wesselhoeft, 1980; Schmidt et al., 1989; Morris & Moore, 1991). The variability of both the SVAS and Williams syndrome phenotypes over time and among individuals contributed to the difficulty in resolving the genetic relation (Morris et al., 1988; Chiarella et al., 1989).

In most families with autosomal dominant SVAS, no one had either developmental delay or mental retardation. This is in sharp contrast to individuals with Williams syndrome. Nevertheless, some individuals with autosomal dominant SVAS had physical features that overlapped those found in individuals with sporadic Williams syndrome. These features included hoarse voice, hernias, and some of the facial features, such as full cheeks, periorbital fullness, and wide mouth.

Most cases of Williams syndrome occur sporadically. However, Morris et al., (1993) identified three families in which the classic Williams syndrome phenotype was transmitted from parent to child. One of these cases involved transmission from father to son, ruling out X-linked inheritance. In all three cases, the parent with Williams syndrome had been identified in childhood as having mental retardation of unknown etiology. The diagnosis of Williams syndrome in the three adults was made only after the diagnosis was established in their child. No history of SVAS was found in any other members of the extended families and, as with other groups of individuals with Williams syndrome, the familial cases demonstrated some phenotypic variability. However, the presence of these families indicates that Williams syndrome is not an "iceberg dominant" of SVAS but rather that Williams syndrome and SVAS must be either allelic or contiguous gene disorders.

Determination of the Genetic Etiology of SVAS and Williams Syndrome

Given these findings, it was apparent that to determine the underlying genetic etiology of SVAS and Williams syndrome, the best strategy would be to employ linkage analysis in families with autosomal dominant SVAS. Dysmorphology examinations were performed by Colleen Morris on members of 10 kindreds with SVAS (175 individuals at risk), looking for Williams syndrome features. In addition, special echocardiographic and Doppler techniques were developed to characterize the variability of the cardiovascular disease in families with SVAS (Ensing et al., 1989). These techniques are highly sensitive and reliable in detecting cardiac lesions, even in individuals who are asymptomatic for SVAS. Linkage between the SVAS phenotype and DNA markers on the long arm of chromosome 7 was demonstrated (Ewart et al., 1993a). A polymorphism at the elastin locus was linked completely, rendering *ELN* a candidate gene. Subsequent studies of three additional SVAS kindreds confirmed that *ELN* mutations cause SVAS. The first kindred included four generations with a 6;7 translocation that disrupted *ELN* at 7q11.23 (Curran et al., 1993; Morris et al., 1993). The second family had a submicroscopical deletion of chromosome 7, which deleted the 3' end of *ELN* between exons 27 and 28 (Ewart et al., 1994). The third family had a 30-kb deletion within *ELN*, deleting exons 2 through 27 (Olson et al., 1995).

The next step in the investigation was to explore the relation between SVAS and Williams syndrome by evaluation of *ELN* in individuals who had Williams syndrome. Because the vascular disease in Williams syndrome is identical to that of SVAS (Perou, 1961; O'Connor et al., 1985), Ewart et al. (1993a) proposed the hypothesis that mutations involving *ELN* also might be responsible for Williams syndrome. Subsequently, submicroscopical deletions of chromosome 7q11.23 resulting in Williams syndrome were discovered (Ewart et al., 1993b). Inherited or de novo deletions of one *ELN* allele were identified in more than 98% of the individuals with Williams syndrome who were studied (Morris et al., 1994; Lowery et al., 1995; Mari et al., 1995). On the basis of this finding, a simple and accurate genetic test for Williams syndrome—fluorescent in situ hybridization (FISH) with probes at *ELN*—was developed.

Significance of the Deletion of one *ELN* Allele

The data suggest that the *ELN* mutation is responsible for the vascular pathology in both Williams syndrome and SVAS. The deletion of one *ELN* allele may result in abnormal production of elastin protein. This genetic error likely affects the formation of elastic fibers that consist of both elastin and microfibrils (Mecham, 1995). Microfibrils, which consist of fibrillin and microfibril-associated glycoprotein, act as the scaffold for elastin. An abnormality of elastic fibers would explain the pathological observation in SVAS: that of the elastic fibers being fragmented and disorganized. Stenosis, caused by fibrosis, is probably a secondary phenomenon, resulting from blood pressure forces acting against a relatively inelastic arterial wall. Peripheral pulmonic stenosis is common in young children with Williams syndrome but usually improves with age, whereas SVAS may worsen. This pattern could be explained by a much lower pressure in the pulmonary circulation, compared with systemic pressures. Other features of Williams syndrome attributable to an abnormality of elastic fibers would include hernias (both inguinal and umbilical), the presence of bladder and bowel diverticulae, the hyperextensibility in the joints of young children, and the occurrence of musculoskeletal problems with aging, including kyphosis, lordosis, and scoliosis. The abnormality of elastin may account in part for some of the soft-tissue components of the Williams syndrome facies, most notably the full jowly cheeks and periorbital fullness. Possibly the hoarse voice is due to abnormalities in elastic fibers affecting the larynx.

Though the *ELN* abnormality explains all the clinical features of SVAS, it does not account for all the features of Williams syndrome, especially the neurobehavioral abnormalities. In fact, *ELN* is expressed only negligibly in the human fetal or adult brain (Frangiskakis et al., 1996). As the deletions in individuals with Williams syndrome extend well beyond *ELN*, other genes that are deleted must account for the cognitive profile, personality profile, and mental retardation that contribute to the Williams syndrome phenotype. Individuals who have especially large deletions of 7q11.23 have an overlapping phenotype with Williams syndrome, but with more severe mental retardation, and do not fit the classic Williams syndrome phenotype (Zackowski et al., 1990; Morris et al., 1993a; Kahler et al., 1995; Meschino & Finegan, 1995). This finding suggests that the critical region of deletion for the complete classic Williams syndrome phenotype has not yet been identified.

Genotype-Phenotype Correlation: SVAS Families with Small Deletions of 7q11.23

The 10 SVAS kindreds studied by Morris (Ewart et al., 1994) included several family members with both SVAS and a history of academic difficulties. Of the 16 members of one of these kindreds (K2049), 10 were found to have a deletion of 7q11.23 (Ewart et al., 1994). The deletion was 83.6

kilobases in length for all 10 individuals, and the breakpoint was near the 3' end of *ELN*. Significant variation of expression of SVAS was found, with some individuals requiring surgery and others being asymptomatic. Five of the 10 affected individuals had some of the facial features found in Williams syndrome. Eight of the 10 individuals, including the 5 with facial features consistent with Williams syndrome, fit the criteria described earlier for the Williams syndrome cognitive profile. (One of the two remaining individuals was considered untestable, owing to a history of multiple seizures.) These eight individuals had auditory short-term memory and language abilities similar to those of unaffected kindred members but had relatively impaired visuospatial constructive abilities. None of the 10 individuals fit the Williams syndrome personality profile or had hypercalcemia. None of the six kindred members who did not have the deletion fit the Williams syndrome medical phenotype, cognitive profile, or personality profile or had hypercalcemia. One affected 4-year-old was developmentally delayed (IQ = 64). All other family members had normal intelligence.

In another kindred (K1895), three of eight members were found to have a deletion of 7q11.23 approximately 300 kilobases in length, which included the entire *ELN* gene but was smaller than typical Williams syndrome deletions, which are approximately 1 megabase in length. All three individuals had SVAS, some facial features consistent with Williams syndrome, and the Williams syndrome cognitive profile. Once again, affected members had auditory rote memory abilities and language abilities similar to unaffected kindred members but had impaired visuospatial constructive cognition. None of the three individuals fit the Williams syndrome personality profile or had hypercalcemia. Of the five kindred members who did not have a deletion, none fit the Williams syndrome phenotype. All family members possessed normal intelligence.

Also studied was third kindred (K1861) in which five of eight family members had SVAS but none had had academic difficulties. In the affected members of this kindred, one *ELN* gene was disrupted by a 6;7 translocation (Morris et al., 1993b). Some of the affected members had connective tissue features consistent with Williams syndrome, such as hoarse voice and inguinal hernia. However, none of the family members fit the Williams syndrome personality profile, and none had hypercalcemia. The two children in the kindred were tested for the Williams syndrome cognitive profile; neither child fit this profile. For both children, visuospatial constructive cognition was a relative strength. All family members possessed normal intelligence.

Eight affected members of three other kindreds (K1790, K2044, and K2260) with autosomal dominant SVAS also were assessed. All eight individuals had point mutations that disrupted one *ELN* allele, and all had SVAS. Five of the eight individuals had some facial features consistent with Williams syndrome, but none fit the Williams syndrome personality profile or the Williams syndrome cognitive profile, and none had hypercalcemia. All had normal intelligence.

The findings from affected members of kindreds K1861, K1790, K2044, and K2260 indicate that abnormalities in *ELN* do not contribute to the impaired visuospatial constructive cognition found in the Williams syndrome cognitive profile. Furthermore, given that the affected individuals from the two SVAS kindreds with small deletions of 7q11.23 show the Williams syndrome cognitive profile, likely a gene or genes contributing to the impaired visuospatial constructive cognition included in that profile is located in the 83.6-kilobase region common to the deletions in kindreds 1895 and 2049 (Morris et al., 1995).

Except for *ELN*, no previously characterized genes had been mapped to the Williams syndrome region of chromosome 7q11.23. To determine whether any other genes were present in the 83.6- region common to the deletion in K1895 and K 2049, the entire region was sequenced (Frangiskakis et al., 1996). Only one gene, *LIM-kinase1* (*LIMK1*), was found. This gene, which is contiguous with *ELN*, was deleted in all affected members of K1895 and K2049 and in all the individuals with Williams syndrome who were tested. However, *LIMK1* was not deleted in any members of the kindreds with isolated autosomal dominant SVAS or in any of the normal controls tested. Thus, hemizygous deletion of *LIMK1* cooccurs with the Williams syndrome cognitive profile. A schematic diagram illustrating the relative locations of *ELN* and *LIMK1*, the deletions found in affected members of K1895 and K2049, and a typical Williams syndrome deletion, is provided in figure 4.19.

To determine the expression of *LIMK1*, we performed Northern analyses using messenger RNA extracted from human fetal and adult tissues. Results indicated that for both fetus and adult, *LIMK1* messenger RNA levels are highest in the brain. These findings, in conjunction with the Williams syn-

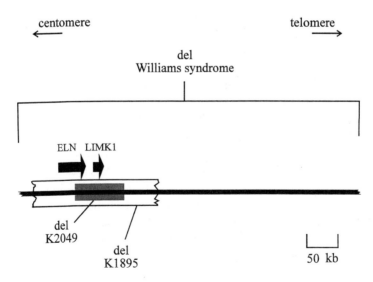

Figure 4.19 Relative locations of *ELN* and *LIMK1*, the deletions found in affected members of K1895 and K2049, and a typical Williams syndrome deletion on chromosome 7q11.23.

drome cognitive profile data for affected and unaffected members of the six kindreds we tested, indicate that *LIMK1* hemizygosity contributes to the impaired visuospatial constructive cognition that occurs in Williams syndrome (Frangiskakis et al., 1996).

CONCLUSION

Individuals with Williams syndrome show a characteristic cognitive profile: relative strengths in auditory rote memory and in language, accompanied by extreme weakness in visuospatial constructive cognition. This profile does not preclude significant relations between abilities in the three domains, however. In fact, correlations in ability levels across domains are very high for individuals with Williams syndrome, even when the effect of CA is controlled statistically. This pattern suggests a strong role for general intelligence (or *g*) in Williams syndrome, even though levels of ability vary dramatically as a function of cognitive domain.

Some 70% of individuals with Williams syndrome have auditory short-term memory abilities in the normal range. These abilities provide an excellent foundation for both vocabulary acquisition and syntactical development. Of course, vocabulary and syntactical development require more than simply good auditory rote memory; conceptual abilities also are critical. Perhaps for this reason, only approximately 60% of the individuals who have Williams syndrome and auditory rote memory ability in the normal range also have vocabulary ability in the normal range. Syntactical ability level is consistent with composite mental ability level and significantly lower than would be expected on the basis of auditory rote memory ability level.

Visuospatial constructive ability is the area of greatest difficulty for individuals with Williams syndrome; only some 20% of the individuals who scored in the normal range on vocabulary ability also scored in the normal range on visuospatial construction. In fact, 57% of the individuals with Williams syndrome obtained the lowest possible scaled score on the DAS pattern construction subtest. Nevertheless, the visuospatial constructive abilities of individuals with Williams syndrome are highly correlated with auditory rote memory abilities, vocabulary ability, and grammatical ability. Furthermore, in at least two important ways, the spatial abilities of individuals with Williams syndrome are similar to those of the general population. First, the low-level spatial organization abilities of individuals with Williams syndrome appear to be normal; grouping by proximity (global processing) takes precedence over processing of individual elements (local processing) of a spatial array. Second, as for the general population, the performance of individuals with Williams syndrome on pattern construction tasks is significantly better when cues are provided regarding how to divide the global design into its local components (individual cubes).

The Williams syndrome cognitive profile of relative strengths in auditory rote memory and language and great weakness in visuospatial constructive abilities is present prior to age 2 and is shown across the entire IQ range of the children and adults with Williams syndrome we have tested: 31 to 90 on the DAS (Elliott, 1990); 40 (the lowest possible IQ) to 104 on the K-BIT (Kaufman & Kaufman, 1990); < 30 to 100 on the BSID-II (Bayley, 1993). The Williams syndrome cognitive profile also is distinctive; it seldom is found in individuals who do not have Williams syndrome. This pattern strongly suggests a role for genetics in the establishment of this profile in Williams syndrome.

Williams syndrome has been shown to involve a hemizygous micro-deletion of chromosome 7q11.23. So far, two genes have been identified in the deleted region: *ELN* and *LIMK1*. The deletion of one *ELN* allele leads to the vascular pathology seen in Williams syndrome and in isolated autosomal dominant SVAS. This deletion, which likely results in abnormal production of elastin protein, accounts for some of the other medical problems demonstrated by many individuals with Williams syndrome, such as hernias and joint problems. Deletion of *ELN* also may account in part for some of the soft-tissue components of the Williams syndrome facies and the characteristic hoarse voice. *ELN* is expressed only neglibly in the brain, however. This finding, combined with the fact that individuals with isolated autosomal dominant SVAS have no difficulty with visuospatial constructive abilities and accordingly do not show the characteristic Williams syndrome cognitive profile, indicates that another gene likely is involved in the visuospatial constructive problems shown by individuals with Williams syndrome. Findings from two kindreds with small deletions of chromosome 7q11.23 indicate the deletion of one *LIMK1* allele. In these families, this deletion cosegregates with relative impairment in visospatial constructive abilities. DNA sequencing of the region involved in the smaller deletion revealed no additional genes. This set of results indicates that the hemizygous deletion of *LIMK1* plays an important role in the visuospatial construction difficulties exhibited by individuals with Williams syndrome.

We plan to continue our strategy of identification and careful clinical, psychological, and molecular genetic study of kindreds with small deletions in other parts of the region typically deleted in Williams syndrome. This strategy should lead to the identification of genes involved in the characteristic Williams syndrome personality, in the mental retardation often found in individuals with Williams syndrome, in the other features characteristic of the Williams syndrome facies, and in hypercalcemia. Continued psychological study of the cognitive strengths and weaknesses of individuals with Williams syndrome and of the strategies adopted by individuals with Williams syndrome to deal with their disability will help us to understand the bases for the wide range of developmental outcomes found among individuals with Williams syndrome. This knowledge should provide a solid foundation for designing more effective intervention strategies for facilitating individuals' attainment of their maximum potential.

ACKNOWLEDGMENTS

This project has been supported by grant HD29957 from the National Institute of Child Health and Human Development, by grant NS35102 from the National Institute of Neurological Disorders and Stroke, and by a grant from the American Heart Association Nevada Affiliate. We thank the National Williams Syndrome Association; the Williams Syndrome Association, Southeast Region; and the Williams Syndrome Association, Far West Region for facilitating our work both by helping to identify potential participants and by permitting us to conduct research at national and regional meetings. Both the individuals who have Williams syndrome and have been involved in this research and their families have been very generous with their time and their commitment to the research; we are grateful to all of them. Sharon Armstrong, Deborah Deckner, Sharon Hutchins, Janell Kalina, Bonnie Klein, Echo Meyer, Bronwyn Robinson, Paul Scott, Natasha Turner, and Sara Voelz were involved in data collection, reduction, and analysis. Stephanie Nelson assisted us with scheduling and field trips. The molecular genetics research described in the genetics section was conducted by the members of Mark Keating's laboratory, especially Amanda Ewart, J. Michael Frangiskakis, and Shannon Odelberg. The research described in the cardiology part of the genetics section was conducted by Gregory Ensing.

REFERENCES

American Guidance Service (1981). *Peabody picture vocabulary test—revised: Supplementary norms tables*. Circle Pines, MN: American Guidance Service.

Akshoomoff, N. A., & Stiles, J. (1996). The influence of pattern type on children's block design performance. *Journal of the International Neuropsychological Society, 2*, 392–402.

Baddeley, A. (1992). Working memory. *Science, 255*, 556–559.

Banken, J. (1985). Clinical utility of considering digits forward and digits backward as separate components of the Wechsler adult intelligence scale–revised. *Journal of Clinical Psychology, 41*, 686–691.

Banks, W. P., & Prinzmetal, W. (1976). Configurational effects in visual information processing. *Perception and Psychophysics, 19*, 361–367.

Bayley, N. (1969). *Bayley scales of infant development*. New York: Psychological Corporation.

Bayley, N. (1993). *Bayley scales of infant development* (2nd ed.). San Antonio, TX: Psychological Corporation.

Bellugi, U., Marks, S., Bihrle, A., & Sabo, H. (1988). Dissociation between language and cognitive functions in Williams syndrome. In D. Bishop & K. Mogford (Eds.), *Language development in exceptional circumstances* (pp. 177–189). London: Churchill Livingstone.

Bellugi, U., Bihrle, A., Neville, H., & Doherty, S. (1992). Language, cognition, and brain organization in a neurodevelopmental disorder. In M. Gunnar & C. Nelson (Eds.), *Developmental behavioral neuroscience: The Minnesota symposium* (pp. 201–232). Hillsdale, NJ: Erlbaum.

Bellugi, U., Wang, P. P., & Jernigan, T. L. (1994). Williams syndrome: An unusual neuropsychological profile. In S. H. Broman & J. Grafman, (Eds.), *Atypical cognitive deficits in developmental disorders: Implications for brain function* (pp. 23–56). Hillsdale, NJ: Erlbaum.

Bennett, F. C., LaVeck, B., & Sells, C. J. (1978). The Williams elfin facies syndrome: The psychological profile as an aid in syndrome identification. *Pediatrics, 61,* 303–306.

Bertrand, J., Mervis, C. B., & Eisenberg, J. D. (1997). Drawing by children with Williams syndrome: A developmental perspective. *Developmental Neuropsychology, 13,* 41–67.

Beuren, A. J. (1972). Supravalvular aortic stenosis: A complex syndrome with and without mental retardation. *Birth Defects Original Article Series, 8(5),* 45–56.

Beuren, A. J., Schulze, C., Eberle, P., Harmjanz, D., & Apitz, J. (1964). The syndrome of supravalvular aortic stenosis, peripheral pulmonary stenosis, mental retardation and similar facial appearance. *American Journal of Cardiology, 13,* 471–482.

Bihrle, A. M., Beelugi, U., Delis, D., & Marks, S. (1989). Seeing either the forest or the trees: Dissociation in visuospatial processing. *Brain and Cognition, 11,* 37–49.

Bishop, D. (1989). *Test for the reception of grammar* (2nd ed.). Manchester, UK: Chapel Press.

Bongiovanni, A. M., Eberlein, W. R., & Jones, I. T. (1957). Idiopathic hypercalcemia of infancy, with failure to thrive. *New England Journal of Medicine, 257,* 951–958.

Carroll, J. B., Davies, P., & Richman, B. (1971). *Word frequency book.* New York: American Heritage.

Chapman, R. (1995). Language development in children and adolescents with Down syndrome. In P. Fletcher & B. MacWhinney (Eds.), *The handbook of child language* (pp. 641–663). Oxford: Blackwell.

Chiarella, F., Bricarelli, F., Lupi, G., Bellotti, P., Domenicucci, S., & Vechio, C. (1989). Familial supravalvular aortic stenosis: A genetic study. *Journal of Medical Genetics, 26,* 86–92.

Curran, M. E., Atkinson, D. L., Ewart, A. K., Morris, C. A., Leppert, M. F., & Keating, M. T. (1993). The elastin gene is disrupted by a translocation associated with supravalvular aortic stenosis. *Cell, 73,* 159–163.

Detterman, D. K. (1987). Theoretical notions of mental retardation and intelligence. *American Journal of Mental Deficiency, 92,* 2–11.

Detterman, D. K., & Daniel, M. H. (1989). Correlations of mental tests with each other and with cognitive variables are highest for low IQ groups. *Intelligence, 13,* 349–359.

Dunn, L. E., & Dunn, L. E. (1981). *Peabody picture vocabulary test–revised.* Circle Pines, MN: American Guidance Services.

Eisenberg, R., Young, D., Jacobson, B., & Boito, A. (1964). Familial supravalvular aortic stenosis. *American Journal of Diseases of Childhood, 108,* 341–347.

Elliot, C. D. (1990). *Differential ability scales.* San Diego: Harcourt, Brace, Jovanovich.

Ensing, G. J., Schmidt, M. A., Hagler, D. J., Michels, V. V., Carter, G. A., & Feldt, R. H. (1989). Spectrum of findings in a family with nonsyndromic autosomal dominant supravalvular aortic stenosis: A Doppler echocardiographic study. *Journal of the American College of Cardiology, 13,* 413–419.

Ewart, A. K., Morris, C. A., Ensing, G. J., Loker, J., Moore, C., Leppert, M., & Keating, M. T. (1993a). A human vascular disorder, supravalvular aortic stenosis, maps to chromosome 7. *Proceedings of the National Academy of Science of the Untied States of America, 90,* 3226–3230.

Ewart, A. K., Morris, C. A., Atkinson, D., Jin, W., Sternes, K., Spallone, P., Stock, A. D., Leppert, M., & Keating, M. T. (1993b). Hemizygosity at the elastin locus in a developmental disorder, Williams syndrome. *Nature Genetics, 5,* 11–16.

Ewart, A. K., Jin, W., Atkinson, D., Morris, C. A., & Keating, M. T. (1994). Supravalvular aortic stenosis associated with a deletion disrupting the elastin gene. *Journal of Clinical Investigation, 93,* 1071–1077.

Finegan, J.-A., Smith, M. L., Meschino, W. S., Vallance, P. L., & Sitarenios G. (1995). *Verbal memory in children with Williams syndrome*. Indianapolis: Society for Research in Child Development.

Frangiskakis, J. M., Ewart, A. K., Morris, C. A., Mervis, C. B., Bertrand, J., Robinson, B. F., Klein, B. P., Ensing, G. J., Everett, L. A., Green, E. D., Proschel, C., Gutowski, N., Noble, M., Atkinson, D. L., Odelberg, S. J., & Keating, M. T. (1996). LIM-kinase1 hemizygosity implicated in impaired visuospatial constructive cognition. *Cell, 86,* 59–69.

Friedman, W. F., & Roberts, W. C. (1966). Vitamin D and the supravalvular aortic stenosis syndrome: The transplacental effects of vitamin D on the aorta of the rabbit. *Circulation, 34,* 77–86.

Garcia, R. E., Friedman, W. F., Kaback, M. M., & Rowe, R. D. (1964). Idiopathic hypercalcemia and supravalvular aortic stenosis. *New England Journal of Medicine, 271,* 117–120.

Gardner, M. F. (1985). *Test of auditory perceptual skills*. Burlingame, CA: Psychological and Educational Publications.

Gosch, A., & Pankau, R. (1994). Social-emotional and behavioral adjustment in children with Williams-Beuren syndrome. *American Journal of Medical Genetics, 53,* 335–339.

Gosch, A., Stading, G., & Pankau, R. (1994). Linguistic abilities in children with Williams-Beuren syndrome. *American Journal of Medical Genetics, 53,* 335–339.

Grimm, T., & Wesselhoeft, H. (1980). Zur Genetik des Williams-Beuren-Syndroms und der isolierten Form der Supravalvularen Aortenstenose: Untersuchungen von 128 Familien. *Zeitschrift fur Kardiologie, 69,* 168–172.

Kemper, S., Kynette, D., Rash, S., & O'Brien, K. (1989). Life span changes to adults' language: Effects of memory and genre. *Applied Psycholinguistics, 10,* 49–66.

Klein, B. P. (1995). *Grammatical abilities of children with Williams syndrome*. Unpublished master's thesis, Emory University, Atlanta, GA.

Klein, B. P., Mervis, C. B., Hutchins, S. S., & Bertrand, J. (1996, July). *Syntactic abilities of children with Williams syndrome*. Presented at the National Professional Conference of the Williams Syndrome Association, King of Prussia, PA.

Joseph, M. C., & Parrott, D. (1958). Severe infantile hypercalcemia with specific reference to the facies. *Archives of Diseases of Childhood, 33,* 385–395.

Kahler, S. G., Adhvaryu, S. G., Helali, N., & Qumsiyeh, M. B. (1995). Microscopically visible deletion of chromosome 7 in a child with features of Williams syndrome. *American Journal of Human Genetics, 57 (suppl.),* A117.

Kaufman, A. S., & Kaufman, N. L. (1990). *Kaufman brief intelligence test*. Circle Pines, MN: American Guidance Service.

Lowery, M. C., Morris, C. A., Ewart, A., Brothman, L., Zhu, X. L., Leonard, C. O., Carey, J. C., Keating, M., & Brothman, A. R. (1995). Strong correlation of elastin deletions, detected by FISH, with Williams syndrome: Evaluation of 235 patients. *American Journal of Human Genetics, 57,* 49–53.

Mari, A., Amati, F., Mingarelli, R., Giannotti, A., Sebastio, G., Colloridi, V., Novelli, G., & Dallapiccola, B. (1995). Analysis of the elastin gene in 60 patients with clinical diagnosis of Williams syndrome. *Human Genetics, 96,* 444–448.

McCarthy, D. (1970). *McCarthy scales of children's abilities*. New York: Psychological Corporation.

Mecham, R. P. (1995). Elastic fiber assembly and organization. *Genetic Counseling, 6,* 157–158.

Merritt, D. A., Palmar, C. G., Lurie, P. R., & Petry, E. L. (1963). Supravalvular aortic stenosis: Genetic and clinical studies [abstract]. *Journal of Laboratory and Clinical Medicine, 62,* 995.

Mervis, C. B., & Bertrand, J. (1997). Developmental relations between cognition and language: Evidence from Williams syndrome. In L. B. Adamson & M. A. Romski (Eds.), *Research on communication and language disorders: Contributions to theories of language development* (pp. 75–106). New York: Brookes.

Mervis, C. B., Robinson, B. F., Bertrand, J., Klein, B. P., & Armstrong, S. C. (1996, April). *Williams syndrome cognitive profile.* San Francisco: Cognitive Neuroscience Society.

Meschino, W. S., & Finegan, J. K. (1995). Deletion of the elastin gene in an atypical case of Williams syndrome. *American Journal of Human Genetics, 57 (suppl.),* A97.

Milani, L., Dall'Oglio, A. M., & Vicari, S. (1995). Spatial abilities in Italian children with Williams syndrome. *Genetic Counseling, 6,* 179–180.

Morris, C. A., Dilts, C., Demsey, S. A., Leonard, C. O., & Blackburn, B. (1988). The natural history of Williams syndrome: Physical characteristics. *Journal of Pediatrics, 113,* 318–326.

Morris, C. A., Greenberg, F., & Thomas, I. T. (1993). Williams syndrome: Autosomal dominant inheritance. *American Journal of Medical Genetics, 47,* 478–481.

Morris, C. A., Leonard, C. O., Dilts, C., & Demsey, S. A. (1990). Adults with Williams syndrome. *American Journal of Medical Genetics Supplement, 6,* 102–107.

Morris, C. A., Mervis, C. B., Bertrand, J., Robinson, B. F., Klein, B. P., Ensing, G. J., Keating, M. T., & Ewart, A. K. (1995, July). *Lumping vs. splitting in Williams syndrome: Supravalvular aortic stenosis families with a phenotype overlapping Williams syndrome.* Presented at the David W. Smith Workshop on Malformation and Morphogenesis, Big Sky, MT.

Morris, C. A., & Moore, C. A. (1991). The inheritance of Williams syndrome. *Proceedings of the Greenwood Genetics Center, 10,* 81–82.

Morris, C. A., Loker, J., Ensing, G., & Stock, A. D. (1993). Supravalvular aortic stenosis co-segregates with a familial 6;7 translocation which disrupts the elastin gene. *American Journal of Medical Genetics, 46,* 737–744.

Morris, C. A., Ewart, A. K., Sternes, K., Spallone, P., Stock, A. D., Leppert, M., & Keating, M. T. (1994). Williams syndrome: Elastin gene deletions. *American Journal of Human Genetics, 55 (suppl.),* A89.

Navon, D. (1977). Forest before trees: The precedence of global features in visual perception. *Cognitive Psychology, 9,* 353–383.

Norman, S., Kemper, S., Kynetter D., Cheung, H., & Anagnopoulos, C. (1991). Syntactic complexity and adults' running memory span. *Journal of Gerontology Psychological Sciences, 46,* 346–351.

O'Connor, W. N., Davis, J. B., Geissler, R., Cottrill, C. M., Noonan, J. A., & Todd, E. P. (1985). Supravalvular aortic stenosis: Clinical and pathologic observations in six patients. *Archives of Pathology and Laboratory Medicine, 109,* 179–185.

Olson, T. M., Michels, V. V., Urban, Z., Csiszar, K., Christiano, A. M., Driscoll, D. J., Feldt, R. H., Boyd, C. D., & Thibodeau, S. N. (1995). A 30 kb deletion within the elastin gene results in familial supravalvular aortic stenosis. *Human Molecular Genetics, 4,* 1677–1679.

Pani, J. R., Mervis, C. B., & Robinson, B. F. (1996, April). *Low level spatial organization in Williams syndrome.* San Francisco: Cognitive Neuroscience Society.

Perou, M. (1961). Congenital supravalvular aortic stenosis. *Archives of Pathology, 71,* 113–126.

Rondal, J. (1995). *An exceptional case of language development in a person with Down syndrome.* Oxford: Blackwell.

Rosch, E. (1973). On the internal structure of perceptual and semantic categories. In T. E. Moore (Ed.), *Cognitive development and the acquisition of language* (pp. 111–144). New York: Academic.

Rosch, E. (1975). Cognitive representations of semantic categories. *Journal of Experimental Psychology: General, 104,* 192–233.

Royer, F. L. (1977). Information processing in the block design task. *Intelligence, 1,* 32–50.

Royer, F. L., & Weitzel, K. E. (1977). Effect of perceptual cohesiveness on pattern recoding in the block design task. *Perception and Psychophysics, 21,* 39–46.

Scarborough, H. S. (1990). Index of productive syntax. *Applied Psycholinguistics, 11,* 1–22.

Scarborough, H. S., Rescorla, L., Tager-Flusberg, H., Fowler, A., & Sudhalter, V. (1991). The relation of utterance length to grammatical complexity in normal and language disordered groups. *Applied Psycholinguistics, 12,* 23–45.

Schmidt, M. A., Ensing, G. J., Michels, V. V., Carter, G. A., Hagler, D. J., & Feldt, R. H. (1989). Autosomal dominant supravalvular aortic stenosis: Large three-generation family. *American Journal of Medical Genetics, 32,* 384–389.

Scott, P., Mervis, C. B., Bertrand, J., Klein, B. P., Armstrong, S. C., & Ford, A. L. (1995). *Semantic organization and word fluency in 9- and 10-year-old children with Williams syndrome.* Indianapolis: Society for Research in Child Development.

Shah, A., & Frith, U. (1993). Why do autistic individuals show superior performance on the block design task? *Journal of Child Psychology and Psychiatry, 34,* 1351–1364.

Spearman, C. E. (1904). "General intelligence" objectively defined and measured. *American Journal of Psychology, 15,* 201–293.

Stapleton, T., MacDonald, W. B., Lightwood, R. (1957). The pathogenesis of idiopathic hypercalcemia in infancy. *American Journal of Clinical Nutrition, 5,* 533–542.

Udwin, O., & Yule, W. (1991). A cognitive and behavioral phenotype in Williams syndrome. *Journal of Clinical and Experimental Neuropsychology, 13,* 232–244.

Wang, P. P., & Bellugi, U. (1994). Evidence from two genetic syndromes for a dissociation between verbal and visual-spatial short-term memory. *Journal of Clinical and Experimental Neuropsychology, 16,* 317–322.

Wechsler, D. (1974). *Wechsler intelligence scale for children—revised.* New York: Psychological Corporation.

Wechsler, D. (1981). *Wechsler adult intelligence scale—revised.* New York: Psychological Corporation.

Wechsler, D. (1991). *Wechsler intelligence scale for children—III.* New York: Psychological Corporation.

Williams, J. C. P., Barratt-Boyes, B. G., & Lowe, J. B. (1961). Supravalvular aortic stenosis. *Circulation, 24,* 1311–1318.

Zackowski, J. L., Raffel, L. F., Blank, C. A., & Schwartz, S. (1990). Proximal interstitial deletion of 7q: A case report and review of the literature. *American Journal of Medical Genetics, 36,* 328–332.

5 Linking Cognition, Brain Structure, and Brain Function in Williams Syndrome

Ursula Bellugi, Debra Mills, Terry Jernigan, Greg Hickok, and Albert Galaburda

Williams syndrome is a rare genetic disorder that carries a distinctive profile of medical, psychological, neurophysiological, and neuroanatomical characteristics. In particular, previous work performed in our and other laboratories has mapped out the cognitive profile of Williams syndrome and its unique identifying features (Bellugi et al., 1992, 1994, 1996a,b; Bellugi & Wang, 1998; Vicari et al., 1996; see also chapter 4). Williams syndrome results in specific dissociations in cognitive functions, both within and across domains: general cognitive deficits but relatively spared linguistic abilities; extreme deficits in spatial cognition but excellent face processing.

In addition, we are now in a position to map out the neural profile of Williams syndrome and to pinpoint aspects of its unique identifying features as well. In this chapter we describe some results from a program project called *Williams Syndrome: Bridging Cognition and Gene*, which involves studies using brain-imaging techniques, including event-related potentials (ERP) magnetic resonance imaging (MRI) and brain cytoarchitectonics. These studies have begun to reveal the functional and structural characteristics of the neural organization of Williams syndrome: neurocognitive characterization of Williams syndrome (U. Bellugi); neurophysiological characterization (D. Mills); neuroanatomical characterization (T. Jernigan); and brain cytoarchitectonic characterization (A. Galaburda). An additional component involves molecular genetic characterization (J. Korenberg). The neural studies have revealed several features characteristic of the Williams syndrome subjects studied and some that may turn out to be unique to Williams syndrome (i.e., they occurred in each Williams syndrome subject studied and did not emerge in any of the other populations examined: individuals with focal lesions, language impairment, or Down syndrome or normals at any age). We argue that these may constitute *neurophysiological markers*, which may prove to characterize Williams syndrome at the neural level.

Further, we can begin to link these two profiles—cognitive and neurobiological—to create an initial picture of the functional neuroarchitecture of the syndrome. This linking can occur in several ways. By drawing on known connections between neurobiological systems and cognitive function, we can begin to match cognitive abnormalities with their probable bases in neurobiological abnormalities. In addition, individual variation within the Williams syndrome population can be used profitably by predicting correlations across individuals between the strength of neurophysiological markers and performance on specific behavioral measures. Finally, distinctive profile characteristics at the neurophysiological level (e.g., abnormal neurophysiological responses to particular language categories) can inform and refine our picture of aspects of the cognitive profile (e.g., unusual linguistic performance). In this chapter, we use all three approaches to focus on linking the cognitive profile of Williams syndrome with recent findings regarding brain structure and brain function in Williams syndrome.

COGNITIVE PROFILE FOR WILLIAMS SYNDROME

Many of the Williams subjects we have studied are classified as mild to moderately mentally retarded, as defined by the American Association on Mental Deficiency. Our subject population of more than 100 individuals with Williams syndrome shows IQ scores ranging from 40 to 100, with a mean IQ of 60; many have difficulty with aspects of general problem solving, and many are not able to achieve independent living. In the context of their cognitive impairment, the Williams syndrome individuals in our studies display characteristic patterns of cognitive performance with peaks and valleys of abilities. Areas that are distinctive, and therefore of theoretical interest, include complex expressive language abilities; disproportionately impaired spatial cognition, particularly at the level of global organization; spared face-processing ability; and abnormal auditory processing, including hyperacusis. Interesting to note is that from studies across populations in different countries, aspects of a characteristic Williams syndrome cognitive profile are emerging.

Spared Expressive Language

The Williams and Down syndrome subjects in our studies had equivalent levels of cognitive impairment as measured by IQ and tended to score equally poorly on other cognitive probes, such as Piagetian tests of conservation (Bellugi et al. 1996). Both Williams syndrome and Down syndrome adolescents failed on cognitive tasks of conservation easily mastered by younger normal children. A major contrast between the two syndrome groups came in their language abilities at all levels. For example, Williams syndrome adolescents performed close to or at ceiling on a linguistic task of comprehension of passive sentences, whereas Down syndrome subjects were close to chance (Bellugi et al., 1996). In addition, Williams adolescents scored significantly higher on word knowledge measures than on the Wechsler Intelligence Scale for Children–Revised (WISC-R) and dramatically better than their Downs counterparts. On a fluency test ("name all the animals you can in 1 minute"), Williams syndrome individuals' scores are indistinguishable

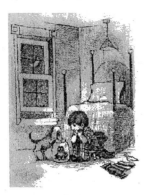

WMS Age 17, IQ 50:

Once upon a time when it was dark at night...the boy had a frog. The boy was looking at the frog...sitting on the chair, on the table, and the dog was looking through...looking up to the frog in a jar. That night he sleeped and slept for a long time, the dog did. But, the frog was not gonna go to sleep. The frog went out from the jar. And when the frog went out...the boy and the dog were still sleeping. Next morning it was beautiful in the morning. It was bright and the sun was nice and warm. Then suddenly when he opened his eyes...he looked at the jar and then suddenly the frog was not there. The jar was empty. There was no frog to be found.

DNS Age 18, IQ 55:

The frog is in the jar. The jar is on the floor. The jar on the floor. That's it. The stool is broke. The clothes is laying there.

Figure 5.1 Relatively spared expressive language in Williams syndrome.

from standardized norms for their chronological age, with many atypical as well as typical exemplars (e.g., *unicorn, ibex, saber-tooth tiger, vulture*). In general, then, compared with age- and IQ-matched Down subjects, the Williams subjects performed far better on tests of grammar comprehension (reversible passives, negation, conditionals) and also on a wide variety of language tasks, including fluency, accessing homonyms, sentence repetition, sentence completion, sentence correction, and elicited narrative tasks (Reilly et al., 1990; Bellugi et al., 1994; Rossen et al., 1996). Figure 5.1 shows examples of the relatively spared expressive language in Williams syndrome subjects as compared to Down subjects, as subjects are asked to tell a story based on a series of wordless pictures (Bellugi et al., 1996).

Impaired Spatial Cognition

On constructive visuospatial tasks, as opposed to language tasks, we have found Williams subjects to be impaired significantly worse than are Down syndrome subjects across all age ranges examined (Jones et al., 1995a). In addition, the Williams syndrome subjects performed more poorly even than children with frank right-hemisphere lesions (Beret et al., 1996). Further, this difficulty with spatial cognition seemed to be especially acute with respect to the global (rather than local) level of spatial organization. Drawings by subjects with Williams syndrome often lacked cohesion or gestalt organization. Williams subjects often had difficulty in maintaining the overall configuration of drawings and focused on internal details, whereas Down subjects tended to show the opposite effect (Bellugi et al., 1990); that is, a drawing of a house by a Williams subject might include windows, a door, and a roof but lack an overall organization of correct spatial relationships (figure 5.2). By contrast, a typical Down subject's drawing might be very simplified but

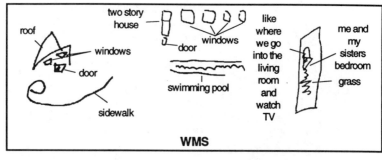

WMS

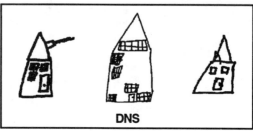

DNS

Free drawings of houses by age- and IQ-matched subjects with Williams syndrome and Down syndrome. Williams syndrome subjects' drawings contain many parts of a house but are not coherently organized, while Down syndrome subjects' drawings are simplified but have the correct overall configuration of a house.

Figure 5.2 Profoundly impaired spatial construction in Williams syndrome.

would show a broad organization of proper Gestalt relationships among elements. Similarly, we found that Williams subjects typically failed to reproduce the correct global organization of blocks in a block design task. They tended to place the blocks in apparently haphazard, noncontiguous arrangements, much like subjects with right-hemisphere damage. Conversely, individuals with Down syndrome typically maintained the overall configuration of a design but failed to replicate the internal pattern. In a process analysis comparing Williams and Down subjects, we found that Williams subjects made far more moves and, almost invariably, moves that were in the direction of continuously fragmented patterns (Bellugi et al., 1994). When asked to reproduce a figure made up of smaller figures (e.g., a large *A* made of small *M*s), a high proportion of the Williams subjects produced only the "local," constituent forms sprinkled across the page and failed to produce the global form, whereas Down subjects tended to show the opposite pattern (Bihrle et al., 1989). In perceptual matching tasks as well, Williams subjects showed a local bias (Bihrle, 1990).

Spared Face Processing

Despite their spatial cognitive dysfunctions, in realms within visuospatial cognition, the Williams subjects displayed selective preservation of abilities.

Benton Face Discrimination versus Line Orientation

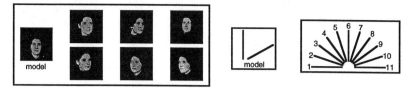

Same Williams syndrome subjects on contrasting spatial tasks.

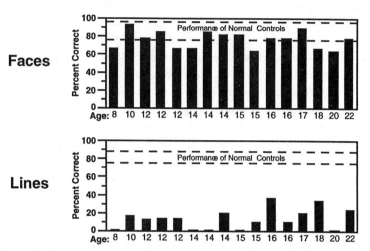

Note the contrast in performance on face discrimination and line orientation discrimination in the same Williams syndrome subjects.

Figure 5.3 Peaks and valleys of abilities in Williams syndrome.

Consider the contrast between two tasks: One is a task of judgment of line orientation, the other is a task of discrimination of unfamiliar faces (figure 5.3). On the line orientation task, all the Williams syndrome subjects were in the range considered *severely deficient* for adults; most of the Williams subjects could not even pass the pretest. However, exactly the same Williams subjects who could not pass the line orientation task demonstrated a pronounced ability to discriminate unfamiliar faces (Bellugi et al., 1992; Wang & Bellugi, 1993, 1994; Rossen et al., 1995a). In fact, across a range of face-processing tasks involving recognition, classification, and memory for faces, many Williams subjects perform in the normal range, despite their general cognitive impairment and in contrast to their depressed abilities in other spatial tasks.

We also examined performance of Williams adolescents on three paradigms involving distinct aspects of face processing: Benton Face Recognition (discrimination of unfamiliar faces), Warrington Recognition Memory for Faces (immediate recall of unfamiliar faces), and Mooney Face Classification (perception of faces from unclosed contours). Williams subjects performed

Bellugi et al.: Linking Cognition and Brain in Williams Syndrome significantly better than did age- and IQ-matched Down controls on all three measures. Moreover, the Williams subjects' results were indistinguishable from those of normal chronological age–matched subjects on the Benton faces task (Rossen et al., 1995a).

Hyperaffectivity

A prime characteristic of many Williams syndrome subjects is their strong impulse toward social contact and affective expression. We have been investigating the intersection of language and affect in Williams subjects through a series of narrative tasks (Reilly et al., 1990; Bellugi et al., 1995; Losh et al., 1997). Subjects are asked to tell a story from a wordless picture book, looking at the pictures as they progress through the book, with no framework provided beyond the pictures themselves. The story is about a multiple-episode search for a runaway pet frog. Not only was the spontaneous language displayed by Williams subjects phonologically and syntactically sophisticated but it was effective in using grammatical devices for narrative purposes (e.g., subordinate clauses to provide foreground and background information). The Williams syndrome (but not the Down syndrome) subjects characteristically provided well-structured narratives: establishing a clear orientation; introducing time of action, characters, and their states and behaviors ("Once upon a time, when it was dark at night"); stating the problem ("Next morning ... there was no frog to be found"); and including a resolution ("They find him [the runaway frog] with a lady").

The most telling distinction, however, between Williams, Down, and matched control subjects is in terms of narrative enrichment devices (figure 5.4). Language may be enriched emotionally through the use of affective prosody as well as through the use of lexically encoded affective devices.

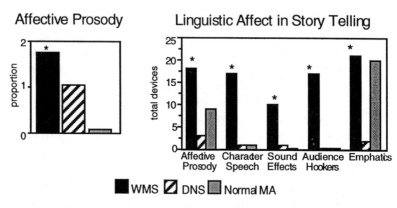

Note the high frequency of affective prosody and linguistic affective devices in Williams syndrome compared to Down syndrome and mental age matched normal subjects.

Figure 5.4 Abnormally high linguistic affect in Williams syndrome.

Affective prosody was tabulated by measuring the use of paralinguistic affective expression, including pitch change, vocalic lengthening, and modifications in volume. In their narrations, Williams subjects were found to use affective prosody far more frequently than did either Down matches or *normal* children of the same mental age. In fact, the Williams subjects continued to use high levels of affective prosody even on second and third retellings of the story. In this respect, their expressivity contrasts markedly with both normal child behavior and that of disordered populations, such as autistic subjects. We now have studies of 50 Williams syndrome children's narratives from 5 years of age through adulthood and can compare development of linguistically encoded affect (Losh et al., 1997; also unpublished manuscript). The affective richness of the Williams narratives is reflected consistently in lexical choices. Their use of exclamatory phrases and other audience-engagement devices is evident throughout many of the stories (e.g., "Suddenly splash! The water came up"; "Lo and behold"; "Gadzooks! The boy and the dog start flipping over"). These devices were far less frequent in normal subjects and were notably absent in the Down subjects' stories. We conclude that despite their cognitive impairments, subjects with Williams are not only sociable and affectively sensitive but show an abundance (or superabundance) of affectivity in both prosody and lexical devices and appear to be able to manipulate affective linguistic devices for the purposes of storytelling (Reilly et al., 1990, 1995; Harrison et al., 1995; Losh et al., 1997). This pattern is strikingly different from that of Down syndrome subjects and also from normal individuals at any age. Moreover, this pattern of abnormally high linguistically encoded affect may be in some ways the polar opposite to that of autistic individuals (Courchesne et al., 1995). Comparisons between individuals with Williams syndrome and those with autism are now beginning to emerge (Karmiloff-Smith et al., 1995; Tager-Flusberg, 1995).

Hyperacusis

One of the sensory characteristics of many individuals with Williams syndrome is an oversensitivity to certain classes of sounds, sometimes called *hyperacusis*. This has been reported consistently by researchers and parents of individuals with Williams syndrome and is prevalent in survey data. In Williams syndrome, this is evidenced as a discomfort or aversion to sounds not uncomfortable to most normal listeners; this reaction to such sounds occurs despite the absence of consistent peripheral auditory pathology (Klein et al., 1990; Marriage, 1995).

FRACTIONATION OF THE COGNITIVE PROFILE

Fractionation of the cognitive profile, a unique constellation of deficit and sparing, raises questions about how these different abilities interrelate, whether they depend on one another or can be dissociated, and whether apparently preserved abilities are subserved by an abnormal underlying organization.

Using correlations across individuals to examine the nature of variability within the syndrome, we in fact have found that the various cognitive abilities of Williams syndrome do not all stand or fall together. For example, though strong, significant intertask associations exist among the face-processing tasks, no significant intertask associations exist between the face-processing tasks and WISC-R IQ or between face processing and other visually based processing tasks, such as a non–faces closure task (Kaufman Assessment Buttery for Children Gestalt Closure), or between face processing and indices of language ability, such as comprehension of grammatical forms (Jones et al., 1995b; Rossen et al., 1995a,b; 1996).

Further, we have found distinct developmental trajectories across cognitive domains in studies involving more than 50 Williams syndrome subjects aged 3 to 23. Williams children, unlike those with Down syndrome, showed developmental trajectories in the cognitive domains of lexical knowledge, spatial cognition, and face processing that are dramatically different from one domain to another. As indicated in figure 5.5, the Down individuals showed essentially a uniform developmental trajectory across the three domains (i.e., uniformly depressed compared to normal). In contrast, the individuals with Williams syndrome showed three distinctly different trajectories (see figure 5.5). On a standardized test of lexical knowledge, the subjects with Williams syndrome began very low but showed a sharp increase with age. On a probe of spatial abilities (copying geometrical shapes), the subjects with Williams syndrome were consistently below the subjects with Down syndrome and plateaued early on. On a task of facial processing (Benton faces), the subjects with Williams syndrome tended to perform well even at a relatively early age (Jones et al., 1995b). Figure 5.5 also shows a significant group by test interaction, with chronological age entered as a covariate (Jones et al., unpublished manuscript).

THE NEUROBIOLOGICAL PROFILE OF WILLIAMS SYNDROME

In addition to the cognitive profile of Williams syndrome, we now are beginning to address the neurobiological profile, using ERPs, structural MRI, and brain cytoarchitectonics. In addition, we make some initial proposals about how these two profiles may be linked.

Neurophysiological Characteristics: Event-Related Potentials

We have undertaken a program of studies using ERP techniques to assess the timing and organization of the neural systems that are active during sensory, cognitive, and linguistic processing in Williams syndrome subjects (Hickok et al., 1995b; Neville et al., 1994, 1995; Mills et al., 1996, 1997). The power

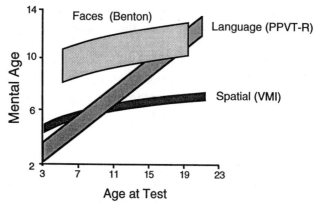

Williams Syndrome

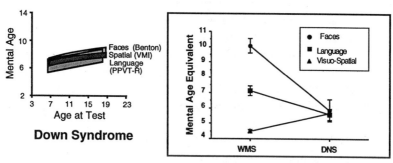

Down Syndrome

A 2 (WMS, DNS) X 3 (Benton, VMI, PPVT) analysis of covariance with chronological age entered as the covariate revealed a significant group X test interaction (p < .0001). (Jones, Rossen & Bellugi, 1995)

Figure 5.5 Contrasts between language, face, and space processing in Williams syndrome.

of this approach is that ERPs provide information about the timing and temporal sequence of neural events and the location of neural activity. Electrodes that detect changes in electrical activity are placed over specific brain areas while subjects are processing information, thus allowing monitoring of the time course of activation on a millisecond-to-millisecond basis. The activity thus recorded occurs well before subjects make an overt response, so this approach bypasses some of the limitations associated with behavioral measures, which may reflect and be influenced by several different, relatively late, response-related aspects of processing. Numerous studies have shown that the ERP technique may be used to index both sensory and cognitive processes and that it is sensitive to specific alterations in related brain systems.

For the studies described later, ERPs have been recorded from 10 subjects with Williams syndrome (in the range of 10–32 years) and have been compared with ERPs from larger samples of normal adults and school-aged children. The results so far suggest the following: (1) Certain ERP patterns are characteristic of all the subjects with Williams and not of the other groups and thus may lead to identification of potential specific electrophysiological markers of the disorder; and (2) the neural systems subserving such cognitive functions as language and face processing in Williams syndrome may be different from normal. Investigations are being carried out to see whether some of the ERP effects may be linked to individual differences in behavioral performance on these cognitive tasks (Mills et al., 1997).

Sensory Processing   Our previous studies have shown that hyperacusis in Williams subjects is not attributable to abnormalities in the peripheral auditory system (Neville et al., 1994). This study explored possible abnormalities in the Williams *cortical* auditory system. Using an *auditory recovery cycle* paradigm, a series of 50-msec tones was presented to the subjects through headphones. Each tone was preceded by a 200-msec, 1000-msec, or 2000-msec interstimulus interval. In normal adults, ERPs to tones display a negativity at approximately 100 msec (N100) followed by a positivity at 200 msec (P200). However, the amplitude of the N100 is markedly attenuated to rapidly presented stimuli. The adult subjects with Williams syndrome showed ERPs that are abnormal in two ways: First, the N100 does not show attenuation to rapidly presented stimuli and, second, the P200 is abnormally large (Neville et al., 1994). We suggest that the abnormal N100/P200 complex is an index of hyperexcitability of the primary auditory cortex. In contrast, auditory brainstem-evoked responses were normal in the Williams syndrome subjects, indicating that the auditory hyperexcitability does not occur at the brainstem level. Taken together, these results suggest that the "hyperacusis" observed in Williams syndrome may be mediated by hyperexcitability specifically within the cortical areas that are used for processing acoustic information.

Language Processing   To investigate on-line processing of grammatical and semantic information in sentences, one paradigm had subjects listen to or read sentences that ended in either a highly semantically probable way or an anomalous way (Neville et al., 1992). Half of the sentences ended with an anomalous last word and half with a word judged to be the best completion. The subject's task was to indicate whether the last word did or did not make sense with the rest of the sentence. In normal adults and children, the anomalous sentence endings elicit a negative component that peaks around 400 msec (N400) (Kutas & Hillyard, 1980). Grammatical and semantic aspects of language are reflected in different patterns of ERPs to open- and closed-class words in the middle of sentences (Neville et al., 1992).

The results from using this paradigm of brain behavior interaction with 10 Williams subjects revealed that the morphology of the ERPs to auditory words was different from that of normal controls (Neville et al., 1994, 1995).

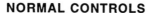

Left Hemisphere, Temporal, Open Class Words

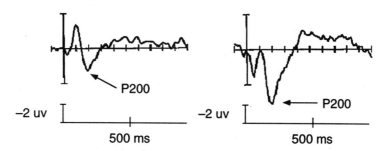

NORMAL CONTROLS   WILLIAMS SYNDROME

P200

−2 uv

500 ms

P200

−2 uv

500 ms

Note large positivity at 200 msec in WMS but not normal controls.

(Mills, Neville, & Bellugi, 1996)

Figure 5.6   Neurophysiological marker of language processing in Williams syndrome.

The Williams subjects showed a characteristic and prominent positivity at 200 msec (P200; figure 5.6). This pattern was characteristic of the subjects with Williams syndrome but was not evident in normal school-age children or in adults (Mills et al., 1996). This effect, apparent only over temporal brain regions, may relate to the Williams syndrome hyperacusis (see previous discussion). Moreover, the expected difference between open- and closed-class words was not evident, as found in normal controls, nor was the left-hemisphere asymmetry for closed-class words. Further, the effect of the semantic anomaly is larger in Williams than in controls and perhaps may be related to the unusual semantic proclivities shown by Williams syndrome subjects in certain tasks. Thus, these ERP differences to anomalous and appropriate sentence endings and to open- versus closed-class words suggest that not only the neural organization but the cognitive functional organization of these aspects of language may be different in Williams subjects as compared to those in controls, despite the apparent relative sparing of language abilities in Williams subjects (Neville et al., 1995).

Face Processing   Studies have shown that face processing is disproportionately spared in many Williams syndrome individuals (Rossen et al., 1995a, 1996; Bellugi et al., 1996b). We studied face processing while recording activity from the scalp in a new paradigm with 10 individuals with Williams syndrome, as compared with normals. Brain activity was recorded as subjects watched photographic pairs of upright or inverted faces presented sequentially on a computer monitor. The subject's task was to indicate whether the second face in the pair was that of the same person or of a person different from the one shown in the first photograph.

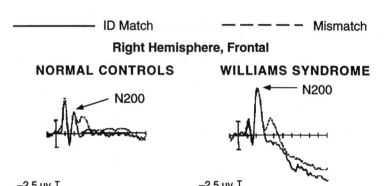

Figure 5.7 Neurophysiological marker of face processing in Williams syndrome.

Results from normal adults showed dramatic differences in the timing and distribution of ERP effects linked to recognition of upright versus inverted faces (Sarfaty et al., 1992; Alvarez & Neville, 1995; Alvarez et al., 1996). In normal adults, ERP differences to matched versus mismatched upright faces consisted of a negativity to the mismatched faces at approximately 320 msec (N320) after the onset of the second stimulus. This N320 effect was largest over anterior regions, specifically of the right hemisphere. In contrast, the mismatch-match effect for inverted faces consisted of a large positive component between 400 and 1000 msec (P500) that was largest over parietal regions and was symmetrical.

In contrast to normal adults, who showed markedly different ERP mismatch effects for upright versus inverted faces, the Williams adults showed an N320 mismatch effect for *both* upright and inverted faces. Moreover, the Williams subjects did not display the N320 right-hemisphere asymmetry observed in the normal adults. Importantly, the Williams subjects also displayed *an abnormally large negativity* at 200 msec (N200) to both upright and inverted faces (approximately four times the amplitude of the N200 component to faces in normal adults; figure 5.7). This abnormally large N200 was observed in all the adult subjects with Williams syndrome but was not observed in controls at any age. These results may be linked to increased attention to faces in subjects with Williams syndrome and appear to be specific to the disorder. Research by others suggests that the N200 may be specific to face processing (i.e., it has been elicited to both upright and inverted *faces* but not to other visual stimuli) in both surface potential recordings (Botzel & Grusser, 1989) and in in-depth recordings in epileptic patients (Allison et al., 1994). The in-depth recordings showed that the N200 was generated from the left and right fusiform and inferior temporal gyri. Both positron emission tomography and functional MRI studies have suggested that the fusiform gyrus is activated during processing of faces but not of other nonface visual stimuli (Haxby et al., 1993, 1996; Nobre et al., 1994). We suggest that the abnormally large negativity at 200 msec, which occurs in all the Williams subjects observed but not in the other groups, may be a brain activity marker linked to their spared face-processing abilities (Mills et al., 1996).

Conclusions

In the neurophysiological studies cited, we found that the Williams syndrome subjects did not display normal hemispheric asymmetry on language-related tasks; priming effects for semantically congruous words were larger than normal in Williams syndrome than in control subjects. Williams syndrome subjects also appear to display auditory hyperexcitability at the cortical level, not characteristic of other groups, and Williams syndrome subjects show an abnormally large N200 evident while they are processing faces. Such studies are providing neurophysiological indices that relate brain and behavior and, furthermore, may result in indices that are phenotypic markers for Williams syndrome (Mills et al., 1996).

NEUROANATOMICAL CHARACTERISTICS

Structural MRI

With the aim of investigating the neural systems that mediate language and cognition in Williams syndrome, we have been engaged also in neuroanatomical studies contrasting Williams and Down syndrome with normal controls (Jernigan et al., 1993; Jernigan & Bellugi, 1994; Jones et al., 1995b; Rossen et al., 1995b). Figure 5.8 shows aspects of the image analytical approach used initially; details are presented in Jernigan and Bellugi (1990, 1994). All analyses were conducted blind to any subject characteristics. Cerebral volumes were defined either manually (primarily the subcortical structures) or stereotaxically (relative to midline corpus callosum landmarks). The cortical gray matter within each hemisphere was parcellated stereotaxically into eight regions. Volumes were normalized by total supratentorial volume to correct for decreased overall brain size in subjects (Jernigan et al., 1993, 1995). The studies have progressed from a characterization of the overall gross morphological differences between the two syndromes to more specifically targeted morphological and physiological investigations underlying the uneven profile of Williams syndrome. Further, we are finding evidence that suggests relationships between regional brain volumes and specific behavioral abilities in Williams subjects.

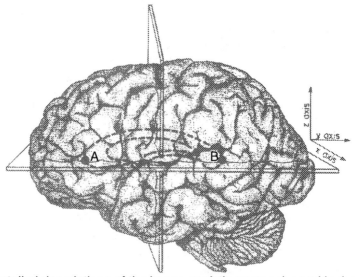

Detailed descriptions of the image-analytic approach used in the
present study are contained in several articles (Jernigan & Bellugi,
1990, 1994; Jernigan, Bellugi, Sowell, Doherty, & Hesselink, 1993).

Figure 5.8 Morphometric volume definition of the brain with magnetic resonance imaging.

Volumetric Findings Despite equivalent overall cerebral hypoplasia in
Williams and Down syndrome, in vivo studies of MRI neuromorphology
suggest other anomalies in the pattern of development (figure 5.9). Nine
subjects with Williams syndrome and 6 subjects with Down syndrome were
studied, all between 10 and 20 years of age, along with 21 normal controls
in the same age range. Proportional volumes were analyzed (i.e., regional
volumes expressed as a proportion of total gray-matter volume; see Jernigan
et al., 1993). Areas of proportional sparing occurred in Down syndrome; subcortical areas, including lenticular nuclei, were proportionally large in Down
syndrome subjects in contrast to those with Williams syndrome and to controls. The Williams frontal cortex appeared to acquire an essentially normal
volume relationship to the posterior cortex. By contrast, in Down syndrome,
the frontal cortex was disproportionately reduced in volume. Limbic structures of the temporal lobe (including uncus, amygdala, hippocampus, and
parahippocampal gyrus) appear proportionately spared in Williams subjects
relative to other cerebral structures, whereas in Down syndrome, such structures were reduced dramatically in volume. Additionally, cerebellar size was
entirely normal in the Williams subjects but were reduced dramatically in
Down subjects. Importantly, in Williams, though paleocerebellar vermal
lobules subtended a smaller area on midsagittal sections than in normals,
neocerebellar lobules were actually larger. In a separate study involving MRI
images from 11 Williams subjects, 7 Down subjects and 18 normal controls
(ages 10–20), neocerebellar tonsils were equal in volume to those of controls

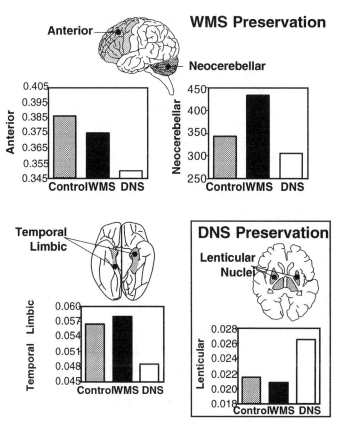

In vivo MRI studies of neuromorphology suggest an anomalous WMS brain-morphological profile consisting of a distinct regional pattern of proportional brain volume deficit and preservation (Bellugi, Klima & Wang, 1996).

Areas of relative preservation in WMS include the neocerebellum and the frontal cortex, the two areas that have undergone the most prominent enlargement in the human brain relative to the brain of primates. Such emerging evidence is consistent with a model where language functions are subserved by a fronto-cortical-neocerebellar system. There is also proportional preservation in the mesial temporal lobe, which in cooperation with certain areas of frontal cortex, is known to mediate important aspects of affective functioning (Bellugi, Wang & Jernigan, 1994).

Figure 5.9 Abnormal brain morphology in Williams and Down subjects.

and significantly larger than those of Down syndrome subjects. In proportion to the cerebrum, tonsils in Williams subjects were larger than in both these groups (Wang et al., 1992).

In a third study, quantitative volumetric analysis of Heschl's gyrus (which maps onto primary auditory cortex) was carried out bilaterally on MRI using Brainvox software (Damasio & Frank, 1992). The absolute volume of Heschl's gyrus in the Williams group did not differ from normal control subjects ($P = .58$) despite significant cerebral hypoplasia evident in the Williams group, whereas compared to a group of Down subjects matched for supratentorial volume, Heschl's gyrus was significantly larger in the Williams group ($P < .003$; figure 5.10). For a tighter control on individual and group differences in brain size, a ratio of primary auditory cortex to a consistently defined, more inclusive portion of the superior temporal gyrus that contains Heschl's gyrus also was calculated. Down and normal control subjects did not differ from one another, but this ratio in the Williams group was significantly *larger* than that of either of the Down and normal subject groups, indicating disproportionate development of Heschl's gyrus in Williams syndrome (Hickok et al., 1995a). A recent study has extended the finding of exaggerated development of Heschl's gyrus in Williams to another auditory area, the planum temporale. Measurements of the planum temporale bilaterally revealed no overall difference in surface area between Williams and normal controls, again despite significant cerebral hypoplasia in the Williams group (Hickok et al., 1995a), suggesting disproportionate growth of the entire posterior supratemporal region in Williams syndrome. The Williams syndrome group did, however, differ from the normal group in terms of the asymmetry of the planum in the left versus the right hemispheres, with the normal leftward asymmetry exaggerated in the Williams group (Hickok et al., 1995a,b). The functional significance of this exaggerated asymmetry is the topic of our current work.

Functional Significance of Volumetric Findings   The differences within cerebral and cerebellar structures previously described suggest that relatively intact linguistic and affective functions in Williams subjects may rely on relatively normal development of some limbic, frontal cortical, and cerebellar structures. Leiner et al., (1993) proposed that a cerebellofrontocortical system has evolved in humans to support the processing demands of fluent speech, pointing out that large increases in the sizes of these structures occur in humans as compared to those in apes (both in relative and absolute terms). Thus, the relative sparing of frontal and cerebellar structures in subjects with Williams syndrome may contribute to their relative linguistic competence. In support of this, a significant correlation was found in MRI data from nine Williams subjects between pooled performance on standardized language measures and a measure of volume of inferior frontal cerebrum normalized by total supratentorial volume. Other regions did not show significant correlations with language performance (Jones et al., 1995b). Further, the volu-

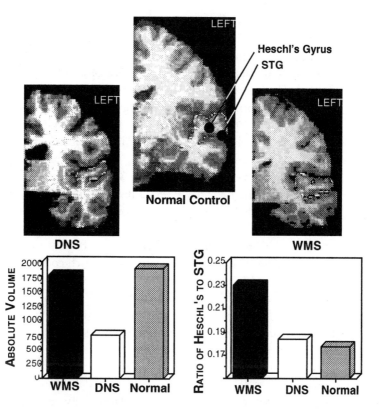

Absolute Volume of Heschl's: Despite equivalently reduced cerebral volume in WMS, absolute volume of A1 in the WMS group did not differ from NC subjects, but was significantly larger than that in DNS subjects (p < .003).

Ratio Volume (Heschl's / STG): A ratio of A1 to a consistently defined portion of the superior temporal gyrus that contains A1 was also calculated. This ratio in WMS subjects was significantly larger than that in both controls, indicating a larger A1 than expected given the volume of adjacent regions. (Hickok, Neville, Mills, Jones, Rossen, & Bellugi, 1995)

Figure 5.10 Abnormally large auditory areas in Williams syndrome individuals.

metric findings on Heschl's gyrus in Williams syndrome subjects relative to Down and normal controls are striking, given that the Williams subjects showed not only a normal volume for this region but, in proportion to surrounding areas, actually show an enlargement of this area (see figure 5.10). This volumetric finding in primary auditory cortex may be related either to hyperacusis or unusual auditory linguistic processing in Williams syndrome or both.

As reviewed, subjects with Williams syndrome are sociable and affectively sensitive, and they use affective linguistic devices at least as frequently as controls do, perhaps even excessively. The present finding of relative volumetric sparing of structures in the limbic system in Williams subjects is interesting in light of these observations. Perhaps a neurodevelopmental course favoring certain limbic structures over other cortical and subcortical structures results in relative prominence of affective strategies in communication. The normal symmetry observed in temporal limbic regions is further evidence of normal maturation and specialization in this system (Jernigan & Bellugi, 1990, 1994; Jernigan et al., 1993). The finding of disproportionately large neocerebellar structures in Williams subjects raises some interesting questions concerning the role of the neocerebellum in aspects of cognition. Neocerebellar vermal lobules VI to VII have been found to be reduced in autism (Courchesne et al., 1995), a disorder in which communication and affect are disordered severely, often involving limited language and extreme difficulty in social interactions, even when general cognition is spared. As noted, Williams syndrome contrasts diametrically with autism: Individuals with Williams syndrome frequently exhibit rich communicative and affective behaviors and frequently are described as excessively social, despite significant general cognitive impairment. Findings that the neocerebellar vermis is enlarged disproportionately in Williams subjects thus suggests an underlying neurobiological basis for Williams syndrome's social and affective characteristics.

Brain morphology also shows a link with face processing in Williams syndrome (Jones et al., 1995b). In vivo MRI data from nine Williams subjects (ages 10–20) revealed a strong correlation between performance on Benton faces and volume of gray matter in inferior posterior medial cortex, including hippocampus, posterior parahippocampal gyrus, and some retrosplenial cortex. Performance on the Warrington Recognition Memory for Faces and Mooney Face Classification also correlated strongly with these volumes. Regional brain volumes were normalized by total supratentorial volume. None of the other cortical regions measured showed significant correlations with these three face-processing measures (figure 5.11). These results are consistent with data from functional imaging (both position emission tomography and functional MRI) on brain areas important for face processing, which implicate these areas. These correlations suggest a neurological underpinning for both the unusual behavioral profile with respect to face processing and the distinctive neurophysiological marker we have described, which appears to be linked to increased attention to faces and to be localized within this brain region. Recall the abnormally large negativity at 200 msec that occurs in all Williams subjects observed when processing faces but not in other groups and not in Williams subjects when processing language or sensory stimuli (see figure 5.7), which may be a brain activity marker linked to spared face-processing abilities.

Particularly relevant to the contrasting brain-anatomical profiles of Williams and Down subjects are the functional distinctions between ventrally and dorsally lying cortical systems that have been described, particularly within the visual system. Form, color, and face-processing functions have been

Inferior Posterior Medial Cortical Gray (IPMCG) correlates strongly with performance across three face processing tasks:

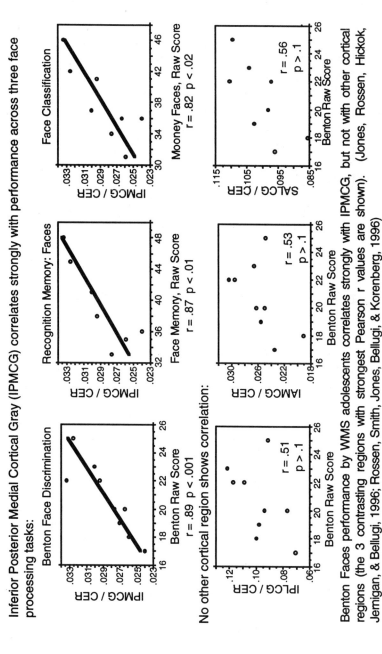

No other cortical region shows correlation:

Benton Faces performance by WMS adolescents correlates strongly with IPMCG, but not with other cortical regions (the 3 contrasting regions with strongest Pearson r values are shown). (Jones, Rossen, Hickok, Jernigan, & Bellugi, 1996; Rossen, Smith, Jones, Bellugi, & Korenberg, 1996)

Figure 5.11   Neuromorphological links to face processing in Williams syndrome.

associated with a ventral cortical system, with predominant input from the parvocellular pathway, whereas spatial integrative and motion-processing functions have been associated with dorsal structures in the temporoparietal junction (related to the magnocellular pathway). In some ways, the spared and impaired visuospatial functions in Williams subjects appear to respect these distinctions. Face processing is spared, whereas spatial integrative functions are impaired markedly. Perhaps cortical systems subserving the slower (but higher-resolution) processes associated with the parvocellular pathway are spared selectively in Williams syndrome, whereas in Down syndrome, both the pathways are affected.

Selective effects on the magnocellular system have been hypothesized to account for dyslexia, another developmental disorder. Ongoing studies with improved higher-resolution methods will permit examination of more specific neuroanatomical structures within these two contrasting syndromes of neurodevelopmental anomaly.

Brain Cytoarchitectonics in Williams Syndrome

Study of Williams syndrome focal cognitive deficits offers an opportunity to link brain findings with cognitive deficits also at the level of brain cytoarchitectonics. Four autopsy brains of individuals with Williams syndrome have been obtained (Galaburda et al., 1994, 1996, and unpublished observations).

Examination of the gross morphology of three of the specimens confirms a fundamentally normal proportional configuration, albeit microencephalic. In the fourth specimen, the parietal, posterior temporal, and occipital regions were markedly reduced in size by comparison to the more rostral portions of the hemispheres (figure 5.12A). The reduction was abrupt and dramatic, as if a band had constricted the posterior portions of the brain. This anomaly could not be explained by a fixation artifact. Remaining to be seen is whether a certain proportion of the Williams syndrome population exhibits this brain morphology characteristic. The curtailment of the dorsal parietal regions and posterior temporal areas may be relevant to the extreme visuospatial deficits in Williams.

Overall sulcal patterns in the four specimens were normal, except for some simplification of tertiary sulcation and a consistently nonopercularized dorsal central sulcus. Normally, the central sulci reach all the way to the interhemispheric fissure and then proceed a short distance farther onto the medial surfaces of the hemispheres. In all the available cases, the central sulcus ended no less than a centimeter lateral to the interhemispheric fissure (figure 5.13). This may indicate abnormal development of the mediodorsal cortices, which have been associated with visuospatial functions.

One specimen has been examined in whole-brain serial histological sections to assess for histopathological and architectonic characteristics. This case showed a large collection of small gliotic intracortical scars affecting

12a.

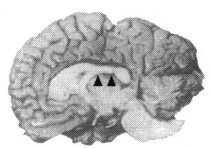

Medial surface of the right hemisphere of an adult Williams syndrome brain showing narrowing of the corpus callosum anterior to the splenium (arrowheads). Note the curtailment of the forebrain posterior to the rolandic sulcus.

12b.

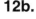
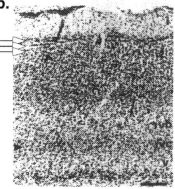
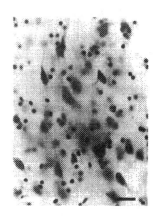

Photomicrograph of the primary visual cortex (Brodmann 17) in WMS. The cortex shows in-creased cell packing density and disordered layering with horizontal, rippled disposition of layers II and III (arrows). Cortical dysplasias appear more severe in the posterior cortical areas.

High-power photo-micro-graph of the subcortical white matter showing a large collection of hetero-topic neurons among oligodendroglial nuclei.

Note increased cell packing density in upper layers.

(Galaburda, Wang, Bellugi, & Rossen, 1994)

Figure 5.12 Brain cytoarchitectonic findings in Williams syndrome.

mainly the dorsal portions of the hemispheres, both rostrally and caudally. None of the lesions are thought to be less than 6 months old, and any or all could have been present since childhood. Stains for myelin did not disclose myelinated scars. Therefore, no hard evidence corroborates that the lesions were present from the time of birth. The dorsal location of the scars is compatible with the visuospatial deficits observed behaviorally. Again, remaining to be seen is whether this finding generalizes across subjects. If so, it may constitute an additional link between neural and cognitive profiles.

The recent finding that Williams syndrome is associated with a hemizygous deletion, including the elastin locus (at chromosome 7q11.23) and contiguous genes (Bellugi & Morris, 1995; Frangiskakis et al., 1996; Korenberg et al., 1996), suggests that some aspects of the brain symptomatology

Bellugi et al.: Linking Cognition and Brain in Williams Syndrome

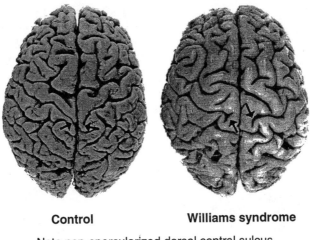

Control　　　　**Williams syndrome**

Note non-opercularized dorsal central sulcus.

Figure 5.13 Unusual sulcal patterns in Williams syndrome brain.

of Williams may be related to abnormal expression of elastin, laminin B1, and acetyl cholinesterase.

Cytoarchitectonic areas appear well developed in the blocks of Williams cerebral cortex that have been examined. All main cytoarchitectonic divisions are identified. However, an increase in cell-packing density of neurons seem apparent, without decrease in cortical thickness, suggesting an overall increase in neuronal numbers. Also, overall increase is seen in cellularity in the glial lines; figure 12B shows the heterotopic neurons and the exaggerated horizontal organization of neurons in area 17. Less common are areas of clustering of neurons and neuron-free areas without gliosis. The observed cell numbers and cell-packing densities suggest early developmental arrest (e.g., prenatally or before the second year) or regressive events occurring postnatally into the middle of the first decade of life (Galaburda et al., 1994, 1996, and unpublished observations).

Taken together, these results suggest that anomalies of brain morphology and microstructure may relate to the extreme visuospatial deficit in Williams syndrome subjects. In general, these findings provide unusual opportunities for linking brain findings to cognitive deficits and their neural underpinnings.

NEW PERSPECTIVES ON BRAIN-BEHAVIOR LINKS IN GENETICALLY BASED SYNDROMES

The original investigations of Williams subjects suggested links related to lateralization of function: the preserved language and the specific visuospatial deficit resembled the profile of right-hemisphere-damaged populations. However, other dominant aspects of the Williams profile have since emerged, including exceptional face processing and preserved linguistic affect, which do not fit with the right hemisphere–damaged profile or with an explanation based on a lateralized model of cognitive functioning in general. Moreover, recent collaborative studies of brain function and brain structure are suggesting new models for understanding the brain bases of the Williams cognitive profile.

First, neurophysiological studies are suggesting that the remarkably well-developed language system characteristic of Williams syndrome may not be lateralized to the left hemisphere as it is in normal populations. Second, in vivo MRI studies of neuromorphology suggest an anomalous Williams brain-morphological profile consisting of distinct regional patterns of proportional deficit and preservation in brain volume. This occurs despite an overall reduction of cerebral volume equivalent to that of the Down syndrome population.

Interestingly, areas of relative preservation in Williams subjects include the neocerebellum and frontal cortex, the two areas that have undergone the most prominent enlargement in the human brain relative to the brain of primates. Such emerging evidence is consistent with a model wherein language functions are subserved by a fronto-cortico-neocerebellar system. The Williams population also shows proportional preservation in mesial temporal lobe, which, in cooperation with certain areas of frontal cortex, is known to mediate important aspects of affective functioning (Jernigan & Bellugi, 1994; Bellugi et al., 1996b). These are some examples of how links across levels may lead to important new information regarding how distributed neural systems may underlie distinct domains of cognitive functioning.

ACKNOWLEDGMENTS

This research was supported in part by grants from the National Institutes of Health (HD26022, HD33113, NS22343, DC01289) and the Oak Tree Philanthropic Foundation. We thank the national and regional Williams Syndrome Associations, the Canadian Association for Williams Syndrome, and the Parents of Down Syndrome Association. We also thank Dr. Margaret Wilson for her helpful comments on the manuscript. We are grateful to the subjects and their families for their participation in these studies. Illustrations copyright Dr. Ursula Bellugi, The Salk Institute for Biological Studies, La Jolla, California.

REFERENCES

Allison, T., McCarthy, G., Nobre, A., Puce, A., & Belger, A. (1994). Human extrastriate visual cortex and the perception of faces, words, numbers, and colors. *Cerebral Cortex, 4*(5), 544–54.

Alvarez, I., Alvarez, P., & Neville, H. (1996). Hemispheric asymmetries to faces presented in the left and right visual fields—an ERP study. *Society for Neuroscience Abstracts, 22,* 1854.

Alvarez, T., & Neville, H. (1995). The development of face discrimination continues into adulthood: An ERP study. *Society for Neuroscience Abstracts, 21,* 2086.

Bellugi, U., Bihrle, A., Jernigan, T., Trauner, D., & Doherty, S. (1990). Neuropsychological, neurological, and neuroanatomical profile of Williams syndrome. *American Journal of Medical Genetics, 6,* 115–125.

Bellugi, U., Bihrle, A., Neville, H., Jernigan, T., & Doherty, S., (1992). Language, cognition, and brain organization in a neurodevelopmental disorder. In M. Gunnar & C. Nelson (Eds.), *Developmental behavioral neuroscience* (pp. 201–232). Hillsdale, NJ: Erlbaum.

Bellugi, U., Hickok, G., Jones, W., & Jernigan, T. (1996a July). *The neurobiological basis of Williams syndrome: Linking brain and behavior.* Presented at the Williams Syndrome Association Professional Conference, King of Prussia, PA.

Bellugi, U., Jones, W., Harrison, D., Rossen, M. L., & Klima, E. S. (1995 March). Discourse in two genetically based syndromes with contrasting brain anomalies. *Paper Presented at the Society for Research in Child Development,* Meeting, Indianapolis, IN.

Bellugi, U., Klima, E. S., & Wang, P. P. (1996b). Cognitive and neural development: Clues from genetically based syndromes. In D. Magnussen (Ed.), *The life-span development of individuals: Behavioral, neurobiological, and psychosocial perspectives. The Nobel Symposium* (pp. 223–243). New York: Cambridge University Press.

Bellugi, U., & Morris, C. A. (Eds.). (1995). Williams syndrome: From cognition to gene. Abstracts from the Williams Syndrome Association Professional Conference [special issue]. *Genetic Counseling, 6*(1), 131–192.

Bellugi, U., & Wang, P. P. (1998). Williams syndrome: From cognition to brain to gene. In G. Edelman & B. H. Smith (Eds.), *Encyclopedia of Neuroscience.* Amsterdam, The Netherlands: Elsevier Science.

Bellugi, U., Wang, P., & Jernigan, T. L. (1994). Williams syndrome: An unusual neuropsychological profile. In S. Broman & J. Grafman (Eds.), *Atypical cognitive deficits in developmental disorders: Implications for brain function* (pp. 23–56). Hillsdale, NJ: Erlbaum.

Beret, N., Bellugi, U., Hickok, G., & Stiles, J. (1996 July). *Integrative spatial deficits in children with Williams syndrome and children with focal brain lesions: A comparison.* Presented at the Williams Syndrome Association Professional Conference, King of Prussia, PA.

Bihrle, A. M. (1990). *Visuospatial processing in Williams and Down syndrome.* Unpublished doctoral dissertation, University of California at San Diego and San Diego State University, CA.

Bihrle, A. M., Bellugi, U., Delis, D., & Marks, S. (1989). Seeing either the forest or the trees: Dissociation in visuospatial processing. *Brain and Cognition, 11,* 37–49.

Botzel, K., & Grusser, O. J. (1989). Electric brain potentials evoked by pictures of faces and nonfaces: A search for face-specific EEG-potentials. *Experimental Brain Research, 77,* 349–360.

Courchesne, E., Bellugi, U., & Singer, N. (1995). Infantile autism and Williams syndrome: Social and neural worlds apart [abstract, special issue]. *Genetic Counseling, 6*(1), 144–145.

Damasio, A. & Frank, J. (1992). Three-dimensional *in vivo* mapping of brain lesions in humans. *Archives of Neurology, 49,* 137–143.

Frangiskakis, J. M., Ewart, A. K., Morris, C. A., Mervis, C. B., Bertrand, J., Robinson, B. F., Klein, B. P., Ensing, G. J., Everett, L. A., Green, E. D., et al. (1996). LIM-kinase1 hemizygosity implicated in imparied visuospatial constructive cognition. *Cell, 86*(1), 59–69.

Galaburda, A. M., Garcia, L. S., & Bellugi, U. (1996). Elastin expression in Williams syndrome cerebellar Purkinje cells. Poster presentation at Williams Syndrome Association Professional Conference, King of Prussia, PA.

Galaburda, A. M., Wang, P. P., Bellugi, U., & Rossen, M. (1994). Cytoarchitectonic findings in a genetically based disorder: Williams syndrome. *Neuroreport, 5,* 758–787.

Harrison, D., Reilly, J., & Klima, E. S. (1995). Unusual social behavior in Williams syndrome: Evidence from biographical interviews [abstract, special issue]. *Genetic Counseling, 6*(1), 181–183.

Haxby, J., Grady, C., Horwitz, B., Salerno, J., Ungerleider, L., Mishkin, M., & Shapiro, M. (1993). Dissociation of object and spatial visual processing pathways in human extrastriate cortex. In B. Gulyas, D. Ottoson, & P. E. Roland (Eds.), *Functional organization of the human visual cortex* (pp. 329–340). Oxford: Pergamon.

Haxby, J. V., Ungerleider, L. G., Horwitz, B., Maisog, J. M., Rapoport, S. I., Grady, C. L. (1996). Face encoding and recognition in the human brain. *Proceedings of the National Academy of Sciences, 93*, 922–927.

Hickok, G., Bellugi, U., & Jones, W. (1995a). Asymmetrical abilities [letter]. *Science, 270*(5234), 219–220.

Hickok, G., Neville, H., Mills, D., Jones, W., Rossen, M., & Bellugi, U. (1995b). Electrophysiological and quantitative MR analysis of the cortical auditory system in Williams syndrome. *Cognitive Neuroscience Society Abstracts, 2*, 66.

Jernigan, T., & Bellugi, U. (1990). Anomalous brain morphology on magnetic resonance images in Williams syndrome and Down syndrome. *Archives of Neurology, 47*, 529–533.

Jernigan, T. L. & Bellugi, U. (1994). Neuroanatomical distinctions between Williams and Down syndromes. In S. Broman & J. Grafman (Eds.), *Atypical cognitive deficits in developmental disorders: Implications for brain function* (pp. 57–66). Hillsdale, NJ: Erlbaum.

Jernigan, T. L., Bellugi, U., Sowell, E., Doherty, S., & Hesselink, J. R. (1993). Cerebral morphological distinctions between Williams and Down syndromes. *Archives of Neurology, 50*, 186–191.

Jernigan, T. L., Wang, P. P., & Bellugi, U. (1995). Neuromorphological characteristics of Williams syndrome [abstract, special issue]. *Genetic Counseling, 6*(1), 145–146.

Jones, W., Rossen, M. L., & Bellugi, U. (1995a). Distinct developmental trajectories of cognition in Williams syndrome [abstract, special issue]. *Genetic Counseling, 6*(1), 178–179.

Jones, W., Rossen, M., Hickok, G., Jernigan, T., & Bellugi, U. (1995b). Links between behavior and brain: Brain morphological correlates of language, face, and auditory processing in Williams syndrome. *Society for Neuroscience Abstracts, 21*(3).

Karmiloff-Smith, A., Klima, E.S., Bellugi, U., Grant, J., & Baron-Cohen, S. (1995). Is there a social module? Language, face processing, and theory-of-mind in subjects with Williams syndrome. *Journal of Cognitive Neuroscience, 7*(2), 196–208.

Klein, A. J., Armstrong, B. L., Greer, M. K., & Brown, F. R. (1990). Hyperacusis and otitis media in individuals with Williams syndrome. *Journal of Speech and Hearing Disorders, 55*(2), 339–344.

Korenberg, J. R., Chen, X-N., Mitchell, S., Sun, Z., Hubert, R., Vataru, E. S., & Bellugi, U. (1996 October). The genomic organization of Williams syndrome. Paper presented at the American Society for Human Genetics, San Francisco, CA.

Kutas, M., & Hillyard, S. (1980). Reading senseless sentences: Brain potentials reflect semantic incongruity. *Science, 207*, 203–205.

Leiner, H. C., Leiner, A. L., & Dow, R. S. (1993). Cognitive and language functions of the human cerebellum. *Trends in Neurosciences, 16*(11), 444–447.

Losh, M., Reilly, J., Bellugi, U., Cassady, C., & Klima, E.S. (1997 October). Linguistically encoded affect is abnormally high in Williams syndrome children. Poster presented at the International Behavioral Neuroscience Society Meeting, San Diego, CA.

Marriage, J. (1995). Central hyperacusis in Williams syndrome [abstract, special issue]. *Genetic Counseling, 6*(1), 152–153.

Mills, D. L., Neville, H. J., & Bellugi, U. (1996). Cerebral organization for spared cognitive functions in adults with Williams syndrome. Presented at the Williams Syndrome Association Professional Conference, King of Prussia, PA.

Mills, D., Neville, H., Appelbaum, G., Prat, C., & Bellugi, U. (1997 October). Electrophysiological markers of Williams syndrome. Poster presented at the International Behavioral Neuroscience Society Meeting, San Diego, CA.

Neville, H., Mills, D., & Bellugi, U. (1995). Functional brain organization in Williams syndrome [abstract, special issue]. *Genetic Counseling, 6*(1), 141–142.

Neville, H., Mills, D., & Lawson, D. (1992). Fractionating language: Different neural subsystems with different sensitive periods. *Cerebral Cortex, 2*, 244–258.

Neville, H., Mills, D. L., & Bellugi, U. (1994). Effects of altered auditory sensitivity and age of language acquistion on the development of language-relevant neural systems: Preliminary studies of Williams syndrome. In S. Broman & J. Grafman (Eds.), *Atypical cognitive deficits in developmental disorders: Implications for brain function* (pp. 67–83). Hillsdale, NJ: Erlbaum.

Nobre, A. C., Allison, T., & McCarthy, G. (1994). Word recognition in the human inferior temporal lobe. *Nature, 372*(6503), 260–263.

Reilly, J. S., Harrison, D., & Klima, E. S. (1995). Emotional talk and talk about emotions [abstract, special issue]. *Genetic Counseling, 6*(1), 158–159.

Reilly, J. S., Klima, E. S., & Bellugi, U. (1990). Once more with feeling: Affect and language in atypical populations. *Development and Psychopathology, 2*, 367–391.

Rossen, M. L., Jones, W., Wang, P. P., & Klima, E. S. (1995a). Face processing: Remarkable sparing in Williams syndrome [abstract, special issue]. *Genetic Counseling, 6*(1), 138–140.

Rossen, M. L., Klima, E. S., Bellugi, U., Bihrle, A., & Jones, W. (1996). Interaction between language and cognition: Evidence from Williams syndrome. In J. H. Beitchman, N. Cohen, M. Konstantareas, & R. Tannock (Eds.), *Language, learning, and behavior disorders: Developmental, biological, and clinical perspectives* (pp. 367–392). New York: Cambridge University Press.

Rossen, M. L., Smith, D., Jones, W., Bellugi, U. & Korenberg, J. (1995b). Spared face processing in Williams syndrome: New perspectives on brain-behavior links in a genetically based syndrome. *Society for Neuroscience Abstracts, 21*(3), 1926.

Sarfaty, T. D., Mills, D. L., Knaudt, P., & Neville, H. J. (1992). Configural and featural processing of faces: ERP and behavioral evidence. *Society for Neuroscience Abstracts, 18*(1), 336.

Tager-Flusberg, H. (1995 March). Language development and the acquisition of a theory of mind: Evidence from autism and Williams syndrome. Paper presented at the Society for Research in Child Development, Meeting, Indianapolis, IN.

Vicari, S., Brizzolara, D., Carlesimo, G. A., Pezzini, G., & Volterra, V. (1996). Memory abilities in children with Williams syndrome. *Cortex, 32*(3), 503–514.

Wang, P. P., & Bellugi, U. (1993). Williams syndrome, Down syndrome and cognitive neuroscience [special contribution]. *American Journal of Diseases of Children, 147*, 1246–1251.

Wang, P. P., & Bellugi, U. (1994). Evidence from two genetic syndromes for a dissociation between verbal and visual-spatial short-term memory. *Journal of Clinical and Experimental Neuropsychology, 16*(2), 317–322.

Wang, P. P., Hesselink, J. R., Jernigan, T. L., Doherty, S., & Bellugi, U. (1992). Specific neurobehavioral profile of Williams syndrome is associated with neocerebellar hemispheric preservation. *Neurology, 42*, 1999–2002.

6 Prader-Willi Syndrome: Toward a Behavioral Phenotype

Elisabeth M. Dykens

CASE VIGNETTE

Mark's mother sighed as she bent to clean under her son's bed. The papers and carefully arranged stacks of old *TV Guides* no longer bothered her, but the candy bar wrappers and soda cans gave her a familiar jolt of apprehension and anger. *How on earth did he get it this time? We watch him constantly, we lock everything, and still he finds a way.*

She sat on the bed and thought again of her son: A handsome boy with a winning smile, a source of both wonder and worry ... always so determined, even as a tiny baby, so floppy but trying so hard to suck, finally gaining weight, but then slow to walk, talk, and learn. Ironic, but now he almost talks too much and is too determined. He's stubborn to the core ... and with a quick temper when things don't go according to plan. Everything always has to be just so with him. Still, that stubbornness was the thing that got him up on a horse last year. That horse was big, even though Mark's so short and carries that extra weight; he just marched right up to that horse and climbed up on him, then grinned ear to ear. He's full of surprises, that's for sure.

First identified more than 40 years ago (Prader et al., 1956), today Prader-Willi syndrome is recognized by most people because of its extraordinary food-related characteristics. As suggested in the case vignette, people with Prader-Willi syndrome have hyperphagia (overeating) and unremitting food-seeking behaviors. Hyperphagia is believed to be due to altered function of the hypothalamus, although the exact anomaly remains unknown (Swaab et al., 1995). People with Prader-Willi syndrome do not have normal feelings of satiety or fullness, and they also have reduced metabolic rates (Holland et al., 1995). These features lead to overeating and to high risks of obesity.

Though many persons with the syndrome often are well-informed about their need to diet, these same individuals may steal food, forage through the garbage, and eat unpalatable items. Without persistent dietary supervision, Prader-Willi syndrome is a life-threatening condition. Even today, complications of obesity are the major causes of morbidity and mortality in this disorder, which otherwise is associated with general good health (Hanchett et al., in press).

Thus, with good reason, food and dietary management long have been major worries in Prader-Willi syndrome. Yet, as the case vignette points out,

Prader-Willi syndrome features many other areas of concern, both physical and behavioral. Physically, babies with Prader-Willi syndrome show central hypotonia that improves with age, a weak cry, and a poor sucking reflex that typically results in a need for gavage or other special feeding techniques (Aughton & Cassidy, 1990). Babies often thus "fail to thrive" for a period of weeks to months. Milestones are delayed, with sitting accomplished at perhaps 12 months and walking at 24 months. Hyperphagia typically has its onset between 2 to 6 years of age. Other physical features evolve over the course of development and include characteristic facial features; short stature; small hands and feet; hypogonadism; sleep disturbance; thick, viscous saliva; decreased vomiting; and temperature control problems (Holm et al., 1993).

As discussed in chapter 7, the genetic cause of Prader-Willi syndrome was not recognized until 1981. Since that time, remarkable progress has been made in the genetic understanding of this syndrome. Briefly, most cases of Prader-Willi syndrome (perhaps 70%) are caused by a deletion on chromosome 15 [del15(q11–13)] that is derived from the father (Ledbetter et al., 1981). The majority of the remaining 30% of cases are caused by maternal uniparental disomy of chromosome 15, in which both members of the chromosome 15 pair come from the mother (Nicholls et al., 1989). Either case demonstrates absence of the active paternal contribution to this region of the genome.

When a similar deletion occurs in the maternally derived chromosome 15 (or when two chromosomes 15 come from the father), an entirely different developmental disorder results (called *Angelman syndrome*). This occurs because different genes are expressed differently, depending on whether they come from the mother or the father, a process known as *genetic imprinting* (Nicholls, 1993). Prader-Willi and Angelman syndromes are the first known human diseases associated with genetic imprinting.

Prader-Willi syndrome thus features dramatic genetic breakthroughs, distinctive physical features, and salient food-related characteristics. Relative to the advances in understanding the genetic etiology of Prader-Willi syndrome, we know surprisingly little about the cognitive or behavioral manifestations of this syndrome. Further, data about Prader-Willi syndrome's behavioral phenotype are scarce relative to other genetic, mental retardation syndromes, such as Down syndrome or fragile X syndrome. To show this, we surveyed behavioral articles published between 1985 and 1995 in seven leading journals representing the fields of mental retardation, child psychiatry, and medical genetics. Of the 254 behavioral articles, 37% were devoted to Down syndrome, 35% to fragile X syndrome, and just 6% to Prader-Willi syndrome (Hodapp & Dykens, 1994; Dykens, 1996).

In this chapter, we review research to data regarding cognition and behavior in persons with Prader-Willi syndrome. Ranges and profiles of cognition and behavior are summarized, as are data on the developmental trajectories of these features. Maladaptive behaviors and psychiatric vulnerabilities also are discussed, including the specificity of these problems to Prader-Willi syndrome. Finally, recommendations are made for future research that both expands and specifies the Prader-Willi behavioral phenotype.

COGNITION

Cognitive Range and Profiles

Although the range of IQ in Prader-Willi syndrome has been well described over the years, researchers only recently have begun to examine other aspects of cognition in this syndrome. These include profiles of cognitive strength and weakness and relations among intelligence and age, degree of obesity, and behavioral problems.

The range of intelligence in persons with Prader-Willi syndrome tends to be high relative to persons with other genetic mental retardation syndromes, such as fragile X syndrome or Down syndrome. The average IQ reported in most studies is near 70 (e.g., Dykens et al., 1992a). Extrapolating IQ data from 575 subjects in 57 published studies, Curfs (1992) found that 34% showed mild mental retardation, 27% had moderate delays, and only 6% showed severe to profound levels of impairment. Notably, 32% were high-functioning, with IQs above 70; 27% showed borderline levels of intelligence (IQ 70–84), and 5% showed average IQ scores. Adaptively, however, even high-functioning individuals rarely function at a level commensurate with their IQs, owing to interference from food-related and other behavioral problems.

Regarding profiles of cognition, early clinical observations suggested that many children with Prader-Willi syndrome showed significant relative strengths in reading and weaknesses in arithmetic (e.g., Holm, 1981; Sulzbacher et al., 1981). These informal observations led to the idea that cognition in Prader-Willi syndrome was best characterized by uneven academic performance, as found in youngsters with learning disabilities. Yet achievement studies do not provide overwhelming support for a learning disability profile. Administering the Kaufman Assessment Battery for Children (KABC; Kaufman & Kaufman, 1984) to 21 adolescents and adults with Prader-Willi syndrome, Dykens et al., (1992a) found a nonsignificant discrepancy in age-equivalent scores in arithmetic versus reading (7.68 years versus 8.55 years, respectively). Further, Taylor (1988) examined an unspecified number of individuals with Prader-Willi syndrome and reported a mean standard achievement test score of 70 in mathematics and 73 in reading. Such findings only hint at uneven academic performance. Future studies must identify to what extent individuals with Prader-Willi syndrome show discrepancies across areas of academic achievement and between achievement and IQ.

Only a handful of studies have moved beyond academic achievement to identify other aspects of cognitive processing in Prader-Willi syndrome. Examining global cognitive patterns with Wechsler-based tests, Borghgraef et al., (1990) reported "great differences" in verbal versus performance IQ

Table 6.1 Summary of cognitive processing studies in people with Prader-Willi syndrome

Study	Tests Administered	Number and Age of Subjects	Salient Findings
Curfs et al., 1991	WISC-R	26 PWS, 7–15 yr	Performance IQ > verbal IQ in 10 subjects; verbal IQ > performance IQ in 3 subjects; block design high in 9 subjects
Dykens et al., 1992a	KABC WISC-R or Stanford-Binet	21 PWS, 13–26 yr 31 PWS, 5–30 yr	Simultaneous > sequential processing strengths: visual-perceptual; weaknesses: visual, motor short-term memory; stable IQ in childhood and adulthood
Gabel et al., 1986	Battery, including Detroit Tests of Learning Aptitude	15 PWS, $M = 12$ yr 15 normal controls	Normals exceeded PWS on all measures For PWS on Detroit, visual recall of objects, letters > auditory recall of words
Taylor, 1988	WISC-R	Unspecified PWS, obese, retarded controls	PWS > controls on block design only
Warren & Hunt, 1981	Pictorial memory tasks	11 PWS, $M = 10.1$ yr, 12 nonspecific matched on age and IQ	PWS < nonspecific in visual short-term memory; PWS had no improvements in performance with increasing age or IQ; PWS on par with nonspecific in long-term memory for well-known information

WISC-R, Wechsler Intelligence Scale for Children–Revised; PWS, Prader-Willi syndrome; KABC, Kaufman Assessment Battery for Children; M, median.

scores in 8 of their 12 subjects with Prader-Willi syndrome. Three of these individuals showed at least a 15-point discrepancy in favor of the verbal IQ. Significant verbal versus performance IQ differences also were found in a study of 26 children with Prader-Willi syndrome (aged 7–15 years), with 10 subjects showing elevations in the performance IQ and 3 in the verbal IQ (Curfs et al., 1991). Findings thus are inconsistent, with perhaps a slight favoring of the performance IQ.

More fine-tuned studies of specific cognitive processes shed some light on these inconsistent findings. Table 6.1 summarizes these studies. Taylor (1988) compared Wechsler subtests in an unspecified number of subjects with Prader-Willi syndrome to a sample of obese, mentally retarded individuals without Prader-Willi syndrome. The two groups showed comparable subtest scores, with just one exception: Relative to the obese controls, subjects with Prader-Willi syndrome showed significantly higher scores on block design, a task tapping visuomotor integration. Similarly, Curfs et al. (1991) found that one-half of their sample showed significant Wechsler Intelligence Scale for Children–Revised subtest scatter, and that 9 of these 13 children had relative strengths in block design. These findings suggest strengths in some individuals in perceptual-spatial organization and visuomotor integration. Consistent with these strengths, some people show an unusual facility with jigsaw puzzles; this skill is noted as a minor finding in the diagnostic criteria for Prader-Willi syndrome (Holm et al., 1993).

Visual processing strengths also are suggested by Gabel et al. (1986), who administered a battery of attentional, visuospatial, and psychomotor tasks to 15 children with Prader-Willi syndrome and 15 age- and gender-matched normal children. Not surprisingly, the Prader-Willi group scored consistently lower than did normal controls, yet they also showed discrepancies in scores on subtests of the Detroit Tests of Learning Aptitude (Baker & Leland, 1967). Prader-Willi subjects had relatively low scores on tasks assessing auditory attention and recall for words and had high scores on tasks measuring visual attention and recall for objects and letters. Gabel et al. (1986) concluded that youngsters with Prader-Willi syndrome may have strengths in visual processing relative to auditory processing.

Further work clarifies and expands certain aspects of the apparent visual processing strength. Administering the KABC to 21 subjects, Dykens et al. (1992a) found that simultaneous processing was better developed than was sequential processing. High scores were noted in tasks assessing perceptual closure, long-term memory, spatial organization, attention to visual detail, and visuomotor integration. Among the sequential processing tasks, which rely on short-term memory, subjects showed particular difficulties with visuomotor and auditory-visual short-term memory. Thus, for some individuals with Prader-Willi syndrome, a profile of relative strengths in perceptual organization and difficulties in visual and other short-term memory tasks is suggested.

Indeed, visual-processing strengths may not always be readily apparent, especially in short-term memory tasks. In a series of studies assessing pictorial short-term memory, Warren and Hunt (1981) compared 11 children with Prader-Willi syndrome to age- and IQ-matched mentally retarded children with nonspecific etiologies. Relative to their mentally retarded counterparts, children with Prader-Willi syndrome showed more difficulties with immediate visual memory, no improvements in recall of stimuli with either increasing mental or chronological age, and a greater loss of information over time. In contrast to their performance on short-term memory deficits, Prader-Willi children performed on par with the nonspecific group in a long-term memory task assessing how quickly subjects recalled well-known information. Interestingly, parents often report that their offspring with Prader-Willi syndrome can recall well-known or more obscure facts with a remarkable level of detail (e.g., where people parked as they arrived for a family party years ago). As suggested by findings by Warren and Hunt (1981), however, this type of recall is not likely to prove unique to Prader-Willi syndrome.

In summary, some individuals with Prader-Willi syndrome show relative strengths in spatial-perceptual organization and visual processing. Further, relative weaknesses may be apparent in short-term memory, including visual, motoric, and auditory short-term processing. Although findings suggest a profile, several warnings are in order. Not all persons with Prader-Willi syndrome show this profile, and studies are needed to identify the range of cognitive variability and possible sources of individual differences in cognitive patterns. Further, cognitive profiles identified to date in Prader-Willi syndrome may be shared among people with other genetic syndromes or with nonspecific etiologies. Prader-Willi cognitive findings do not seem as distinctive or striking as do profiles in other genetic conditions, such as Williams syndrome (see chapters 4 and 5), or Down syndrome (Hodapp, 1996). Additional comparative studies thus are necessary to settle the question of whether Prader-Willi syndrome is associated with a unique or even distinctive profile of cognitive or academic strength or weakness.

Additional research is needed also regarding the language of people with Prader-Willi syndrome. Although only two studies have examined this issue, neither one finds a distinctive linguistic profile. Branson (1981) found no common features in the language profiles of 21 children with Prader-Willi syndrome. Similarly, a variety of linguistic profiles were observed in 18 children by Kleppe et al., (1990). Differences were seen across subjects' severity of speech and language problems and in the range of their intelligibility, fluency, and voice problems. Kleppe et al. (1990) however, did find some common speech-language characteristics, primarily hypernasality, errors with certain speech sounds and complex syntax, and reduced vocabulary skills relative to age expectations. Speech and articulation difficulties likely are associated with hypotonia and (perhaps) thick, viscous saliva (Kleppe et al., 1990). Speech problems, primarily with articulation and intelligibility, also were noted by 33 of 43 parents of children with Prader-Willi syndrome aged 4 to 19 years (Dykens & Kasari, 1997). In addition, as implied in the case vignette, individuals with Prader-Willi syndrome often talk too much and verbally perseverate on a narrow range of topics (Dykens et al., 1996). Remaining unknown, however, is how perseveration relates to such linguistic features as pragmatics, discourse, and the social uses of language.

Cognitive Development and Correlates

Recent work has begun to describe how IQ relates to age and to such features as weight and behavioral problems. An early study of eight children with Prader-Willi syndrome reported that IQ declines in early childhood (Dunn, 1968). What was unclear, however, was whether these declines were assessed by formal IQ tests or by a failure to achieve certain developmental milestones. Using standardized IQ scores, Dykens et al. (1992a) conducted both cross-sectional and longitudinal analyses of IQ change in children and adults. IQ scores were cross-sectionally examined in 21 adolescents and adults, and longitudinal analyses included 31 subjects (ages 5–30 years) who had been given the same IQ test twice. IQ scores showed nonsignificant fluctuations in both cross-sectional and longitudinal analyses, with no evidence of IQ declines in childhood or early adulthood. Though longitudinal studies in very young children or older adults have not yet been done, overall IQ scores appear relatively stable in school-age children and young adults. Further longitudinal work is needed to clarify this stable trajectory, as it differs from the trajectories of intelligence seen in some other genetic syndromes, such as Down syndrome (Hodapp & Zigler, 1990) or fragile X syndrome (Dykens et al., 1994).

Other early work in Prader-Willi syndrome suggested a significant, inverse correlation between IQ and weight (Crnic et al., 1980), with lower IQ scores associated with increased weight. Indeed, it was suggested that prevention of obesity also might prevent mental retardation. Yet, common lore in the Prader-Willi syndrome community actually suggests the opposite relation— that brighter individuals may be more clever or ingenious about obtaining food and thus are at increased risk of obesity. Recent data do not support either hypothesis. Dykens et al. (1992a) found no significant relations between IQ and body mass indices (a measure of obesity). Persons with relatively high versus low IQ scores thus seem similarly vulnerable to the syndrome's problems of obesity and weight control.

A final correlate of IQ concerns behavior problems. The central issue here is whether high IQs might serve as a protective factor against some of the syndrome's more troublesome maladaptive behaviors. Comparing 43 subjects with relatively high IQs (mean IQ, 79) to 43 subjects with lower IQs (mean IQ, 59), Dykens and Cassidy (1995) found no significant differences in either the type or severity of maladaptive behavior across groups. These data, which are consistent with clinical observations, have important service delivery implications. In particular, state or other agencies that use low IQ scores (usually below 70) as a service eligibility requirement may exclude higher-functioning persons who have similar treatment needs as lower-functioning persons. Thus, in Prader-Willi syndrome, IQ may be a less meaningful entry point into state or other systems of care than are the behavioral needs of the person being served.

MALADAPTIVE BEHAVIOR AND PSYCHOPATHOLOGY

Range and Correlates of Maladaptive Behavior

Young children with Prader-Willi syndrome often are described as pleasant, friendly, and somewhat placid (Cassidy, 1984). These features do not necessarily disappear yet, as implied in the case vignette, older children and adults routinely are described as showing a host of negative or maladaptive behaviors. Often, managing these behaviors is more difficult than food seeking and poses multiple challenges to families, teachers, and clinicians (Dykens & Hodapp, in press).

Characteristic behavior problems are noted as a minor criterion in the consensus diagnostic criteria for Prader-Willi syndrome (Holm et al., 1993), with often-noted problems, including temper tantrums, stubbornness, oppositionality, rigidity, lying, and stealing. Many persons with Prader-Willi syndrome are also described as quite clever and manipulative, especially in regard to obtaining food. The frequency and severity of maladaptive behaviors

Table 6.2 Percentages of subjects showing selected maladaptive behaviors on the Child Behavior Checklist or the Reiss Screen

Child Behavior Checklist (N = 43; 4–19 yr)	
Skin picking	95%
Argues a lot	95%
Stubborn	93%
Underactive	91%
Obsessions	88%
Tantrums	88%
Disobeys	81%
Overeating	80%
Mood changes	77%
Speech problems	76%
Talks too much	74%
Excessive sleep	74%
Impulsive	74%
Teased by peers	72%
Overweight	70%
Compulsions	86%
Prefers being alone	68%
Lies, cheats	67%
Kids don't like	65%
Steals at home	58%
Reiss Screen (N = 61; 13–46 yr)	
Temper tantrums	84%
Eating problem	81%
Impulsivity	74%
Hostile	73%
Aggressive	64%
Stealing	60%
Social inadequacies	56%
Low energy	53%
Attention seeking	53%
Sleep problem	53%

were examined recently in more detail in two separate samples of subjects with Prader-Willi syndrome. Dykens and Kasari (1997) administered the Child Behavior Checklist (CBCL) (Achenbach, 1991) to parents of 43 children (ages 4–19 years), and Dykens and Cassidy (1995) used the Reiss Screen for Maladaptive Behavior in 61 adolescents and adults (ages 13–49 years). Table 6.2 summarizes the frequencies of salient maladaptive behaviors from both studies. Of note is the consistency across samples in rates of certain behaviors, such as temper tantrums, impulsivity, and stealing (primarily food or money for food).

Further, the majority of subjects in both studies showed scores that reached clinically significant levels. Among the 43 children and adolescents, 72% had CBCL T-scores consistent with Achenbach's (1991) clinically referred sample (Dykens & Kasari, 1997). Among the 61 adolescents and adults, 85% had one or more clinically elevated subtest scores on the Reiss Screen, with most (72%) showing two or more clinical elevations (Dykens & Cassidy, 1995). Maladaptive behaviors thus often reach a point where further clinical evaluation and interventions are necessary (Dykens & Hodapp, 1997).

IQ level and gender do not appear significantly associated with maladaptive behaviors. Maladaptive behaviors are, however, significantly related to heightened levels of familial stress (Dykens et al., 1996; Hodapp et al., 1997). In particular, nonfood behavior problems in offspring with Prader-Willi syndrome (especially such "externalizing" problems as tantrums and aggression) may be the best predictors of familial stress, even as compared to other features, such as the offspring's age, gender, IQ level, or degree of obesity. Further, stress in families with offspring with Prader-Willi syndrome is high relative to stress in families with offspring with other types of mental retardation (Hodapp et al., 1997).

In addition, maladaptive behavior may be related to weight but in a way that is opposite to general expectations. Dykens and Cassidy (1995) found that thinner adults (i.e., with lower body mass indices) had maladaptive behavior scores significantly higher than those in heavier persons (i.e., with higher body mass indices). Specifically, thinner subjects showed more distressful affect and problems in thinking: confused and distorted thinking, anxiety, sadness, fearfulness, and crying. Although preliminary to further work, these findings may be related to the stress of losing weight, and to changes in brain chemistry and physical activity level.

Development of Maladaptive Behavior

It is not yet entirely clear how maladaptive features in persons with Prader-Willi syndrome shift and change over the course of development. The beginning of hyperphagia in early childhood often is associated with the onset or worsening of behaviors, such as temper tantrums and aggression. These behaviors then seem fairly stable across the developmental years. Dykens and Cassidy (1995) found similar rates of tantrums and other externalizing behaviors in young children aged 4 to 7 years and in older children aged 8 to 12 years. Yet, advancing age in these same children was correlated with heightened internal distress and features of depression, including withdrawal, isolation, negative self-image, and pessimism.

Due to growing physical and psychosocial pressures, some clinical reports note that behavioral problems increase in the adolescent and adult years

(Greenswag, 1987; Whitman & Accardo, 1987). In contrast, others observe clinically that behavioral and emotional problems lessen with advancing age and that older adults with Prader-Willi syndrome may be more amenable to intervention (Waters, 1990).

Changes in maladaptive behavior also may not follow a simple linear function. Instead, these behaviors may wax and wane throughout adulthood (Dykens et al., 1992b; Dykens & Cassidy, 1995). Though some behaviors increase with age, others may improve or remain fairly stable. Examining 21 adolescents and adults cross-sectionally with the CBCL, Dykens et al. (1992b) found that underactivity and fatigue increased with age, whereas certain externalizing difficulties (e.g., running away and destroying property) decreased from adolescence to adulthood. Still other behaviors seemed to be fairly stable, such as temper tantrums, stubbornness, skin picking, and hoarding (Dykens et al., 1992b). Longitudinal studies are needed to clarify these preliminary cross-sectional findings.

The waxing and waning of behavioral features sometimes may be associated with specific psychosocial stressors. Many young adults, for example, experience increased behavioral difficulties when they leave home and move into a group home setting or when they transition from one job to another. In other persons, however, psychosocial precipitants for behavioral shifts are not apparent.

Psychiatric Features

Most research in dual diagnosis (i.e., in persons with mental retardation and psychiatric illness) uses heterogeneous groups of subjects with mixed etiologies (Dykens, 1996). These mixed groups typically are examined by their levels of cognitive impairment (e.g., mild, moderate, severe) or by their age, gender, or residential status (Borthwick-Duffy, 1994; Hodapp & Dykens, 1994). Thus, with few exceptions, more is known about psychiatric illness in mentally retarded subjects with mixed etiologies than in persons with specific syndromes.

Partly due to this mixed-group approach, little is yet known about the prevalence rates of psychiatric disorders in the population of persons with Prader-Willi syndrome. Although population-based prevalence studies have yet to be done, clinically we find that certain psychiatric disorders occur infrequently. For example, although many people with Prader-Willi syndrome steal food and are impulsive and distractible, rates seem low for full-blown conduct disorder or attention deficit hyperactivity disorder. Tic disorders, dementia, schizophrenia, and autism also appear relatively infrequently in this population. Recently, however, Clarke (1993) and Clarke et al., (1995) reported on psychotic episodes in four young adults with Prader-Willi syndrome; all cases showed a paternal deletion of chromosome 15. These patients had a sudden onset of hallucinations and other psychotic symptoms, with no obvious precipitating events. All showed good outcome after milieu and pharmacological treatment. These cases suggest a need for large-scale studies that identify whether Prader-Willi syndrome involves a particular vulnerability to schizophrenia-spectrum disorders, above and beyond the risk associated with mental retardation.

Further, Prader-Willi syndrome does not appear to include a heightened risk of autism or pervasive developmental disorder beyond the risk due to mental retardation. Of the handful of patients with Prader-Willi syndrome and co-occurring autism or PDD-NOS that we have seen in the clinical setting, however, all had maternal disomy of chromosome 15. These clinical observations are consistent with Rogan et al. (1994), who suggested increased risks of autism or other, rare disorders in Prader-Willi cases involving maternal disomy of chromosome 15.

In contrast to low-frequency problems, several psychiatric disorders may occur with increased frequency in persons with Prader-Willi syndrome. These include affective disorders and obsessive-compulsive disorder. Depressive features, such as sadness and low esteem, and anxiety, fears, and worries have been noted in several studies on maladaptive behavior in Prader-Willi syndrome (e.g., Whitman & Accardo, 1987; Dykens et al., 1992b; Stein et al., 1994; Dykens & Cassidy, 1995). Dykens and Kasari (1997), for example, found that 77% of 43 Prader-Willi syndrome children (ages 4–19 years) showed mood lability on the CBCL (Achenbach, 1991). Further, parents noted that 54% of these children were worried and that 42% were unhappy, sad, or depressed.

Yet, no research has examined these or other maladaptive features using formal DSM-IV (American Psychiatric Association, 1994) or ICD-10 diagnostic criteria for depressive or anxiety disorders. Thus, what remains unknown is the point at which the sadness or worry shown by some persons with the syndrome might lead to full-blown affective disorder. Also unclear are the factors that might predispose some persons with the syndrome to be more or less susceptible to affective disorders.

Increased risks of obsessive-compulsive disorder also are quite likely in persons with Prader-Willi syndrome. Compulsive-type symptoms long have been hallmark features of Prader-Willi syndrome, primarily skin picking, food preoccupations, and repetitive food-seeking behaviors (e.g., Dykens et al., 1992b; Holm et al., 1993; Hellings & Warnock, 1994; Stein et al., 1994). Yet many persons show repetitive thoughts and compulsive behaviors not related to skin picking or food.

Recently, Dykens et al. (1996) identified a wide range of nonfood obsessions and compulsions in 91 children and adults with Prader-Willi syndrome. As measured by the Yale-Brown Obsessive-Compulsive Scale (Goodman et al., 1989), prominent compulsions in this sample included hoarding (e.g., paper, pens, trash, toiletries) and rewriting; needs to tell, ask, or know; and concerns with symmetry, exactness, ordering, and arranging. Table 6.3 summarizes the percentage of subjects showing these various symptoms.

Table 6.3 Percentages of 91 subjects with Prader-Willi syndrome showing specific compulsive symptoms on the Yale-Brown Obsessive Compulsive Scale

Compulsions	Percentage
Cleaning	24
Checking	15
Repeating rituals	37
Counting	17
Ordering and arranging	40
Symmetry and exactness	35
Hoarding	58
Need to tell, ask, or know	53

Source: Adapted from Dykens et al., 1996.

As in the case of Mark in the case vignette, who carefully arranged old *TV Guides*, subjects in this study often ordered and arranged toys or objects according to specific rules based on size, shape, color, or simply until they were "just right." Many subjects rewrote letters or words until they were just right; others could not tolerate papers not cut exactly on the line or slight imperfections in the environment. More than half of the subjects also had to tell, ask, or say things, often perseverating on a narrow range of topics. Relatively fewer subjects had cleaning, contamination, or checking symptoms.

Further, as specified in DSM-IV criteria for obsessive-compulsive disorder (American Psychiatric Association, 1994), a remarkably high proportion of subjects had moderate to severe levels of obsessive and compulsive symptomatology. Indeed, 64% showed at least a moderate level of symptom-related distress, and 80% had symptom-related adaptive impairment. Other ties between Prader-Willi syndrome and obsessive-compulsive disorder were found by comparing 43 adults with Prader-Willi syndrome to age- and gender-matched nonretarded adults with obsessive-compulsive disorder (Dykens et al., 1996). The matched Prader-Willi and obsessive-compulsive groups showed similar levels of symptom severity, similar numbers of compulsions, and more areas of symptom similarity than difference.

Increased risks of obsessive-compulsive disorder thus are indicated strongly in persons with Prader-Willi syndrome; these individuals exhibit a wide range of severe symptoms and are similar to nonretarded adults with obsessive-compulsive disorder. In contrast, studies with heterogenous groups of persons with mental retardation find only 1% to 3% who meet criteria for obsessive-compulsive disorder (e.g., Meyers, 1987; Vitiello et al., 1989). Possibly one or more genes associated with this increased vulnerability to obsessive-compulsive disorder are found in the Prader-Willi critical region on chromosome 15, or possibly the pathogenesis of Prader-Willi syndrome in some way predisposes to obsessive and compulsive behaviors.

Further work is needed to identify the extent to which Prader-Willi syndrome also involves heightened risks of affective, impulse control, or psychotic disorders above and beyond the risks associated with mental retardation per se. Also still unknown is how any of these psychiatric features relate to molecular genetic status. Behavioral or cognitive differences generally have not been found between subjects with chromosome 15 paternal deletion versus maternal disomy (Cassidy et al., 1997). Though deletion cases may be more prone to repetitive skin picking and perhaps other compulsive symptoms (Cassidy, 1995) and maternal disomy cases may be more prone to autism or PDD symptoms (Rogan et al., 1994), more research is needed to clarify these preliminary observations.

Specificity of Maladaptive Features

Although considerable work remains, the psychiatric and maladaptive features of Prader-Willi syndrome are becoming increasingly better understood. However, studies have yet to compare these features to other persons with mental retardation. In particular, we do not know which psychiatric and maladaptive features are specific to Prader-Willi syndrome, which are shown by many persons with mental retardation, and which are shared by only a few other etiologies of mental retardation.

At first glance, hyperphagia appears a unique aspect of Prader-Willi syndrome. Though some people with mental retardation show increased interests in food or propensities to being overweight (Prasher, 1995), generally it is not to the same degree as that exhibited in Prader-Willi syndrome. Other behaviors, such as temper tantrums, argumentativeness, or stubbornness, are seen in many persons with mental retardation in general.

Although not unique in all aspects of maladaptive behavior, certain behaviors may be more common in persons with Prader-Willi syndrome relative to others with mental retardation. Dykens and Kasari (1997) compared 43 subjects with Prader-Willi syndrome (ages 4–19 years) to age- and gender-matched subjects with Down syndrome and nonspecific mental retardation. As measured by the CBCL (Achenbach, 1991), subjects with Prader-Willi syndrome were more apt to overeat and be overweight and to show skin picking, verbal perseveration, obsessions, compulsions, sleep problems, underactivity, and other behaviors. Table 6.4 summarizes mean CBCL scores across these and other behaviors in the Prader-Willi syndrome, Down syndrome, and nonspecific groups.

A discriminant function analysis of these CBCL data suggested a relatively distinct Prader-Willi behavioral phenotype, with 91% of Prader-Willi cases correctly classified and just 3 of the 86 comparison group subjects mistakenly assigned to the Prader-Willi group. Seven behaviors best discriminated the three groups, with the Prader-Willi group being singularly high in skin picking, fatigue, obsessions, and talking too much. Thus, a blend of certain maladaptive behaviors appear quite distinctive to Prader-Willi syndrome and

Table 6.4 Means, standard deviations, and F-values of 15 behaviors showing significant Child Behavior Checklist differences across groups

	Prader-Willi Syndrome		Down Syndrome		Nonspecific		
	M	SD	M	SD	M	SD	F*
PWS > DS, NS							
Skin picking	1.63	(.58)	.26	(.54)	.21	(.51)	67.10
Argues a lot	1.51	(.59)	.79	(.67)	.95	(.84)	7.05
Obsessions	1.44	(.70)	.60	(.73)	.60	(.85)	10.83
Underactive	1.33	(.64)	.42	(.63)	.35	(.61)	23.42
Overeating	1.26	(.79)	.40	(.69)	.30	(.64)	17.85
Talks too much	1.26	(.85)	.44	(.67)	.86	(.97)	6.31
Excessive sleep	1.19	(.82)	.14	(.41)	.14	(.47)	30.68
Overweight	1.14	(.86)	.40	(.66)	.26	(.62)	13.05
Overtired	1.12	(.66)	.26	(.44)	.26	(.49)	20.93
Gets teased	1.05	(.79)	.30	(.51)	.42	(.66)	8.72
Compulsions	.98	(.80)	.40	(.62)	.60	(.85)	6.61
Steals at home	.70	(.67)	.09	(.37)	.09	(.37)	17.17
PWS, DS > NS							
Speech problem	1.37	(.85)	1.30	(.83)	.65	(.81)	10.70
Rather be alone	.84	(.69)	.77	(.68)	.33	(.57)	8.12
PWS, DS < NS							
Hyperactive	.23	(.48)	.47	(.70)	.86	(.80)	6.53

PWS, Prader-Willi syndrome; DS, Down syndrome; NS, nonspecific.
*$P < .002$ for all comparisons.

highly predictive of this disorder. Overeating, food obsessions, and sleep disturbances are salient in Prader-Willi syndrome, yet other obsessions and repetitive, compulsive-type behavior also seem to be central distinguishing features of this syndrome.

TOWARD A BEHAVIORAL PHENOTYPE

In considering behavioral work in Prader-Willi syndrome, this chapter highlights the need for future work on cognitive profiles and trajectories and on the prevalence of various behavioral features and psychiatric disorders. Yet, other research approaches are needed to show both the variability and the distinctiveness of the Prader-Willi behavioral phenotype.

In particular, a behavioral phenotype is best regarded as an increased *probability* or *likelihood* that people with a given syndrome will exhibit certain behavioral or developmental sequelae as compared to those without the syndrome (Dykens, 1995). Viewing phenotypes in this way opens the door for two avenues of future work. First, more studies are needed to compare subjects with Prader-Willi syndrome to persons with other types of mental retardation. Such comparisons identify the specificity of the Prader-Willi behavioral phenotype, or those aspects of the syndrome that are unique versus shared.

Second, if phenotypes are viewed in probabilistic terms, not all persons with Prader-Willi syndrome will show the syndrome's characteristic features to the same extent or at the same point. Vast individual differences exist within Prader-Willi syndrome, and more studies are needed to identify possible sources of this variability. Development is one promising source of within-syndrome variability, as maladaptive behaviors and hyperphagia seem to wax and wane over the life span. Psychosocial variables, such as self-esteem or family stress and support, also likely mediate the variable expression of behavior in Prader-Willi syndrome. Further, genetic status likely will account for some syndromic variability. Clinical observations, for example, suggest some behavioral differences across subjects with chromosome 15 paternal deletion versus maternal uniparental disomy. Studies are underway to test more rigorously these informal observations.

Finally, behavioral work has focused almost exclusively on the maladaptive characteristics of Prader-Willi syndrome. Indeed, many of these features, such as hyperphagia, compulsions, or skin picking, are quite compelling and immediately capture our attention with their clinical urgency (Dykens & Hodapp, 1997). Of equal importance, however, are future studies on the competencies and strengths of persons with Prader-Willi syndrome. What, for example, allowed the youngster in the case vignette to surprise his mother and spontaneously get up on a horse? Specific studies are needed to explore personality strengths, adaptive skills, and social competencies and how all these features shift and change over the life span. Such data round out Prader-Willi syndrome's behavioral phenotype, thereby shedding new light on ways of optimizing success in persons with this complex disorder.

ACKNOWLEDGMENT

The author thanks Robert M. Hodapp, Ph.D., for his helpful comments on an earlier draft of this manuscript.

REFERENCES

Achenbach, T. M. (1991). *Manual for the child behavior checklist/4–18 and 1991 profile*. Burlington, VT: University of Vermont Department of Psychiatry.

American Psychiatric Association (1994). *Diagnostic and statistical manual of mental disorders* (4th ed.). Washington, DC: American Psychiatric Association.

Aughton, D. A., & Cassidy, S. B. (1990). Physical features of Prader-Willi syndrome in neonates. *American Journal of Diseases in Childhood, 144*, 1251–1254.

Baker, H. J., & Leland, B. (1967). *Detroit tests of learning aptitude*. Indianapolis: Bobbs-Merrill.

Borghgraef, M., Fryns, J. P., & Van Den Berghe, H. (1990). Psychological profile and behavioral characteristics in 12 patients with Prader-Willi syndrome. *Genetic Counseling, 38*, 141–150.

Borthwick-Duffy, S. A. (1994). Epidemiology and prevalence of psychopathology in people with mental retardation. *Journal of Consulting and Clinical Psychology, 62,* 17–27.

Branson, C. (1981). Speech and language characteristics of children with Prader-Willi syndrome. In V. A. Holm, S. Sulzbacher, & P. Pipes (Eds.), *Prader-Willi syndrome* (pp. 179–183). Baltimore: University Park Press.

Cassidy, S. B. (1984). Prader-Willi syndrome. *Current Problems in Pediatrics, 14,* 1–55.

Cassidy, S. B. (1995, June). *Complexities of clinical diagnosis of Prader-Willi syndrome.* Paper presented to the Second Prader-Willi Syndrome International Conference, Sormarka, Oslo, Norway.

Cassidy, S. B., Forsythe, M., Heeger, S., Nicholls, R. D., Schork N., Benn, P. & Schwartz, S. (1997). Comparison of phenotype between patients with Prader-Willi syndrome due to deletion 15q and uniparental disomy 15. *American Journal of Human Genetics, 68,* 433–440.

Clarke, D. J. (1993). Prader-Willi syndrome and psychoses. *British Journal of Psychiatry, 163,* 680–684.

Clarke, D. J., Webb, T., & Bachmann-Clarke, J. P. (1995). Prader-Willi syndrome and psychotic symptoms: Report of a further case. *Irish Journal of Psychological Medicine, 12,* 27–29.

Crnic, K. A., Sulzbacher, S., Snow, J., & Holm, V. A. (1980). Preventing mental retardation associated with gross obesity in the Prader-Willi syndrome. *Pediatrics, 66,* 787–789.

Curfs, L. G. (1992). Psychological profile and behavioral characteristics in Prader-Willi syndrome. In S. B. Cassidy (Ed.), *Prader-Willi syndrome and other 15q deletion disorders* (pp. 211–222). Berlin: Springer.

Curfs, L. G., Wiegers, A. M., Sommers, J. R., Borghgraef, M., & Fryns, J. P. (1991). Strengths and weaknesses in the cognitive profile of youngsters with Prader-Willi syndrome. *Clinical Genetics, 40,* 430–434.

Dunn, H. G. (1968). The Prader-Labhart-Willi syndrome: Review of the literature and report of nine cases. *Acta Paediatrica Scandanavia, 186,* 1–38.

Dykens, E. M. (1995). Measuring behavioral phenotypes: Provocations from the "new genetics". *American Journal on Mental Retardation, 99,* 522–532.

Dykens, E. M. (1996). DNA meets DSM: Genetic syndromes' growing importance in dual diagnosis. *Mental Retardation, 34,* 125–127.

Dykens, E. M., & Cassidy, S. B. (1995). Correlates of maladaptive behavior in children and adults with Prader-Willi syndrome. *American Journal of Medical Genetics, 60,* 546–549.

Dykens, E. M., & Hodapp, R. M. (1997). Treatment issues in genetic mental retardation syndromes. *Professional Psychology: Research and Practice, 28,* 263–270.

Dykens, E. M., Hodapp, R. M., & Leckman, J. F. (1994). *Behavior and development in fragile X syndrome.* Newbury Park, CA: Sage.

Dykens, E. M., Hodapp, R. M., Walsh, K., & Nash, L. J. (1992a). Profiles, correlates and trajectories of intelligence in individuals with Prader-Willi syndrome. *Journal of the American Academy of Child and Adolescent Psychiatry, 31,* 1125–1130.

Dykens, E. M., Hodapp, R. M., Walsh, K., & Nash, L. J. (1992b). Adaptive and maladaptive behavior in Prader-Willi syndrome. *Journal of the American Academy of Child and Adolescent Psychiatry, 31,* 1131–1136.

Dykens, E. M., & Kasari, C. (1997). Maladaptive behavior in children with Prader-Willi syndrome, Down syndrome and non-specific mental retardation. *American Journal on Mental Retardation, 102,* 228–237.

Dykens, E. M., Leckman, J. F., & Cassidy, S. B. (1996). Obsessions and compulsions in Prader-Willi syndrome. *Journal of Child Psychology and Psychiatry, 37,* 995–1002.

Gabel, S., Tarter, R. E., Gavaler, J., Golden, W., Hegedus, A. M., & Mair, B. (1986). Neuropsychological capacity of Prader-Willi children: General and specific aspects of impairment. *Applied Research in Mental Retardation, 7,* 459–466.

Goodman, W. K., Price, L. H., Rasmussen, S. A., Mazure, C., Fleischmann, R. L., Hill, C. L., Heninger, G. R., & Charney, D. S. (1989). The Yale-Brown Obsessive-Compulsive Scale: Development, use and reliability, *Archives of General Psychiatry, 46,* 1006–1011.

Greenswag, L. R. (1987). Adults with Prader-Willi syndrome: A survey of 232 cases. *Developmental Medicine and Child Neurology, 29,* 145–152.

Hanchett, J. M., Butler, M., Cassidy, S. B., Holm, V., Parker, K. R., Wharton, R., & Zipf, W. (in press). Age and causes of death in Prader-Willi syndrome patients. *American Journal of Medical Genetics.*

Hellings, J. A., & Warnock, J. K. (1994). Self-injurious behavior and serotonin in Prader-Willi syndrome. *Psychopharmacology Bulletin, 30,* 245–250.

Hodapp, R. M. (1996). Cross-domain relations in Down syndrome. In J. A. Rondal, J. Perera, L. Nadel, & A. Comblain (Eds.), *Down syndrome: Psychological, psychobiological, and socioeducational perspectives* (pp. 65–79). London: Whurr Publications.

Hodapp, R. M., & Dykens, E. M. (1994). Mental retardation's two cultures of behavioral research. *American Journal on Mental Retardation, 98,* 675–687.

Hodapp, R. M., Dykens, E. M., & Masino, L. (1997). Stress and support in families of persons with Prader-Willi syndrome. *Journal of Autism and Developmental Disorders, 27,* 11–23.

Hodapp, R. M., & Zigler, E. (1990). Applying the developmental perspective to individuals with Down syndrome. In D. Cicchetti & M. Beeghly (Eds.), *Children with Down syndrome: A developmental perspective* (pp. 1–28). New York: Cambridge University.

Holland, A. J., Treasure, J., Coskeran, P., & Dallow, J. (1995). Characteristics of the eating disorder in Prader-Willi syndrome: Implications for treatment. *Journal of Intellectual Disability Research, 39,* 373–381.

Holm, V. A. (1981). The diagnosis of Prader-Willi syndrome. In V. A. Holm, S. Sulzbacher, & P. L. Pipes (Eds.), *Prader-Willi syndrome* (pp. 27–44). Baltimore: University Park Press.

Holm, V. A., Cassidy, S. B., Butler, M. G., Hanchett, J. M., Greenswag, L. R., Whitman, B. Y., & Greenberg, F. (1993). Prader-Willi syndrome: Consensus diagnostic criteria. *Pediatrics, 91,* 398–402.

Kaufman, A. S., & Kaufman, N. L. (1984). *Kaufman assessment battery for children.* Circle Pines, MN: American Guidance Service.

Kleppe, S. A., Katayama, K. M., Shipley, K. G., & Foushee, D. R. (1990). The speech and language characteristics of children with Prader-Willi syndrome. *Journal of Speech and Hearing Disorders, 55,* 300–309.

Ledbetter, D. H., Riccardi, V. M., Airhart, S. D., Strobel, R. J., Keenen, S. B., & Crawford, J. D. (1981). Deletion of chromosome 15 as a cause of Prader-Wili syndrome. *New England Journal of Medicine, 304,* 325–329.

Meyers, B. A. (1987). Psychiatric problems in adolescents with developmental disabilities. *Journal of the American Academy of Child and Adolescent Psychiatry, 26,* 74–79.

Nicholls, R. D. (1993). Genomic imprinting and uniparental disomy in Angelman and Prader-Willi syndrome: A review. *American Journal of Medical Genetics, 46,* 16–25.

Nicholls, R. D., Knoll, J. H., Butler, M. G., Karam, S., Lalande, M. (1989). Genetic imprinting suggested by maternal heterodisomy in nondeletion Prader-Willi syndrome. *Nature, 16,* 281–285.

Prader, A., Labhart, A. & Willi, A. (1956). Ein syndrom von aidositas, kleinwuchs, kryptorchismus und oligophrenie nach myotonieartigem zustand im neugeborenenalter. *Schweizerische Medizinische Wochenschrift, 86,* 1260–1261.

Prasher, V. P. (1995). Overweight and obesity amongst Down syndrome adults. *Journal of Intellectual Disability Research, 39,* 437–441.

Rogan, P. K., Mascari, J., Ladda, R. L., Woodage, T., Trent, R. J., Smith, A., Lai, W., Erickson, R. P., Cassidy, S. B., Peterson, M. B., Mikkesen, M., Driscoll, D. J., Nicholls, R. D., & Butler, M. G. (1994, July). *Coinheritance of other chromosome 15 abnormalities with Prader-Willi syndrome: Genetic risk estimation and mapping.* Paper presented to the Sixteenth Annual PWS (USA) National Scientific Day, Atlanta, GA.

Stein, D. J., Keating, K., Zar, H. J., & Hollander, E. (1994). A survey of the phenomenology and pharmacotherapy of compulsive and impulsive-aggressive symptoms in Prader-Willi syndrome. *The Journal of Neuropsychiatry and Clinical Neuroscience, 6,* 23–29.

Sulzbacher, S., Crnic, K., & Snow, J. (1981). Behavioral and cognitive disabilities in Prader-Willi syndrome. In V. A. Holm, S. Sulzbacher, & P. Pipes (Eds.), *Prader-Willi syndrome* (pp. 147–169). Baltimore, MD: University Park.

Swaab, D. F., Purba, J. S., & Hofman, M. A. (1995). Alterations in the hypothalamic paraventricular nucleus and its oxytocin neurons (putative satiety cells) in Prader-Willi syndrome: A study of 5 cases. *Journal of Clinical Endocrinology and Metabolism, 80,* 573–579.

Taylor, R. L. (1988). Cognitive and behavioral features. In M. L. Caldwell & R. L. Taylor (Eds.), *Prader-Willi syndrome: Selected research and management issues* (pp. 29–42). New York: Springer.

Vitiello, B., Spreat, S., & Behar, D. (1989). Obsessive-compulsive disorder in mentally retarded patients. *Journal of Nervous and Mental Disease, 177,* 232–236.

Warren, J., & Hunt, E. (1981). Cognitive processing in children with Prader-Willi syndrome. In V. A. Holm, S. Sulzbacher, & P. Pipes (Eds.), *Prader-Willi syndrome* (pp. 161–177). Baltimore: University Park.

Waters, J. (1990). Prader-Willi syndrome. In J. Hogg, J. Sebba, & L. Lambe (Eds.), *Profound mental retardation and multiple impairment: Vol 3. Medical and physical care and management* (pp. 54–67). London: Chapman and Hall.

Whitman, B. Y., & Accardo, P. (1987). Emotional problems in Prader-Willi adolescents. *American Journal of Medical Genetics, 28,* 897–905.

7 Cognition, Behavior, Neurochemistry, and Genetics in Prader-Willi Syndrome

Travis Thompson, Merlin G. Butler, William E. MacLean, Jr., Beth Joseph, and Dawn Delaney

Prader-Willi syndrome is a genetic developmental disability characterized by a cluster of specific behavioral features of which a voracious and insatiable appetite is the most striking. Prader-Willi syndrome is the most common known genetic cause of obesity. The eating disorder associated with Prader-Willi syndrome can be so severe as to be life-threatening, including eating to the point of stomach rupture. Though a cluster of commonly covarying clinical features are exhibited by people with this syndrome, only the eating disorder is common to all affected individuals.

Much has been written about the anatomical, endocrine, metabolic, and genetic characteristics of people with Prader-Willi syndrome, but relatively less attention has been paid to the equally striking behavioral features. Prader-Willi syndrome shares important behavioral and psychological features with other disorders and disabilities, such as autism and obsessive compulsive disorder, but only Prader-Willi syndrome includes the unique combination of features that distinguish this extraordinary syndrome. In this chapter, we review what is known about the behavioral, cognitive, and other psychological features of Prader-Willi syndrome and to pose some questions for further consideration.

HISTORY AND PREVALENCE

The Prader-Willi syndrome was first described in nine people by Prader et al., (1956). Since that time, more than 800 cases have been reported in the literature (Butler et al., 1986; Butler, 1990, 1994; Greenswag & Alexander, 1995). The cardinal features of the syndrome included hypotonia during infancy, with improvement by 9 months of age, obesity with onset between 6 months and 6 years of age, and an average age of onset by 2 years. Obesity is considered the most significant health problem, but hypogonadism and under-development of sex organs in both genders are additional features. Both men and women are considered infertile. Male subjects present with an under-developed scrotum and undescended testicles or cryptorchidism. Though people with Prader-Willi syndrome have a developmental disability, they do not necessarily have mental retardation. Slightly fewer than half of the people with Prader-Willi syndrome function in the low-average range of intellectual functioning, and somewhat more than half test in the mild to moderate range of mental retardation. Additional findings include short stature (particularly in adulthood), small hands and feet, hypopigmentation, a particular facial appearance, and a partial deletion of chromosome 15 in some 70% of Prader-Willi syndrome individuals. The diagnosis is easier to make in male than in female subjects, particularly during infancy; therefore more male persons are reported with this disorder. Prader-Willi syndrome is one of the most common chromosome deletion syndromes and affects about one in every 10,000 to 20,000 individuals (Butler, 1990; Greenswag & Alexander, 1995). This syndrome has been reported in all races and ethnic groups, although it is reported disproportionately more in whites. Still not known is whether this reflects differences in reporting by different racial and ethnic groups or whether it reflects actual base-rate differences.

This syndrome has been reported rarely to recur in a family. At least 10 families reported in the literature have more than one affected member (Butler, 1990). The chance for recurrence appears to be less than 1%, particularly in those patients with the chromosome 15 deletion.

PREGNANCY AND DELIVERY

Reduced fetal movement or activity is noted in the majority of Prader-Willi syndrome pregnancies. Some one-fourth of babies with Prader-Willi syndrome present at delivery in an unusual position, such as breech presentation. Perhaps one-half of babies with Prader-Willi syndrome are born either 2 weeks earlier or later than anticipated by the delivery due dates. An overrepresentation is seen of babies with Prader-Willi syndrome born in the autumn months, particularly October.

BIRTH AND EARLY INFANCY

Because of generalized hypotonia, these babies have a floppy appearance. Prader-Willi syndrome can be mistaken for other disorders (e.g., Werdnig-Hoffman syndrome) affecting the brain and central nervous system (CNS). Extensive medical evaluations, including muscle biopsies and brain imaging studies, frequently are performed and are either normal or not diagnostic for a specific syndrome. Most infants with Prader-Willi syndrome seem to lack a distinctive facial expression, have a weak cry, and display little spontaneous movement, excessive sleep, and a poor suck reflex, which may necessitate tube feedings or a gastrostomy to treat the feeding difficulties. Failure to thrive and poor weight gain are common features of infants with Prader-Willi syndrome. These babies also may have temperature instability, and their body temperature may rise or fall for no known reason. This change in body temperature and abnormal appetite may be due to a hypothalamic

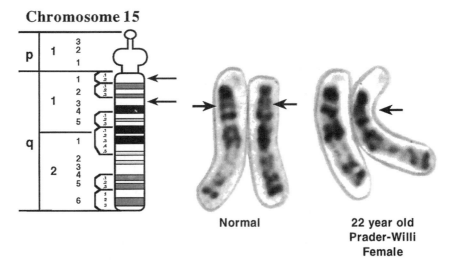

Chromosome 15

Normal

22 year old
Prader-Willi
Female

Figure 7.1 Representative high-resolution chromosome 15 pair from a normal individual (chromosome 15 pair on left) and a 22-year-old Prader-Willi syndrome individual with a chromosome 15q11q13 deletion of one of the chromosome 15s (pair on right). The arrows show the nondeleted chromosome 15q11q13 region in the normal chromosome in each chromosome 15 pair. A chromosome 15 idiogram (850 band level) is shown on the left with the breakpoints at q11 and q13 designated by arrows.

abnormality, although gross neuropathological studies to date have not identified a brain lesion in this area. Recently, preliminary brain imaging studies (e.g., positron emission tomography) evaluating brain metabolism showed decreased glucose metabolism in the parietal lobes and hypothalamus in a Prader-Willi syndrome patient (Butler & Kessler, 1992). Neuroimaging studies in Prader-Willi syndrome are discussed later.

Mild dysmorphic features are seen during infancy, including a narrow forehead; small upturned nose; thin upper lip and down-turned corners of the mouth; a long, narrow-appearing head (dolichocephaly); upward slanting of the palpebral fissures; sticky saliva; fair skin and hair color; and small hands and feet (Butler et al., 1986; Butler, 1989, 1990).

GENETICS

In 1980, Ledbetter et al. (1980) reported a small deletion of the proximal long arm of chromosome 15 involving the 15q11q13 region using newly developed high-resolution chromosome methods (figure 7.1). Butler and Palmer (1983) reported that parental chromosomes generally were normal but that the chromosome 15 deletion originated with the father in all Prader-Willi syndrome families studied. This puzzling observation later was characterized with newer molecular genetic techniques. In addition, Strakowski and Butler (1987) found an overrepresentation of fathers working in hydrocarbon-exposed occupations at the time of conception, compared with the general population. The chromosome 15 deletion was seen in approximately 60 percent of people with Prader-Willi syndrome, whereas the remaining patients showed normal chromosomes 15, or translocations or other anomalies involving chromosome 15.

Butler et al. (1986) found clinical differences in individuals who had Prader-Willi syndrome and normal chromosomes and those with the chromosome 15 deletion. Individuals with the chromosome 15 deletion showed lighter hair and eye color, fairer complexion than that of other similarly aged family members, and sun sensitivity. The people who had Prader-Willi syndrome and showed visible deletions were more homogeneous in their clinical features than were the individuals who had Prader-Willi syndrome but did not have chromosome 15 deletions.

Additional genetic findings were discovered by Nicholls et al. (1989), using then-new molecular genetic techniques, in individuals who had Prader-Willi syndrome and had normal-appearing chromosomes. They reported that for people who had Prader-Willi syndrome and normal chromosomes 15, both members of the chromosome 15 pair were donated by the mother and no chromosome 15 was found from the father. This interesting phenomenon was called *maternal uniparental disomy* of chromosome 15.

Thus, two genetic causes exist for Prader-Willi syndrome: (1) a deletion of the 15q11q13 region of the father's chromosome 15 or (2) two copies of chromosome 15 from the mother, which is observed in perhaps 25% of people with Prader-Willi syndrome (Mascari et al., 1992). The molecular genetic research showed a difference in gene activity or expression of the proximal long arm of chromosome 15 in male and female subjects (Nicholls, 1994). An intact chromosome 15q11q13 region is required from the father to prevent the findings recognized as Prader-Willi syndrome. If this chromosome region was deleted or if the entire chromosome 15 from the father were absent, Prader-Willi syndrome will result. Figures 7.1 and 7.2 show

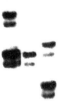

Figure 7.2 Polymerase chain reaction (PCR) amplification studies were undertaken using DNA sequences to produce large DNA fragments from each of the two chromosome 15s from a Prader-Willi syndrome (PWS) family. Sequence data from a known DNA segment from the 15q11q13 region (e.g., D15S128 locus) were used in the PCR reaction. The mother showed two signals, each representing her different chromosome 15s (left lane); the PWS individual showed only one signal generated from one of the mother's chromosome 15s (middle lane) and the father showed two signals, each representing his different chromosome 15s (right lane). The PWS child had only one signal (from the mother's chromosome 15) demonstrating a deletion of the DNA segment or locus (for example, D15S128) from the 15q11q13 region donated by the father.

molecular genetic testing of two Prader-Willi syndrome families (one with a 15q11q13 deletion in the Prader-Willi syndrome patient and the second with maternal disomy 15) using polymerase chain reaction amplification of DNA segments from the chromosome 15q11q13 region.

In the late 1980s, several people were reported to have the same apparent chromosome 15q11q13 region deleted but did not have the classic features of Prader-Willi syndrome. These individuals had ataxia, seizures, and a wide-appearing head, nose, and mouth; they lacked speech, had severe mental retardation, and often displayed peculiarly inappropriate laughter. This condition is called *Angelman syndrome*, named after Dr. H. Angelman, who, in 1965, first described people with these findings (Angelman, 1965). DNA studies of chromosome 15 showed the deletion, when present (70% of people with Angelman syndrome having a 15q11q13 deletion and the remaining people having normal-appearing chromosomes 15), was maternal in origin and the intact chromosome 15 was from the father (Williams et al., 1989; Zackowski et al., 1993). A small percentage of individuals with Angelman syndrome (perhaps 5%) had paternal disomy of chromosome 15 (both chromosomes 15 from the father and no chromosome 15 identified from the mother). Thus, Prader-Willi and Angelman syndromes represent the first examples in humans of *genetic imprinting*, or the differential expression of genetic information whether inherited from the mother or from the father. Therefore, a gene may be functional only on one member of a chromosome pair. This newly reported genetic phenomenon may play a significant role in other poorly understood genetic conditions.

Increasing evidence indicates that in most instances of Prader-Willi syndrome, the cluster of features comprising the syndrome may be determined by more than one gene from the chromosome 15q11q13 region (i.e., a *contiguous gene syndrome*). There are several recently identified candidate genes on chromosome 15 that appear to contribute different features of Prader-Willi syndrome. The locations and names of candidate genes on chromosome 15 from the 15q11q13 region and their possible role in Prader-Willi syndrome are shown in figure 7.3. One important candidate gene is small-nuclear ribonucleoprotein polypeptide N (*SNRPN*) a paternally expressed gene (not active on the mother's chromosome 15) which is found in the smallest deletions recognized in Prader-Willi syndrome patients (Ozcelik et al., 1992; Buiting et al., 1995). This gene functions in brain tissue of normal individuals and assists other genes to function properly in the brain. The human *SNRPN* gene is one of a gene family that encodes proteins involved in pre-mRNA splicing. The gene is paternally expressed as demonstrated by the use of cell lines from Prader-Willi syndrome patients (with maternal chromosome 15q11q13 alleles only) and Angelman syndrome patients (with paternal chromosome 15q11q13 alleles only). This gene is expressed predominantly in brain tissue and especially in central neurons but can be found in a wide range of somatic tissues and is an important candidate gene for Prader-Willi syndrome. Tissue-specific expression patterns suggest

Figure 7.3 Polymerase chain reaction amplification studies were performed from a Prader-Willi syndrome (PWS) family using sequence data from a DNA segment from the 15q11q13 region (e.g., *GABRB3* gene). The father (left lane), the PWS individual (middle lane), and the PWS mother (right lane) each showed two signals representing intact nondeleted chromosome 15s and the presence of two copies of the *GABRB3* gene. In comparison of the DNA patterns, the PWS individual's patterns are identical to the mother's, but no DNA signal was produced from the chromosome 15 from the father. Therefore, the PWS individual had two chromosome 15s, and both were from the mother; no chromosome 15 came from the father, indicating uniparental maternal disomy of chromosome 15.

the involvement of a class of these ribonucleoprotein particles in tissue-specific mRNA splicing. Thus, an abnormality in the expression of *SNRPN* could affect alternative splicing of important gene transcripts in the brain leading to developmental or functional derangements of the nervous system.

DNA methylation analysis of the *SNRPN* gene in a variety of human tissues have demonstrated the presence or absence of the *SNRPN* gene product and could provide a quick and highly reliable diagnostic assay for both Prader-Willi syndrome and Angelman syndrome. The putative transcription start site for this gene is extensively methylated on the repressed maternal allele and is unmethylated on the expressed paternal allele, thus showing genetic imprinting. These findings are consistent with a key role for DNA methylation in the imprinted inheritance and subsequent gene expression of the human *SNRPN* gene as a key player in the development of Prader-Willi syndrome (Ozcelik et al., 1992; Glenn et al., 1996). Additional studies are needed to identify and characterize genes from the 15q11q13 region that may cause Prader-Willi syndrome and also Angelman syndrome (see figure 7.4).

EATING DISORDER

The most striking feature of children and youth with Prader-Willi syndrome is their voracious appetite and persistent eating. Children with Prader-Willi syndrome report being continuously hungry, seemingly never satiating and rarely vomiting. The metabolic rate of children with Prader-Willi syndrome is 40% lower than normal and, with decreased physical activity and an increased food intake, rapid weight gain develops (Hill et al., 1990). The resulting obesity is substantial and highly resistant to change (Holm, 1981), primarily when dietary management techniques alone are employed. Estimates posit that as many as one-third of Prader-Willi syndrome patients weigh more than 200% of ideal body weight (Schoeller et al., 1988; Meaney & Butler, 1989).

II. Syndromes with Known Genetic Etiologies

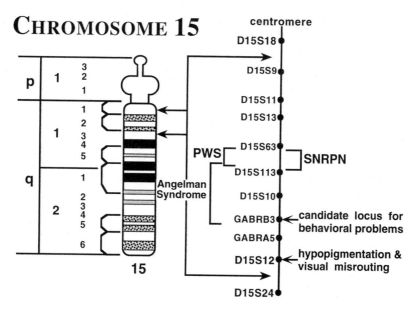

Figure 7.4 High-resolution chromosome 15 idiogram or drawing showing the chromosome bands and the numbers assigned to the band and to the chromosome breakpoints, designated by arrows at 15q11q13, leading to the 15q11q13 deletion commonly seen in Prader-Willi syndrome (PWS) patients. An expanded view of the 15q11q13 region with assigned locations of DNA loci or markers including known genes in the region. An approximate position for the gene(s) for PWS is shown in the drawing along with the location of *SNRPN*, a paternally expressed candidate gene for PWS. The approximate site designated the site of the gene(s) that cause Angelman syndrome, an entirely different clinical condition with a similar 15q11q13 deletion but of maternal origin. Other DNA loci that may cause additional features in both PWS or Angelman syndrome also are given.

The unremitting food searching and consumption often lead to behavior problems and other psychosocial dysfunction. Food-related behavior problems often become prominent at approximately age 4. Temper tantrums related to attempts to satisfy an insatiable appetite are common. Researchers and clinicians describe temper tantrums when food is denied (e.g., Bray et al., 1983), characterized as "rages" by Cassidy (1984). Holm (1981) reported that 74% of the sample of children and adults with Prader-Willi syndrome had "violent outbursts" related to obtaining food. This lack of satiety is complicated by the inability to vomit if they overeat or are ill. As a result, for a person with Prader-Willi syndrome to have uncontrolled access to food is unhealthy. These individuals can weigh 250 pounds or more by late teens if not controlled, and they generally are short in relationship to family background (Butler et al., 1989). They do not experience the growth spurt observed in the average adolescent. The average adult male subject is 155 centimeters or 61 inches tall, and 148 centimeters or 58 inches characterizes male subjects affected with the syndrome.

Additional problems during adolescence and adulthood include sleep disturbances and sleep apnea, which may correlate with the degree of obesity.

Scoliosis or curvature of the spine and osteoporosis also may occur, and these patients should be monitored for these findings and treated.

People with Prader-Willi syndrome may have 40% to 50% body fat, which is two or three times more than in normal individuals, whereas the lean body mass is lower than in normal individuals. A sex-reversed fatness pattern (i.e., male subjects having more fat than female subjects) also is observed (Meaney and Butler, 1989). The heaviest deposition of subcutaneous fat is in the truncal region and limbs.

Avoidance of physical exercise is widely described as a pervasive aspect of Prader-Willi syndrome (e.g., Greenswag, 1987; Schoeller et al., 1988; Hill et al., 1990). People with Prader-Willi syndrome not only need fewer calories to maintain their weight than do lean people; they require fewer calories for maintenance than do others who are equally obese (Cassidy, 1984). Schoeller et al. (1988) reported that even after weight loss, children with Prader-Willi syndrome could consume no more than an average of 60% of a typical diet and still maintain their weights. Early diagnosis and intervention with dietary restrictions, increased physical activity, and family counseling are needed to control the obesity and its life-threatening complications.

BEHAVIORAL AND COGNITIVE DEVELOPMENT

Childhood

Delayed motor milestones are seen by early childhood in most children with Prader-Willi syndrome. Infants with Prader-Willi syndrome typically sit independently at 11 to 12 months, crawl at 15 to 16 months, walk independently at 24 to 27 months, use their first word at 23 to 28 months, and have 10-word vocabularies at 38 to 39 months (Dunn et al., 1981; Butler et al., 1986; Greenswag, 1987). The delay in achieving motor milestones appears to be due in large part to slowed psychomotor development and not to excessive weight. Language appears to be the most delayed of the developmental milestones. Within children with Prader-Willi syndrome, an analysis of persons with chromosome 15 deletion as compared with nondeletion did not reveal significant differences in milestone attainment (Butler et al., 1986).

Perhaps one-half of children with Prader-Willi syndrome develop behavior problems (e.g., temper tantrums, stubbornness, depression) between 3 and 5 years of age, and these problems may be pronounced by late childhood and adolescence. Behavioral problems commonly are precipitated by withholding of food; however, increasing evidence indicates that many behavior problems may not be food-related. Controlling food intake, managing the obesity, and behavioral problems often are very difficult for parents. Hypopigmentation (particularly in those with the chromosome 15 deletion), speech articulation defects, eye problems (e.g., strabismus), and dental problems (e.g., enamel hypoplasia, cavities) are observed frequently.

Adolescence and Adulthood

Adolescents with Prader-Willi syndrome do not mature sexually as rapidly as their peers. External signs of adulthood, such as beard growth, underarm and pubic hair, and enlargement of breasts (in girls) may not be apparent or are delayed. Approximately one-third of appropriately aged female subjects with Prader-Willi syndrome have menstrual periods, although not regularly. Adolescent female subjects are unlikely to become pregnant, and male subjects with Prader-Willi syndrome do not produce sperm. Some female and male subjects have undergone hormone therapy with some success in developing secondary sexual characteristics. Typical adolescent rebelliousness often is exaggerated in these individuals, with a constant struggle with parents and other adults over access to food. People with Prader-Willi syndrome can eat large quantities of food at one sitting if undisturbed.

Emergence of Psychiatric Symptoms

The early literature on psychiatric symptoms in Prader-Willi syndrome relied heavily on anecdotal case reports using retrospective interviews and symptom questionnaires. These findings emphasize a variety of personality problems manifested as frequent temper tantrums, stubbornness, manipulative behavior, depression, emotional lability, arguing, worrying, compulsive behavior, skin picking, difficulty in adapting to new situations, difficulty in relating to peers, poor social relationships, low self-esteem, and difficulty in detecting social cues from other people (Hall & Smith, 1972, Hermann, 1981; Holm, 1981; Peri et al., 1984; Sulzbacher et al., 1981; Cassidy, 1984; Greenswag, 1987; Whitman & Accardo, 1987).

Several studies have included comparison groups. Turner and Ravacabu (1981) compared the maladaptive behavior of 10 institutionalized mentally retarded persons with Prader-Willi syndrome and 10 controls matched for age, gender, and intellectual level but not obesity status. The Prader-Willi syndrome subjects were more verbally aggressive, self-assaultive, and regressive but less sexually inappropriate than were the controls. Taylor and Caldwell (1983) compared Prader-Willi syndrome subjects and a group of intellectually similar, obese persons on part II (Maladaptive Behavior) of the American Association of Mental Deficiency Adaptive Behavior Scale. The subjects were significantly more self-abusive, exhibited less stereotyped behavior, and were less sexually aberrant than were the controls, although these latter differences did not reach the $P < .05$ confidence level.

Curfs et al. (1995) compared 28 children with Prader-Willi syndrome matched with regular schoolchildren on gender and age (but not intellectual level) using a Dutch translation of the California Child Q-set, a measure of behavior and personality characteristics. Children with Prader-Willi syndrome were significantly less agreeable, less conscientious, less open to new ideas and experiences, less motorically active, more irritable, and more dependent than were those in the comparison group. However, it is not clear to what degree the obtained findings were influenced by differences in functioning level and not Prader-Willi syndrome per se. The personality dimensions were not related systematically to the presence or absence of a 15q11q13 deletion. Recent studies have used objective behavior rating scales to describe the behavioral adaptation of people with Prader-Willi syndrome. (These studies are reviewed in detail in chapter 6.)

Cognitive Characteristics

Decreased intellectual functioning, or hypomentia, was among the four original defining characteristics of Prader-Willi syndrome (Prader et al., 1956; Dunn, 1968; Zellweger & Schneider, 1968). IQs have ranged from 12 to 100 in those studies in which individual test results or ranges have been reported (Zellweger & Schneider, 1968; Jancar, 1971; Hall & Smith, 1972; Crnic et al., 1980; Dunn et al., 1981; Butler et al., 1986; Dykens et al., 1992). The average IQ typically is in the mild range of mental retardation (55–70). The distribution includes very few cases within the average range of intelligence or profound range of mental retardation.

Variation in IQ results has been examined with regard to several correlates. For example, IQ has been correlated with chronological age (CA). Early reports suggested that IQ values declined with age in cross-sectional studies (Crnic et al., 1980) and longitudinal studies (Dunn et al., 1981). However, another study failed to find a decrease in IQ over time in either cross-sectional or longitudinal analyses (Dykens et al., 1992). On the contrary, test scores were remarkably similar over testing sessions 3 years apart for subjects ages 3 to 30 years.

Other correlates of IQ in this population include body weight and chromosomal factors. Crnic et al. (1980) reported that individuals with Prader-Willi syndrome who never were obese had IQs significantly higher (mean = 80.2) than those of Prader-Willi syndrome subjects who currently were obese (mean = 57.3) or had been obese and had lost weight while participating in a comprehensive weight management program at the University of Washington (mean = 59.9). Differences in the groups were not due to differences in parent education. However, as Dykens et al. (1992) pointed out, Crnic et al. (1980) did not account for variability in height of their subjects. The relation between obesity, assessed as body mass index, and IQ in 18 persons with Prader-Willi syndrome was $r = -0.21$ and statistically nonsignificant in their study. Butler et al. (1986) compared IQs of their patients on the basis of presence or absence of a chromosome 15 deletion and found that subjects with the deletion had IQs higher (mean = 69.6) than those in patients without the deletion (mean = 59.2). No previous study has determined whether gender accounts for variance in these scores.

Some consideration has been given to relative strengths and weaknesses in intellective or cognitive abilities among people with Prader-Willi syndrome. Typically, these analyses are based on psychological test profiles and include comparisons of verbal and performance portions of intelligence tests, variation in subtest scores, and styles of cognitive processing, such as the simultaneous and sequential scores from the Kaufman Assessment Battery for Children (KABC). Comparisons of verbal and performance portions of intelligence tests reveal that many people with Prader-Willi syndrome score significantly higher on the performance subtests (Curfs et al., 1991), but this has not been a universal finding (Gabel et al., 1986). Comparisons of Wechsler subtest scores reveals block design to be a significant strength for some subjects (Curfs et al., 1991) and suggests an ability to recognize and evaluate figural relations. Dykens et al. (1992), using the KABC, found significant weakness in sequential processing relative to simultaneous processing —a finding consistent with the view that people with Prader-Willi syndrome have strengths in tasks requiring the integration of stimuli in a spatial mode. Anecdotal reports of superior puzzle-solving ability in Prader-Willi syndrome patients also are consistent with this hypothesis (Holm, 1981).

Warren and Hunt (1981) compared cognitive capabilities of adults with Prader-Willi syndrome and controls matched on mental age and IQ. The Prader-Willi syndrome subjects had difficulty with short-term memory processing and lost more information from memory over time as compared with controls. Warren and Hunt speculated that stimulus encoding may be limited. No significant differences were found in long-term memory.

Gabel et al. (1986) compared children with Prader-Willi syndrome and controls matched for gender and CA. Prader-Willi syndrome subjects did not perform as well on an abbreviated form of the Wechsler Intelligence Scale for Children (Revised), Trails B, Symbol Digit, Porteus Mazes, Grooved Pegboard (one measure of motor impersistence), and the Talking Pen (a motor accuracy test) as compared with children with average intelligence test scores. The groups did not differ on Trails A (although the Prader-Willi syndrome group took nearly twice as long as nonretarded controls) and two measures of impersistence. Lack of appropriate controls of comparable intellectual ability render it impossible to determine whether differences observed are unique to Prader-Willi syndrome.

Branson (1981) reported that 52% of her sample of 21 children with Prader-Willi syndrome demonstrated language comprehension and production abilities commensurate with overall cognitive level. The remaining children had uneven receptive language (comprehension) profiles relative to their expressive (production) abilities. Seventeen of 21 children exhibited atypical speech-sound production skills, with considerable variability ranging from unintelligible speech in some cases to extremely subtle difficulties in others. These difficulties included nasal air emission, oral-motor difficulties, and other articulation deficits. Branson suggested a lack of common features in the speech and language abilities of children with Prader-Willi syndrome and recommended individualized assessment and therapy (where necessary). A study by Kleppe et al., (1990) revealed multiple articulation errors (dysarthria), reduced intelligibility, and delayed language skills (vocabulary, syntactical, and morphological abilities).

Academic Achievement

Early studies suggested that children with Prader-Willi syndrome may have concomitant learning disabilities, given their frequent placement in learning disabilities educational programs (Sulzbacher et al., 1981). Such placements apparently were based on the observed variability in relative skills and deficits in academic performance. Reading abilities were reported generally to be better developed than were arithmetic abilities. A subsequent analysis of 232 persons with Prader-Willi syndrome conducted by Greenswag (1987) found that 75% of the participants had received special education services. These persons typically performed at the sixth-grade level or lower in reading and the third-grade level or lower in mathematics. Still unclear, however, is the degree to which referral for special education services was based primarily on delayed cognitive functioning versus presentation of behavior problems (e.g., tantrums, food stealing, skin picking, and other self-injury).

Studies that included standardized achievement testing generally support the view that Prader-Willi syndrome subjects have reading scores somewhat higher than mathematics scores, although the magnitude of the differences is small (Taylor & Caldwell, 1983; Dykens et al., 1992). Contrary to the learning disabilities hypothesis, Taylor and Caldwell reported no differences in level of academic achievement between the Prader-Willi syndrome subjects and a comparison group of intellectually similar, obese persons. Moreover, the achievement test scores were fairly consistent with the intelligence scores. Dykens et al. (1992) reported among 21 adolescents and adults with Prader-Willi syndrome a significant difference in academic achievement sections of the KABC as compared with the sequential and simultaneous processing components of the test. However, the difference was due to the overall academic achievement scores being greater than the ability measures. Such findings raise questions concerning a learning disabilities description.

Adaptive Behavior

Very little formal assessment has been directed at adaptive behavior functioning in persons with Prader-Willi syndrome. Taylor (1988) reported AAMD Adaptive Behavior Scale (ABS) data from an unpublished study conducted by Taylor and Caldwell (1983). ABS scores of adults with Prader-Willi syndrome were compared with those of a group of intellectually similar, obese individuals without the syndrome. The only significant difference between the groups on part I of the ABS was in the physical development category, whereas the subjects with Prader-Willi syndrome had scores that were 34 percentile points below those of the control group.

In an attempt to establish the developmental profile of adaptive behavior in 21 adolescents and adults with Prader-Willi syndrome, Dykens et al. (1992) used the Vineland Adaptive Behavior Scales. Adaptive strengths were apparent for the group as a whole in daily living skills, and a relative weakness was seen in socialization, particularly in coping skills. Dykens et al. (1992) also reported that daily-living skills become more of a strength with increasing age. They suggested that the strengths in this area might be related to experience with food-oriented behaviors and accessibility to kitchen areas.

FOOD PREFERENCE, FOOD MOTIVATION, AND PUTATIVE NEUROCHEMICAL MECHANISMS

Several lines of evidence suggest that genetic material on chromosome 15 may alter synthesis, release, metabolism, binding, intrinsic activity, or reuptake of specific neurotransmitters or may alter the receptor numbers or distribution, involved in modulating hunger and satiation. Among the likely candidates are endogenous opioids and GABAergic or serotoninergic mechanisms. These same neurochemical systems are known to be involved in a variety of emotional and cognitive functions.

Possible Opioid Mechanisms and Feeding

Several lines of animal laboratory evidence implicate opiate brain mechanisms in feeding (Holtzman, 1974; Morley & Levine, 1985). Opioids stimulate short-term feeding, and opioid antagonists decrease food intake by laboratory animals (Sanger, 1981; Reid, 1985). Opioid receptor mechanisms appear to have selective effects on specific macroconstituent consumption, depending on food preferences. Marks-Kaufman (1982) found that though morphine had little effect on protein intake by rats, carbohydrate intake decreased and fat intake increased. Shor-Posner et al., (1986) found that increased preference for fats induced by morphine was observed only in food-deprived rats and found that food-satiated rats consumed more protein. Gosnell et al., (1990) found that morphine selectively increased fat consumption by fat-preferring rats and increased carbohydrate consumption by carbohydrate-preferring animals. In other words, opioid mechanisms primarily amplify the rewarding value of whatever food a given individual already prefers, while having little effect on consumption of other foods.

Other data specifically suggest that endogenous opioids may be involved in the eating disorder associated with Prader-Willi syndrome. Elevated cerebrospinal β-endorphin has been reported in Prader-Willi syndrome (Krotkiewski et al., 1983). On the basis of these and the foregoing observations, several investigators administered naloxone, a parenteral opiate antagonist, to people with Prader-Willi syndrome in an effort to reduce food intake. The results with naloxone have been inconsistent but generally not encouraging (Kyriakidews et al., 1980; Krotkiewski et al., 1983; Zipf & Berntson, 1987). Considering that naloxone's half-life in blocking the narcotic agonist effects is short, still unclear is whether opiate receptor blockade would have occurred long enough to reduce the feeding-inducing effect associated with endogenous opioid agonist binding. Zlotkin et al., (1986) administered the longer-acting opioid antagonist naltrexone to four adolescents with Prader-Willi syndrome and found no net reduction in calorie intake during an unrestricted eating period of 7 days. Zlotkin et al. noted that the duration of naltrexone treatment may have been too short to have been effective in reducing caloric intake. Assuming that individuals being treated with opioid antagonists had a long history of consuming high-carbohydrate and high-fat foods, they would not be expected to stop suddenly or markedly to reduce their consumption of such foods, even if their physiological or neurochemical preference were shifted. Possibly, the individual may have to consume repeatedly the previously highly preferred food over several occasions to discover that eating that food no longer is satisfying.

Possible Serotoninergic Mechanisms in Food Intake

That serotonin influences eating has been known for a very long time (Leibowitz, 1980; Silverston & Goodall, 1986; Garattini et al., 1988). Laboratory animal and human clinical evidence indicates that serotoninergic agonists and uptake blockers reduce food intake and lead to weight loss. Luo and Li (1990, 1991) found that fluoxetine, a serotoninergic agonist, selectively reduced consumption of a high-carbohydrate—low-protein diet. Kanarek et al., (1991) also found weight loss and food intake reduction by rats treated with fluoxetine, but the effects on a high-fat diet were greater than on a high-carbohydrate diet. Pijil et al. (1991) treated 23 healthy, nondepressed obese women with 60 mg/day of fluoxetine and, over a 2-week period, observed mean weight loss of 3.5 kg, as compared with a 0.5-kg weight gain for placebo-treated subjects. McGuirk and Silverston (1990) administered 60 mg/day of fluoxetine to healthy male subjects of normal body weight, and observed a 1.07 kg weight loss over 2 weeks as compared with an 0.15-kg gain for placebo-treated controls. Similar findings have been reported by other investigators in obese and nonobese people without cognitive handicaps (e.g., Levine et al., 1987, 1989). Dech and Budow (1991) treated a 17-year-old youth who had mild mental retardation and Prader-Willi syndrome with fluoxetine and reported a marked improvement in weight control and some improvement in other compulsive behavior. Selikowitz et al. (1990) treated 15 people who had Prader-Willi syndrome (average age, 27 years) for 6 weeks with another serotoninergic agonist, fenfluramine, and obtained significant weight loss and decreased food-related emotional behavior but no change in skin picking (a common feature of Prader-Willi syndrome).

Possible GABAergic Mechanisms in Feeding

Several genes that code for components of the GABA receptor are located in the 15q11q13 region and are deleted or disomic in individuals with Prader-Willi syndrome (Wagstaff et al., 1991). If, as a result, binding of GABA to GABA receptors is decreased, owing to a reduction in the presence of a subunit of the GABA receptor, a compensatory increase may occur in GABA release. Ebert et al., (1997) found elevated plasma levels of GABA in people with Prader-Willi syndrome as compared to age- and weight-matched controls. High densities of GABA-A receptors are found in the anterior and medial hypothalamus, and more modest levels are seen throughout the entire hypothalamic region (Wagstaff et al., 1991). As the ventromedial hypothalamus is a satiety center and the lateral hypothalamus is a hunger center (Wagstaff et al., 1991), a reasonable suspicion might be that alterations of the GABA-A receptor distributions in these regions may result in elevated GABA levels. Such alterations could reduce satiety or increase feeding (Dahir & Butler, 1991).

Evidence of Other Neurochemical and Neurohumoral Dysregulation in Prader-Willi Syndrome

Many appetite-regulating factors are involved in hunger and satiation, including cholecystokinin (cck), bombesin, gastrin-releasing peptide, insulin, pancreatic glucagon, glucagonlike peptide 1, calcitonin, neuropepide Y, satietin, ceruletide, leptin (Ob protein), pancreatic polypeptide, and several separate protein receptors in the brain. Some of these factors have been understudied in Prader-Willi syndrome subjects and in human obesity in general. Holland et al. (1993) studied behavioral, cognitive, and metabolic response to 1-hour food intake sessions in 13 adults with Prader-Willi syndrome and in 10 matched controls. Increases in plasma glucose levels were correlated inversely with changes in hunger ratings in the Prader-Willi syndrome group but not the control group. The increase seen in the serum cck levels during the meal in the Prader-Willi syndrome group was significantly greater than that in the controls, indicating that in Prader-Willi syndrome, failure of peripheral CCK release in response to food was not the explanation for the impaired satiety response.

Most of the findings seen in Prader-Willi syndrome (e.g., mental deficiency, hyperphagia, behavioral problems, hypogonadism) could result from brain abnormalities. However, computed tomography or magnetic resonance imaging brain scan has revealed no consistent brain abnormalities in patients with this syndrome (Butler, 1990).

Neuropsychiatric features seen in Prader-Willi syndrome patients include such obsessive-compulsive symptoms as excessive appetite, trichotillomania, pressured and loquacious speech, incessant skin picking, compulsive stealing, hoarding, and fears. Other behavioral disturbances are impulsivity and aggression ranging from agitated depression to acute psychosis. Understanding the nature of these behaviors and neuropsychiatric features will be an important step in improving the quality of life in these patients.

Sieg et al. (1991) performed single-photon emission computed tomography on two Prader-Willi syndrome patients and showed increased metabolism in the left frontal cortex and decreased metabolism in the temporal and parietal regions bilaterally in both patients. To confirm whether brain metabolic disturbances exist in Prader-Willi syndrome patients, Butler and Kessler (1992) performed brain positron emission tomography using 18F-labeled 2-fluorodeoxyglucose on one adult male and two adult female subjects with this diagnosis. Their brain glucose metabolism patterns were compared with those of normal adult subjects. Fifteen transaxial slices were obtained simultaneously with in-place resolution of 7 mm and an axial resolution of 8 mm. One of the patients (a 34-year-old white man) showed decreased metabolic activity in the anteroinferior portion of the temporal lobe, in the inferior frontal lobes, and in the basal ganglia bilaterally, compared with the cortex. The two adult women showed minor or no detectable metabolic disturbances in the brain, as compared with controls.

Brain electrical activity mapping (BEAM) was used by Sieg et al. (1992) to delineate the electrophysiological status of the brain in six Prader-Willi syndrome patients. Topographical surface distribution maps of electroencephalographic (EEG) frequency bands and evoked potential data provide a way to detect abnormalities that conventional methods may fail to identify. Topographical EEG frequency components generated from the six patients showed increased frontal delta activity in three patients and increased frontal theta activity in the remaining patients. Increased posterior alpha activity was observed in four subjects. Significant P300 abnormalities were observed in auditory evoked potentials in the subjects, with the most remarkable being increased bifrontal positivity. In four subjects, decreased bitemporal activity of the P300 also was observed. Overall, their results demonstrated consistent topographical EEG and auditory evoked potential P300 abnormalities. Increased frontal delta, frontal theta, and posterior alpha activity also have been reported in subjects with obsessive-compulsive disorder.

The BEAM techniques measure processes that critically affect CNS blood flow and metabolism. The new technology of functional magnetic resonance imaging should be helpful in monitoring blood flow to the regions of the brain that correlate with a metabolic active state of regions of the brain. Certain elements of chromosome 15 (15q11q13) region must have a role in CNS development, and motivation and abnormal gene expression appear to be the ultimate pathogenic substrate resulting in abnormal brain physiology and function in Prader-Willi syndrome.

The β_3-adrenergic receptor gene was proposed as another candidate gene for obesity. This receptor is considered a major factor in the regulation of metabolism. The loss of this gene in mice causes decreased metabolism, hypothermia, and excessive fat deposits. Characterizing this receptor gene in obese humans (including Prader-Willi syndrome) may lead to a better understanding of obesity. Studies of the resting metabolic rate in Prader-Willi syndrome subjects and similarly aged obese and nonobese controls indicate decreased metabolism in Prader-Willi syndrome subjects in relationship to their lean body mass (Hill et al., 1990). These studies further support a possible role of a gene that regulates metabolism, such as the β_3-adrenergic receptor gene in Prader Willi syndrome.

CHROMOSOME 15 LINK BETWEEN PRADER-WILLI SYNDROME AND OTHER CHROMOSOME 15 CONDITIONS

Chromosome 15 abnormalities also have been implicated in a variety of distinct phenotypes, separate or in conjunction with Prader-Willi syndrome or Angelman syndrome. Specifically, several patients with autistic characteristics, mental retardation, and seizures have been reported with an extra marker chromosome 15. In the majority of these patients, conventional and molecular cytogenetic studies confirmed the chromosomal origin of the extra supernumerary chromosome to be a duplicated region of chromosome 15 extending to at least the 15q13 band of the long arm of chromosome 15. DNA marker studies suggested a maternal origin of the extra duplicated chromosome 15 from the 15q11q13 region (Flejter et al., 1996).

Recently, obsessive-compulsive behavior has been reported as a common finding in Prader-Willi syndrome subjects, further supporting a major gene for this behavioral finding in chromosome 15q11q13 (Whitman & Accardo, 1987). Whether obsessive compulsive behavior is correlated with a specific genetic lesion or subtype (i.e., deletion, disomy, duplication) is not known at present. Interestingly, several genes have been reported in the 15q11q13 region other than the *SNRPN* gene and may be candidates for clinical findings associated with Prader-Willi syndrome, including the lack of inhibition, hyperphagia (possibly related to the GABA-A receptor subunit gene) and hypopigmentation (*p* gene or oculocutaneous albinism type II gene located at the D15S12 locus). Additional research is needed to correlate the phenotype with the genotype for both Prader-Willi syndrome and Angelman syndrome patients to delineate further the clinical variation seen in affected individuals and to compare with appropriately matched controls.

CONCLUSION

Parents of children with Prader-Willi syndrome describe their children as "trapped" in a food-oriented world, a life in which nearly every moment of every day revolves around a struggle to prevent the child from overeating (Well, 1988). Many families have concluded that placing their child with mild or moderate mental retardation in an institutional setting is the only alternative available to them, inappropriate as it is (Thompson et al., 1988).

Capable young women and men end up living in highly restrictive settings surrounded by people with severe and profound mental retardation and very severe behavior problems (violent aggression and self-injurious behavior). This is an unacceptable choice to be forced to make, but it is the only available alternative for many.

Possibly one or more of the abnormal metabolic or neurochemical processes involved in Prader-Willi syndrome may be shared with other eating disorders, such as forms of bulimia, anorexia nervosa, pica, or other types of genetically regulated obesity. As obesity is one of the major health problems facing the United States, any contribution to preventing these eating and weight-control problems could be a significant public health contribution.

Finally, emotional and behavior disorders associated with developmental disabilities account disproportionately for the cost of care of people with mental retardation in the United States. Destructive behavior is a burden on health care and on the educational and social service systems, to say nothing of the burden on the individuals and families involved. The eating disorder associated with Prader-Willi syndrome is related to specific genetically mediated neurochemical or metabolic problems. The same is likely to be true of other developmental disabilities commonly associated with self-injury and aggressive behavior (e.g., autism, de Lange syndrome, fragile X syndrome). Arriving at a more thorough understanding of Prader-Willi syndrome will provide a strategy that could serve as a model for understanding other genetically mediated behavior disorders associated with developmental disabilities.

ACKNOWLEDGMENTS

This research was supported in part by a program project grant PO1 HD 30329 from the National Institute of Child Health and Human Development to the John F. Kennedy Center of Vanderbilt University. This manuscript is based in part on an article written by Travis Thompson, Merlin G. Butler, William MacLean, and Beth Joseph—"Prader-Willi Syndrome: Genetics and Behavior"—which appeared in the *Peabody Journal of Education*, 1996, 71(4), 187.

REFERENCES

Angelman, H. (1965). "Puppet" children: A report on three cases. *Developmental Medical Child Neurology, 7,* 681–688.

Branson, C. (1981). Speech and language characteristics of children with Prader-Willi syndrome. In V. Holm, S. Sulzbacher, & P. Pipes (Eds.), *Prader-Willi syndrome.* Baltimore: University Park Press.

Bray, G. A., Dahms, W. T., Swerdloff, R. S., Fiser, R. H., Atkinson, R. L., & Carrel, R. E. (1983). The Prader-Willi syndrome: A study of 40 patients and a review of the literature. *Medicine, 62*(2), 59–80.

Buiting, K., Saitoh, S., Gross, S., Dittrich, B., Schwartz, S., Nicholls, R. D., & Horsthemke, B. (1995). Inherited microdeletions in the Angelman and Prader-Willi syndromes define an imprinting centre on human chromosome 15. *Nature Genetics, 9,* 395–400.

Butler, M. G. (1989). Hypopigmentation: A common feature of Prader-Labhart-Willi syndrome. *American Journal of Human Genetics, 45,* 140–146.

Butler, M. G. (1990). Prader-Willi syndrome: Current understanding of cause and diagnosis. *American Journal of Medical Genetics, 35,* 319–332.

Butler, M. G. (1994). Prader-Willi and Angelman syndromes: Examples of genetic imprinting in man. In P. K. Seth & S. Seth (Eds.), *Human Genetics: New Perspectives*: New Delhi, India: Omega Scientific Publishers.

Butler, M. G., Haynes, J. L., & Meaney, F. J. (1989). Intra-familial and midparental PWS child correlations and heritability estimates of anthropometric measurements in Prader-Willi syndrome families. *Dysmorphology and Clinical Genetics, 4,* 2–6.

Butler, M. G., & Kessler, R. M. (1992). Positron emission tomography of three adult patients with Prader-Willi syndrome. *Dysmorphology and Clinical Genetics, 6,* 30–31.

Butler, M. G., Meaney, F. J., & Palmer, C. G. (1986). Clinical and cytogenetic survey of 39 individuals with Prader-Labhart-Willi syndrome. *American Journal of Medical Genetics, 23,* 793–809.

Butler, M. G., & Palmer, C. G. (1983). Parental origin of chromosome 15 deletion in Prader-Willi syndrome. *Lancet, 1,* 1285–1286.

Cassidy, S. B. (1984). Prader-Willi syndrome. *Current Problems in Pediatrics, 14,* 1–55.

Crnic, K. A., Sulzbacher, S., Snow, J., & Holm, V. A. (1980). Preventing mental retardation associated with gross obesity in the Prader-Willi syndrome. *Pediatrics, 66,* 787–789.

Curfs, L. M. G., Hoondert, V., Van Lieshout, C. F. M., & Fryns, J.-P. (1995). Personality profiles of youngsters with Prader-Willi syndrome and youngsters attending regular schools. *Journal of Intellectual Disability Research, 39,* 241–248.

Curfs, L. M. G., Wiegers, A. M., Sommers, J. R. M., Borghgraef, M., & Fryns, J. P. (1991). Strengths and weaknesses in the cognitive profile of youngsters with Prader-Willi syndrome. *Clinical Genetics, 40,* 430–434.

Dahir, G. A., & Butler, M. G. (1991). Is GABA-A receptor B-3 subunit abnormality responsible for obesity in Prader-Willi syndrome individuals? *Dysmorphology and Clinical Genetics, 5,* 112–113.

Dech, B., & Budow, L. (1991). The use of fluoxetine in an adolescent with Prader-Willi syndrome. *Journal of American Academy of Child and Adolescent Psychiatry, 30,* 298–302.

Dunn, H. G. (1968). The Prader-Willi syndrome: Review of the literature and the report of nine cases. *Acta Pediatrica Scandinavia, Supplement, 186,* 1–38.

Dunn, H. G., Tze, W. J., Alisharan, R. M., & Sulzbacher, M. (1981). Clinical experience with 23 cases of Prader-Willi syndrome. In V. A. Holm, S. Sulzbacher, P. L. Pipes (Eds.), *Prader-Willi syndrome* (pp. 69–88). Baltimore: University Park Press.

Dykens, E. M., Hodapp, R. M., Walsh, K., & Nash, L. J. (1992). Profiles, correlates, and trajectories of intelligence in Prader-Willi syndrome. *Journal of the American Academy of Child and Adolescent Psychiatry, 31*(6), 1125–1130.

Ebert, M. H., Schmidt, D. E., Thompson, T., & Butler, M. G. (1997). Elevated plasma gamma-amino butyric acid (GABA) levels in individuals with Prader-Willi or Angelman syndromes. *Journal of Neuropsychiatry and Clinical Neuroscience, 9,* 75–80.

Flejter, W. L., Bennett-Baker, P. E., Ghaziuddin, M., McDonald, M., Sheldon, S., & Gorski, J. L. (1996). Cytogenetic and molecular analysis of inv dup(15) chromosomes observed in two patients with autistic disorder and mental retardation. *American Journal of Medical Genetics, 61,* 182–187.

Gabel, S., Tarter, R. E., Gavaler, J., Golden, W. L., Hegedus, A. M., & Maier, B. (1986). Neuropsychological capacity of Prader-Willi children: General and specific aspects of impairment. *Applied Research in Mental Retardation, 7,* 459–466.

Garattini, S., Bizzi, A., Caccia, S., Mennini, T., & Samanin, R. (1988). Progress in assessing the role of serotonin in the control of food intake. *Clinical Neuropharmacology, 11*(suppl.)1, 18–32.

Glenn, C. C., Saith, S., Jong, M. T. C., Filbrandt, M. M., Surti, U., Driscoll, D. J., & Nicholls, R. D. (1996). Gene structure, DNA methylation, and imprinted expression of the human SNRPN gene. *American Journal of Human Genetics, 58,* 335–346.

Gosnell, B. A., Krahn, D. D., & Majchrazak, M. J. (1990). The effects of morphine on diet selection are dependent upon baseline diet preferences. *Pharmacology, Biochemistry and Behavior, 37,* 207–212.

Greenswag, L. R. (1987). Adults with Prader-Willi syndrome: A survey of 232 cases. *Developmental Medicine and Child Neurology, 29,* 145–152.

Greenswag, L. R., & Alexander, R. C. (1995). *Management of Prader-Willi syndrome.* New York: Springer.

Hall, B. D., & Smith, D. W. (1972). Prader-Willi syndrome. *Journal of Pediatrics , 81,* 286–293.

Hermann, J. (1981). Implications of Prader-Willi syndrome for the individual and family. In V. A. Holm, J. J. Sulzbacher, & P. L. Pipes (Eds.), *Prader-Willi syndrome* (pp. 229–244). Baltimore: University Park Press.

Hill, J. O., Kaler, M., Spetalnick, B., Reed, G., & Butler, M. G. (1990). Resting metabolic rate in Prader-Willi syndrome. *Dysmorphic Clinical Genetics, 4,* 27–32.

Holland, A. J., Treasure, J., Coskeran, J., Dallow, J., Milton, N., & Hillhouse, E. (1993). Measurement of excessive appetite and metabolic changes in Prader-Willi syndrome. *International Journal of Obesity, 17,* 527–532.

Holm, V. A. (1981). The diagnosis of Prader-Willi syndrome. In V. A. Holm, S. Sulzbacher, P. L. Pipes (Eds.), *Prader-Willi syndrome* (pp. 27–44). Baltimore: University Park Press.

Holtzman, S. G. (1974). Behavioral effects of separate and combined administration of naloxone and D-amphetamine. *Journal of Pharmacology and Experimental Therapeutics, 189,* 51–60.

Jancar, J. (1971). Prader-Willi syndrome (hypotonia, obesity, hypogonadism, growth and mental retardation). *Journal of Mental Deficiency Research, 15,* 20–29.

Kanarek, R. B., Glick, A. L., & Marks-Kaufman, R. (1991). Dietary influences on the acute effects of anorectic drugs. *Physiology and Behavior, 49*(1), 149–152.

Kleppe, A. A., Katayama, K. M., Shipley, K. G., & Foushee, D. R. (1990). The speech & language characteristics of children with Prader-Willi syndrome. *Journal of Speech and Hearing Disorders, 55*(2), 300–309.

Krotkiewski, M., Fagerberg, B., Bjorntrop, P., & Terenius, L. (1983). Endorphines in genetic human obesity. *International Journal of Obesity, 7,* 595–598.

Kyriakidews, M., Silverston, T., Jeffcoate, W., & Laurence, B. (1980). Effect of naloxone on hyperphagia in Prader-Willi syndrome. *Lancet, 1*(8173), 876–877.

Ledbetter, D. H., Riccardi, V. M., Youngbloom, S. A., Strobel, R. J., Keenan, B. S., Crawford, J. D., & Louro, J. M. (1980). Deletion (15q) as a cause of the Prader-Willi syndrome (PWS). *American Journal of Human Genetics, 32*, 77A.

Leibowitz, S. F. (1980). Neurochemical systems of the hypothalamus in control of feeding and drinking behavior behavior and water and electrolyte excretions. In P. Morgane & J. Panskepp (Eds.), *Handbook of the hypothalamus* (pp. 299–243). New York: Decker.

Levine, L. R., Enas, G. G., Thompson, W. L., Byyny, R. L., Dauer, A. D., Kirby, R. W., Kreindler, T. G., Levy, B., Lukas, C. P., McIlwain, H. H., & Nelson, E. B. (1989). The use of fluoxetine, a selective serotonin-uptake inhibitor, in the treatment of obesity: A dose-response study. *International Journal of Obesity, 13*, 635–645.

Levine, K., Rosenblatt, R. & Bosomworth, C. (1987). Use of a serotonin re-uptake inhibitor, fluoxetine, in the treatment of obesity. *International Journal of Obesity, 11*(suppl.)3, 185–190.

Luo, & Li. (1990). Food intake and selection pattern of rats treated with dexfenfluramine, fluoxetine and RU 24969. *Brain Research Bulletin, 24*, 729–733.

Luo, & Li. (1991). Effects of repeated administration of serotonergic agonists on diet selection and body weight in rats. *Pharmacology Biochemistry and Behavior, 3*, 495–500.

Marks-Kaufman, R. (1982). Increased fat consumption induced by morphine administration in rats. *Pharmacology, Biochemistry and Behavior, 16*, 949–955.

Mascari, M. J., Gottlieb, W., Rogan, P. K., Butler, M. G., Weller, D. A., Armour, J. A. L., Jeffreys, A. J., Ladda, R. L., & Nicholls, R. D. (1992). The frequency of uniparental disomy in Prader-Willi syndrome: Implications for molecular diagnosis. *New England Journal of Medicine, 326*, 1599–1607.

McGuirk, J. & Silverston, S. (1990). The effect of the 5-HT re-uptake inhibitor fluoxetine on food intake and body weight in healthy male subjects. *International Journal of Obesity, 14*, 361–72.

Meaney, F. J., & Butler, M. G. (1989). Characterization of obesity in Prader-Labhart-Willi syndrome: Fatness patterning. *Medical Antrhropology Quarterly, 3*, 294–305.

Morley, J. E., & Levine, A. S. (1985). Pharmacology of eating behavior. *Annual Review of Pharmacology and Toxicology, 25*, 127–146.

Nicholls, R. D. (1994). New insights reveal complex mechanisms involved in genomic imprinting [editorial]. *American Journal of Human Genetics, 54*, 733–740.

Nicholls, R. D., Knoll, J. H. M., Butler, M. G., Karam, S., & Lalande, M. (1989). Genetic imprinting suggested by maternal heterodisomy in non-deletion Prader-Willi syndrome. *Nature, 342*, 281–285.

Ozcelik, T., Leff, S., Robinson, W., Donlan, T., Lalande, M., Sanjines, E., Schinzel, A., & Francke, U. (1992). Small nuclear ribonucleoprotein polypeptide N (SNRPN), an expressed gene in the Prader-Willi syndrome critical region. *Nature Genetics, 2*, 265–269.

Peri, G., Molinari, E., & DiBlasio, P. (1984). Psychological observations on patients with PWS. *Acta Medica Auxologica, 161*, 29–43.

Pijil, H., Koppeschaar, H. P., Willekens, F. L., Op-de-Kamp, I., & Velduis, H. D. (1991). Effect of serotonin re-uptake inhibition by fluoxetine on body weight and spontaneous food choice in obesity. *International Journal of Obesity, 15*, 237–242.

Prader, A., Labhart, A., & Willi, H. (1956). Ein Syndrome von Adipositas, Kleinwuchs, Kryptochismus und Oligophrenie nach myatonieartigem Zustand in Neugeborenenalter. *Schweizerische Medizinische Wochenschrift, 86*, 1260–1261.

Reid, L. D. (1985). Endogenous opioid peptides and regulation of drinking and feeding. *American Journal of Clinical Nutrition, 42,* 1099–1132.

Sanger, D. J. (1981). Endorphinergic mechanisms in the control of food and water intake. *Appetite, 2,* 193–208.

Schoeller, D. A., Levitsky, L. L., Bandini, L. G., Dietz, W. W., & Walczak, A. (1988). Energy expenditure and body composition in Prader-Willi syndrome. *Metabolism, 37,* 115–120.

Selikowitz, M., Sunman, J., Pendergast, A., & Wright, S. (1990). Fenfluramine in Prader-Willi syndrome: A double blind, placebo controlled trial. *Archives of Disease in Childhood, 65,* 112–114.

Shor-Posner, G. I., Azar, A. P., Filart, R., Tempel, D., & Leiboweitz, S. F. (1986). Morphine-stimulated feeding: Analysis of macronutrient selection and paraventricular nucleus lesions. *Pharmacology, Biochemistry and Behavior, 24,* 921–939.

Sieg, K. G., Gaffney, G. R., & Harty, J. R. (1992). Topographic EEG and auditory evoked potential P300 abnormalities in Prader-Willi syndrome. *Dysmorphology and Clinical Genetics, 6,* 31.

Sieg, K. G., Gaffney, G. R., Preston, D. F., & Erickson, H. M. (1991) SPECT brain imaging of Prader-Willi syndrome using technetium-99m-hexamethylpropylene-amine oxime. *American Journal of Medical Genetics, 41,* 529.

Silverston, I. E., & Goodall, E. (1986). Serotoninergic mechanisms in human feeding: The pharmacological evidence. *Appetite, 7*(suppl), 85–97.

Strakowski, S. M., & Butler, M. G. (1987). Paternal hydrocarbon exposure in Prader-Willi syndrome. *Lancet, 2,* 1458.

Sulzbacher, S., Crnic, K., & Snow, J. (1981). Behavioral and cognitive disabilities in Prader-Willi syndrome. In V. Holm, S. Sulzbacher, & P. Pipes (Eds.), *Prader-Willi syndrome.* Baltimore: University Park Press.

Taylor, R. L. (1988). Cognitive and behavioral characteristics. In M. L. Caldwell & R. L. Taylor (Eds.), *Prader-Willi syndrome.* New York: Springer.

Taylor, R., & Caldwell, M. L. (1983, November). Psychometric performances of handicapped obese individuals with and without Prader-Willi syndrome. Paper presented at the Meeting of the American Association on Mental Deficiency, Dallas, TX.

Thompson, D. G., Greenswag, L. R., & Eleazer, R. (1988). Residential programs for individuals with Prader-Willi syndrome. In L. R. Greenswag, & R. C. Alexander (Eds.), *Management of Prader-Willi syndrome* (pp. 205–222). New York: Springer.

Turner, R., & Ravakabu, R. H. A. (1981). A retrospective study of the behavior of Prader-Willi syndrome versus the institutionalized retarded person. In V. Holm, S. Sulzbacher, & P. Pipes (Eds.), *Prader-Willi syndrome.* Baltimore: University Park Press.

Wagstaff, J., Knoll, J. H. M., Fleming, J., Kikuess, E. F., Martin-Gallardo, A., Greenberg, F., Graham, J., Menninger, J., Ward, D., Venter, J. C., & Lalande, M. (1991). Localization of the gene encoding GABA-A receptor B3 subunit to the Angelman/Prader-Willi region of human chromosome 15. *American Journal of Human Genetics, 49,* 330–337.

Warren, J., & Hunt, E. (1981). Cognitive processing in children with Prader-Willi syndrome. In V. Holm, S. Sulzbacher, & P. Pipes (Eds.), *Prader-Willi syndrome.* Baltimore: University Park Press.

Wett, M. (1988). A national parent network: The Prader-Willi Syndrome Association. In L. R. Greenswag, & R. C. Alexander (Eds.), *Management of Prader-Willi syndrome* (pp. 223–230). New York: Springer.

Whitman, B., & Accardo, P. (1987). Emotional symptoms in Prader-Willi syndrome adolescents. *American Journal of Medical Genetics, 28,* 897–905.

Williams, C. A., Gray, B. A., Hendrickson, J. E., Stone, J. W., & Cantu, E. S. (1989). Incidence of 15q deletion in the Angelman syndrome: A survey of twelve affected persons. *American Journal of Medical Genetics, 32,* 339–345.

Zackowski, J. L., Nicholls, R. D., Gray, B. A., Bent-Williams, A., Gottlieb, W., Harris, P. J., Waters, M. F., Driscoll, D. J., Zori, R. T. & Williams, C. A. (1993). Cytogenetic and molecular analysis in Angelman syndrome. *American Journal of Medical Genetics, 46,* 7–11.

Zellweger, H., & Schneider, H. J. (1968). Syndrome of hypotonia-hypomentia-hypogonadism-obesity (HHHO) or Prader-Willi syndrome. *American Journal of Diseases of Children, 115,* 588–598.

Zipf, W. B., & Bernston, G. G. (1987). Characteristics of abnormal food-intake patterns in children with Prader-Willi syndrome and study of effects of naloxone. *American Journal of Clinical Nutrition, 46,* 277–281.

Zlotkin, S. H., Fettes, I. M., & Stallings, V. A. (1986). The effects of naltrexone, an oral β-endorphine antagonist, in children with Prader-Willi syndrome. *Journal of Clinical Endocrinology and Metabolism, 63*(5), 1229–1232.

8 Developmental Deficits in Children with Down Syndrome

Marian Sigman

One of the central questions asked about children with neurodevelopmental disorders is whether their development is simply delayed or actually is different from the development of normal children (Zigler & Balla, 1977; Weisz & Zigler, 1979). This question is conceptualized in terms of two different issues. The first issue concerns the extent to which the development of a particular diagnostic group of children follows a progression with age that is similar to the developmental progression of normal children. The second issue is whether development in different domains, such as cognition and affect or language, is parallel. To address the second issue, researchers compare the associations between different skills of the developmentally disabled children and typically developing children or match the two groups on a particular skill and determine whether they show equivalent abilities in another domain.

Several reasons suggest the importance of determining whether specific deficits are associated with particular syndromes. First, a precise depiction of the abilities and disabilities associated with a syndrome is crucial to understanding the functioning of individuals who suffer from this syndrome. This information allows us to know what difficulties the individual is likely to face, the extent to which these difficulties can be mastered, and alternative pathways that may be available to replace lines of development that are blocked. Such descriptions can be achieved only by using a developmental framework, as abilities and disabilities may change, depending on the child's stage of development.

The identification of specific deficits also may contribute to our understanding of the neurobiological and genetic substrates of the disorder. To the extent that psychological functions have been localized in particular cerebral areas, the identification of deficits and strengths may point to nervous system areas that are affected by the syndrome. In addition, the parallel identification of psychological, genetic, and cerebral abnormalities in a neurodevelopmental disorder may broaden our understanding of the relations between genetic factors and their brain and behavioral expressions. The investigation of neurodevelopmental disorders opens a window onto the associations between functional characteristics and neurogenetic factors, especially if behavioral and biological abnormalities are specific and limited.

For certain syndromes, the answer to the question of developmental delay or difference is very obvious. For example, autistic children show clear deficits in their development (Sigman & Capps, 1997). Their development does not follow the stages shown by normal children. They are far more knowledgeable about objects than about people, their perceptual and cognitive abilities outstrip their communicative capacities, and their understanding of other people is impaired regardless of their level of intellectual functioning. Developmental difference is manifested in both types of comparisons: first, comparisons of the associations between their various skills and those of normal individuals and, second, comparisons of mental age–matched individuals on social and communication skills. Children with other syndromes manifest this uneven pattern of development, although the areas of strength and weakness vary from one syndrome to the next. For example, children with Williams syndrome have strengths in language and weaknesses in perceptual skills.

The evidence regarding developmental delay versus difference is less clear in the case of children with Down syndrome. The extent to which the children are seen as developmentally delayed or deficient varies with the age of the child, the domains examined, and the manner in which one measures coherence of development. Thus, in the same volume on children with Down syndrome, one set of authors (Hodapp & Zigler, 1990) stresses the deficits of children with Down syndrome, whereas another set of authors (Cicchetti & Beeghly, 1990) stresses the similarities of developmental paths and integration across domains in children with Down syndrome and typically developing children.

The one area of development in which Down syndrome children and adults show obvious deficits is in expressive language (see Gibson, 1978; Chapman, 1995; Miller, 1987 for reviews). Individuals with Down syndrome converse in a very limited fashion. Many individuals with Down syndrome never acquire conversational skills that are more advanced than those shown by normal preschool children, even though their other cognitive abilities progress beyond this level (Fowler, 1990). Syntactical abilities seem particularly impaired in those individuals with enough language to manifest such disabilities. In younger or less developed individuals, lexical skill also are quite limited (Miller, 1988).

In an interesting series of studies, Mervis (Mervis, 1988, 1990) demonstrated that the conceptual and language development of young children with Down syndrome is both similar to and different from the conceptual and language development of young normal children. Like normal children, children with Down syndrome assume that a person pointing to an object is identifying the whole object rather than a part of the object. The first words acquired by children with Down syndrome are similar to those acquired initially by normal children. Finally, both groups of children form the same basic conceptual categories, which do not always correspond to the conceptual categories of adults (see also Tager-Flusberg, 1986). However, children with

Down syndrome acquire vocabulary more slowly than do normal children. Mervis (1988) suggested that the vocabulary spurt manifested by normal children occurs more slowly in children with Down syndrome. The deficit in semantic acquisition may be due to the limited information-processing and memory skills of children with Down syndrome and to caregiver styles of communication that are less than optimal for enhancing the language development of these children.

The research program reviewed in this chapter has investigated the social and communicative characteristics of children and caregivers, which may affect the early language acquisition of children with Down syndrome. We examined social behaviors, nonverbal communication, object use, and affect because of the theoretical and empirical links between such skills and normal language acquisition. Two major aims have been the focus of this research program. The first aim addressed the question of developmental deficit versus delay with comparisons of the behaviors and responses of children with Down syndrome and normal children matched for mental and language age. These studies, which are reviewed first in this chapter, have identified deficiencies in the children with Down syndrome in nonverbal communication, attention, and mastery behaviors but not in emotional responsiveness. The second aim was to identify correlates and predictors of language acquisition in children with Down syndrome. Both child abilities and caregiver behaviors were found to be associated with concurrent language abilities and with gains in language skills over the course of a year. The second part of this chapter discusses the findings of these correlational studies in the light of their significance for interventions.

COMPARISONS OF CHILDREN WITH DOWN SYNDROME AND NORMAL CHILDREN

Preverbal Communicative Skills

Well before they can speak, normally developing children learn ways to communicate with other people. To begin with, this communication is dyadic, involving the infant in an interchange with the caregiver with no outside point of reference. Starting in the second half of the first year, communication becomes triadic, so that another person or object becomes the subject of the communication. Communication at this age may involve requests or demands relative to the outside focus or may be a simple bid for shared attention to this object or other person.

The need to communicate manifested in the learning of appropriate gestures and of the skills that are learned seem to serve as prerequisites for the acquisition of verbal communicative capacities. A child who is either unmotivated or unable to use preverbal communicative gestures or responses may be less likely to learn language easily and quickly. Part of what drives the child's acquisition of language may be a desire to explore and master objects and experiences that are out of reach of the child and require adult assistance. Another part may be the desire to share these experiences with caregivers and familiar peers.

A fair amount of evidence suggests that young children with Down syndrome use nonverbal requests for objects or assistance with objects less frequently than do normal children of similar mental age. Deficits in nonverbal requesting behaviors have been identified in two different samples of children with Down syndrome in our laboratory (Mundy et al., 1988, 1995). These children were less likely to point to an object out of reach or to hand to an experimenter a wind-up toy that had wound down. The children did not outgrow this deficit: Children with both lower and higher mental ages exhibited less requesting of objects and assistance than did normal children. Similar results also were reported by Wetherby et al., (1989). In addition, children with Down syndrome have been found to use verbal requests less than do normal mental age–matched children during interactions with their mothers (Beeghly et al., 1990). However, not all studies of the nonverbal and verbal communicative behaviors of children with Down syndrome have identified a deficit in requesting (Greenwald and Leonard, 1979; Lobato et al., 1981; Smith and von Tetzchner,1986). If children with Down syndrome are less motivated or less able than normal children to request objects or experiences that are out of reach, this might partly account for their lag in expressive language.

In terms of nonverbal gestures aimed at promoting joint attention (also called *declarative gestures*) and responses to others' bids for joint attention, some studies show deficits in children with Down syndrome, whereas others do not. Our most recent analyses of the data from all the subjects whom we have studied do not reveal differences between children with Down syndrome and normal children in initiating or responding to joint attention (Sigman & Ruskin, unpublished manuscript), confirming the results of our first study (Mundy et al., 1988). Smith and von Tetzchner (1986) found that children with Down syndrome less frequently used a combined sound and gaze shift to get the adult to attend to an object did than normal children but used simpler joint attention behaviors quite frequently. Similarly, the study by Greenwald and Leonard (1979) found that the declarative aims of normal children were implemented more in the use of verbalizations and combined gestures and verbalizations than was true for the children with Down syndrome, who tended to resort solely to gestural communication. Thus, children with Down syndrome seem as likely to initiate shared attention with others. However, they use less advanced means to do so and may be less able to coordinate their attention with the attention of others, an issue discussed later.

Attention to People and Objects

In contrast to individuals in triadic interactions involving objects and other people, children with Down syndrome initiate dyadic interactions as much as other children of the same developmental level. In fact, in our first study, the children with Down syndrome engaged in more turn taking and made more invitations for social interaction to the experimenter than did the typically developing children. To understand this behavioral pattern more fully, Kasari et al. (1990) coded attention to the experimenter's face and hands and to the focal and nonfocal toys. Children with Down syndrome were more attentive than the normal children to the experimenter's face and less attentive to the toy that was out of reach.

These results confirm the findings from studies of younger children with Down syndrome (Berger & Cunningham, 1981; Gunn et al., 1982). In a study of 8- to 19-month-old children, Jones (1980) found that children with Down syndrome looked at their caregiver for longer periods than did normal children. Similarly, Landry and Chapieski (1989, 1990) reported that 12-month-old children with Down syndrome looked more to their caregivers than did a preterm control group. The cooccurrence of looking at the same object by the child and mother also was less for the children with Down syndrome than for the preterm control children.

These findings suggest that children with Down syndrome are more likely to attend to other people in situations in which normal children might look at objects. Several factors could account for this difference in behavior. First, the children with Down syndrome could have some difficulties in attending to stimuli and in shifting attention. This would explain the observation by Krakow and Kopp (1983) that children with Down syndrome were more likely to focus on toys that were near them and less at people who were sitting at some distance than was true for other mentally retarded children. Thus, some of the differences in findings between studies may result from different physical arrangements that make the objects or people more focal. In other words, as evidenced in the studies by Jones (1980) and Landry and Chaprieski (1989), children with Down syndrome may choose to look at certain objects because of the difficulties demonstrated by children with Down syndrome in shifting attention from people to objects.

Infants with Down syndrome look at stimuli for longer durations than do other infants, perhaps partly because of limitations in their ability to take in information and partly because of their hypotonia. Miranda and Fantz (1974) showed that children with Down syndrome showed less preference than did normal children for novel stimuli using a fixed familiarization time. Similarly, Cohen (1981) demonstrated slower habituation and less dishabituation to a novel stimulus in infants with Down syndrome than in normal infants. Recent studies using sonograms show that fetuses with Down syndrome habituate more slowly to sounds while in utero.

My own experience dramatically confirmed these research findings. In 1975, Coles and I conducted a study of eye-movement patterns during habituation of normal infants in Jerome Bruner's laboratory at Oxford (Coles & Sigman, 1987). We had a serious problem with losing data. Our recorder was very sensitive to the changes in the image of the back-lit pupil. Because the infants looked very briefly and kept moving around as they habituated, the recording device could not keep up with the variations in focus of the photographed image. At one point, Vicki Lewis, who was studying habituation patterns in infants with Down syndrome and was not experiencing difficulties with losing data, invited me to observe one of her testing sessions. When I saw the behavior of her subject, I could see why she was not having our problems. The infant with Down syndrome whom she was studying looked at the target stimulus for very long periods and hardly moved. His lack of restlessness and overly sustained attention was dramatic; he did not seem to habituate to an unchanging stimulus. Thus, some of the differences observed in the focus of attention of children with Down syndrome may stem from their limitations in cognition, attention, and motor control.

Social Referencing and Emotional Responsiveness

To understand the ways in which children with Down syndrome use their attention to gain information about the world, our second study included a number of paradigms designed to assess the issue directly. As part of this study, the social referencing of children with Down syndrome was observed when a small robot entered the room and the mother and experimenter showed either fear or joy (Kasari et al., 1995). As mentioned, joint attention behaviors were observed also in the more neutral play interaction with the experimenter. Although the children with Down syndrome showed no deficits in initiating joint attention during play (i.e. they alternated looks between the toy and experimenter with frequency equal to that in normal children), they shifted attention between the robot and the adult showing emotion much less frequently than did the nonhandicapped children. The children with Down syndrome looked for equal length of time at the person (either mother or experimenter) and the robot, whereas the nonhandicapped children looked at the robot for twice as long as at the person. In this situation, the robot and the adults were nearly equidistant from the subject.

The infrequency of gaze shifts between person and robot may be due to the attention limitations already discussed, except that no differences were observed in the more neutral play situation. An alternative explanation is that the children with Down syndrome may not understand that social referencing can be used for appraising situations. Normal children look at other people in ambiguous situations to make sense of the situations. For example, the normal infant will look at the mother when a stranger enters the room and then will either smile or frown, depending on the mother's facial expression. Children with Down syndrome may take longer to realize that they can use the facial expressions of others to guide their own reactions.

This raises the question of whether the children with Down syndrome understand the facial expressions of others (Kasari & Sigman, 1996). Assessing understanding of emotional expression is difficult in nonverbal children because the children cannot be asked to label facial expressions. For this reason, some studies have relied on measuring the affective responses of young children with Down syndrome to stimuli of varying emotional impact. Very young infants with Down syndrome tend to show less positive affect in interaction with caregivers than is true for normal infants (Cicchetti & Sroufe, 1978; Emde et al., 1978; Brooks-Gunn & Lewis, 1982). Fewer studies of this kind have been conducted with children with Down syndrome who are older than 1 year. However, the anthor's research group has conducted many studies in which Down syndrome children were part of a larger group of mentally retarded children. The children's attention, behavior, and affect in response to adults' show of distress, pleasure, fear, or anger were videotaped and coded. The responses of the mentally retarded children (ages approximately 3–5 years) were not very different from those of the normal group (Sigman et al., 1986, 1992). Moreover, in a study of the responses of children with Down syndrome to an experimenter pretending to have hurt her finger, children with Down syndrome appeared to be more distressed than did the normal children (Kasari et al., 1990). Thus, children with Down syndrome appear to be as responsive emotionally as are nonhandicapped children after the first year of life.

Emotional understanding can be assessed directly in older children who have the verbal abilities to label emotions. However, most studies have examined children with mental retardation without particular reference to Down syndrome. A recent study by Kasari et al., (1994) found that 4- to 6-year-old children with Down syndrome were as capable as were normal children (matched for mental age) of verbalizing, recognizing, and identifying emotions on a series of tasks employing puppets in situations chosen to depict affect-arousing events. Thus, the greater attention paid to the emotions of others in social referencing situations probably is not due to a lack of understanding of these emotions.

Preference for Social Interactions and Mastery Motivation

Another reason for the protracted attention to others in triadic situations might be that children with Down syndrome have a heightened interest in social interactions in comparison to object interactions. To test this directly, 40 children with Down syndrome and 25 normal subjects in our second study were presented with alternating toy situations and social situations during two testing sessions (Ruskin et al., 1994). The experimenter sat opposite the child at a small table, and toys were placed on a small shelf in view of the child. In the toy situations, the subjects were presented with commercially available toys whereas, in the social situations, the experimenter sang different songs in an animated fashion. Children with Down syndrome looked at the singing experimenter more than did the normal children, who were matched for mental and language age. In comparison to the control group, the children with Down syndrome were three times more likely to participate in singing the songs and twice as likely to reject the toy by pushing it away from themselves. The children with Down syndrome also smiled less than did the normal children during toy mastery.

These findings suggest that the children with Down syndrome are more interested in interacting with other people and less interested in interacting with toys than are normal children of the same mental and language age. However, matching the stimulus qualities of social and nonsocial stimuli is very difficult. Legerstee & Bowman (1989) reported that infants with Down syndrome did not differ in their interest in people and objects if the activity level of the people and objects was controlled. Therefore, the children with Down syndrome in this study may have preferred the social interactions because the experimenter was more active than were the toys. On the other hand, the difference in activity level did not affect the preferences of the normal children. These children were less interested in the experimenter and more interested in toys than were the children with Down syndrome, despite the higher activity level of the experimenter.

To investigate the object-focused behaviors of children with Down syndrome more fully, the videotapes were recoded to examine both high-level goal-directed mastery and lower-level object exploration, such as manipulating, examining, or banging the toys (Ruskin et al., 1994). The ratio of exploration to goal-directed mastery behaviors did not differ for the two groups. However, the typically developing children engaged in longer consecutive strings of goal-directed mastery behaviors than did the children with Down syndrome. Moreover, the normal children showed more positive affect while playing with the toys. The group difference was particularly strong for positive affect that cooccurred with goal-directed mastery. The normal children expressed much more pleasure during goal-directed mastery than during exploration, whereas the children with Down syndrome were equally positive during both activities.

Overall, 2- to 3-year-old children with Down syndrome were less interested in mastering objects, although they were able to generate as many mastery behaviors as normal children. In contrast, 6- to 12-month-old infants with Down syndrome used less effective means to explore objects, but their total mastery behavior did not differ from that of control subjects (Vietze et al., 1983; MacTurk et al., 1985). This developmental difference from the first year to the subsequent years is similar to the difference reported for affective engagement. In characterizing the behaviors and reactions of children with Down syndrome, developmental stage clearly is an important determinant.

Associations Between Requesting Behaviors, Focus of Attention, and Task Mastery

To summarize, children with Down syndrome aged between 2 and 4 years seem very different from normal children matched on developmental level in several ways. First, they are less likely to request objects or assistance with objects. Second, their attention is directed differently. In contrast to normal children, they look more at the faces of other people and less at objects, coordinate attention to objects with others less, and alternate looks between ambiguous objects and people less. Finally, they seem relatively uninterested in mastering objects and more interested in social engagements.

One issue is the universality of these deficits in the Down syndrome group. If a small subgroup of children with Down syndrome is accounting for all these results, strong intercorrelations should be seen between the behaviors measured. Some children with Down syndrome might request objects infrequently because they were uninterested in mastering these objects, or they might be so involved in social interactions with a partner that they might not care much whether a wind-up toy was activated. Although we have not investigated associations among all these behaviors, a great deal of overlap is not apparent in those characteristics that have been examined. The shared variance between the frequency of requesting behaviors and any of the task mastery behaviors was only some 5%. Similarly, whereas children with Down syndrome who looked for long durations at the experimenter's face tended to request objects less, the correlation did not reach significance ($r(13) = -0.46$). Given the limited overlap in behaviors, the deficits do not seem confined to just a subgroup of the children with Down syndrome.

THE UNIQUENESS OF THE DEVELOPMENTAL DEFICITS OF CHILDREN WITH DOWN SYNDROME

The preceding discussion suggests that the development of attention, nonverbal communication, and interest in inanimate objects and task mastery is fundamentally different in children with Down syndrome and normal children. Thus, the evidence supports the notion that Down syndrome involves some forms of developmental difference and delay. At the same time, the evidence does not prove that these developmental differences are unique to Down syndrome.

The only way to determine whether a developmental deficit is unique to a syndrome is to compare the skills of children with that syndrome with the skills of children who suffer from other syndromes. Without such evidence, differences between children with a neurodevelopmental disorder and normal children may be a consequence of some other factor, such as mental retardation or experiences involved in having a neurological deficit. As in autism, the evidence shows not only that children with autism differ from normal children in joint attention but that they differ from children with Down syndrome and from children with other forms of developmental delays and learning disabilities. The uniqueness of deficits in children with Down syndrome has been addressed infrequently because of the difficulty of locating enough children with other disorders at the same chronological age. Children with Down syndrome undergo diagnosis earlier than children with other forms of developmental delay, except for children with severe motor problems that limit the extent to which they can be assessed.

Because our research group has been studying young children with autism, Down syndrome, and other forms of developmental delay for close to 20 years, we now have sufficient data to compare all these children to normally developing children. This comparison shows that all the developmentally delayed groups initiate behavior regulation less than do the normal children. Moreover, the children with Down syndrome initiate behavior regulation as frequently as do the developmentally delayed and autistic children. Thus, the deficit in behavior regulation appears to characterize all mentally retarded children rather than being unique to children with Down syndrome.

We do not have similar data on attention and task mastery, so we do not know whether the deficits discussed are unique to Down syndrome or characterize children with other neurodevelopmental disorders. However, our impression from studies of high-risk and disabled children is that both attention and task mastery generally are impaired as a function of developmental delay.

NONVERBAL BEHAVIORS AS CORRELATES AND PREDICTORS OF LANGUAGE SKILLS

As discussed at the outset of this chapter, deficits in nonverbal communication behaviors are particularly interesting because of the hypothesized associations between nonverbal and verbal communicative skills. Children with deficits in nonverbal communication are expected to have problems with verbal communication. In fact, the frequency with which children with Down syndrome initiate joint attention and social interaction predict gains in expressive language skills over the course of a year (Sigman & Ruskin, unpublished manuscript). Moreover, a trend is seen in the frequency of requesting behaviors for predicting gain in expressive language skills, a finding that corroborates earlier results reported by Smith and Von Tetzchner (1986). They found a predictive association between requesting behaviors and expressive language in a sample of 24-month-old Norwegian children who had Down syndrome and whose language was assessed 1 year later.

Nonverbal communication skills reflected in initiating joint attention and requesting may be particularly crucial for the earliest form of language acquisition, the use of holophrastic or one-word speech, rather than for the elaboration of more complex language skills. Evidence for this is that in our first study, which had a more cognitively advanced sample than did our second study, relations between nonverbal and verbal communication skills only held for the low mental age subjects, who tended to have either no expressive language or used one-word speech. In the second study, with a less advanced sample, the associations held for the entire sample.

Expressive language skills also were predicted by particular patterns of attention and affect shown by the children with Down syndrome. Children who looked less at the experimenter, referenced ambiguous objects more, had longer consecutive strings of goal-directed behavior, and showed more positive affect both to people and to toys that were being mastered had expressive language scores concurrently and predictively higher than those of children who showed less of these behaviors. Thus, children with Down syndrome are more likely to begin to speak if they show interest in objects and discriminating attention to people. Like nonverbal communicative gestures, these behaviors tend to be associated with early language acquisition rather than with gains in language after the one-word period.

CAREGIVER-CHILD INTERACTION AND LANGUAGE GAINS

The caregiving environment of the child may be the place to look for gains in the more advanced language capacities of children with Down syndrome. Caregivers of children with Down syndrome appear to communicate differently from caregivers of normal children (Beeghly et al., 1984; Miller, 1987). Caregivers of children with Down syndrome have been reported to give more directives and to be less responsive to the verbal input of their children. As an example, Mervis (1990) has shown that mothers of children with Down syndrome focus on their children, using words that are appropriate for adult conceptual categories, more frequently than do mothers of normal children who tend to accept the early use of words to fit child categories. Thus, one mother continued correcting her Down syndrome child's use of the word *kitty* to refer to a picture of a tiger, a correction made much less frequently by mothers of normal children.

To identify communicative characteristics of mothers of children with Down syndrome, mother-child play patterns were observed in each of our two studies. In the first study, mother-child interaction was videotaped during a 12-min play session (Kasari et al., 1990). The session began with a 4-min free play episode followed by four 2-min episodes of doll play, puzzle play, social game, and cleanup. Children's nonverbal communicative gestures were observed and coded. Mothers' responsiveness to these bids, frequency of positive statements, and the duration of mutual play also were coded. In addition, the frequency with which mothers either indicated an object by pointing or showing or requested an object or assistance was recorded. The mothers of children with Down syndrome were equally or more responsive than were the mothers of typically developing children. Mothers in both groups were very responsive to communicative acts by their children, rarely failing to respond to either nonverbal or verbal bids. Mothers of the low-mental-age children with Down syndrome made more positive comments to their children and requested objects or assistance with objects more often than did the mothers of children in any of the other three groups.

Some maternal behaviors were associated with the nonverbal and verbal communicative abilities of their children. Mutual play between caregiver and child was more protracted with children who had higher nonverbal communicative and receptive language skills. Mothers tended to request objects and assistance more frequently from children of lower abilities. The associations between maternal and child behaviors seemed quite general and equally likely to reflect the child's influence on the mother as was the mother's influence on the child.

In our second study, Kasari and Harris (Harris et al., 1996) designed a behavioral coding system aimed at assessing the amount of shared attention between the caregiver and child, the extent to which the caregiver or child selects the topic of shared attention, and whether the caregiver maintains or changes the topic. This coding system was based on those used in several previous studies by other investigators (Tomasello & Farrar, 1986; Tannock, 1988; Landry & Chapieski, 1989). Children and their mothers were videotaped during a 5-min free-play situation, and this coding system was applied to the videotaped observations. In both groups, children selected the topics of shared attention more than did caregivers. Caregivers maintained and redirected attention to the child-selected topic about equally, but they maintained attention to a topic that they had selected more than they redirected. Children with Down syndrome and their caregivers spent more time sharing attention to an object than did normal children and their caregivers. Overall, caregivers of children with Down syndrome maintained attention to topics more than did caregivers of normal children, although the difference between groups was significant only for caregiver selected topics.

The amount of shared attention and extent to which the caregiver maintained attention to topics were predictive of receptive language gains for both groups of children 1 year later. The extent to which the caregiver followed the child's lead in topic selection seemed more important for the children with Down syndrome than for the normal children. Gains in receptive language were predicted only by the extent of caregiver maintenance of *child-selected* topics for the Down syndrome group. The amount of variance in language gains accounted for by this caregiver behavior was considerable. For the normal, only the predictive relation between maintenance of *caregiver-selected* topics and language gains was significant, although a nonsignificant trend was seen in the association between maintenance of child-selected topics and language gains. In line with this, redirecting the child's attention seemed particularly deleterious to the language development of the children with Down syndrome.

The gains were significant for both groups only in language comprehension, not in the productive use of language. This was true as well for predictions of language gains from the amount of shared attention between caregiver and children; the only significant associations were with language comprehension. Interpretation of this finding is complicated by the fact that the associations of caregiver characteristics with language comprehension and production are not all that different in magnitude.

To summarize, caregivers of children with Down syndrome seemed to be nearly as skillful in communicating with their children as were caregivers of normal children. Some of the differences in findings between our results and those of other studies may stem from the caregiver behaviors investigated. As an example, Mervis (1990) reported differences in the extent to which the caregivers stressed the use of mature conceptual categories, a factor not examined in this study. However, the results of our study indicate that some caregivers of Down syndrome are very skillful language facilitators, at least in the ways that we have measured.

Caregiver behaviors do seem to be important predictors of language development in these children. Caregivers who are sensitive to the problems in attention shifting discussed earlier seem to be most successful in enhancing the language development of their children. Accepting the child's selection of a topic and maintaining this topic appears to be particularly crucial for the conceptual and language development of children with Down syndrome.

CONCLUSION

In summary, children with Down syndrome appear to show developmental differences, not merely delays, in the kinds of gestural communication, attention, and mastery behaviors that typically appear in the preverbal period of development. Their communicative development does not follow the same course as that of normal children. At an age when they are able to initiate joint attention, they are less likely to request objects or assistance with objects. In comparison to normal children, their attention is more focused on people and less on objects, and they show less interest and pleasure in mastery. Within the Down syndrome groups, children who show more serious deficits in these areas are less able to understand and use language and are likely to make smaller gains in language over time.

The extent to which these deficits in requesting, attention, and mastery behavior are maintained as the children grow up has not been addressed. These deficits may be short-lived and confined only to the early years of life even if they have indirect consequences for language acquisition. Research is needed that investigates the presence of such deficits in school-age children and adolescents with Down syndrome.

As mentioned, language acquisition seems particularly tied to the development of communicative capacities and interests of these children. However, some plasticity seems evident in that environmental factors can shape the children's understanding of verbal concepts. Caregivers who are sensitive to the limitations of their children with regard to attention to objects are able to advance the language comprehension of these children. Clearly, the specific deficits of children with Down syndrome are less dramatic than are those of children with other developmental disorders, such as autism and Williams syndrome. Differences between behaviors in children with Down syndrome and those in control children are smaller and vary considerably within the group of children with Down syndrome as regards the severity of specific deficits. On the other hand, deficits in language development are more significant. For example, in our second study, the mean language age of the children with Down syndrome advanced only 4 to 5 months over the course of a year, whereas their overall mental age gained 8 months. Given this serious deficit in language development, the identification of child and caregiver characteristics that may influence language learning remains a very important goal for research.

ACKNOWLEDGMENT

The research reported in this chapter was supported by grant HD17662 from the National Institute of Child Health and Human Development. Connie Kasari, Ph.D., Peter Mundy, Ph.D., Ellen Ruskin, Ph.D, and Nurit Yirmiya, Ph.D. contributed to this research. This chapter is dedicated to the memory of Joanne (Nan) Krakow, Ph.D., among whose many accomplishments was her research on the development of young children with Down syndrome.

REFERENCES

Beeghly, M., Weiss, B., & Cicchetti, D. (1984, April). *Structure and style of free play behavior in Down syndrome and non-handicapped children.* Paper presented at the International Conference on Infant Studies, New York.

Beeghly, M., Weiss-Perry, B., & Cicchetti, D. (1990). Beyond sensorimotor functioning: Early communicative and play development of children with Down syndrome. In D. Cicchetti & M. Beeghly (Eds.), *Children with Down syndrome: A developmental perspective* (pp. 329–368). New York: Cambridge University Press.

Berger, J., & Cunningham, C. (1981). The development of eye contact between mothers and normal versus Down's syndrome infants. *Developmental Psychology, 17,* 678–689.

Brooks-Gunn, J., & Lewis, M. (1982). Affective exchanges between normal and handicapped infants and their mothers. In T. Field & A. Fogel (Eds.), *Emotion and early interaction* (pp. 161–212). Hillsdale, NJ: Erlbaum.

Chapman, R. (1995). Language development in children and adolescents with Down syndrome. In P. Fletcher & B. MacWhinney (Eds.), *The handbook of child language* (pp. 641–663). Oxford: Blackwell.

Cicchetti, D., & Beeghly, M. (1990). An organizational approach to the study of Down syndrome: Contributions to an integrative theory of development. In D. Cicchetti & M. Beeghly (Eds.), *Children with Down syndrome: A developmental perspective* (pp. 29–62). Cambridge: Cambridge University Press.

Cicchetti, D., & Sroufe, L. A. (1978). An organizational view of affect: Illustrations from the study of Down's syndrome infants. In M. Lewis & L. A. Rosenblum (Eds.), *The development of affect.* New York: Plenum.

Cohen, L. B. (1981). Examination of habituation as a measure of aberrant infant development. In S. L. Friedman & M. Sigman (Eds.), *Preterm birth and psychological development* (pp. 241–253). New York: Academic Press.

Coles, P., & Sigman, M. (1987). Infant saccadic eye movement during habituation to a geometric pattern. In J. K. O'Regan & A. Levy-Schoen (Eds.), *Eye movements: From physiology to cognition.* New York: North Holland/Elsevier.

Emde, R., Katz, E., & Thorpe, J. (1978). Emotional expression in infancy: II. Early deviations in Down's syndrome. In M. Lewis & L. A. Rosenblum (Eds.), *The development of affect* (pp. 351–360). New York: Plenum.

Fowler, A. (1990). Language abilities in children with Down syndrome: Evidence for a specific syntactic delay. In D. Cicchetti & M. Beeghly (Eds.), *Children with Down syndrome: A developmental perspective* (pp. 302–328). Cambridge: Cambridge University Press.

Gibson, D. (1978). *Down's syndrome: The psychology of mongolism.* Cambridge: Cambridge University Press.

Greenwald, C. A., & Leonard, L. B. (1979). Communicative and sensorimotor development of Down's syndrome children. *American Journal of Mental Deficiency, 84,* 296–303.

Gunn, P., Berry, P., & Andrews, R. (1982). Looking behavior of Down syndrome infants. *American Journal of Mental Deficiency, 87,* 344–347.

Harris, S., Kasari, C., & Sigman, M. (1996). Joint attention and language gains in children with Down syndrome. *American Journal on Mental Retardation 100,* 608–619.

Hodapp, R. M., & Zigler, E. (1990). Applying the developmental perspective to individuals with Down syndrome. In D. Ciccetti & M. Beeghly (Eds.), *Children with Down syndrome: A developmental perspective* (pp. 1–28). Cambridge: Cambridge University Press.

Jones, O. L. M. (1980). Prelinguistic communication skills in Down's syndrome and normal infants. In T. Field (Ed.), *High-risk infants and children: Adult and peer interactions* (pp. 205–225). New York: Academic.

Kasari, C., Freeman, S., Mundy, P., & Sigman, M. (1995). Attention regulation by children with Down syndrome: Coordinated joint attention and social referencing. *American Journal on Mental Retardation, 100,* 128–136.

Kasari, C., Hughes, M., & Freeman, S. (1994, June). *Emotion recognition in children with Down syndrome.* Paper presented at the International Conference on Behavioral Development, Amsterdam.

Kasari, C., Mundy, P., & Sigman, M. (1990, April). *Empathy in toddlers with Down syndrome.* Paper presented at the Society for Research in Child Development, Seattle, WA.

Kasari, C., Mundy, P., Yirmiya, N., & Sigman, M. (1990). Affect and attention in children with Down syndrome. *American Journal on Mental Retardation, 95*(1), 55–67.

Kasari, C., & Sigman, M. (1996). Expression and understanding of emotion in atypical development: Autism and Down syndrome. In M. Lewis & C. Sullivan (Eds.), *Emotional Development in Atypical Children* (pp. 109–130). Hillsdale, NJ: Erlbaum.

Krakow, J. B., & Kopp, C. B. (1983). The effects of developmental delay on sustained attention in young children. *Child Development, 54,* 1143–1155.

Landry, S. H., & Chapieski, M. L. (1989). Joint attention and infant toy exploration: Effects of Down syndrome and prematurity. *Child Development, 60,* 103–118.

Landry, S. H., & Chapieski, M. L. (1990). Joint attention of six-month-old Down syndrome and preterm infants: I. Attention to toys and mother. *American Journal on Mental Retardation, 94,* 488–498.

Legerstee, M., & Bowman, T. G. (1989). The development of responses to people and toys in infants with Down syndrome. *Infant Behavior and Development, 12,* 465–477.

Lobato, D., Barrera, R. D., & Feldman, R. S. (1981). Sensorimotor functioning and prelinguistic communication of severely and profoundly retarded individuals. *American Journal of Mental Deficiency, 85,* 489–494.

MacTurk, R. H., Vietze, P. M., McCarthy, M. E., McQuiston, A. T., & Yarrow, L. J. (1985). The organization of exploratory behavior in Down syndrome and nondelayed infants. *Child Development, 56,* 573–581.

Mervis, C. B. (1988). Early lexical development: Theory and application. In L. Nadel (Ed.), *The psychobiology of Down syndrome* (pp. 101–143). Cambridge: MIT Press.

Mervis, C. B. (1990). Early conceptual development of children with Down syndrome. In D. Cicchetti & M. Beeghly (Eds.), *Children with Down syndrome: A developmental perspective* (pp. 252–301). Cambridge: Cambridge University Press.

Miller, J. F. (1987). Language and communication characteristics of children with Down syndrome. In S. Paschel, C. Tingey, J. Rynders, A. Crocker, & C. Crutcher (Eds.), *New perspectives on Down syndrome* (pp. 233–262). Baltimore: Brooks Publishing.

Miller, J. F. (1988). The developmental asynchrony of language development in children with Down syndrome. In L. Nadel (Ed.), *The psychobiology of Down syndrome* (pp. 167–198). Cambridge: MIT Press.

Miranda, S. B., & Fantz, R. L. (1974). Recognition memory in Down's syndrome and normal infants. *Child Development, 54,* 1168–1175.

Mundy, P., Kasari, C., Sigman, M., & Ruskin, E. (1995). Nonverbal communication and early language acquisition in children with Down syndrome and in normally developing children. *Journal of Speech and Hearing Research, 38,* 154–167.

Mundy, P., Sigman, M., Kasari, C., & Yirmiya, N. (1988). Nonverbal communication skills in Down syndrome children. *Child Development, 59,* 235–249.

Ruskin, E., Kasari, C., Mundy, P., & Sigman, M. (1994). Attention to people and toys during social and object mastery in children with Down syndrome. *American Journal on Mental Retardation, 99*(1), 103–111.

Ruskin, E., Mundy, P., Kasari, C., & Sigman, M. (1994). Object mastery motivation of children with Down syndrome. *American Journal on Mental Retardation, 98*(4), 499–509.

Sigman, M., & Capps, L. (1997). *Children with autism; A developmental perspective.* Cambridge: Harvard University Press.

Sigman, M., Kasari, C., Kwon, J. H., & Yirmiya, N. (1992). Responses to the negative emotions of others by autistic, mentally retarded and normal children. *Child Development, 63,* 796–807.

Sigman, M., Mundy, P., Sherman, T., & Ungerer, J. (1986). Social interactions of autistic, mentally retarded and normal children and their caregivers. *Journal of Child Psychology and Psychiatry, 27,* 647–655.

Smith, L., & von Tetzchner, S. (1986). Communicative, sensorimotor, and language skills of young children with Down syndrome. *American Journal of Mental Deficiency, 91,* 57–66.

Tager-Flusberg, H. (1986). Constraints on the representation of word meaning: Evidence from autistic and mentally retarded children. In M. Barrett & S. A. I. Kuczaj (Eds.), *The development of word meaning* (pp. 69–81). New York: Springer.

Tannock, R. (1988). Mothers' directiveness in their interactions with their children with and without Down syndrome. *American Journal of Mental Retardation, 93,* 154–165.

Tomasello, M., & Farrar, M. J. (1986). Joint attention and early language. *Child Development, 57,* 1454–1463.

Vietze, P. M., McCarthy, M., McQuiston, S., MacTurk, R., & Yarrow, L. (1983). Attention and exploratory behavior in infants with Down syndrome. In T. Field & A. Sostek (Eds.), *Infants born at risk: Physiological, perceptual, and cognitive processes* (pp. 251–268). New York: Grune & Stratton.

Weisz, J., & Zigler, E. (1979). Cognitive development in retarded and nonretarded persons: Piagetian tests of the similar sequence hypothesis. *Psychological Bulletin, 90,* 153–178.

Wetherby, A., Yonclas, D., & Bryan, A. (1989). Communication profiles of preschool children with handicaps: Implications for early identification. *Journal of Speech and Hearing Disorders, 31,* 148–158.

Zigler, E., & Balla, D. (1977). Personality factors in the performance of the retarded. *Journal of the American Academy of Child Psychiatry, 16,* 19–27.

9 Down Syndrome in Cognitive Neuroscience Perspective

Lynn Nadel

In the past, the study of normal cognitive development has been greatly enriched by the careful examination of select cases of abnormal development. Following a tradition established in the nineteenth century in the study of language and other cognitive functions, psychologists have sought insight into the maturation of specific abilities through the study of infants and children whose development is distorted by a variety of genetic, epigenetic, or experience-driven abnormalities. In recent years, this approach has benefited from knowledge provided by new methods in both molecular and systems neuroscience. As a consequence, a field of study most properly termed *developmental cognitive neuroscience* is now emerging, bringing together the expertise of developmental psychologists, neuropsychologists, and developmental neuroscientists. This field offers the promise of shedding light on normal and abnormal development of both mind and brain. Thoughtful analysis of the consequences of abnormal development, and its neural underpinnings, should lead to new insights about normal mind-brain relations. Equally important, such analyses could lead to treatment and prevention approaches that were unimaginable as recently as a decade ago. In this regard, work is desirable on as large a variety of developmental syndromes as possible, because each syndrome brings to the field its own special issues and possibilities.

Down syndrome is characterized by several unique features that make it an excellent model case. It is perhaps the most prevalent neurodevelopmental disorder, occurring in approximately 1 of 800 live births throughout the world. In nearly all infants affected with Down syndrome, the etiology and date of onset of the syndrome are known: A third chromosome 21 is present from the moment of conception. The exceptions involve individuals with limited triplication of only parts of chromosome 21, referred to as *mosaics*, or *translocations*. These patients account for approximately 5% of the total cases and can be readily identified cytogenetically. This group offers a unique study population within which one can look at the implications of triplication of only specific segments of chromosome 21. Notwithstanding the common starting point for those with trisomy 21, the range of outcomes in individuals with Down syndrome is astounding. Thus, Down syndrome offers a case study in the variability with which genotypes are translated into phenotypes.

Finally, individuals with Down syndrome probably comprise the majority of infants and children with *mental retardation*. However, in contrast to what used to be assumed, this retardation is *not* an across-the-board phenomenon; it manifests itself more severely in some areas of mental function than in others. As a consequence, Down syndrome offers a unique opportunity to link together specific abnormalities in neural maturation with particular problems in cognitive development. To do so, we need data on neural and cognitive development in individuals with Down syndrome and a clear understanding of the ways in which these differ from the normal case. In this chapter, we review existing data with an eye toward promoting this linkage; it will be clear, however, that we are far from an understanding of exactly what is wrong, and what is right, in development in Down syndrome. We will draw parallels, where possible, between specific cognitive and neural defects but elsewhere will have to be content simply to document what is known.

Much of the work on individuals with Down syndrome has focused on their abilities in the domain of language, and a number of excellent recent reviews of this work are available (e.g., Rondal, 1994, 1995; Miller, 1995). In this chapter, we focus instead on aspects of learning and memory in individuals with Down syndrome, in a framework provided by an analysis of the neural systems known to underlie various forms of learning and memory. We suggest that difficulties in both the acquisition of information (learning) and the long-term storage and retrieval of information (memory) are a part of the phenotype of Down syndrome.

It is now clear that multiple learning and memory systems exist (see Nadel, 1992, 1994, for recent reviews) and, in most clinical syndromes (such as Down syndrome, Alzheimer disease, Parkinsonism, and Huntington's disease), impairments of learning and memory predominantly affect some (but rarely all) of these forms of learning and memory. To the extent that one wishes to develop intervention strategies for infants and children with Down syndrome, one must understand which learning and memory systems are disproportionately impaired and which are not. Important also is an understanding of which, if any, of these impairments can be ameliorated and which cannot. This latter issue requires careful attention to the underlying neural correlates of the impairment and to the cognitive structure of the various kinds of learning.

Accordingly, we begin with a discussion of the various kinds of learning and memory, briefly reviewing some of the data that have demonstrated the existence and nature of these multiple systems. We then continue with a review of what is known about the neural impairments associated with Down syndrome and how these might affect the various types of learning and memory discussed in the opening section. After this, we review current knowledge about learning and memory in individuals with Down syndrome, from a wide range of learning situations. In the final section, we draw some conclusions about the range of effects one sees in learning and memory performance in individuals with Down syndrome and about the kinds of information that we still lack and sorely need if we are to understand fully this syndrome's impact on learning and memory. We conclude with some thoughts about mind-brain maturation, given the insights derived from study of this particular developmentally disabled population.

THE NATURE OF LEARNING AND MEMORY

In recent years, it has become clear that learning and memory functions cannot be characterized in a singular fashion, either in terms of their behavioral and cognitive properties or in terms of the neural systems on which they rest. Initially in work with animals (e.g., Nadel & O'Keefe, 1974; O'Keefe & Nadel, 1978) and subsequently in work with humans (e.g., Cohen & Squire, 1980), researchers have proved the existence of multiple learning and memory systems with distinct properties and neural bases; these distinctions are critically important in understanding the precise nature of various clinical syndromes such as amnesia, Alzheimer disease, and, as will be argued here, Down syndrome. Understanding the nature and specific roles of multiple memory systems is relevant to the proper characterization of Down syndrome because the neural dysfunctions observed in this and most other syndromes are not spread evenly throughout the brain. Rather, they affect some parts of the brain more than others. To the extent that different brain regions are essential for very different forms of learning and memory, determining what kinds of learning and memory exist, what brain regions are responsible for each type, and what brain regions are particularly compromised in Down syndrome is critical. Only when we have answers to all these questions will we be able to state with some assurance just what aspects of learning and memory are especially at risk in this syndrome.

TYPES OF LEARNING AND MEMORY

Some time ago, O'Keefe and Nadel (1978) proposed that a particular part of the brain, the hippocampus, was involved in a highly specific form of learning and memory that we called *cognitive mapping*. We contrasted the kind of learning carried out by this brain region (and its collaborating neighbors) with other forms of learning that did not have the same maplike qualities. Table 9.1 indicates the key features of the two main classes of learning that we postulated, which we called *locale* and *taxon* learning. The names *locale* and *taxon* were chosen to reflect central distinguishing features of these two types of learning: Locale learning incorporates information about the location of objects and events. Taxon learning, by contrast, does not incorporate such contextual information, focusing instead on the conceptual and categorical information obtained through experiences in the environment. As Table 9.1 shows, these two types of learning differ in many important respects. Locale learning is assumed to be rapid, one-trial, easily changed,

Table 9.1 Two types of learning and their properties

Property	Locale learning	Taxon learning
Speed of learning	Rapid, one-trial	Slow, incremental
Persistence	Easily changed	Highly persistent
Flexibility	High	Low
Contextual links	Bound to context	Free of context
Motivation	Curiosity	Biological reward
Representation	Map/relational	Categorical

flexible in use, related to the context in which it is obtained (e.g., episodic), and acquired without regard to standard biological motivations such as food, water, and safety. Taxon learning, on the other hand, is assumed generally to be relatively slow, incremental, persistent and changed only with difficulty, inflexible in use, not related to the context in which it is obtained, and typically acquired in relation to the action of biological rewards.

Locale and taxon learning systems are distinguished also by the nature of the representations they establish—that is, the way in which they store acquired information. Within the locale system, information is stored in a maplike representation (hence, the use of the term *cognitive map* to describe the hippocampus) such that all parts of an acquired memory stand in some relation to all other parts. In this way, one part of an episode memory can serve as a retrieval cue for another part. Further, this form of relational storage permits inferences between and among parts of the memory that might never have occurred together. For example, we can figure out the relations between two parts of a city even though we have never gone from one to the other because they are both part of a larger relational structure. In the same vein, we can use this structure to generate new "paths" from one place to another, whether we are talking about real places in the environment or just figurative places in some learned representation. The term *map* is used here not to imply that there is a literal map in the brain but rather that the underlying neural system—in this case, in the hippocampus—functions as though it had the properties of maps as just described.

In contrast, within the taxon system, information is stored by virtue of categorical relations, with links between categories established through pairwise associations. We have likened this form of representation to a "route" to contrast it with the weblike nature of maps. These routelike representations do not have the kind of flexibility and do not permit the same sort of inferences as do maps. Hence, the kind of learning, and what can be done with the information acquired, varies in important ways between the locale and taxon systems.

On the basis of our work with animal models (Nadel & O'Keefe, 1974), and others' work with humans (Schacter & Tulving, 1994), we argued that these two kinds of learning were subserved by different regions in the brain and, indeed, that the properties that distinguish them derive in large measure from the underlying computational structure of the neural systems involved. As noted previously, we supposed that locale learning depended on the hippocampus and neighboring structures in the medial temporal lobe of the brain. Taxon learning was supposed to be dependent on other parts of the cerebral cortex, basal ganglia, and various other subcortical structures. We pointed out that there were many types of taxon learning and that different types were likely to be subserved by different brain regions. Taxon learning includes not only the category learning noted earlier but also the learning of skills, habits, and procedures, which can be viewed as motor "concepts."

Of course, these two separate learning systems are not independent of one another. We postulated that information flowed into the hippocampal learning system through the taxon system and that using the maplike information in the hippocampus required activation of appropriate information in these other brain areas. I have further speculated, with others, that the rapidly formed memories in the hippocampal system contribute to the consolidation of memories in other brain regions (Squire et al., 1984; McClelland et al., 1992; Nadel & Moscovitch, 1997) and that, in the absence of the hippocampus, there might be problems with this consolidation process. I return to this important point later.

More recent work by numerous other investigators in a range of species has largely confirmed the notion that essentially two types of learning systems exist and that these are to be distinguished along the lines of the properties spelled out in Table 9.1 (Mishkin et al., 1984; Sutherland & Rudy, 1989; Squire, 1992; Cohen & Eichenbaum, 1993; Schacter & Tulving, 1994; Nadel, 1992, 1994). This emerging synthesis on the nature of multiple learning and memory systems does not mean that all agree on all the details, of course, but there is sufficient agreement to permit those with clinical interest in syndromes in which there are learning and memory difficulties to make certain predictions about the nature of those problems if those predictions can be based on knowledge of the underlying neural defects. Considerable evidence now points to the notion that in a variety of syndromes, impairments in memory reflect these distinctions among types of memory.

Insofar as one can be certain of the neural concomitants of Down syndrome, and insofar as one can be confident about the kinds of learning and memory to which the affected neural regions are central, one ought to be able to make specific predictions about the learning and memory abilities and disabilities of individuals with Down syndrome. This is, to be sure, a very simplistic way to approach the matter, for although every individual with Down syndrome who is trisomic for chromosome 21 starts from the same point, the range of abilities in this population, and the range of neural dysfunctions (as previously noted) is staggering. This range, paradoxically, implies cause for great hope because, if some individuals can attain great things, then achievement of great things must, in some theoretical sense at least, be possible for all. (For further discussion of this point, see Rondal, 1994, 1995.)

NEURAL SEQUELAE OF DOWN SYNDROME

What, then, do we currently know of the precise neural sequelae of Down syndrome? Answering this question is more difficult than one might imagine at first glance, because we are dealing with a moving target. Data from a wide range of studies indicate that, at birth, apparently little distinction can be made between the brains of normal and Down syndrome individuals (Brooksbank et al., 1989; Wisniewski & Schmidt-Sidor, 1989; Florez et al., 1990; Schmidt-Sidor et al., 1990; Bar-Peled et al., 1991; Pazos et al., 1994). Yet both postmortem studies and various, more recent, noninvasive neuro-imaging studies have demonstrated rather clear differences between normal and Down syndrome individuals as early as 6 months of age. Whence do these differences emanate, and what is their significance?

An immediately obvious difference is that the brains of individuals with Down syndrome are typically smaller than those of age-matched controls, at least after 6 months of age. However, one possibility that has been given in-sufficient attention in the past, but which must be attended more carefully, is that this difference is merely a consequence of the fact that Down syndrome individuals are smaller overall: That is, the differences in brain size could be a matter of *allometry*. This possibility, together with the fact that there is no clear relation between brain size and "intelligence," suggests that the mental retardation observed in Down syndrome likely results from something other than gross differences in brain size.

It is not simply that the brains of Down syndrome individuals are smaller overall but that certain brain areas are disproportionately affected whereas others are affected quite minimally. This differential impact is not predicted by allometry and must be considered very carefully in any attempt to draw conclusions from the study of neuropathology. Before we discuss these spe-cific problems, another factor must be taken into account: the probability that brain development is influenced in highly important ways by experience. If this is true, and increasing reasons from a range of basic neurobiological studies exist to argue that it is, then the study of the brains of individuals with Down syndrome who have recently come to postmortem evaluation might be highly misleading. Most of these individuals did not benefit from the kinds of early stimulation regimens that now are available and indeed prevalent and that might have a direct impact on brain development. Cur-rently, this is a highly speculative but very important area; as noted earlier, such brain plasticity is one of the best hopes for bringing about significant improvements in the development of individuals with Down syndrome. At this time, we do not know, from either a theoretical or an empirical perspec-tive, the extent to which experience can cause changes in normal brain de-velopment. We do not know whether normal possibilities for brain plasticity exist in individuals with Down syndrome. We do not know the extent to which changes in brain development that are promoted by specific stimula-tion regimens can translate into meaningful behavioral and cognitive improvements. We do not know which kinds of changes would be beneficial and which would not. Obviously, a great deal is still unknown in this area, and we can be certain of very little, except that further research on these issues is of the utmost importance. Though one does not wish to raise false hopes, it is noteworthy that we now know the brain to be much more malleable than was previously thought.

Having registered these caveats, what can we say about nervous system development and function in Down syndrome? Data bearing on this question come from a number of sources; for present purposes, we emphasize what is known about neural development, but some discussion of neural function in adolescents and adults helps to illuminate the developmental story. We will begin with a discussion of what the nervous system is like at or before birth, to get a sense of the starting point. We then discuss what the nervous system is like as the individual with Down syndrome develops through childhood and adolescence and into adult life. For some time, we have known that as individuals with Down syndrome reach "old age," signs of neuropathology emerge much earlier in this population than in the normal population. This fact may help us understand some of the developmental abnormalities observed in Down syndrome.

Information about neural function and development comes from three primary sources: neuroanatomical studies of brains from individuals with Down syndrome who died at various ages, neurophysiological studies of the dynamic properties of the brains of individuals with Down syndrome at various ages, and neuroimaging studies of the metabolic activity of the brains of individuals with Down syndrome, typically in adulthood.

Early Development

A wide range of studies points to the already-noted conclusion that the brain of an individual with Down syndrome at or shortly before birth is, in many respects, indistinguishable from the brain of a normal individual (Brooksbank et al., 1989; Wisniewski & Schmidt-Sidor, 1989; Florez et al., 1990; Schmidt-Sidor et al., 1990; Bar-Peled et al., 1991; Pazos et al., 1994). Normal values have been reported for brain and skull shape, brain weight, proportion of specific cerebral lobes, size of cerebellum and brainstem, and the emergence of most neurotransmitter systems. The fact that relative normalcy exists at birth is potentially of the greatest significance, as it seems to create the opportunity to do something about the not-yet-created differences that clearly do emerge during the period immediately after birth.

Evidence exists, however, that some changes begin to emerge as early as 22 weeks' gestational age (Schmidt-Sidor et al., 1990), and by the age of 6 months a number of important differences already are obvious. Some of these differences are expressed in terms of the proportion of individuals with Down syndrome who show abnormal values of brain region size, rather than in terms of a uniform abnormality in all instances. This too is important, as it highlights the variability in this population, a variability that attests to the critical role of environmental (epigenetic) factors in determining the phenotype in Down syndrome, given the uniform genotypic feature of trisomy 21.[1] One very noticeable difference concerns a postnatal delay in myelination (Wisniewski, 1990), global at first but then manifested primarily in nerve tracts that are myelinated especially late in development, such as the fibers linking the frontal and temporal lobes; this delay is observed in nearly 25% of Down syndrome infants between the ages of 2 months and 6 years. Though we should not underestimate the impact of this myelination delay, it certainly is worth noting that in all cases, myelination is within normal range at birth, whereas in 75% of the cases, it is within normal range throughout early development. Delayed myelination has also been observed in a study employing magnetic resonance imaging on a single infant (18 months of age) with Down syndrome (Koo et al., 1992).

Neuropathological differences after 3 to 5 months of age include a shortening of the fronto-occipital length of the brain, which appears to result from a reduction in growth of the frontal lobes, a narrowing of the superior temporal gyrus (observed in approximately 35% of cases), diminished size of the brainstem and cerebellum (observed in most cases), and a significant reduction (20%–50%) in the number of cortical granular neurons (see Crome et al., 1966; Benda, 1971; Blackwood & Corsellis, 1976). The data provide some indication of a relation between the occurrence of neuropathological abnormalities and other problems in Down syndrome, such as congenital heart disease. Notwithstanding these differences, however, the overall picture in infancy is one of relative normalcy, although individuals with Down syndrome tend to fall toward the bottom of the normal range (or outside it) on most measures.

Investigations of neural function (as opposed to structure) in early infancy suggest some abnormalities: In particular, evidence exists of either delayed or aberrant auditory system development (Jiang et al., 1990) that might contribute to the widespread hearing disorders observed in Down syndrome. Obviously, such a disorder, if organic, could be related to many of the subsequent difficulties seen in the learning of language. In addition, evidence of a more widespread abnormality in electroencephalographic (EEG) coherence seems to reflect a generally impoverished dendritic environment. This difference, like many of the others, emerges only sometime after birth (McAlaster, 1992). It appears that this effect is predominant in posterior, rather than anterior, brain regions and in the left more than the right hemisphere.

Later Development and Adulthood

The evidence of neuropathological sequelae in Down syndrome is more extensive for the middle rather than the early stage of life. Data from both postmortem studies and studies of brain function in select populations indicate that the changes beginning to emerge early in life become more prominent and prevalent by early adolescence. Thus, Becker et al. (1986) showed that dendritic arborizations in the visual cortex of individuals with Down syndrome were paradoxically greater than normal early in infancy but then considerably less than normal by the age of 2 years. These authors speculate that the initial overabundance might result from a compensatory response to the absence of adequate synapse formation, but the basic point remains that by early childhood the neocortex is impoverished. This increasing deficit in neocortical microstructure has been confirmed by Wisniewski and Schmidt-Sidor (1989) and, as we have already observed, myelination is delayed in a significant number of children with Down syndrome.

Relatively few studies have concentrated on brain function in adolescents and young adults with Down syndrome, and the existing data are somewhat equivocal. Devinsky et al. (1990) reported relatively normal EEG α-activity in young adults (< 40 years of age), and Schapiro et al. (1992) reported relatively normal brain metabolism in a similar group, using positron emission tomography (PET) measures of glucose uptake and regional blood flow. They did report some disruption of normal neuronal interactions between the frontal and parietal lobes, possibly including the language area of Broca. Overall, they concluded that in younger subjects with Down syndrome, generally cerebral atrophy does not extend beyond what would be predicted by the smaller cranial vault and stature of these subjects. On the other hand, in those cases in which dementia can be observed in younger subjects, clear signs of abnormal cerebral atrophy and metabolic deficiencies are seen. Enlargement of the ventricles is a standard sign in these cases. In an earlier study looking at glucose uptake, these investigators found abnormal interactions between the thalamus and neocortex, in particular the temporal and occipital lobes, speculating that, as a result, there might be a problem with "directed attention" (Horwitz et al., 1990). A study of EEG coherence (McAlaster, 1992) reported abnormal development of EEG profiles in subjects with Down syndrome, again with a particular emphasis on the posterior cortical regions.

A recent PET study of seven young adults with Down syndrome (mean age, 28 years) without dementia (Haier et al., 1995) confirmed previous findings that the overall cortical glucose metabolic rate is *higher* in subjects with Down syndrome (and in other mentally retarded subjects) than in normal controls. This seemingly paradoxical increase typically is interpreted as a sign of "inefficiency."[2] When one looks at specific areas more closely, decreases in metabolic rate are observed in medial frontal and medial temporal lobes in the Down syndrome subjects and some evidence exists of dysfunction in the basal ganglia.

Overall, the evidence from the study of subjects in midlife still is inconclusive. Though clear problems exist in some cases, with some evidence for localized neuropathology, the general picture is highly diffuse. This, however, is not the case when one looks at studies focused on somewhat older subjects.

For some years, it has been clear that neuropathology resembling that seen in Alzheimer disease is prevalent in individuals with Down syndrome after the age of approximately 35 years. Many studies have concentrated on this issue, documenting the ways in which the neuropathology seen in Down syndrome is similar to, or different from, that seen in Alzheimer disease. A very important fact emerging over the last 5 years of careful study is that though virtually 100% of individuals with Down syndrome show neuropathology similar to that associated with Alzheimer disease, fewer than 50% show the dementia invariably seen with Alzheimer disease. This uncoupling of the neuropathology from the dementia has, of course, occasioned considerable interest, with an initial emphasis on attempts to determine whether there might be subtle differences between the cases of Down syndrome and Alzheimer disease that could explain the dissociation observed in Down syndrome but not in Alzheimer disease. It has not been possible to pinpoint any such difference that could be said, with confidence, to account for this fact (e.g., Cork, 1990). Recently, H. Wisniewski (personal communication) has shown that there is a critical difference between Down syndrome and Alzheimer disease with regard to the nature of the amyloid deposits found in the plaques characteristic of the neuropathology common in these two conditions. Dementia is observed only when insoluble amyloid, which causes the formation of fibrous tangles, is present. This type of amyloid rarely is seen in Down syndrome until one is more than 50 years of age, regardless of the extent of gross neuropathology.

Four recent articles provide an up-to-date view on the neuropathology observed in adults with Down syndrome (Weis, 1991; Lögdberg & Brun, 1993; Kesslak et al., 1994; Raz et al., 1995). Weis (1991) applied stereological techniques in combination with magnetic resonance imaging (MRI) scans to estimate the size of various brain regions in a group of seven adults (30–45 years of age) with Down syndrome. The volume of the whole brain was smaller in subjects with Down syndrome. When the data were normalized and then considered as a ratio of the volume of the cranial cavity, specific differences were observed in cortex and white matter overall, with a not-quite-significant difference in cerebellum ($P < .06$). The study by Kesslak et al. (1994) looked at 13 adults with Down syndrome, using MRI to assess the size of various brain regions. Two additional subjects with clinically diagnosed dementia also were studied. The main findings in the group without dementia were a decrease in the size of the hippocampus and neocortex and a paradoxical increase in the size of the parahippocampal gyrus. No significant differences were observed in the superior temporal lobe, the middle and inferior temporal lobes, the lateral ventricles, or cortical or subcortical areas. In these Down syndrome subjects, only two significant age-related changes were observed: With aging, ventricle size increased and hippocampal size decreased. In the two subjects with dementia, considerable brain atrophy and an enlargement of the ventricles were seen, in general creating a picture similar to that observed in Alzheimer disease but absent from the subjects with

Down syndrome who were not clinically demented, even those as old as 51 years.

The next study (Raz et al., 1995) evaluated 25 adults, 13 with Down syndrome, also using MRI. Most critically, these researchers' results were adjusted for body size, so they took into account differences resulting simply from allometry. The authors found that a number of brain regions were smaller in the Down syndrome subjects, including the hippocampal formation, the mammillary bodies, and parts of the cerebellum and cerebral hemispheres. They also replicated the increase in size of the parahippocampal gyrus observed by Kesslak et al. (1994). There was some shrinkage of other brain regions, including the dorsolateral prefrontal cortex, the anterior cingulate cortex, the pericalcarine cortex, the inferior temporal and parietal cortex, and the parietal white matter. No differences at all were observed in orbitofrontal cortex, precentral and postcentral gyri, and the basal ganglia. The last study, by Lögdberg and Brun (1993), applied morphometric analyses to the brains of seven subjects with Down syndrome (mean age, 25.3 years) and demonstrated a significant decrease in gyri size in the frontal lobe.

These observed changes confirm earlier reports of decreased volume of cerebellum (Jernigan & Bellugi, 1990) and of decreased dendritic spines and volume in hippocampus (Ferrer & Gullotta, 1990). Reports have also been made of neuropathology in the amygdala (Mann & Esiri, 1989; Murphy et al., 1992), particularly in those subregions most closely associated with the hippocampus (Murphy & Ellis, 1991).

The earliest neuropathological changes with aging in Down syndrome seem to appear in parts of the hippocampal formation, especially the entorhinal cortex, but also involving the dentate gyrus, CA_1, and the subiculum (Mann & Esiri, 1989; Hyman, 1992). There is extensive cell loss in the locus coeruleus (Mann et al., 1990), a brainstem nucleus that projects to the hippocampal formation; this was most noticeable in cases of severe dementia.

In sum, widespread signs of neuropathology are seen in older Down syndrome subjects, but there is a selectivity in terms of where signs are seen first and where they are most prominent. In this regard, changes in hippocampal formation (Ball & Nuttal, 1981, Sylvester, 1983; Ball et al., 1986), temporal lobe in general (Deb et al., 1992; Spargo et al., 1992), and cerebellum (Cole et al., 1993) stand out.

Work with animal models of Down syndrome is consistent with this picture and adds some measure of confidence to the conclusions drawn from the human data. The trisomy 16 mouse (Ts16) has generally been viewed as a plausible model of trisomy 21 in humans (e.g., Holtzman et al., 1995). These animals, however, do not survive birth, and study of the postnatal neural and behavioral consequences of this trisomy has awaited the development of a partial Ts16 mouse that survived into adulthood and that had triplicates of most of the human chromosome 21 genes. Recently, this goal has been accomplished with the development of Ts65Dn mice (Davisson et al., 1993). Recent behavioral work with these mice, using a variety of paradigms, is highly consistent with the idea that damage in the hippocampus is a major part of Down syndrome (Escorihuela et al., 1995; Coussons-Read & Crnic, 1996). In both of these studies, the Ts65Dn mice showed behavioral profiles highly similar to those observed after experimental damage in the hippocampus in mouse and rat studies. Thus, the Ts65Dn mice were hyperactive, defective in spatial learning, but normal in other forms of learning not dependent on the hippocampus. The development of new kinds of partially trisomic mice, with triplication restricted to other segments of the critical chromosomes, should help greatly in unraveling the relation between the genetic defect and neural dysfunction.

Overall, study of neuropathology in early and later life points to effects in certain regions of the cortex, including most prominently the temporal lobe[3] and hippocampal formation (Wisniewski et al., 1986) and in the cerebellum. In analyzing learning and memory difficulties, then, we should be particularly alert to those kinds of changes that might reflect particular problems with these neural systems. In the present context, we should focus on the potential impact on development of abnormalities in these specific systems.

LEARNING AND MEMORY IN INDIVIDUALS WITH DOWN SYNDROME

In considering the learning and memory abilities of individuals with Down syndrome, the two major concerns already discussed must be taken into account: First, learning and memory must be considered as involving a number of separate systems and, second, attention must be paid to the abilities of individuals at various stages of life. A review of existing studies make clear that some brain systems are affected more than others and that these brain systems are responsible for only some—not all—kinds of learning.

At this juncture, let us focus on one of the conclusions drawn from this review—that is, parts of the medial temporal lobe, particularly the hippocampus, seem disproportionately affected in Down syndrome. The evidence for this is now very clear in older subjects, if only suggestive in younger subjects. Work with animals models, as we have seen, supports this view. As noted earlier, the hippocampal system is involved in spatial cognition in particular, flexible learning in general, and the normal consolidation of what has already been learned. Therefore, we should expect selective difficulties with this kind of learning. It is known that the hippocampal system is not crucial for much learning about categories and concepts, nor is it necessary for skill learning; hence, we should expect relatively normal performance in these domains.

Unfortunately, we do not have as clear a picture of the precise functions of the cerebellum, another brain region prominently affected in subjects with Down syndrome. Some evidence suggests that the cerebellum is involved in motor skills, but other indications are that it might be critical in the acquisition of conditioned responses—for example, the so-called nictitating membrane response. We will see later some evidence that this form of conditioning indeed is impaired in older subjects with Down syndrome.

Before attributing particular problems with learning and memory to specific neuropathologies, we must take into account difficulties that individuals with Down syndrome might have in sensory and perceptual function that could contribute to or account for these learning problems. As we have already noted, indications exist of an organic basis for hearing difficulties that could certainly compromise language learning (Marcell & Cohen, 1992). In addition, a defect in visual acuity (Courage et al., 1994) could contribute to problems with learning in situations where visual information is critical. Such indications suggest that early stimulation programs must be sensitive to sensory and perceptual function, to promote the maximization of capacities in these areas that might otherwise be suboptimal, thereby imposing a limit on the learning process. Difficulties on the motor side also must be taken into account in evaluating learning ability (Henderson, 1985).

Once these more peripheral difficulties have been considered, what evidence do we have of further difficulties in learning and memory, and how might these relate to underlying neural dysfunction?

Early Learning

In general, infants with Down syndrome show relatively normal abilities in learning and memory [but see Hepper & Shahidullah (1992) for a report of impaired habituation in two fetuses with Down syndrome]. This does not mean, however, that either they, or indeed normally developing infants, have the full adult range of learning and memory abilities at birth. In fact, this is not the case, as some parts of the brain mature postnatally, and the forms of learning and memory dependent on them are not available until some time after birth. The medial temporal lobe, and particularly the hippocampus, as well as parts of the cerebellum, are included in this category. The fact that these late-developing structures are apparently especially at risk in Down syndrome probably is of considerable importance (see Nadel, 1986). Although insufficient evidence exists to permit certainty about exact ages, there is little doubt that in humans, as in most other animals, the hippocampus is not fully functional until many months after birth, perhaps as many as 16 to 18 months (see Nadel & Zola-Morgan, 1984; Nadel & Willner, 1989). This means that the kinds of learning and memory that depend on this system are not available to infants.

In an early series of studies, Ohr and Fagen (1991, 1993) looked at the ability of infants to acquire behaviors based on learning about the *contingencies* between their own movements (leg kicking) and reinforcement. They reported that 3-month-old infants with Down syndrome were entirely normal at this task, including initial learning, acquisition speed, and retention. In a later report (Ohr & Fagen, 1994), these same authors showed that 9-month-old infants with Down syndrome were impaired, as a group, in learning about the contingency between arm movements and reinforcement. However, they noted that *some* infants with Down syndrome were able to learn. They concluded that after 6 months there is a relative decline in conditionability in infants with Down syndrome as compared to normally developing infants. This is in agreement with the general picture emerging from studies of brain maturation, which also show relative normalcy at birth but increasing abnormality after 6 months.

Mangan (1992) tested control infants and infants with Down syndrome on a variety of spatial tasks, one of which (a place-learning task) was designed especially to assess the state of function of the hippocampal system. This place-learning task does not emerge in normal development until approximately 18 months of age, which matches current estimates of when the hippocampus itself becomes functional (Mangan & Nadel, 1990). Two other spatial tasks were used, one involving response learning, in which the child had to make a consistent body-turn, and the other involving cue learning, in which the child had to approach a specific cue. In all three tasks, the child was searching for a toy hidden in a hole. After learning, the infants were removed from the apparatus for a delay interval, then were given a "memory" test. Mangan tested children at the age of 16 to 20 months on the response and cue tasks and at the age of 26 to 30 months on the place task. He found that children with Down syndrome were somewhat impaired in the learning of all three tasks, although they did manage to learn them all. On the critical memory probes, children with Down syndrome performed similarly to the normal children on the response and cue tasks but were severely impaired on the place task. This pattern of results is consistent with diffuse, but mild, neuropathology combined with much more extensive pathology localized to the hippocampus.

In another study of spatial abilities, Uecker et al. (1994) showed that children with Down syndrome experienced difficulties in a task requiring the mental rotation of a stick figure, as compared with another group of learning-disabled children. Although capable of representing the stimulus in imagery, the children with Down syndrome were impaired at the spatial-transformational task of rotating that image. How, if at all, this relates to the spatial defect observed in place learning remains to be determined.

A great deal of work on learning within the language domain has been carried out in children with Down syndrome (see Rondal, 1994). We know that difficulties in the acquisition of language can be quite severe, particularly in the phonological and syntactical domains (see Tager-Flusberg, 1999), but cases also are seen in which language capacity is within normal range or even at the upper end of that range. Infants with Down syndrome show many of the normal features of prelanguage behavior, including babbling and imitation, although some subtle (but possibly important) differences are observed between Down syndrome and normally developing infants in this regard (Oller & Siebert, 1988; Lynch et al., 1990; Steffens et al., 1992). Sigman and her colleagues (Mundy et al., 1988; see also chapter 8) have shown deficits in the use of nonverbal requests in young children with Down syndrome. Similar deficits in requesting behavior have been demonstrated in other studies, including one assessing verbal requests (Beeghly et al., 1990), but a number of studies have failed to detect a deficit (e.g., Greenwald & Leonard, 1979). Though pinpointing the precise defect at the root of the typical language problem is difficult, there is little to suggest that the difficulty is primarily one of learning or memory. Sigman (chapter 8) stresses as precursors to language problems defective requesting behavior, less-than-optimal caregiver behavior, and a diminished capacity to initiate joint attention. Tager-Flusberg (1999) focuses on auditory working memory, which certainly could account for the observed phonological defects. The fact that the disproportionate difficulties are observed in grammatical development is consistent with the idea that learning and memory problems are not at the root of language defects in Down syndrome.

Vocalization appears to be under contingent control in infants with Down syndrome (Poulson, 1988), and these infants' ability to acquire words seems normal also, albeit slow (Hopmann & Nothnagle, 1994). As the focus of this chapter is on learning and memory, we will not consider in further detail the acquisition of language.

In a series of longitudinal studies, Wishart (1993) has carefully examined the performance of children with Down syndrome in contingency detection tasks, on standard intelligence tests, and in terms of the development of the "object concept." Here this work is only briefly summarized. Contingency learning was studied in a situation in which infants could produce rotation of a brightly colored mobile by a kick that would break a light beam. Normally developing infants can learn the contingency by 2 months of age, which involves kicking at a rate of $1.5 \times$ baseline (taken as the kicking rate during a period when the contingency was not in effect). Children with Down syndrome were impaired in acquiring this task but, beyond that, differences in how they performed are very revealing. Wishart (1993) used several different reward schedules that varied in the extent to which subjects received "free" (noncontingent) rewards. Counterintuitively, such rewards diminished the extent to which children with Down syndrome participated in controlling the rotation of the mobile themselves. Although these children maintained an interest in the task well beyond the age at which normally developing children ceased being interested, this interest was satisfied by passive acceptance of free rewards as readily as by active participation in gaining the rewards. Relating this intriguing finding to any of the known neural difficulties observed in Down syndrome is difficult.

In a characteristic fashion, young children develop notions about the continuing existence and properties of objects. Children with Down syndrome have typically been shown to acquire this basic object concept more slowly than do normal children (e.g., Rast & Meltzoff, 1995) but, with extensive training, they can acquire it at more or less the same time as normally developing infants (Wishart, 1993). However, a different kind of problem emerges in this task situation: instability of acquisition. Although the typical subject with Down syndrome solved various levels of the tasks used to assess the object concept at ages not very far from the norm, performance after acquisition could be highly variable and apparently beset by motivational difficulties. Once again, these problems, if representative of the learning style of children with Down syndrome, are extremely important in considering effective intervention. The results of Wishart's studies using standard intelligence test batteries suggests that they are indeed representative. Test-retest reliability was very low because successes gained in one test might not appear on retesting as soon as 2 weeks later. New skills show up, only to disappear shortly thereafter. One could speculate that evidence of such apparently rapid forgetting is consistent with damage in the hippocampal formation, but considerably more data are required before this conclusion can be accepted.

The motivational difficulties and developmental instabilities observed in Wishart's work strongly suggest that young children with Down syndrome are not merely delayed in mental development but actually follow a somewhat different path. As Wishart (1993, p. 392) points out, this view "has the substantial merit of being consistent with data from the neurosciences showing DS [Down syndrome] to be associated with fundamental differences in the morphology and functioning of the brain."

To summarize the situation in infants and children, evidence exists of relatively normal learning of certain types, especially in the youngest subjects. The kinds of learning that appear normal fall into the category labeled as *taxon* learning: simple conditioning, for example, and deferred imitation (Rast & Meltzoff, 1995). Evidence also is available for some highly specific learning deficits, which typically emerge only some months or even years after birth. The evidence is consistent with a specific problem in the hippocampal formation spatial-cognitive system. Thus, early development of learning and memory in Down syndrome seems selectively rather than generally impaired.

The learning and memory problems that begin to emerge in late infancy become considerably more noticeable as the infant grows to childhood and adolescence. Most of our knowledge for this period comes from the learning of language, but some information is available about other kinds of learning and memory. The major point to be stressed from these data has less to do with the inability of children with Down syndrome to acquire words or linguistic constructions or other non verbal material and more to do with their inability to "stabilize" the information that they do manage to acquire. Wishart (1993) and Fowler (1988) stress this point, which might reflect, among other factors, impairments in the consolidation function earlier attributed to the hippocampal system.

In a recent study, Carlesimo et al. (1997) have demonstrated a specific memory impairment in Down syndrome. Their subjects included 15 persons with Down syndrome (mean chronological age, 16.7; mean mental age, 9.1),

15 persons with non–Down syndrome mental retardation (mean chronological age, 17.1; mean mental age, 9.7) and 30 normal children matched for mental age with the two experimental groups. Subjects were tested on a variety of implicit and explicit memory paradigms, including word-stem completion, list learning, and prose recall. Robust and comparable priming effects were seen in all groups in the stem-completion task, indicating that implicit memory was intact in both groups of mentally retarded individuals. However, deficits were observed in both explicit memory tasks. Performance on these kinds of explicit memory paradigms has been linked to function of the hippocampal system; hence, the defects suggest differential impairment in hippocampal function and thereby converge with data from the study of spatial cognition.

Adulthood and Aging

A great deal of recent research has focused on the deterioration of learning, memory, and other cognitive capacities as individuals with Down syndrome reach the age of 35 or older. From the perspective of the present chapter, this work is important for two reasons. First, it adds weight to the conclusions reached from work with younger subjects. Second, it allows us to consider data that address the issue of possible long-term consequences of systematic treatments during development. As noted earlier, beyond the age of 35 one can be reasonably certain that at least some signs of neuropathology will be present in the brain of most or all individuals with Down syndrome. The relation between this pathology and the onset of dementia and, eventually, Alzheimer disease is being actively studied. Here more than anywhere else, the notion that we are studying a "moving target" is relevant. As more individuals with Down syndrome reach older ages in relatively good health, and as a higher proportion of these individuals will have enjoyed the benefits of early intervention programs and increased expectations, the picture of Down syndrome capabilities might change. Given our earlier comments about brain plasticity, it is even possible that the certainty of neuropathology will change. Clearly, we need to find ways to identify, prospectively if possible, those aging subjects with Down syndrome who are most at risk for developing the clinical signs of Alzheimer disease.

One sign of this possibility is emerging in the work of Wisniewski's group. Their current work on visual and auditory memory in high-functioning subjects between 27 and 57 years of age leads them to conclude that "declines in functioning, particularly in memory, in older mildly and moderately mentally retarded adults with DS [Down syndrome] are not a necessary occurrence within the age range sampled" (Devenny et al., 1992).

Other studies, however, report a loss of learning and memory capacities that seems to affect most areas of cognitive function in aging individuals with Down syndrome (e.g., Caltagirone et al., 1990), although not in a uniform way. Language seemed particularly impaired in this latter study of subjects with a mean age of approximately 35 years, and the profile that was observed was not the same as that seen in Alzheimer disease. Hemdal et al. (1993), on the other hand, report that a group of subjects with a mean age of approximately 24 years demonstrated deficits in olfactory identification that seemed very like those observed in Alzheimer disease patients. Similarly, Woodruff-Pak et al. (1994, 1996) showed that Down syndrome subjects older than 35 years were likely to have deficits in eye-blink conditioning similar to those observed in Alzheimer disease patients. However, these deficits were not complete, and extra training permitted most of the subjects to achieve the criterion. The authors suggested that this latter result is perhaps more indicative of defective hippocampal than defective cerebellar functioning.

Ellis et al. (1989) tested a group of subjects with a mean age of 26.8 years on a task that assessed memory for pictures and for their location in a book. These subjects were very poor at recalling the pictures and were significantly worse at remembering the pictures' location. Interestingly, the distribution of the subjects with Down syndrome was bimodal: Some did very well on the location task, whereas others did very poorly.

Overall, evidence from the study of older individuals with Down syndrome is consistent with the view that these subjects' learning and memory deficits are not global. However, insufficient data exist to support precise statements about what is more impaired and what is less impaired. We also have evidence that in old age, as in infancy and childhood, a very wide range of outcomes is possible. The fact that, with aging, individuals with Down syndrome are increasingly likely to develop cognitive signs similar to, if not identical with, those in Alzheimer disease patients certainly suggests that some underlying similarities exist in the neuropathological profiles of these conditions. That many older individuals with Down syndrome do not develop a full-blown Alzheimer profile is cause for hope and also reason to be cautious in accepting the view that these syndromes are virtually identical in old age.

CONCLUSIONS

Learning and memory are disrupted in Down syndrome, and progress is being made in defining exactly what the deficit is. Most indications suggest that the impairment is not spread across all learning and memory systems equally but instead selectively affects only some systems. At this time, clear evidence implicates the forms of learning and memory dependent on the hippocampus; suggestive evidence also implicates the cerebellum.

Our review of neuropathology suggests that major differences between normally developing children and children with Down syndrome emerge only some months after birth. The corollary to this is the relatively normal, though restricted, learning observed in early infancy. Important deficits emerge within the first year, and they take on a very specific character. Some deficits occur in learning specific kinds of information, such as about places or particular features of language, and some deficits are of a more abstract nature, such as the seeming instability of material that has apparently been learned, only to be "forgotten" shortly thereafter.

Throughout childhood and adolescence, serious learning impairments exist, restricting to a very modest level the achievement of the vast majority of individuals with Down syndrome. At this stage, one sees considerable instability as well as long periods during which little or no progress is made, only to be followed by new acquisitions. Nonetheless, there are exceptions to this pattern; some individuals achieve considerable heights, and their progress offers hope for the future. A thorough neuropsychological analysis of the learning and memory capacities of children with Down syndrome is required, guided by knowledge of how various tasks can be used to assess the functional status of specific learning and memory systems in the brain.

With advancing age, it is virtually certain that individuals with Down syndrome will develop neuropathology that is similar to that seen in Alzheimer disease. However, it now is well documented that only some of these subjects actually will develop the dementia characteristic of Alzheimer disease. Though no accepted explanation for this uncoupling of the neuropathology and dementia yet exists, it is a fact of considerable practical and theoretical importance. The most recent neuropsychological work only strengthens the view that the two are somehow critically different. Determining why a large proportion of individuals with Down syndrome apparently avoid the sequelae of Alzheimer disease is an important task for research in the coming years.

In sum, we slowly are unraveling the enigma that is the mental retardation associated with Down syndrome. Knowledge of which particular learning systems are affected and which are preferentially spared will help in the design of more effective early intervention programs. If current indications that the hippocampal system is particularly subject to disruption hold up, approaching children with Down syndrome in a way not unlike that used for amnesic patients (see Glisky & Schacter, 1989)—that is, by concentrating on learning and memory systems that are more or less intact—might be appropriate. Advantages of this approach are, first, that the children would experience success rather than frustration much of the time and, second, that it might be possible for children to build on the knowledge gained through these systems to acquire skills usually dependent on the other systems. On the other hand, early stimulation of the at-risk hippocampal system (and possibly the cerebellar system as well) could both improve its status in infancy and childhood and diminish the likelihood of Alzheimer disease–like neuropathology during aging. Clearly, there are good reasons to focus on both sides of the equation and to approach intervention with due regard to the complex nature of the learning and memory deficit.

ACKNOWLEDGMENTS

Portions of this chapter were written while the author was on a sabbatical from, and supported by, the University of Arizona. It is adapted from Nadel (1996). Support for this work was provided also by Cognitive Neuroscience Program grants from the McDonnell Foundation and the Flinn Foundation.

NOTES

1. It seems entirely probable that, for most characteristics (including mental functions), there is a "normal" distribution of values—a typical bell curve—in both normally developing infants and infants with Down syndrome.

2. Although this interpretation of inefficiency makes intuitive sense, it does make one pause when considering results from *all* PET studies, in which increases in activity usually are interpreted as signs of normal, not inefficient, function.

3. In an intriguing study of perceptual capacity, Bihrle et al. (1989) have shown that adolescents with Down syndrome are considerably more impaired in analysis of *local* features as compared to *global* features. This result strongly points to the inferotemporal cortex and, perhaps more precisely, to the dorsal region. (See Horel, 1994, for an analysis of the role of this area in local versus global perception.)

REFERENCES

Ball, M. J., & Nuttall, K. (1981). Topography of neurofibrillary tangles and granovacuoles in the hippocampi of patients with Down's syndrome: Quantitative comparison with normal ageing and Alzheimer's disease. *Neuropathology and Applied Neurobiology, 7*, 13–20.

Ball, M. J., Schapiro, M. B., & Rapoport, S. I. (1986). Neuropathological relationships between Down syndrome and senile dementia Alzheimer type. In C. J. Epstein (Ed.), *The neurobiology of Down syndrome* (pp. 45–58). New York, Raven Press.

Bar-Peled, O., Israeli, M., Ben-Hur, H., Hoskins, I., Groner, Y., & Biegon, A. (1991). Developmental patterns of muscarinic receptors in normal and Down's syndrome fetal brain—an autoradiographic study. *Neuroscience Letters, 133*, 154–158.

Backer, L. E., Armstrong, D. L., & Chan, F. (1986). Dendritic atrophy in children with Down's syndrome. *Annals of Neurology, 20*, 520–526.

Beeghly, M., Weiss-Perry, B., & Cicchetti, D. (1990). Beyond sensorimotor functioning: Early communicative and play development of children with Down syndrome. In D. Cicchetti & M. Beeghly (Eds.), *Children with Down syndrome: A developmental perspective* (pp. 329–368). New York: Cambridge University Press.

Benda, C. E. (1971). Mongolism. In J. Minckler (Ed.) *Pathology of the nervous system* (Vol. 2, p. 1867). New York: McGraw-Hill.

Bihrle, A. M., Bellugi, U., Delis, D., & Marks, S. (1989). Seeing the forest or the tress: Dissociation in visuospatial processing. *Brain and Cognition, 11*, 37–49.

Blackwood, W., & Corsellis, J. A. N. (1976). *Greenfield's neuropathology* (pp. 420–421). Chicago: Year Book Medical.

Brooksbank, B. W. L., Walker, D., Balazs, R., & Jorgenesen, O. S. (1989). Neuronal maturation in the foetal brain in Down syndrome. *Early Human Development, 18*, 237–246.

Caltagirone, C., Nocentini, U., & Vicari, S. (1990). Cognitive functions in adult Down's syndrome. *International Journal of Neuroscience, 54,* 221–230.

Carlesimo, G. A., Marotta, L., & Vicari, S. (1997). Long-term memory in mental retardation: Evidence for a specific impairment in subjects with Down's syndrome. *Neuropsychologia, 35,* 71–79.

Cohen, N. J., & Eichenbaum, H. (1993). *Memory, amnesia, and the hippocampal system.* Cambridge, MA: MIT Press.

Cohen, N. J., & Squire, L. R. (1980). Preserved learning and retention of a pattern-analyzing skill in amnesia: Dissociation of knowing how and knowing that. *Science, 210,* 207–210.

Cole, G., Neal, J. W., Singhrao, S. K., Jasani, B., & Newman, G. R. (1993). The distribution of amyloid plaques in the cerebellum and brain stem in Down's syndrome and Alzheimer's disease: A light microscopical analysis. *Acta Neuropathologica, 85,* 542–552.

Cork, L. C. (1990). Neuropathology of Down syndrome and Alzheimer disease. *American Journal of Medical Genetics Supplement, 7,* 282–286.

Courage, M. L., Adams, R. J., Reyno, S., & Kwa, P.-G. (1994). Visual acuity in infants and children with Down syndrome. *Developmental Medicine and Child Neurology, 36,* 586–593.

Coussons-Read, M. E., and Crnic, L. S. (1996). Behavioral assessment of the Ts65Dn mouse, a model for Down syndrome: Altered behavior in the elevated plus maze and open field. *Behavior Genetics, 26,* 7–13.

Crome, L., Cowie, V., & Slater, E. (1966). A statistical note on cerebellar and brain-stem weight in Mongolism. *Journal of Mental Deficiency, 10,* 69–72.

Davisson, M. T., Schmidt, C., Reeves, R. H., Irving, N. G., Akeson, E. C., Harris, B. S., & Bronson, R. T. (1993). Segmental trisomy as a mouse model for Down syndrome. In C. J. Epstein (Ed.), *The phenotypic mapping of Down syndrome and other aneuploid conditions* (pp. 117–133). New York: Wiley-Liss.

Deb, S., de Silva, P. N., Gemmell, H. G., Besson, J. A. O., Smith, F. W., & Ebmeier, K. P. (1992). Alzheimer's disease in adults with Down's syndrome: The relationship between regional cerebral blood flow equivalents and dementia. *Acta Psychiatrica Scandinavica, 86,* 340–345.

Devenny, D. A., Hill, A. L., Patxot, O., Silverman, W. P., & Wisniewski, K. E. (1992). Ageing in higher functioning adults with Down's syndrome: An interim report in a longitudinal study. *Journal of Intellectual Disability Research, 36,* 241–250.

Devinsky, O., Sato, S., Conwit, R. A., & Schapiro, M. B. (1990). Relation of EEG alpha background to cognitive function, brain atrophy, and cerebral metabolism in Down's syndrome. *Archives of Neurology, 47,* 58–62.

Ellis, N. R., Woodley-Zanthos, P., and Dulaney, C. L. (1989). Memory for spatial location in children, adults, and mentally retarded persons. *American Journal on Mental Retardation, 93,* 521–527.

Escorihuela, R. M., Vallina, I. F., Baamonde, C., Montero, J. J., Dierssen, M., Fernández-Teruel, A., Tobeña, A., & Flórez, J. (1995). Evaluation of Ts65Dn mice, a putative Down syndrome model, in sensorimotor, emotional and spatial learning tasks. *Society for Neuroscience Abstracts, 21,* 200.

Ferrer, I., & Gullotta, F. (1990). Down's syndrome and Alzheimer's disease: Dendritic spine counts in hippocampus. *Acta Neuropathologica, 79,* 680–685.

Florez, J., del Arco, C., Gonzalez, A., Pascual, J., & Pazos, A. (1990). Autoradiographic studies of neurotransmitter receptors in the brain of newborn infants with Down syndrome. *American Journal of Medical Genetics Supplement, 7,* 301–305.

Fowler, A. (1988). Determinants of rate of language growth in children with DS. In L. Nadel (Ed.), *The psychobiology of Down syndrome* (pp. 215–245). Cambridge, MA: MIT Press.

Glisky, E. L., & Schacter, D. L. (1989). Extending the limits of complex learning in organic amnesia: Computer training in a vocational domain. *Neuropsychologia, 27*, 107–120.

Greenwald, C. A., & Leonard, L. (1979). Communicative and sensorimotor development of Down's syndrome children. *American Journal of Mental Deficiency, 84*, 296–303.

Haier, R. J., Chueh, D., Touchette, P., Lott, I., Buchsbaum, M. S., MacMillan, D., Sandman, C., LaCasse, L., and Sosa, E. (1995). Brain size and cerebral glucose metabolic rate in non-specific mental retardation and Down syndrome. *Intelligence, 20*, 191–210.

Hemdal, P., Corwin, J., & Oster, H. (1993). Olfactory identification deficits in Down's syndrome and idiopathic mental retardation. *Neuropsychologia, 31*, 977–984.

Henderson, S. E. (1985). Motor skill development. In D. Lane & B. Stratford (Eds.), *Current approaches to Down's syndrome*. Eastbourne, UK: Holt, Rinehart and Winston.

Hepper, P. G., & Shahidullah, S. (1992). Habituation in normal and Down's syndrome fetuses. *The Quarterly Journal of Experimental Psychology, 44B*, 305–317.

Holtzman, D. M., Kilbridge, J., Chen, K. S., Rabin, J., Luche, R., Carlson, E., Epstein, C. J., & Mobley, W. C. (1995). Preliminary characterization of the central nervous system in partial trisomy 16 mice. In C. J. Epstein, T. Hassold, I. T. Lott, L. Nadel, & D. Patterson (Eds.), *Etiology and pathogenesis of Down syndrome* (pp. 227–240). New York: Wiley-Liss.

Hopmann, M. R., & Nothnagle, M. B. (1994, April). *A longitudinal study of early vocabulary of infants with Down syndrome and infants who are developing normally.* Poster presented at the International Down Syndrome Research Conference, Charleston, SC.

Horel, J. A. (1994). Local and global perception examined by reversible suppression of temporal cortex with cold. *Behavioural Brain Research, 65*, 157–164.

Horwitz, B., Schapiro, M. B., Grady, C. L., & Rapoport, S. I. (1990). Cerebral metabolic pattern in young adult Down's syndrome subjects: Altered intercorrelations between regional rates of glucose utilization. *Journal of Mental Deficiency Research, 34*, 237–252.

Hyman, B. T. (1992). Down syndrome and Alzheimer disease. In L. Nadel & C. J. Epstein (Eds.), *Down syndrome and Alzheimer disease* (pp. 123–142). New York: Wiley-Liss.

Jernigan, T. L., & Bellugi, U. (1990). Anomalous brain morphology on magnetic resonance images in Williams syndrome and Down syndrome. *Archives of Neurology, 47*, 529–533.

Kesslak, J. P., Nagata, S. F., Lott, I., & Nalcioglu, O. (1994). Magnetic resonance imaging analysis of age-related changes in the brains of individuals with Down's syndrome. *Neurology, 44*, 1039–1045.

Koo, B. K. K., Blaser, S., Harwood-Nash, D., Becker, L., & Murphy, E. G. (1992). Magnetic resonance imaging evaluation of delayed myelination in Down syndrome: A case report and review of the literature. *Journal of Child Neurology, 7*, 417–421.

Lögdberg, B., & Brun, A. (1993). Prefrontal neocortical disturbances in mental retardation. *Journal of Intellectual Disability Research, 37*, 459–468.

Lynch, M., Oller, K., Eilers, R., & Basinger, D. (1990, June). *Vocal development of infants with Down's syndrome.* Presented at the Symposium for Research on Child Language Disorders, Madison, WI.

Mangan, P. A. (1992). *Spatial memory abilities and abnormal development of the hippocampal formation in Down syndrome.* Unpublished doctoral dissertation, University of Arizona, Tucson.

Mangan, P. A., and Nadel, L. (1990). Development of spatial memory in human infants. *Bulletin of the Psychonomic Society, 28,* 513.

Mann, D. M. A., & Esiri, M. M. (1989). The pattern of acquisition of plaques and tangles in the brains of patients under 50 years of age with Down's syndrome. *Journal of the Neurological Sciences, 89,* 169–179.

Mann, D. M. A., Royston, M. C., & Ravindra, C. R. (1990). Some morphometric observations on the brains of patients with Down's syndrome: Their relationship to age and dementia. *Journal of the Neurological Sciences, 99,* 153–164.

Marcell, M. M., & Cohen, S. (1992). Hearing abilities of Down syndrome and other mentally handicapped adolescents. *Research in Developmental Disabilities, 13,* 533–551.

McAlaster, R. (1992). Postnatal cerebral maturation in Down's syndrome children: A developmental EEG coherence study. *International Journal of Neuroscience, 65,* 221–237.

McClelland, J. L., McNaughton, B. L., O'Reilly, R., & Nadel, L. (1992 November). Complementary roles of hippocampus and neocortex in learning and memory. Paper Presented at the Meeting of the Society for Neuroscience, Anaheim, CA.

Miller, J. F. (1995). Individual differences in vocabulary acquisition in children with Down syndrome. In C. J. Epstein, T. Hassold, I. T. Lott, L. Nadel, & D. Patterson (Eds.), *Etiology and pathogenesis of Down syndrome* (pp. 93–103). New York: Wiley-Liss.

Mishkin, M., Malamut, B., & Bachevalier, J. (1984). Memories and habits: Two neural systems. In J. L. McGaugh, G. Lynch, & N. M. Weinberger (Eds.), *The neurobiology of learning and memory.* New York: Guildford Press.

Mundy, P., Sigman, M., Kasari, C., & Yirmiya, N. (1988). Nonverbal communication skills in Down syndrome children. *Child Development, 59,* 235–249.

Murphy, G. M., Jr., & Ellis, W. G. (1991). The amygdala in Down's syndrome and familial Alzheimer's disease: Four clinicopathological case reports. *Biological Psychiatry 30,* 92–106.

Murphy, G. M., Jr., Ellis, W. G., Lee, Y.-L., Stultz, K. E., Shrivastava, R., Tinklenberg, J. R., & Eng, L. F. (1992). Astrocytic gliosis in the amygdala in Down's syndrome and Alzheimer's disease. In A. C. H. Yu, L. Hertz, M. D. Norenberg, E. Sykova, & S. G. Waxman (Eds.), *Progress in Brain Research* (Vol. 94, 475–483). Amsterdam: Elsevier Science Publishers.

Nadel, L. (1986). Down syndrome in neurobiological perspective. In C. J. Epstein (Ed.), *The neurobiology of Down syndrome* (pp. 239–251). New York: Raven Press.

Nadel, L. (1992). Multiple memory systems: What and why. *Journal of Cognitive Neuroscience, 4,* 179–188.

Nadel, L. (1994). Multiple memory systems: What and why. An update. In D. Schacter & E. Tulving (Eds.), *Memory systems 1994* (pp. 39–63). Cambridge, MA: MIT Press.

Nadel, L. (1996). Learning, memory and neural function in Down's syndrome. In J. Perera, J. Rondal, & L. Nadel (Eds.), *Down's syndrome. Psychological, psychobiological, and socio-educational perspectives.* London: Whurr Publishers.

Nadel, L., & Moscovitch, M. (1997). Memory consolidation, retrograde amnesia and the hippocampal complex. *Current Opinion in Neurobiology, 7,* 217–227.

Nadel, L. & O'Keefe, J. (1974). The hippocampus in pieces and patches: An essay on modes of explanation in physiological psychology In R. Bellairs and E. G. Gray (Eds.), *Essays on the nervous system. A Festschrift for J. Z. Young.* Oxford: Clarendon Press.

Nadel, L., & Willner, J. (1989). Some implications of postnatal maturation in the hippocampal formation. In V. Chan-Palay & C. Köhler (Eds.), *The hippocampus: New vistas.* New York: Alan R. Liss.

Nadel, L., & Zola-Morgan, S. (1984). Infantile amnesia: A neurobiological perspective. In M. Moscovitch (Ed.), *Infant memory*. New York: Plenum Press.

Ohr, P. S., & Fagen, J. W. (1991). Conditioning and long-term memory in three-month-old infants with Down syndrome. *American Journal on Mental Retardation, 96*, 151–162.

Ohr, P. S., & Fagen, J. W. (1993). Temperament, conditioning, and memory in 3-month-old infants with Down syndrome. *Journal of Applied Developmental Psychology, 14*, 175–190.

Ohr, P. S., & Fagen, J. W. (1994). Contingency learning in 9-month-old infants with Down syndrome. *American Journal on Mental Retardation, 99*, 74–84.

Oller, K., & Siebert, J. M. (1988). Babbling in prelinguistic retarded children. *American Journal on Mental Retardation, 92*, 369–375.

O'Keefe, J., & Nadel, L. (1978). *The hippocampus as a cognitive map*. Oxford: Clarendon Press.

Pazos, A., del Olmo, E., Diaz, A., del Arco, C., Rodriguez-Puertas, R., Pascual, J., Palacios, J. M., & Florez, J. (1994, April). *Serotonergic (5-HT_{1A} and 5-HT_{1D}) and muscarinic cholinergic receptors in DS brains: An autoradiographic analysis*. Poster presented at the International Down Syndrome Research Conference, Charleston, SC.

Poulson, C. L. (1988). Operant conditioning of vocalization rate of infants with Down syndrome. *American Journal on Mental Retardation, 93*, 57–63.

Rast, M., & Meltzoff, A. N. (1995). Memory and representation in young children with Down syndrome: Exploring deferred imitation and object permanence. *Development and Psychopathology, 7*, 393–407.

Raz, N., Torres, I. J., Briggs, S. D., Spencer, W. D., Thornton, A. E., Loken, W. J., Gunning, F. M., McQuain, J. D., Driesen, N. R., & Acker, J. D. (1995). Selective neuroanatomical abnormalities in Down syndrome and their cognitive correlates: Evidence from MRI morphometry. *Neurology, 45*, 356–366.

Rondal, J. A. (1994). Exceptional language development in mental retardation: The relative autonomy of language as a cognitive system. In H. Tager-Flusberg (Ed.), *Constraints on language acquisition: Studies of atypical children* (pp. 155–174). Hillsdale, NJ: Erlbaum.

Rondal, J. A. (1995). *Exceptional language development in Down syndrome: Implications for the cognitive-language relationship*. Cambridge: Cambridge University Press.

Schacter, D. L., & Tulving, E. (1994). *Memory systems 1994*. Cambridge, MA: MIT Press.

Schapiro, M. B., Haxby, J. V., & Grady, C. L. (1992). Nature of mental retardation and dementia in Down syndrome: Study with PET, CT, and neuropsychology. *Neurobiology of Aging, 13*, 723–734.

Schmidt-Sidor, B., Wisniewski, K., Shepard, T. H., & Sersen, E. A. (1990). Brain growth in Down syndrome subjects 15 to 22 weeks of gestational age an birth to 60 months. *Clinical Neuropathology, 9*, 181–190.

Spargo, E., Luthert, P. J., Janota, I., and Lantos, P. L. (1992). β4A deposition in the temporal cortex of adults with Down's syndrome. *Journal of the Neurological Sciences, 111*, 26–32.

Squire, L. R. (1992). Memory and the hippocampus: A synthesis of findings with rats, monkeys, and humans. *Psychological Review, 99*, 195–231.

Squire, L. R., Cohen, N. J., & Nadel, L. (1984). The medial temporal region and memory consolidation: A new hypothesis. In H. Weingartner & E. Parker (Eds.), *Memory consolidation*. Hillsdale, NJ: Erlbaum.

Steffens, M. L., Oller, K., Lynch, M., & Urbano, R. (1992). Vocal development in infants with Down syndrome and infants who are developing normally. *American Journal on Mental Retardation, 97*, 235–246.

Sutherland, R. J., & Rudy, J. W. (1989). Configural association theory: The role of the hippocampal formation in learning, memory, and amnesia. *Psychobiology, 17,* 129–144.

Sylvester, P. E. (1983). The hippocampus in Down's syndrome. *Journal of Mental Deficiency Research, 27,* 227–236.

Tager-Flusberg, H. (1999). Language development in atypical children. In M. Barrett (Ed.), *The development of language* (pp. 311–348). London: UCL Press.

Uecker, A., Obrzut, J. E., & Nadel, L. (1994). Mental rotation performance by learning disabled and Down's syndrome children: A study of imaginal development. *Developmental Neuropsychology, 10,* 395–411.

Weis, S. (1991). Morphometry and magnetic resonance imaging of the human brain in normal controls and Down's syndrome. *The Anatomical Record, 231,* 593–598.

Wishart, J. (1993). The development of learning difficulties in children with Down syndrome. *Journal of Intellectual Disability Research, 37,* 389–403.

Wisniewski, K. E. (1990). Down syndrome children often have brain with maturation delay, retardation of growth, and cortical dysgenesis. *American Journal of Medical Genetics Supplement, 7,* 274–281.

Wisniewski, K. E., Laure-Kamionowska, M., Connell, F., & Wen, G. Y. (1986). Neuronal density and synaptogenesis in the postnatal stage of brain maturation in Down syndrome. In C. J. Epstein (Ed.), *The neurobiology of Down syndrome* (pp. 29–44). New York: Raven Press.

Wisniewski, K., & Schmidt-Sidor, B. (1989). Postnatal delay of myelin formation in brains from Down syndrome infants and children. *Clinical Neuropathology, 8,* 55–62.

Woodruff-Pak, D. S., Papka, M., & Simon, E. W. (1994). Eyeblink classical conditioning in Down's syndrome, fragile X syndrome, and normal adults over and under age 35. *Neuropsychology, 8,* 14–24.

Woodruff-Pak, D. S., Romano, S., & Papka, M. (1996). Training to criterion in eyeblink classical conditioning in Alzheimer's disease, Down's syndrome with Alzheimer's disease, and healthy elderly. *Behavioral Neuroscience, 110,* 22–29.

10 Turner Syndrome: A Cognitive Neuroscience Approach

Joanne Rovet and Lori Buchanan

Turner syndrome is a disorder of sex chromosome complement that affects only female individuals and has a distinctive set of physical and psychological features. Turner syndrome is caused by the loss of some material from the X chromosome, usually an entire X chromosome. Physical manifestations, including short stature, gonadal dysgenesis, mild skeletal abnormalities, and a defect in lymphatic clearance, exist with considerable variability as to the severity and type of physical stigmata. This variability in both the physical and psychological profiles of girls with Turner syndrome can be found in the two case studies we describe here.

CASE REPORT 1

BL is a lovely 14-year-old daughter of a dentist and an accountant. The only obvious physical symptom of Turner syndrome is her short stature (approximately 4 ft 7 in.). BL's mother reports an uneventful pregnancy with BL, who was described as an easy-going infant with mild colic and no feeding disorders. All early motor and language developmental milestones were reached at appropriate times and, with the exception of a tonsillectomy and adenoidectomy at 7, BL has never been hospitalized for illness, and her health and vision are normal. Academically, she is entering grade 9 and has been a very successful student to this point, with achievements placing her near the top of her class. Socially, BL is very popular at school, and she has several close friends and one long-standing "best" friend. She appears to be both cheerful and positive in her outlook, exuding abundant self-confidence.

BL's scholastic achievements reflect the combination of high commitment and a bright-average intelligence that was demonstrated during her testing session. Her Weschler Intelligence Scale (3rd edition) full-scale IQ score was 109, with a verbal IQ of 118 and a performance IQ of 98. BL performed above the eightieth percentile on all tests of verbal ability. In contrast, the visual performance subtests resulted in a considerable scatter, with scores ranging from the ninety-fifth percentile on the maze subtest to a low of sixth percentile on symbol search subtest.

BL was brought in for this assessment because her parents were concerned that she may have some of the mathematics impairments often noted in children with Turner syndrome. Consequently, BL's mathematics skills were tested using the Wide Range Achievement Test–Revised (WRAT-R) and the KEYMATH test of mathematics abilities. She scored at the fifty-fifth percentile on the mathematics subtest of the WRAT-R which, though normal, is in sharp contrast to her score at the ninety-ninth percentile on reading and at the eighty-fourth percentile on spelling. The KEYMATH pen and paper mathematics test was used to provide a more fine-grained analysis of mathematics skills, and BL scored at the eighty-fourth percentile on tests of basic concept knowledge of geometry and rational numbers, above the seventy-fifth percentile on the arithmetic application subtests (i.e., measurement, time and money, estimation, data interpretation, and problem solving) and at the sixty-third percentile on tests of basic knowledge of numeration. Her mental computation scores were all at or above the seventy-fifth percentile. However, weaknesses were evident in division and multiplication (i.e., sixteenth percentile and thirty-seventh percentiles, respectively). Her overall score on the KEYMATH was at the eighty-eighth percentile. Thus, although BL does have some difficulties with multiplication and division, her mathematics abilities certainly are within normal range.

BL's memory was assessed using the Wide Range Assessment of Memory and Learning and the Denman Neuropsychology Memory Scale. On the former, she produced a score that placed her at the fifty-fifth percentile overall, but she demonstrated a relative strength in the verbal domain, with a score at the ninety-second percentile for memory of verbal information and a score at the tenth percentile for memory for visual information. Similarly, on the Denman, BL scored at the seventh percentile on nonverbal memory.

In summary, BL is a healthy, very well-adjusted 14-year-old girl with a bright-average intelligence and strengths in verbal abilities. Relative weaknesses, although still in the normal range, were observed on some tests of mathematics computations and in visual memory.

CASE REPORT 2

WL, a 13-year-old daughter of separated parents, lives with her mother and two younger siblings. Her physical features are typical of Turner syndrome: She has a very high upper palate, resulting in an unusually small upper jaw, a webbed neck, and short stature (approximately 4 ft 6 in.). She is presently in grade 7 at school and has had an adequate academic career to this point. However, her mother and teachers have noted a recent decline in performance, and WL is concerned about her performance in mathematics and French. She worries that she may not pass these courses. Socially, WL is not very popular in her school, has no close friends, and appears to be somewhat depressed and lacking in self-confidence. Her relationship with her siblings is also strained.

WL's mother reported an uneventful pregnancy, and WL's infancy was described as unremarkable aside from minor feeding problems associated with having a high upper palate. All early motor milestones were reached at appropriate times, but WL did not begin using phrases until after being enrolled in speech therapy at approximately 3 years of age. WL has an enlarged heart and an accompanying abnormality in rhythm, which was corrected with the insertion of a pacemaker at age 8. Her kidney is horseshoe-shaped, and she has had numerous urinary tract infections.

During the testing session, WL showed a positive attitude and was very inquisitive. Although she often claimed an inability to perform tasks, with coaxing she was able to perform them quite well. She displayed considerable intuition and self-awareness, particularly with respect to her scholastic limitations and her tendency toward acting immaturely and being overly anxious. Her mother's report agrees, for the most part, with WL's self-assessment, with the exception that mother claims that WL is somewhat disruptive and hyperactive, though WL does not believe this to be true.

WL's scholastic difficulties likely reflect a combination of psychological difficulties (i.e., her slight depression and lack of self-confidence) and a low-average intelligence that was demonstrated during her testing session. Her performance on the full-scale Weschler Intelligence Scale–Revised resulted in an overall full-scale IQ score of 84, with a verbal IQ of 98 and a performance IQ of 72. Within both the verbal and performance domains, little scatter was observed.

WL was referred for this assessment because both her mother and her teachers were concerned about recent difficulties in school, in particular with mathematics and French. WL's school achievement was assessed using the WRAT-R, and she scored at the forty-fifth percentile in arithmetic, the seventy-ninth percentile in reading, and the sixty-fourth percentile on the spelling. On the KEYMATH, she scored at the thirteenth percentile overall, showing difficulties in multiplication (second percentile) and division (ninth percentile). Relative strengths were found on arithmetic application (i.e., measurement, time and money, estimation, data interpretation, and problem solving), all of which were scored at near the fiftieth percentile. Memory was assessed using the Denman Neuropsychology Memory Scale, on which she obtained a full-scale memory quotient of 66, with scores of 77 for verbal memory and 59 for nonverbal memory.

In summary, WL's health and physical appearance are both, to a large extent, affected by her Turner syndrome. She is of low average intelligence, with clear disabilities in both mathematics and memory for nonverbal information. Her social skills are impaired, and she suffers from a lack of confidence in her academic abilities.

The preceding case studies illustrate the symptom variability and the commonalties that are present within the Turner syndrome population. Both girls are very short, but they differ in terms of the severity of other symptoms. WL showed the classic features of facial dysmorphology, webbed neck, and cardiac and kidney problems, whereas BL was healthy, quite attractive, and normal-appearing. Cognitively, both girls showed a significant discrepancy between verbal and nonverbal abilities, and both were less proficient in mathematics than in reading. However, as BL had above average verbal abilities, her relatively poorer nonverbal abilities were in the normal range. This stands in contrast to WL, whose poorer nonverbal abilities were in the borderline range. She also had fewer coping mechanisms, and her low self-esteem contributed to her academic difficulties. Although both girls showed the cognitive pattern suggestive of a nonverbal learning disability, (Rovet, 1995), as with their physical features, considerable variability separated them in degree and extent of cognitive impairment.

IDENTIFYING THE CORE COGNITIVE DEFICITS IN TURNER SYNDROME

Since the discovery of the cytogenetic basis for the physical stigmata characterizing Turner syndrome (Ford, 1956), individuals with this condition have been the focus of several attempts to identify the genetic basis of the associated neuroanatomical and neurobehavioral characteristics. Because Turner syndrome may result in abnormal estrogen levels, this group also has been the focus of studies of sex hormones and abilities (Nyborg, 1990). However, the etiological basis of their deficits and adequate explanations for the source of variability have not yet been determined. These questions remain despite efforts of several laboratories, including ours and that of Ross. Also lacking is proper theoretical justification for their pattern of deficit.

This chapter describes our reanalysis of these questions in light of empirical and theoretical advances in other areas of psychology, particularly with regard to the visual system. Recent work in cognitive neuroscience has demonstrated two distinct neuroanatomical pathways for the processing of visuospatial information. These include (1) a dorsal stream that projects from the magnocellular cells in the thalamus to the occipital cortex and the posterior parietal lobe and (2) a ventral stream that projects from the thalamus's parvocellular cells through to the inferior temporal cortex (see Kosslyn, 1980 for a description of both neurological and cognitive discussions of these pathways). The first pathway is associated with the processing of spatial location information and has come to be known as the *where* pathway; the second is associated with processing object identity information and is known as the *what* pathway (Haxby et al., 1991; Sergent et al., 1992a,b; Kosslyn et al., 1993).

We propose that this pathway distinction provides a useful theoretical framework for studying visuospatial deficits in Turner syndrome. The basis of this framework is our assumption that the physiological distinction between *what* and *where* pathways translates into functional dissociations that may be at the heart of the variability in the cognitive strengths and weaknesses in the disorder. This has led us to investigate how children and adolescents with Turner syndrome perform according to *what* and *where* processing distinctions. Recent studies of Turner syndrome and other disorders also have produced a discussion of a third type of nonverbal processing (Ross et al., 1995; see also chapter 4), which is assumed to mediate visuoconstructive processing (the *how* processes). Though this third process type does not enjoy the same-well defined physiological descriptions as those in the *what* and *where* processes, it does appear, nonetheless to be a distinct form of visuospatial processing. Our goal was to identify which of these three pathways or processes may be disrupted in Turner syndrome and to determine how this relates to mathematics and social processing deficits in affected individuals. A future goal was to identify the genetic bases for difficulties along one or more streams.

This chapter reviews the extant psychological findings regarding Turner syndrome and shows some of the shortcomings of traditional approaches to understanding the problem. We then provide preliminary findings from two studies, which deploy a process analysis approach. These studies involve (1) a retrospective reanalysis of clinical data obtained about subjects with Turner syndrome and matched controls and (2) the development and use of an experimental reaction-time paradigm that taps the dissociation between *what* and *where* processes. Our aim is to show that this approach offers a promising methodology for better understanding the genetic (and possibly hormonal) determinants of behavior in Turner syndrome. The implications of these findings for other syndromes and disorders also is discussed.

THE PHYSICAL, BEHAVIORAL, AND NEUROLOGICAL CHARACTERISTICS OF TURNER SYNDROME

Physical Characteristics

Turner syndrome affects between 1 in 2000 (Nielsen et al., 1977) and 1 in 5000 (Hook & Warburton, 1983) female persons, with similar representation among different ethnic and racial groups. Though some 60% of individuals are missing one of the two X chromosomes that characterize normal female subjects, others have (1) a structural abnormality or rearrangement of one or both X chromosomes, (2) the presence of part of a Y chromosome, (3) the loss of *part* of a second X chromosome, or (1) mosaicism involving both a normal and an abnormal cell line. The single X or 45,X condition occurs during gamete production prior to fertilization and can be maternal or paternal in origin; in 70% of the cases, it appears that the paternal sex chromosome is absent (Mather et al., 1991). An individual with mosaicism may have one or several different cell populations, such as the usual mosaic karyotype in which some cells contain the classic 45,X makeup, whereas others contain a normal 46,X makeup. Further variations of mosaicism exist such that as many as seven different cell lines can occur in a single individual. Mosaicism normally takes place after fertilization of the ovum during early mitosis.

The physical phenotype of Turner syndrome is characterized by a generalized growth defect, ovarian failure, and the variable presence of certain somatic features. Growth failure begins in utero, with infants being perhaps 3 cm shorter than normal at birth (Giovannelli & Balestrazzi, 1996) and having further loss in height between 3 and 12 years of age. The final adult height of women with Turner syndrome is 4 ft, 9 in., depending on country of origin (Ranke, 1996). Studies of biosynthetic growth hormone on children with Turner syndrome indicate considerable variability as to final outcome and ultimate benefit (Albertsson-Wikland & Ranke, 1995).

Ovarian failure occurs from a massive loss of oocytes in utero and after birth, which results in streak or dysgenetic ovaries. Although ovarian dysgenesis is a normal process in all female subjects, for some unknown reason this is highly accelerated in individuals with Turner syndrome (Singh & Carr, 1966). For the vast majority of women with Turner syndrome, this results in a lack of secondary sexual development and infertility. With modern advances in assisted reproduction, however, a few women with Turner syndrome have given birth to healthy normal children.

The somatic abnormalities include skeletal deformities, such as an unusual carrying angle of the elbows (cubitus valgus), shield chest, short fourth metacarpals, short neck, and spinal abnormalities. Atypical facies reflecting micrognathia, reduced facial skeleton size, and a high, arched palate leading to feeding difficulties (Mathiesen et al., 1992) also can occur. Abnormalities of the facial bone structures are associated with an elevated incidence of ear infections and hearing loss. Another common abnormality is a basic defect in the lymphatic clearance system, which is associated with aortic coarctation (Lippe, 1982), ptosis, and neck webbing (Giovannelli & Balestrazzi, 1996). Individuals with Turner syndrome also may have multiple pigmented nevi (Simpson, 1975).

The genetic phenomenon known as *X inactivation* (Lyon, 1962) signifies that for the vast majority of genes on the X chromosome, only one of the two X copies is expressed—hence the greater number of similarities than of differences among female subjects with Turner syndrome and normal female persons. However, now several sites on the X chromosome are known to escape X inactivation, and these are thought to be the sources for the somatic (and psychological) features of Turner syndrome. Indeed, current thinking holds that as many as five sites on the X chromosome contribute to the phenotype (Page, 1995). Because individuals with Turner syndrome have one instead of two alleles of these particular genes, they will have reduced expression of the associated proteins (Zinn et al., 1993). The decreased production of these proteins is thought to contribute to the Turner syndrome stigmata and to other endocrine and environmental factors (Ross, 1990).

Behavioral Characteristics

Global Intelligence   Numerous studies based primarily on adult women with Turner syndrome have reported a reduction in global IQ (e.g., Grumbach et al., 1955) but no apparent increase in mental subnormality. In a review of 19 studies describing the findings from 226 cases, a mean IQ of 94.6 was observed as compared with 103.9 for controls (Rovet, 1990). Lower IQ was associated with selective impairment in the nonverbal, visuospatial processing domain (Garron, 1977; Shaffer, 1962) and reflected a 12-point difference between verbal and performance IQ, favoring verbal (Rovet, 1990). At least one chromosomal abnormality in Turner syndrome, known as a *ring chromosome*, is associated with increased risk of mental retardation (Migeon et al., 1994).

Two studies have examined the relation between somatic features and intelligence. Money and Granoff (1965) reported no relationship between number or type of physical anomaly and IQ or the visual minus performance IQ discrepancy. Garron (1977) reported that IQ was not associated with cubitus valgus, neck webbing, moles, or finger or cardiac defects, but individuals with more than three stigmata had visual and performance IQ scores lower overall than those of individuals with fewer stigmata.

Temple and Carney (1993) compared IQ test results of two groups of subjects with Turner syndrome. In one group, all subjects had the classic 45,X karyotype, whereas in the other, the subjects had other karyotypes, which included a partial deletion, mosaicism, an isochromosome, and ring mosaicism. Although the groups did not differ in overall IQ, only the "pure" group showed a significant advantage for verbal over performance subtests of the IQ test, whereas this discrepancy between verbal and performance scores also was noted in the individuals with an isochromosome karyotype.

Specific Abilities Studies have shown that individuals with Turner syndrome do poorly on a wide variety of visuospatial and visuomotor tasks including construction (Murphy et al., 1994); design copying (Waber, 1979); directional sense (Alexander et al., 1964); extrapersonal space perception (Alexander & Money, 1966); mazes (Nielsen et al., 1977); mental rotation (Rovet & Netley, 1982); nonverbal memory (Ross et al., 1995); part-whole perception (Silbert et al., 1977); the rod-and-frame task (Nyborg, 1990); rotor pursuit (Ross et al., 1996); spatial reasoning (Money & Alexander, 1966); spatial working memory (Romans et al., 1997); visual discrimination (Silbert et al., 1977); visual memory (Murphy et al., 1994); visual reasoning (Murphy et al., 1994), visual sequencing (Robinson et al., 1986); and visuomotor integration (Lewandowski et al., 1985). Although one investigator has suggested that these subjects exhibit "space-form blindness" (Money, 1963), in their everyday lives they do drive cars and navigate adequately in their environments. Downey et al. (1991) described individuals with Turner syndrome as competent in using new equipment, assembling objects from parts, arranging objects, and interpreting graphs and charts, but they have a greater-than-usual difficulty at "picturing the outcome of a construction project." Visuospatial abilities appear to be lower in subjects with Turner syndrome, regardless of karyotype (Murphy, et al., 1994); and Ross et al. (1996) reported that their deficits in motor tasks are restricted to those involving spatial components.

In examining visuospatial deficits across several domains, Ross et al. (1995) reported that female subjects with Turner syndrome had the most difficulty on tasks examining "how things go together" as compared to tasks of visual or spatial processing. Also, the *where* aspects of visual processing were more impaired than were the *what* aspects. Girls with Turner syndrome did not differ in confrontation naming, sentence repetition or verification, verbal fluency, face perception, facial memory, and oral reading (Murphy et al., 1994). In one of the only studies to use experimentally based reaction time tasks in subjects with Turner syndrome, Rovet and Netley (1982) observed differences between Turner syndrome and matched controls on selective reaction time parameters of a mental rotation task. In particular, the Turner syndrome group had significantly larger slope values, suggesting slower mental transformation rates, but they did not differ from controls in their intercept values, suggesting equivalent visual discrimination skills.

Although their language skills are generally intact (Rovet & Netley, 1982), those individuals with high arched palates or hearing loss may have early speech and language difficulties (Robinson et al., 1986). Problems in early motor development and subsequent clumsiness also have been reported (Bender et al., 1984). Difficulties with executive functioning have been described in the areas of fluency, planning, and flexibility (Waber, 1976), as have problems with short-term memory (Berch, 1996); attention (Ross et al., 1995); temporal analysis (Silbert et al., 1977); numerical computation (Rovet, 1993); face affect processing (McCauley et al., 1987); facial recognition (Waber, 1979; Ross et al., 1995); and auditory sequencing (Silbert et al., 1977).

Behavior and Personality A characteristic behavioral profile reflecting both a specific profile of traits and immature personality development has been shown in children with Turner syndrome (El Abd et al., 1995). They tend to be prone to hyperactivity (Rovet, 1995), to have poorer social skills and peer relations (McCauley, 1990; Rovet & Ireland, 1994), to prefer younger children (Rovet & Ireland, 1994), and to have low self-esteem (Rovet, 1995), particularly with respect to physical and athletic self-esteem (Ross et al., 1996). Skuse et al. (1994) pointed out an increased incidence of psychiatric disorders, which is equivalent to referred cases requiring clinical intervention. Interestingly, the incidence of psychiatric disorders was higher in cases with mosaicism than in those with a pure 45,X karyotype (Skuse et al., 1994). A large study of unselected adolescents with Turner syndrome indicated that they were not at serious risk of psychopathology but that they were more vulnerable to problems with social relationships (McCauley et al., unpublished manuscript). In contrast, Mambelli et al. (1996) reported an increased incidence of phobias, anxiety crises, obsessive traits, and depression in preadolescent and adolescent groups, which reflects their poorer socialization and less adequate means of dealing with their anxieties.

Women with Turner syndrome are described as being happy, more extroverted or more introverted than normal, very talkative, less able to postpone gratification, and more phlegmatic than usual, and to show lower-than-normal levels of arousal (Money & Mittenthal, 1970), increased stress tolerance, social immaturity, poor interpersonal relationships, and low self-esteem (Mambelli et al., 1996). Low self-esteem appears to be associated with number and severity of physical stigmata (Pavlidis et al., 1995) and with family factors (Kagan, unpublished manuscript). In a qualitative analysis of the reports of three women regarding their experience of having Turner syndrome, Kagan found wide differences in acceptance and self-worth, which reflected perceived physical attractiveness and family acceptance. In summarizing this literature, McCauley (1990) has reported that adults with Turner syndrome are not at increased risk for severe psychopathology but that they are more prone to mild depression (McCauley, 1990). According to Mambelli et al. (1996), their affective disabilities can inhibit their cognitive development, keeping them at a concrete level of thinking and unable to engage in divergent thinking and introspection or to entertain ambivalent and conflictual thoughts.

In a study at our laboratory, we examined the behavioral characteristics of a large sample of children with Turner syndrome who were not selected on the basis of height and genetic karyotype. These results were obtained at baseline, prior to entry into a Canada-wide trial of growth hormone therapy in this population (Rovet & Ireland, 1994). Poor social competence was observed to be linked to extremely short stature, whereas their behavior problems reflected specific karyotypes. Specifically, children with a chromosomal rearrangement, presence of some Y chromosome material, or a partial deletion of one X chromosome had more behavioral problems than did children with a 45,X karyotype, mosaicism, or an isochromosome. The specific behavior problems that were observed reflected increased withdrawal or depression and conduct, social, thought, and attention problems. However, noteworthy is that 34% were unaffected socially and 71% were unaffected behaviorally (Rovet, 1995).

Overall, these results suggest an increased incidence of behavior problems reflecting more immaturity and hyperactivity in girls with Turner syndrome. A classic personality profile was not found, however, presumably owing in part to the complexity of factors contributing to the variability in presentation of the syndrome and to family and peer factors. Low self-esteem is common and appears to reflect degree of short stature and possibly other phenotypic features (Kagan, unpublished manuscript). According to Mambelli et al. (1996), these behavioral characteristics may have an inhibitory effect on cognitive functioning.

Achievement   Children with Turner syndrome are at increased risk of problems at school, in greater need of special education services, and more likely to fail a grade (Rovet, 1993). However, not all children are affected to the same degree, and not all have problems. Academically, they are excellent and avid readers, and they have few difficulties with mechanical reading and reading comprehension. Although their spelling and written language skills are adequate, parents report they have more than usual difficulty in completing tasks and difficulty with written work (Rovet, 1995). Nevertheless, the majority do show difficulties with mathematics, ranging from moderate to severe. Using criteria for subtyping from Rourke and Strang (1983), we assigned children with Turner syndrome and controls into different learning disability groups. We found that 55% had a learning disability, as compared with 26% of controls (Rovet, 1993). In Turner syndrome, this always involved an arithmetical disability, alone or in combination with reading problems, but never only a reading disability, unlike controls who showed this pattern. Problems in arithmetical processing involved primarily computational skills, whereas geometry was affected less severely.

In a study from our laboratory (Rovet et al., 1994), error analyses were conducted on the responses by girls with Turner syndrome to selected items of the WRAT-R and the KEYMATH Diagnostic Arithmetic Test. These analyses were based on the model of McCloskey et al., (1985) for mathematics processing that was derived from patients who became acalculic after localized brain injury, and on Temple's (1989, 1991) procedures for analyzing arithmetic errors in children with dyscalculia. Arithmetic test items were subdivided into number-processing or computational domains, with the latter reflecting fact retrieval or procedural knowledge processes. Using 45 girls with Turner syndrome (aged 7–16 years) and 93 chromosomally normal matched female controls, we found in the Turner syndrome group an increased incidence of fact retrieval problems on the WRAT-R and procedural knowledge problems on both the WRAT-R and KEYMATH (the lack of fact retrieval problems on the KEYMATH was attributed to the fact that it was an untimed test). Error analyses revealed that the girls with Turner syndrome were more likely to confuse component steps and less likely to complete or separate intermediate steps than were controls, but the two groups did not differ in their knowledge of subprocesses, such as carrying and borrowing. Analyses by age revealed that in the girls with Turner syndrome, difficulties in fact retrieval reflected lags in development with catchup, whereas their problems in procedural knowledge reflected true deficits.

Developmental Changes Developmental changes in Turner syndrome are poorly understood. Indeed, with one exception (Bender et al., 1984), no longitudinal studies have targeted population, and few have even examined findings cross-sectionally by age. However, in Bender's studies, results from children with Turner syndrome were combined with results from children with other sex chromosome anomalies and were never examined from a developmental perspective exclusively within a Turner syndrome group. Thus, even in this study, discerning the developmental features of Turner syndrome was difficult. In the majority of studies, the age range of the sample has been too broad to allow an assessment of differences occurring only at specific ages.

Several studies have compared girls with Turner syndrome and controls who were at different age levels. In an early comparison of preadolescent and adolescent girls with Turner syndrome, we found that only preadolescents showed the classic discrepancy between verbal and nonverbal skills. In contrast, young adolescents below age 16 showed lower verbal skills and low nonverbal abilities as compared to older adolescents (> 16 years), for whom the discrepancy reappeared. Though this finding suggests that verbal abilities may be vulnerable to a lack of pubertal changes during early adolescence in this population, it also may reflect increasing difficulty and demands on abstract verbal thinking at the upper limits of intelligence testing for children. Ross et al. (1995) have provided valuable information with respect to the developmental trajectory of various visuospatial and visuomotor deficits in children with Turner syndrome (see chapter 11); but an upper age limit of 14.9 years in their study indicates clearly that much remains to be examined with respect to older girls. However, in more recent studies by Romans et al. (1997), this same group showed that attentional and executive processing deficits on tasks involving high spatial working memory demands were deficient in girls with Turner syndrome regardless of age. In contrast (and in support of our findings), an age-related increment in verbal fluency failed to occur in subjects between ages 12 and 17.

Summary   Turner syndrome is associated with a wide range of physical and behavioral characteristics. Individuals with Turner syndrome show cognitive impairments primarily in the visuospatial domain, though problems in executive functioning, memory, and attention also have been observed. One investigator has reported that a problem in working memory may be the core deficit underlying Turner syndrome subjects' poor visuospatial performance (Berch, 1996). Though the findings are relatively consistent across studies, within studies considerable variability in the presentation of associated deficits has been observed (Pennington et al., 1985). The principle factors contributing to this variability have not been identified. Moreover, many of the studies are methodologically limited, owing to small sample sizes, wide age ranges, and lack of controls (Rovet, 1990; El Abd, et al., 1995) and further research is needed, particularly research grounded in accepted theory. Recent advances from the field of cognitive neuroscience offer a useful approach for explaining the visuospatial processing deficit in this population (see later).

Neurobiological Characteristics

A number of studies have been conducted on children and adults with Turner syndrome to determine the presence of unique neuroanatomical characteristics and whether these account for the behavioral features previously described. The findings show little consistency as to either lateralizing or localizing effects (Rovet, 1990). The present consensus supports a more diffuse involvement than originally conceived (Money, 1963) and that differences may by organizational and functional, not structural.

Neuropathological Findings   Three autopsy descriptions of patients with Turner syndrome have reported considerable neuroanatomical heterogeneity in this population. One case had a neuronal migration defect (Kolb & Heaton, 1975); another exhibited a neurodevelopmental abnormality in the posterior right hemisphere (Reske-Nielsen et al., 1982); and the third showed neither of these brain pathologies and had no previous cognitive impairment (Reske-Nielsen et al., 1982).

Clinical Tests Studies based on neuropsychological test batteries have provided varying results, ranging from a focal right parietal dysfunction (Money, 1973) to more extensive posterior right-hemisphere dysfunction (McGlone, 1985) to dysfunction involving the entire right hemisphere (Silbert et al., 1977) or the parietal and frontal regions of both hemispheres (Waber, 1979). This research typically is limited by relatively small sample sizes. Murphy et al. (1994) reported that the X chromosome may affect the development of both cerebral hemispheres, particularly the association neocortices, whereas hormonal factors may serve to modify development of particular brain regions, such as the right parietal lobes.

Cerebral Lateralization Studies At least seven studies have attempted to determine whether atypical hemispheric specialization and organization explain the characteristic neurocognitive profile in Turner syndrome. These studies have used dichotic listening procedures with verbal stimuli (Waber, 1979; Gordon & Galatzer, 1980; Netley & Rovet, 1982; Lewandowski et al., 1985) or a visual T-scope presentation with both verbal and nonverbal information (McGlone, 1985). One study reported the results on four laterality tasks (Rovet, 1990).

Across studies, the results indicated that subjects with Turner syndrome showed weaker-than-normal left-hemisphere biases for verbal information but no difference in right-hemisphere bias for nonverbal material. In contrast, girls with Turner syndrome showed a greater-than-normal tendency to use their left hemispheres in the processing of nonverbal information. Degree of lateralization appeared to vary with type of stimulus and mode of presentation.

Electrophysiological Studies Although electroencephalographic studies have reported atypical recordings in many subjects with Turner syndrome (Poenaru et al., 1970; Tsuboi & Nielsen, 1976), no single problem has been identified and considerable variability exists among individuals and across studies. Portellano-Perez et al. (1996) used brain maps based on electroencephalographic measurements to show that the brain structures activated during different cognitive processes may differentiate Turner syndrome and controls. For example, reading activated the right hemisphere to a greater degree in girls with Turner syndrome than in controls, whereas arithmetic activated the left parietal lobe in controls and the right hemisphere in girls with Turner syndrome.

Two studies have used event-related potential (ERP) paradigms in girls with Turner syndrome. Shucard et al. (1992) observed that subjects with Turner syndrome produced a profile suggestive of less adequate processing of ongoing irrelevant or competing information by the right hemisphere. Johnson and Ross (1994) examined ERPs in two age groups of adolescents with Turner syndrome, none of whom were treated with hormones, while they performed two different tasks. In one—the "oddball" task—subjects had to discriminate between high- and low-pitched tones. In the second, they were required to identify whether line drawings of hands in varying orientations represented a right or a left hand. Two distinct cognitive deficits were observed: one suggestive of a congenital abnormality and the other suggestive of a maturational abnormality (Johnson et al., 1993). Regarding the congenital problem, girls with Turner syndrome in both young and old age groups differed from their respective controls on an early ERP wave component during the visual discrimination task. This finding suggested a problem in stimulus analysis in all subjects with Turner syndrome. On the auditory oddball task, however, only the old Turner syndrome group differed from their age-matched controls. This disparity was observed specifically in the O-wave component, which is known to develop during midpuberty and reflects stimulus orientation and the ability to change contexts. Thus, the girls with Turner syndrome failed to show this late cognitive development. At a functional level, this deficit suggests that they have greater-than-normal difficulty in placing events in their proper context and show a tendency to overrate the impact of events.

Johnson and Ross (1994) also studied ERP components in a subject who had Turner syndrome and had normal endogenous estrogen levels and in Turner syndrome subjects who received estrogen therapy during late adolescence. The subject with normal estrogen levels showed a performance remarkably similar to, and a wave profile to comparable those in normal female subjects, whereas the subjects receiving their estrogen therapy late failed to show a normal responses. These results suggest a possible critical period for estrogen, without which normal adolescent maturation of selective brain systems fails to occur.

Neuroimaging Studies   At least four studies of Turner syndrome subjects have involved neuroimaging techniques. Using position emission tomography (PET), Clark et al., (1990) found that glucose uptake was reduced in the parietal occipital lobes of women with Turner syndrome. In a volumetric magnetic resonance imaging (MRI) study of 8- to 14-year-old girls with Turner syndrome, Ross et al., (1993) reported an increased bilateral ventricular volume that was attributed to a generalized process operating during neurodevelopment affecting both white and gray matter formation. These researchers also studied a set of 10-year-old twins discordant for Turner syndrome (Reiss et al., 1993). The twin with Turner syndrome typically did not do as well on tests of visuospatial ability, attention, and executive functioning but did not differ from her sister in mathematics. MRI scans revealed significantly reduced gray matter volume in the left parietal perisylvian and right prefrontal regions for the twin with Turner syndrome, whereas her cerebrospinal fluid was increased in the right posterior parieto-occipital area. Finally, in a study comparing MRI scans of women with a pure 45,X karyotype, women with a mosaic karyotype, and healthy controls, all subjects in the groups with Turner syndrome had significantly smaller MRI volumes in the hippocampus, caudate, lenticular, and thalamic nuclei and in parietooccipital brain matter on both sides (Murphy et al., 1993). Murphy et al. attributed their findings to the role of the X chromosome in the development and aging of gray matter in the striatum, diencephalon, and cerebral hemispheres.

Summary These findings suggest specific neuroanatomical abnormalities associated with Turner syndrome. Although these neurodevelopmental modifications appear to be genetically modulated, reflecting how much X chromosomal material is missing and the specific sites that are lost, functional differences may be associated with hormonal dysfunction (Ross et al., 1993). Regardless of methodology, abnormalities in the occipital and parietal lobes of the right hemisphere appear to be primary. According to Murphy et al. (1994), right posterior abnormalities reflect the abnormal hormonal milieu, whereas the association cortices are affected by the atypical X chromosome complement.

A COGNITIVE NEUROSCIENCE APPROACH TO STUDYING VISUOSPATIAL PROCESSING DEFICITS

Recent advances in cognitive neuroscience have identified the existence of distinct and unique neuroanatomical pathways for processing visuospatial information (Kosslyn, 1980). One pathway projects from parvocellular layers of the thalamus through the occipital cortex to the inferotemporal cortex, and the other proceeds from the magnocellular layers of the thalamus through the occipital cortex to the posterior parietal cortex. The first pathway, which is assumed to subserve object identification, is known as the *what* stream, whereas the second, which is assumed to subserve object location, is known as the *where* stream. According to Merigan and Maunsell (1993), the *where* or dorsal stream pathway may develop earlier than does the *what* or ventral stream pathway.

These pathway distinctions originally were discovered in primates in whom ablations to the temporal region disrupted the ability to discriminate objects, whereas ablations to the parietal cortex disrupted the ability to discriminate spatial locations (Mishkin et al., 1983). The findings also have been upheld in studies of patients who had localized brain damage (De Renzi, 1982; Bauer & Reubens, 1985) and in whom lesions in the temporal cortex were associated with difficulty with color and form discrimination (agnosia), visual memory, and facial recognition (prosapagnosia; Levine et al., 1985), and lesions in the parietal cortex with hemifield neglect, disruption of visuomotor orientation, left–right confusion, impaired visual reaching, and markedly impaired spatial ability (Levine et al., 1985).

Using PET scan methodology, several studies have examined dissociations in the normal visuospatial processing system (Haxby et al., 1991; Sergent et al., 1992a,b). The findings have confirmed that separate areas of the brain were activated when *what* and *where* processing tasks were contrasted.

McIntosh et al. (1994) used structural equation modeling techniques to map functional networks of cortical visual pathways obtained with PET. Finally, researchers have manipulated the dissociations between visual and spatial processing using experimental reaction-time paradigms in college students (Tresch et al., 1993).

Summary and Implications for Research on Turner Syndrome

These results suggest that the magnocellular-parietal stream is sensitive to processing spatial information, whereas the parvocellular-temporal stream is sensitive to processing visual information. The possibility that these streams represent two independent pathways that develop at different rates and are potentially affected by different factors assumes that girls with Turner syndrome may be differentially affected in one but not in the other pathway. Functionally, we know that they are more affected in the spatial analysis than in the visual detail component of visuospatial processing (Rovet & Netley, 1982; Leneman et al., 1996) and that neurobiologically, they are more likely to be impaired along the parietal pathway than along the infero-temporal. Also, Ross (1995) has suggested that they may have difficulty along an additional *how* dimension, which has not been described physiologically. This lack of physiological specificity likely is a reflection of the fact that this kind of processing involves a number of different components of the visual system, including the integration of several neurocognitive pathways (see chapter 4).

Given recent studies of an association between a gene on the long arm of the X chromosome (in the fragile X site) that is restricted to the development of magno cells (Chaudhuri, personal communication), we predicted that girls with Turner syndrome would be affected more in the *where* than in the *what* pathway. After Ross et al. (1995), we also predicted an impairment on *how* processes. In the next section, we describe two preliminary findings from studies applying this cognitive neuroscience approach to children and adolescents with Turner syndrome.

Application of a Cognitive Neuroscience Approach in Turner Syndrome

We recently conducted two studies on children and adolescents with Turner syndrome. The first is a retrospective reanalysis of clinical data that were classified according to the three processes of interest (i.e., *what*, *where*, and *how*). The second study deploys an experimental paradigm that we developed to dissociate *what*-versus-*where* processing in immediate and delayed conditions.

Study 1:   Clinical Retrospective Analysis   This study compared six children with Turner syndrome (ages, 9.5–13.1 years) with six age- and verbal

Table 10.1 Pathway assignments for clinical tests

What
Denman: faces
Rey: visual detail analysis score

Where
Picture completion
Rey: spatial analysis score

How
Block design
Denman: Rey copy
Beery

IQ–matched (±5 points) female controls. The Turner syndrome group was derived from our clinical files, whereas the controls were identified from our control pool of subjects participating in other studies in our laboratory. All subjects received (1) the picture completion subtest of the Weschler Intelligence Scales for Children–Revised, in which they had to determine the missing features from a line drawing of a familiar object; (2) the block design subtest of the same Weschler test, in which they manipulated red and white blocks to reproduce designs of increasing difficulty shown on cards; (3) the faces subtest of the Denman Neuropsychological Memory Scale, in which they recognized previously studied faces; (4) the immediate Rey-figure of the Denman Neuropsychological Memory Scale, in which they copied a very complex line drawing of an unfamiliar object; and the Beery Visual Motor Integration test, a pen-and-paper copying task in which the 24 geometrical forms ranged from easy to very complex. Based on a previous study in which visuospatial subtests of 58 normal controls were factor-analyzed, the following subtests were assigned to *what, where,* and *how* pathways (as shown in table 10.1). Additionally interesting to us was the Rey-Ostereith figure-copying task, which was provided as a subtest of the Denman Memory Inventory. We used a new method for scoring that reflected the *what* and *where* distinctions: *What* processing was evaluated by examining the integrity of feature based details in the child's reproduction, whereas *where* processing was scored by examining the extent to which the child's reproduction was faithful to the original with respect to spatial relations (see Leneman et al., 1996 for a more detailed discussion of these scoring procedures). As a control measure, subjects also were compared on the Denman Immediate Story Recall subtest.

Results on spatial tasks first were converted to z-scores and were combined across processing domains as set out in Table 10.1. Scores on *t*-tests comparing Turner syndrome and control groups on the three domain composites were highly significant, reflecting the poorer performance by the Turner syndrome group (figure 10.1). The slightly lower level of significance for *what* ($P = .005$) than for *where* ($P = .001$) or *how* ($P = .0003$) tasks sug-

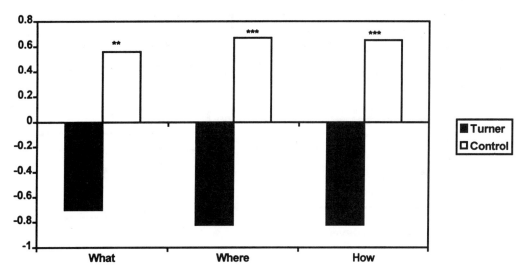

Figure 10.1 Mean pathway composite scores.

gested to us that girls with Turner syndrome might be less affected in visual than in spatial processing. However, a repeated-measures analysis of variance across domains indicated that though the groups were highly different from one another, no differential effect was seen for any pathway (i.e., no interaction between group and domain factors). Notably, on the Denman memory task, girls with Turner syndrome performed significantly better than did controls (Turner syndrome, 13; control, 7.5; $P < .002$). Though these results suggest that all visuospatial pathways may be affected in Turner syndrome, because the clinical measures we used were not pure indices of processing in each pathway, they might not be sensitive to differential pathway effects. For this reason, a set of experimental procedures was developed as described later.

Study 2: Experimental Approach This study compared performance of nine girls with Turner syndrome to seven age- and verbal IQ–matched controls. The goal was to examine the separation of *what* and *where* processes and the contribution of working memory deficits to the visuospatial impairments in Turner syndrome [see Buchanan et al., (1998) for a complete description]. The primary questions of interest were whether one or both types of processing are impaired in Turner syndrome and, if so, what role working memory played.

A set of computer-based experiments was designed to address these questions (figure 10.2). In these experiments, two stimuli that varied on two dimensions (e.g., identity and location) were presented on a computer display, and participants were required to judge whether the two stimuli had the same shape or same location as specified by the examiner. For example, if a triangle appeared in both displays, the correct answer for a shape judgment

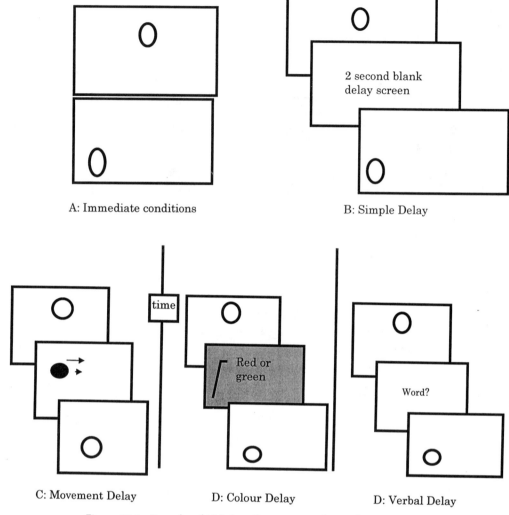

Figure 10.2 Examples of trials from the experimental procedure.

was yes, whereas if these triangles appeared in different locations, the correct answer for a location judgment was no. By using stimulus location and stimulus identity as the two varying dimensions in this paradigm, we had hoped to tease apart the *what*-versus-*where* components of visual processing. Specifically, a comparison of shape versus location decisions was expected to supply information about the relative functioning of the *what* and *where* processes in girls with Turner syndrome versus those in controls. Contrary to prediction, we found that those with Turner syndrome did not differ from the controls with respect to either type of decision (figure 10.3), although a general slowing across all conditions was seen in the girls with Turner syndrome.

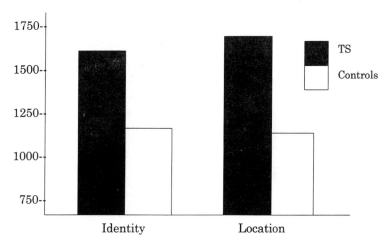

Figure 10.3 Reaction times for Turner syndrome (TS) group and control group as a function of decision.

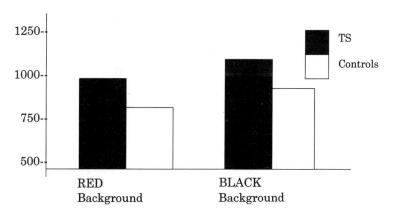

Figure 10.4 Reaction times for Turner syndrome (TS) group and control group as a function of background manipulation.

In addition to the location-shape conditions, two other manipulations were carried out. The first manipulation took advantage of the color-processing abilities of the parvocellular and magnocellular pathways. Because color is processed by only the parvocellular pathway, the presentation of stimuli at equiluminance should favor the parvocellular pathway, thus equating the Turner syndrome group and the controls *if* the deficit in Turner syndrome is limited to the magnocells. In one condition, stimuli were presented in white on a black background, whereas in the second condition, they were presented in green on a red background. Despite our expectations, the groups did not differ with respect to this background manipulations (figure 10.4), which indicates that the deficit may arise later in the visuospatial processing system.

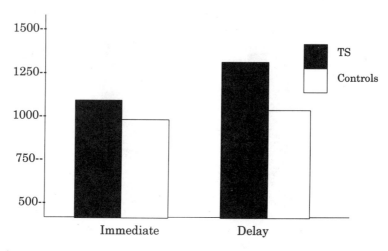

Figure 10.5 Reaction times for Turner syndrome (TS) group and control group as a function of delay.

Our next question of interest was whether visuospatial deficits in the Turner syndrome population could be explained on the basis of working memory impairments. To answer this we included a time-lag manipulation in which decisions were made to stimuli presented simultaneously in one condition and with a 2-sec delay between presentation of the two stimuli in the second condition. Although the group X delay interaction did not reach significance ($F < 1$), this manipulation did appear to affect the Turner syndrome group more than it did the controls (figure 10.5). As this suggested to us that working memory may play a role in the visuospatial deficits in Turner syndrome, we further examined the involvement of working memory deficits in Turner syndrome.

Working memory was studied by introducing a secondary-interference task manipulation during the 2-sec delay between the presentation of the first and the second shapes; figure 10.2C–E depict these conditions. In these conditions, children had to maintain information about the target shapes in memory while also making supplementary decisions on either visual (detecting either color or movement in a display) or verbal information (deciding whether a letter string is a real word). As Figure 10.6 shows, the Turner syndrome group was at a distinct disadvantage when the secondary task involved visuospatial discrimination but not verbal discrimination. As this was not true for the control group, we interpreted these findings as indicating that a visuospatial working memory impairment is a core deficit in Turner syndrome.

As a supplementary goal, we sought to determine whether performance on the experimental task could be predicted by the karyotype of the girls with Turner syndrome. To accomplish this goal, we calculated a measure of score for visuospatial memory interference; this score was determined by comparing the difference between reaction times for the verbal and the

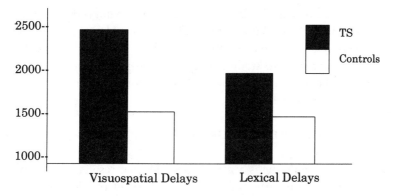

Figure 10.6 Reaction times for Turner syndrome (TS) group and control group as a function of secondary task manipulation.

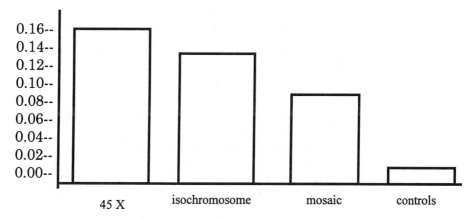

Figure 10.7 Visual interference scores for Turner syndrome group (by karyotype) and controls.

visuospatial interference tasks and dividing that difference by overall reaction time for each individual. Although our numbers were limited, a trend did appear in the data, with karyotype groups involving 45,X, mosaicism, and isochromosome differing with respect to this visuospatial interference score (figure 10.7). The same was not true for general processing speed, as grouping by karyotype did not reveal any trends in overall reaction time data despite the fact that the Turner syndrome group was consistently slower in every condition.

In summary, our experimental data show a general processing slowness in the Turner syndrome group relative to controls. This general slowing was not predicted by karyotype. In contrast, a specific deficit in visuospatial working memory was predicted by karyotype. These findings suggest to us the possibility of two core deficits in Turner syndrome: a reduction of processing speed and a difficulty in managing competing visuospatial information in short-term or working memory. However, as preliminary data showed that the location task was not more difficult than was the shape task for the girl with Turner syndrome, our initial hypothesis of a pathway deficit was not supported. Furthermore, the background manipulation condition that was used to study performance when the parvo pathway alone was in use showed no difference between groups, again failing to support our working hypothesis.

GENERAL CONCLUSIONS

Turner syndrome is a genetic disorder that results in a distinctive profile of cognitive strengths and weaknesses. Particularly affected in individuals with this disorder is their ability to process information in the visuospatial domain, which may predispose them to a classic nonverbal learning disability that ultimately leads to considerable difficulty with math. Nevertheless, considerable variability exists among individuals as to who are affected and as to the degree and severity of deficit. No study has as yet provided adequate explanations for this variability, although promising leads have come from several laboratories.

Recent advances in the field of cognitive neuroscience offer increased precision for understanding the functional deficit in Turner syndrome and its neuroanatomical underpinnings. On the basis of behavioral, neuropsychological, and neuroimaging findings, we proposed that individuals with Turner syndrome would be affected selectively in one of the major pathways underlying visuospatial processing: the pathway associated with the processing of *where*, or spatial location information. However, our findings from two preliminary studies supported this hypothesis only minimally. Our study involving a retrospective reanalysis of clinical data showed that the subjects' deficit was widespread, affecting *what*, *where*, and *how* processes. In contrast, our experimentally based study involving computerized assessments of object identity and spatial location information suggested that subjects' deficits may be secondary to an impairment in visuospatial working memory.

Further research capitalizing on a cognitive neuroscience approach such as this would be invaluable in characterizing the deficit in this population and clarifying other disorders showing a similar profile of cognitive disabilities. We propose that characterizing different subtypes of nonverbal learning disabilities in the general population along these lines would have tremendous potential for designing effective intervention and remediation.

REFERENCES

Albertsson-Wikland K., & Ranke, M. (1995). *Turner syndrome in a lifespan perspective: Research and clinical aspects.* Amsterdam: Elsevier.

Alexander, D., & Money, J. (1966). Turner's syndrome and Gerstmann's syndrome: Neuropsychologic comparisons. *Neuropsychologia, 4,* 265–273.

Alexander, D., Walker, H., & Money, J. (1964). Studies in direction sense. *Archives of General Psychiatry, 10,* 337–339.

Bauer, R. M., & Rubens, A. B. (1985). Agnosia. In K. M. Heilman and E. Valenstein (Eds.), *Clinical neuropsychology* (2nd ed., pp. 187–241). New York: Oxford University Press.

Bender, B., Puck, M., Salbenblatt, J., & Robinson, A. (1984). Cognitive development of unselected girls with complete and partial X monosomy. *Pediatrics, 73,* 175–182.

Berch, D. B. (1996). Memory. In J. Rovet (Ed.), *Turner syndrome across the lifespan.* Toronto: Klein Graphics.

Buchanan, L., Pavlovic, J., & Rovet, J. (1998). A Reexamination of visuospatial deficits in Turner syndrome: Contributions of working memory. *Developmental Neuropsychology, 14,* 341–367.

Clark, C., Klonoff, H., & Hayden, M. (1990). Regional cerebral glucose metabolism in Turner syndrome. *Canadian Journal of Neurological Sciences, 17,* 140–144.

De Renzi, E. (1982). Memory disorders following focal neocortical damage. *Philosophical Transactions of the Royal Society of London–Series B: Biological Sciences, 298*(1089), 73–83.

Downey, J., Elkin, E., Ehrhardt, E., Meyer-Bahlburg, A., Bell, H., & Akira, J. (1991). Cognitive ability and everyday functioning in women with Turner syndrome. *Journal of Learning Disabilities, 24,* 32–39.

El Abd, S., Turk, J., & Hill, P. (1995). Annotation: Psychological characteristics of Turner syndrome. *Journal of Child Psychology and Psychiatry, 36,* 1109–1124.

Ford, C. E., & Hamerton, J. L. (1956). The chromosomes of man. *Acta Genetica et Statistica Medica, Basel, 6(2),* 264–265.

Garron, D. (1977). Intelligence among persons with Turner's syndrome. *Behavior Genetics, 7,* 105–127.

Giovennilee, G., & Balestrazzi, P. (1996). Turner syndrome: Phenotypic variability. In J. Rovet (Ed.), *Turner syndrome across the lifespan.* Toronto: Klein Graphics.

Gordon, H., & Galatzer, A. (1980). Cerebral organization in patients with gonadal dysgenisis. *Psychoneurendocrinology, 5,* 235–244.

Grumbach, C. H., Van Wyck, J. J., & Wilkens, L. (1955). Chromosomal sex in gonadal dysgenesis relationship to male pseudohermaphorditism and theories of human sex differentiation. *Journal of Clinical Endocrinology, 15,* 1161–1193.

Haxby, J., Grady, C., Ungerleider, L., & Horwitz, B. (1991). Mapping the functional neuroanatomy of the intact human brain with brain work imaging. *Neuropsychologia, 29,* 539–555.

Hook, E. B., & Warburton, D. (1983). The distribution of chromosomal genotypes associated with Turner's syndrome: Livebirth prevalence rates and evidence for diminished fetal mortality and severity in genotypes associated with structural abnormalities or mosaicism. *Human Genetics, 64,* 24–27.

Johnson, R., & Ross, J. (1994). Event-related potential indications of altered brain development in Turner syndrome. In S. Broman & J. Grafman (Eds.), *Atypical cognitive deficits in developmental disorders: Implications for brain function* (pp. 217–242). Hillsdale, NJ: Erlbaum.

Johnson, R., Rohrbaugh, J., & Ross, J. (1993). Altered brain development in Turner's syndrome. *Neurology, 43,* 801–808.

Kolb, J., & Heaton, R. (1975). Lateralized neurologic deficits and psychopathology in a Turner syndrome patient. *Archives of General Psychiatry, 32,* 1198–1200.

Kosslyn, S. E. (1980). *Image and mind.* Cambridge MA: Harvard University Press.

Leneman, M., Buchanan, L., Pavlovic, J., & Rovet, J. (1996). *"What", "where" and "how": Visuo-spatial impairments in congenital hypothyroidism.* Presented at the Annual International Neuro-psychology Society Meeting, Chicago, IL.

Levine, D. N., Warach, J., & Farah, M. J. (1985). Two visual systems in mental imagery: Dissociations of "what" and "where" in imagery disorders due to bilateral posterior cerebral lesions. *Neurology, 35,* 1010–1018.

Lewandowski, L., Costenbader, V., & Richman, R. (1985). Neuropsychological aspects of Turner syndrome. *International Journal of Neuropsychology, 1,* 144–147.

Lippe, B. M. (1982). Primary ovarian failure. In S. A. Kaplan (Ed.), *Clinical pediatric and adolescent endocrinology* (pp. 325–366). Philadelphia: Saunders.

Lyon, M. F. (1962). Sex chromatin and gene action in the mammalian X-chromosome. *American Journal of Human Genetics, 14,* 135–148.

Mambelli, M. C., Perulli, L., Casella, G., Leventaki, R., Perini, C., Gozzi, G., Panizzolo, C., Rigon, F., & Condini, A. (1996). Difficulties and experiences in dealing with the needs of patients with Turner syndrome and their families: The usefulness of a multidisciplinary approach. In J. Rovet (Ed.), *Turner syndrome across the lifespan.* Toronto: Klein Graphics.

Mather, A., Stekol, L., Schatz, D., MacLaren, N., Scott, M., & Lippe, B. (1991). The parental origin of the single X chromosome in Turner syndrome: Lack of correlation with parental age or clinical phenotype. *The American Journal of Human Genetics, 48,* 682–686.

Mathiesen, B., Reilly, S., & Skuse, D. (1992). Oral motor dysfunction and feeding disorders in infants with Turner syndrome. *Developmental Child Neurology, 34,* 141–149.

McCauley, E., (1990). Pychosocial and emotional aspects of Turner syndrome. In D. Berch & B. Bender (Ed.), *Sex chromosome abnormalities and human behavior: Psychological studies* (pp. 78–99). Boulder, CO: Westview Press.

McCauley, E., Kay, T., Ito, J., & Treder, R. (1987). The Turner's syndrome: Cognitive deficits, affective discrimination and behavior problems. *Child Development, 58,* 464–473.

McCloskey, M., Caramazza, A., & Basili, A. (1985). Cognitive mechanisms in number processing and calculation: Evidence from dyscalenlia. *Brain and Cognition, 4,* 171–196.

McGlone, J. (1985). Can spatial deficits in Turner's syndrome be explained by focal CNS dysfunction or atypical speech lateralization? *Journal of Clinical and Experimental Neuropsychology, 7,* 375–394.

McIntosh, A. R., Grady, C. L., Ungerleider, L. G., Haxby, J. V., Rapoport, S. I., & Horwitz, B. (1994). Network analysis of cortical visual pathways mapped with PET. *The Journal of Neuroscience, 14,* 655–666.

Merigan, W. H., & Maunsell, J. H. (1993). How parallel are the primate visual pathways? *Annual Review of Neuroscience, 16,* 369–402.

Migeon, B. R., Luo, S., Jani, M., & Jeppesen, P. (1994). The severe phenotype of females with tiny ring X chromosomes is associated with inability of these chromosomes to undergo X inactivation. *American Journal of Human Genetics, 55,* 497–504.

Mishkin, M., Ungerleider, L. G., & Macko, K. A. (1983). Object vision and spatial vision: Two cortical pathways. *Trends in Neuroscience, 6,* 414–417.

Money, J. (1963). Cytogenetic and psychosexual incongruities with a note on space-form blindness. *American Journal of Psychiatry, 119,* 820–827.

Money, J., & Alexander, D. (1966). Turner's syndrome: Further demonstration of the presence of specific cognitional deficiencies. *Journal of Medical Genetics, 3,* 47–48.

Money, J., & Granoff, D. (1965). IQ and the somatic stigmata of Turner's syndrome. *American Journal of Mental Deficiency, 70,* 69–77.

Murphy, D., Allen, G., Haxby, J., Largay, K., Daly, E., White, B., Powell, C., & Schapiro, M. (1994). The effects of sex steroids, and the X chromosome, on female brain function: A study of the neuropsychology of adult Turner syndrome. *Neuropsychologia, 32,* 1309–1323.

Murphy, D., DeCarli, C., Daly, E., Haxby, J., Allen, G., White, B., McIntosh, A., Powell, C., Horwitz, B., Rapoport, S., & Schapiro, M. (1993). X-chromosome effects on female brain: A magnetic resonance imaging study of Turner's syndrome. *Lancet, 342,* 1197–1200.

Nielsen, J., Nyborg, H., & Dahl, G. (1977). Turner's syndrome: A psychiatric-psychological study of 45 women with Turner's syndrome, compared with their sisters and women with normal karyotypes, growth retardation, and primary amenorrhea. *Acta Jutlandica, 45,* (Medicine Series 21), 190.

Nyborg, H. (1990). Sex hormones, brain development, and spatio-perceptual strategies in Turner syndrome. In D. Berch & B. Bender (Eds.), *Sex chromosomes abnormalities and human behavior: Psychological studies* (pp. 100–129). Boulder, CO: Westview Press.

Page, D. C. (1995). Mapping and targeting Turner genes. In K. A. Albertsson-Wikland & M. B. Ranke (Eds.), *Turner syndrome in a life span perspective: Research and clinical aspects* (pp. 297–308). Amsterdam: Elsevier.

Pavlidis, K., McCauley, E., & Sybert, V. (1995). Psychosocial and sexual functioning in women with Turner syndrome. *Clinical Genetics, 47,* 85–89.

Pennington, B. F., Heaton, R. K., Karzmark, P., Pendelton, R., Lehman, R., & Shucard, D. W. (1985). The neuropsychological phenotype in Turner's syndrome. *Cortex, 21,* 391–404.

Poenaru, S., Stanesco, V., Poenaru, L., & Stoian, D. (1970). EEG dans le syndrome de Turner. *Acta Neurologica Belgica, 70,* 509–522.

Portellano-Perez, J., Bouthelier, R., & Asensio-Monge, I. (1996). New neurophysiological and neuropsychological contributions about Turner syndrome. In J. Rovet (Ed.), *Turner syndrome across the lifespan.* Toronto: Klein Graphics.

Ranke, M. (1996). Growth and predicting growth in Turner syndrome. In J. Rovet (Ed.), *Turner syndrome across the lifespan.* Toronto: Klein Graphics.

Reiss, A. L., Freund, L., Plotnick, L., Baumgartner, T., Green, K., Sozer, A. C., Raeder, M., Boehm, & Denkla, M. (1993). The effects of X monosomy on brain development: Monozygotic twins discordant for Turner's dsyndrome. *Annals of Neurology, 34,* 97–105.

Reske-Nielsen, E., Christensen, A., & Nielsen, J. (1982). A neuropathological and neuro-psychological study of Turner's syndrome. *Cortex, 18,* 181–191.

Robinson, A., Bender, B., Borelli, J., Puck, M., Salbenglatt, J., & Winter, J. (1986). Sex chromosomal aneuploidy: Prospective and longitudinal studies. In S. Ratcliffe & N. Paul (Eds.), *Prospective studies on children with sex chromosome aneuploidy* (pp. 23–73). New York: Alan R. Liss.

Romans, S., Roeltgen, D., Kushner, H., & Ross, J. (1997). Executive function in girls with Turner's syndrome. *Developmental Neuropsychology, 13,* 24–40.

Ross, J. L. (1990). Disorders of the sex chromosomes: Medical overview. In: C. S. Holmes (Ed.), *Psychoendocrinology, brain, behavior and hormonal interactions.* New York: Springer.

Ross, J. L., Kushner, H., & Roeltgen, D. P., (1996). Developmental changes in motor function in girls with Turner syndrome. *Pediatric Neuropsychology, 15,* 317–322.

Ross, J. L., Reiss, A. L., Freund, L., Roeltgen, D., & Cutler, G. B., Jr. (1993). Neurocognitive function and brain imaging in Turner syndrome: Preliminary results. *Hormone Research, 39,* 65–69.

Ross, J. L., Roeltgen, D., & Cutler, G. B. (1995). The neurodevelopmental transition between childhood and adolescence in girls with Turner syndrome. In K. A. A!bertsson-Wikland & M. B. Ranke (Eds.), *Turner syndrome in a life span perspective: Research and clinical aspects* (pp. 297–308). Amsterdam: Elsevier.

Rourke, B. & Strang, J. D., (1983). Subtypes of reading and arithmetic disabilities: a neuropsychological analysis. In M. Rutter (Ed.), *Developmetal neuropsychiatry*. New York: Guilford Press.

Rovet, J. (1990). The cognitive and neuropsychological characteristics of children with Turner syndrome. In D. Berch & B. Bender (Eds.), *Sex chromosome abnormalities and human behavior: Psychological studies* (pp. 38–77). Boulder, CO: Westview Press.

Rovet, J. (1993). The psychoeducational characteristics of children with Turner syndrome. *Journal of Learning Disabilities, 26,* 333–341.

Rovet, J. (1995). Behavioral manifestations of Turner syndrome in children: a unique phenotype. In K. A. Albertsson-Wikland & M. B. Ranke (Eds.), *Turner syndrome in a life span perspective: Research and clinical aspects* (pp. 297–308). Amsterdam: Elsevier.

Rovet, J., & Ireland, L. (1994). The behavioral phenotype of children with Turner syndrome. *Journal of Pediatric Psychology, 19,* 779–790.

Rovet, J., & Netley, C. (1982). Processing deficits in Turner's syndrome. *Developmental Psychology, 18,* 77–94.

Rovet, J., Szekely, C., & Hockenberry, M. (1994). Specific arithmetic deficits in children with Turner syndrome. *Journal of Clinical and Experimental Neuropsychology, 16,* 820–839.

Sergent, J., Ohta, S., & MacDonald, B. (1992a). Functional neuroanatomy and object processing. A positron emission tomography study. *Brain, 1,* 15–36.

Sergent, J., Zuck, E., Levesque, M., & MacDonald, B. (1992b). Positron emission tomography study of letter and object processing: Empirical findings and methodological considerations. *Cerebral Cortex, 2,* 68–80.

Shaffer, J. W. (1962). A specific cognitive deficit observed in gonadal aplasia (Turner syndrome). *Journal of Clinical Psychology, 18,* 403–406.

Shucard, D. W., Shucard, J. L., Clopper, R. J., & Schacter, M. (1992). Electrophysiological and neuropsychological indices of cognitive processing deficits in Turner syndrome. *Developmental Neuropsychology, 8,* 299–323.

Silbert, A., Wolff, P., & Lilienthal, J. (1977). Spatial and temporal processing in patients with Turner's syndrome. *Behavior Genetics, 7,* 11–21.

Simpson, J. (1975). Gonadal dysgenisis and abnormalities of the human sex chromosomes: Current status of phenotypic-karyotpic correaltions. In D. Bergsma (Ed.), *Birth Defects: Original article Series 11* (pp. 23–55). New York: Stratton Intercontinental Medical Book Corp.

Singh, R., & Carr, H. (1966). The anatomy and histology of human embryos and fetuses. *Anatomy Research, 155,* 369–384.

Skuse, D., Percy, E., & Stevenson, J. (1994). Psychosocial functioning in Turner syndrome: A national survey. In B. Stabler & L. Underwood (Eds.), *Growth, stature, and adaptation: Behavioural, social and cognitive aspects of growth delay.* Chapel Hill: University of North Carolina Press.

Temple, C. (1989). Digit dyslexia: A catagory specific disorder in developmental dyscalculia. *Cognitive Neuropsychology, 6,* 93–116.

Temple, C. (1991). Procedural dyscalculia and number fact dyscalculia: A double dissociation in developmental dyscaluculia. *Cognitive Neuropsychology, 8,* 155–176.

Temple, C., & Carney, R. (1993). Intellectual functioning of children with Turner syndrome: A comparison of behavioural phenotypes. *Developmental Medicine and Child Neurology, 35,* 691–698.

Tresch, M. C., Sinnamon, H. M., & Seamon, J. G. (1993). Double dissociation of spatial and object visual memory: Evidence from selective interference in intact human subjects. *Neuropsychologia, 31,* 211–219.

Tsuboi, T., & Nielsen, J. (1976). Electroencephalographic examination of 50 women with Turner's syndrome. *Acta Neurologica Scandinavica, 54,* 359–365.

Waber, D. (1979). Neuropsychological aspects of Turner syndrome. *Developmental Medicine and Child Neurology, 21,* 58–70.

Zinn, A., Page, D., & Fisher, E. (1993). Turner syndrome: The case of the missing sex chromosome. *Trends in Genetics, 9,* 90–93.

11 Turner Syndrome: Potential Hormonal and Genetic Influences on the Neurocognitive Profile

Judith L. Ross and Andrew Zinn

Turner syndrome (TS), or monosomy X, is the complex human phenotype of female individuals from whom the second sex chromosome is completely or partially absent. Common X chromosome abnormalities in TS include complete monosomy X (45, X), X isochromosomes (46, X, i[Xq]), ring X chromosomes (46, X, r[X]), and X deletions (46, X, del[Xp] or 46, X, del[Xq]), with mosaicism for a second cell line (e.g., 45, X/46, X, i[Xq]) present in anywhere from 28% to 67% of subjects in several large series (Held et al., 1992).

The incidence of sex chromosome abnormalities that include monosomy X has been estimated to be approximately 1 in 3000 to 5000 liveborn girls, but the disorder may be present in as many as 2% of all conceptions. Fewer than 1% of all 45, X embryos survive to term (Hook & Warburton, 1983; Hassold, 1986). The ovaries in girls with TS apparently form normally initially but involute prematurely at 4 to 5 months' gestation (Held et al., 1992). As a result of this so-called gonadal dysgenesis, the children, as a rule, lack ovarian estrogen production, do not undergo spontaneous pubertal maturation, and are infertile (Hassold, 1986). Extragonadal TS features include short stature and congenital malformations such as webbing of the neck, shield chest, horseshoe kidney, and coarctation of the aorta (Hook & Warburton, 1983). In addition, these children manifest a particular neurocognitive and social profile. This chapter addresses the following questions about the neurocognitive profile in girls and women with TS:

1. What is the "typical" or most characteristic neurocognitive profile, and how does it evolve between childhood and adolescence?

2. What is the role of estrogen replacement therapy in influencing the typical neurocognitive profile?

3. What are the potential genetic determinants of this neurocognitive profile?

CHARACTERISTIC COGNITIVE AND BEHAVIORAL PROFILE IN TURNER SYNDROME

Most studies have found that verbal ability (particularly verbal IQ) is similar in TS girls versus control girls (McCauley et al., 1987; Ratcliffe et al., 1991;

Robinson et al., 1991; Rovet, 1991, 1993; Stewart et al., 1991; Ross et al., 1995). Consistently, visuospatial or spatial-perceptual abilities are impaired in children and adolescents with TS (Money, 1973; Waber, 1979; Netley & Rovet, 1982; Pennington et al., 1985; Williams et al., 1992; Swillen et al., 1993; Murphy et al., 1994). TS patients perform less well than do controls on spatial, attentional, and short-term memory tasks (Williams et al., 1991; Rovet, 1993). Other neuropsychological domains in which differences between TS subjects and controls (normal or matched for short stature) have been identified include affect discrimination (in particular, comprehension or discrimination of facial affective expression), performance IQ, and dichotic listening (McCauley et al., 1987; Nyborg, 1991). Significant differences in motor function have also been demonstrated in girls with TS versus control girls (Levandonski et al., 1985; Salbenblatt et al., 1987; Bender et al., 1993). Executive function, defined as planning, organizing, and time-management skills, also is impaired (Waber, 1979; Pennington et al., 1985; Bender et al., 1993; Romans et al., 1997) in TS subjects.

These neurocognitive alterations in TS patients have suggested to some investigators an anomalous hemispheric maturation, such that the right hemisphere is underdeveloped relative to the usual asymmetry seen in normal, age-matched control subjects (Money, 1973; Netley & Rovet, 1982). Hier and Crowley (1982) and Pennington et al. (1985) support an alternative hypothesis for the etiology of the cognitive profile of TS patients that is consistent with a more diffuse brain abnormality. Pennington et al. (1985) compared TS subjects to patients with left hemispheric lesions, right hemispheric lesions, and diffuse brain injury. They found cognitive differences between the TS group and normal control subjects that most resembled diffusely head-injured patients. In addition, they found great variability in the pattern of cognitive performance in TS subjects.

Recent neurophysiological and neuroanatomical studies have demonstrated significant differences between TS patients and normal controls. Data exist that support an early, sustained abnormality in cerebral substrate, either as a primary genetic factor or secondary to the endocrine or environmental influences. In electrophysiological studies, Johnson et al. (1993) have shown that in girls with TS ages 7 to 18 years, evoked potentials differ from those of normal controls in attention and orientation responses. Tsuboi et al. (1988) showed electroenecphalographic (EEG) differences between TS subjects, ages 6 to 47 years, and normal control subjects. In studies of regional cerebral glucose metabolism in TS, decreased metabolism has been found bilaterally, in the occipital and parietal cortex (Clack et al., 1990). Autopsy studies of the brains of three TS women have demonstrated heterogeneous abnormalities, including mild cortical dysplasia and brain atrophy bilaterally and small gyri in the temporal and occipital lobes (Reske-Nielson et al., 1982). Previous neuroanatomical studies of adult women with TS demonstrated some left and greater right-sided reduction of parietal-occipital brain matter (Murphy et al., 1993). Recently, Reiss et al. (1993, 1995) performed detailed neuroanatomical magnetic resonance imaging (MRI) studies of 30 girls with TS and female controls and in an unusual set of monozygotic twin girls discordant for TS. These investigators reported differences in the right posterior regions (parietal and temporal) and the left parietal-perisylvian region in the TS subjects.

In addition to cognitive differences, social-behavioral between girls with TS and normal girls have been described (Waber, 1979; Netley & Rovet, 1982; Bender et al., 1984, 1993; Pennington et al., 1985; McCauley et al., 1987; Rovet, 1991). Children with TS exhibit more frequent behavioral problems, mature more slowly, and experience greater difficulties in social relationships than do control subjects of short stature (McCauley et al., 1995). The TS girls, on average, have fewer friends, need more structure in socialization, and experience greater difficulty in understanding social cues than do peers matched for age, height, IQ, and socioeconomic status (McCauley et al., 1986, 1995; Downey et al., 1991; Rovet & Ireland, 1994). We recently reported a decline in psychological well-being between the ages of 9 and 12 years in adolescent girls with TS (McCauley et al., 1995). Social dysfunction in childhood appears to be predictive of social, psychological, academic, and occupational dysfunction in adolescence and adulthood (Cowen et al., 1973). This has been confirmed in studies demonstrating that adult women with TS manifest increased psychiatric difficulties and poor self-esteem (McCauley et al., 1984; Downey et al., 1991). Such dysfunction has important implications for attaining adult socioeconomic success.

The pathogenesis of impaired cognitive development in TS is unknown. Observed deficits could be due to environmental, endocrine, or genetic factors, either alone or in combination. For example, girls with TS are shorter than their peers and may have unusual facial characteristics, factors that might affect the way that they are treated and, thus, their cognitive and behavioral development. Alternatively, cognitive deficits could result from the deficiency of prepubertal sex steroids owing to severe premature ovarian failure. Early estrogen exposure from a functioning ovary in early infancy may affect impact these changes. Additionally, pubertal replacement of estrogen in adolescence may also influence or ameliorate certain deficits, as will be discussed later. Finally, the genetic abnormality in TS, determined by the absence of one or more genes on the X chromosome, could affect brain development directly; this, too, will be discussed later.

Previous studies have not looked at large numbers of children with TS across a wide range of childhood years and generally have not controlled for verbal IQ or socioeconomic status. We previously investigated whether the most commonly described TS neurocognitive pattern is found across all age ranges in young girls with TS. This issue is important because short stature and absent puberty may affect adolescent girls more than younger girls. We tested the hypothesis that deficits would be more pronounced in older than in younger TS subjects.

Table 11.1 Demographic data

	Younger		Older		P value (TS vs. Control)
	TS	Control	TS	Control	
N	35	50	21	50	
Chronological age	8.8 ± 1.3	8.7 ± 0.9	12.3 ± 0.5	12.2 ± 0.8	0.25
SES*	46 ± 16	48 ± 12	43 ± 13	49 ± 13	0.10

*Socioeconomic status (SES) was determined according to the Hollingshead Two-Factor Index of Social Status.
Note: Values are mean ± standard deviation.

A total of 56 TS subjects (younger, 6–10.9 years old; older, 11.0–14.9 years old) were studied with a specifically constructed neurocognitive battery designed to focus on neurocognitive deficits previously noted in TS girls. The karyotypes of these subjects included nonmosaic 45, X (65%); mosaic 45, X/ 46, XX, 45, X/46, Xi(Xq), 45, X/46, XX/47, XXX, 45X/46Xdel(X), 45X/46X, r (X), or complex mosaics (26%); and nonmosaic partial X deletions 46, X, i(Xq) or 46, X, del(X) (9%). In addition, we evaluated an age-matched group of control girls (table 11.1). The racial composition of the TS and control groups was similar: 86% white for both groups. Two subjects with verbal IQs of less than 70 were excluded from the analyses and results because they were globally impaired. None of the TS subjects received any prior treatment with estrogen, and approximately 40% were being treated with growth hormone in a double-blind study design.

Subjects were individually administered a battery of neuropsychological tests specifically designed to assess several domains of cognitive function, including memory, visuospatial abilities, visuomotor skills, language, and attention. Our intent was to assess a broad range of cognitive abilities, encompassing some domains known to be impaired as well as some domains thought to be normal in TS.

The Wechsler Intelligence Scale for Children was employed as a measure of intelligence because it provides a valid and reliable index of global intelligence [the full-scale IQ (FSIQ)] and estimates of specific abilities, such as verbal- and performance-based skills [verbal IQ (VIQ) and performance IQ (PIQ), respectively]. This measure serves as a useful frame of reference for comparison with other neurocognitive tests and was administered according to standardized procedures. We also computed the Kaufman's Freedom From Distractibility (FFD) and Perceptual Organization Factors (POF), each of which are composite scores of three subtests: arithmetic, digit span, and coding for FFD and picture completion, object assembly, and block design for POF, respectively. The reading subtest from the Wide-Range Achievement Test–Revised was employed as a brief measure of academic achievement in reading. To examine phonological decoding skills more directly, the nonword reading subtest from the Battery of Linguistic Analysis for Writing and Reading was employed. Both VIQ and reading were predicted to be normal in the TS children. This finding was influenced, to some extent, by eliminating from analyses girls with VIQs of less than 70.

The Rey-Osterrieth Complex Figure Test was employed to assess nonverbal memory. Four tasks were employed to assess various functions related to visuospatial ability. The Motor-Free Visual Perception Test includes five subtests that assess various visuoperceptual analyses and synthesis. Aspects of spatial cognition also were assessed using the Judgment of Line Orientation Task. This task requires that the child judge the directional orientation of lines and is thought to be sensitive to spatial skills mediated by the right hemisphere in right-handed individuals. The Money Street Map Test was employed to assess aspects of spatial cognition related to the ability to discriminate left-right orientation and to follow a simple street map (Reiss et al., 1995). The fourth test was the Test of Facial Recognition, which requires the subject to match a face with a series of target faces and assesses visual discrimination of the complex, nonverbal stimuli associated with facial features.

Visuomotor skills were assessed using measures of both graphomotor ability and constructional ability. The Developmental Test of Visual-Motor Integration (VMI) was employed as a reliable and rapid assessment of developmental visual motor skills. The Rey-Osterrieth Complex Figure Test also was employed as a measure of visuomotor skill that requires more spatial skills and organizational abilities than the VMI. An additional measure of visuomotor ability was derived from the Kaufman POF. These spatial memory and visuospatial-perceptual domains were predicted to be impaired in the TS girls but not the control girls.

We employed three separate measures to examine aspects of attention and impulsivity. The Test of Variables of Attention, a visual, continuous-performance test, was employed to look at sustained attention and vigilance. In addition, the Kaufman factor (FFD) was used as a measure of short-term auditory memory and attention. The Matching Familiar Figures Test also was employed to assess impulsive reactions to simple visual stimuli. Errors are believed to be a useful measure of impulsive reactions to stimuli. The attention domain was predicted to be impaired in the TS girls but not control girls.

We observed diffuse impairment of nonverbal cognitive domains involving visuoperceptual, visuomotor, and visuospatial abilities and of attention in non-estrogen-treated girls with TS, 6 to 14.9 years old (tables 11.2 and 11.3). VIQ and verbal skills were normal in the TS subjects (see table 11.2). These results are compatible with multifocal or diffuse right hemisphere dysfunction and, in general, were similar in the younger and the older age groups. Dysfunction of the anterior region is suggested by evidence of impairment on attention tasks. The existence of posterior right hemisphere dysfunction is suggested by untreated TS girls' performance on a variety of visuoperceptual tasks. Recent controlled trials (McCauley et al., 1987; Reiss et al., 1995) also argue for impairment of similar cognitive domains, including visuospatial

Table 11.2 General cognitive function

Domain	Test	Younger TS	Younger Control	Older TS	Older Control
Intelligence	VIQ	103 ± 14	107 ± 11	103 ± 10	104 ± 10
	PIQ	92 ± 14[c]	107 ± 11	93 ± 11[c]	106 ± 14
	FSIQ	98 ± 14[c]	108 ± 11	98 ± 9[c]	105 ± 12
	VIQ-PIQ	11 ± 11[c]	0 ± 12	10 ± 14[c]	2 ± 11
WISC-R subtests	Information	10.1 ± 2.9	10.9 ± 1.8	9.7 ± 1.9	10.2 ± 2.2
	Similarities	11.7 ± 3.3	12.0 ± 2.9	12.0 ± 1.9	11.6 ± 2.4
	Arithmetic	9.0 ± 2.3[c]	11.1 ± 2.5	9.9 ± 2.7	10.6 ± 2.7
	Vocabulary	11.0 ± 3.1[a]	10.7 ± 3.1	10.3 ± 1.9	10.3 ± 2.0
	Comprehension	11.1 ± 2.4	11.2 ± 2.5	10.7 ± 2.4	10.7 ± 2.7
	Digit span	8.0 ± 3.1[c]	11.4 ± 2.7	7.9 ± 3.2[b]	10.6 ± 3.2
	Picture completion	8.7 ± 2.4[c]	11.0 ± 2.2	8.1 ± 2.0[a]	10.0 ± 2.9
	Picture arrangement	10.1 ± 3.4	11.5 ± 2.5	9.9 ± 2.8	11.0 ± 2.8
	Block design	9.0 ± 3.3[a]	10.9 ± 3.2	9.2 ± 2.1	10.7 ± 3.6
	Object assembly	8.3 ± 2.8[c]	10.5 ± 2.3	8.2 ± 2.8[a]	10.4 ± 3.1
	Coding	8.2 ± 3.1[c]	10.1 ± 3.1	9.7 ± 3.3[b]	12.3 ± 3.0
Academic	Wide Range Achievement Test– Reading Standard Score	95 ± 17[b]	105 ± 12	95 ± 22[a]	107 ± 15
	Nonword reading	40 ± 13[b]	47 ± 17	55 ± 13	59 ± 13

TS, Turner syndrome; VIQ, verbal IQ; PIQ, performance IQ; FSIQ, full-scale IQ; WISC-R, Wechsler Intelligence Scale for Children–Revised.
P value (ANOVA, TS vs. control): [a]$p \leq .05$; [b]$p \leq .006$; [c]$p \leq .0001$.
$P < .05$ may not be significant after the Bonferroni adjustment for multiple comparisons.
Note: Values are mean ± standard deviation.

skills, visuomotor skills, spatial memory (Matsumoto et al., 1991), attention, and facial affect recognition (Bender et al., 1984, 1993; Rovet, 1991; Williams et al., 1991, 1992). We examined two different age groups of TS girls (6–10.9 and 11.0–14.9 years) who had not received any estrogen replacement and found few differences in the pattern of impairment in each age group as compared to their respective controls. This is consistent with a well-controlled study in which adult TS women were compared to their sisters and to short normal women (Downey et al., 1991). The IQ patterns in the adult TS women differed from those of controls and resembled those typically described in TS children.

In summary, the TS subjects showed evidence compatible with right cerebral brain dysfunction and deficits generally involving nonverbal skills. The neuromaturational abnormality in TS may result from the X chromosome monosomy or from hormone deficiencies secondary to gonadal dysgenesis, or from both. The remainder of this chapter explores the contributions of estrogen deficiency and the missing X chromosome to cognitive development in TS.

Table 11.3 Nonverbal abilities

Domain	Test	Young		Old	
		TS	Control	TS	Control
Memory	Rey-imm (visual)	21 ± 14^a	27 ± 13	26 ± 11^a	36 ± 17
	Rey-del	20 ± 14	26 ± 12	23 ± 11^b	37 ± 15
Perception	Facial recog	37 ± 6^a	40 ± 4	40 ± 5^b	44 ± 4
Spatial	JLO	12.8 ± 5.1	14.5 ± 5.6	18.6 ± 6.5	20.1 ± 6.0
	MSM	15.5 ± 3.8	13.1 ± 4.9	14.6 ± 5.3^b	8.4 ± 5.9
	MVPT	102 ± 13^b	111 ± 11	115 ± 8	117 ± 8
	MVPT-t	175 ± 96^a	140 ± 57	194 ± 120^c	98 ± 40
Visuomotor	VMI	89 ± 11^c	107 ± 12	84 ± 11^c	105 ± 14
	Rey-copy	39 ± 20^c	53 ± 11	53 ± 11^c	65 ± 6
	POF	9.0 ± 2.2^c	11.0 ± 1.8	8.8 ± 1.9^b	10.5 ± 2.3
Attention	TOVA	10.7 ± 6.8	9.2 ± 5.2	9.9 ± 6.4^b	5.7 ± 4.2
	TOVA-t	697 ± 186	676 ± 104	482 ± 65^a	536 ± 80
	MFFT	4.9 ± 2.4^a	6.4 ± 2.8	6.9 ± 2.6	7.9 ± 2.7
	MFFT-t	108 ± 77	148 ± 145	153 ± 82	161 ± 107
	FFD	8.4 ± 2.1^c	11.2 ± 1.5	9.2 ± 2.3^b	11.2 ± 2.1

Rey = Rey-Osterrieth Complex Figure, immediate (imm) and delayed (del) recall; Facial recog = Test of Facial Recognition; JLO = Judgment of Line Orientation; MSM = Money Street Map (toward plus away) errors; MVPT = Motor-Visual Perception Test; MVPT-t = MVPT time; VMI = Test of Visual-Motor Integration; Rey-copy = Rey-Osterrieth Complex Figure, copy; POF = perceptual organization factor (Kaufman, WISC-R subtests, picture completion, object assembly, and block design); TOVA = Test of Variables of Attention, commission errors; TOVA-t = response time; MFFT = Matching Familiar Figures Test; MFFT-t = MFFT time; FFD = Freedom from Distractibility.

P value (ANOVA, TS vs. control): $^a p \leq .05$; $^b p \leq .006$; $^c p \leq .0001$.

$P < .05$ may not be significant after the Bonferroni adjustment for multiple comparisons.

INFLUENCE OF ESTROGEN REPLACEMENT ON COGNITION AND BEHAVIOR IN TURNER SYNDROME

The cognitive and behavioral deficits in TS could be due, at least in part, to absent ovarian estrogen production. Sex hormones (estrogen and androgen) appear to influence brain development in fetal life and through puberty. However, the mechanism of these effects is not known. Sex steroids may function (1) transiently as neuromodulators by potential mechanisms such as occupying receptors and initiating an enzyme cascade, modifying uptake of neurotransmitters, or altering neuronal electrical activity; (2) permanently by altering synapse formation and remodeling; or (3) by both of these mechanisms (McEwen et al., 1987; Matsumoto et al., 1991).

The ovaries in normal girls produce very small amounts of estrogen and, possibly, androgen before puberty in levels that are difficult to measure in the usual assays. The production of estrogen by the ovaries increases significantly throughout puberty, until adult levels are reached. Postmortem studies of infants with normal ovarian development in the first 2 years of life indicate that female infants also appear to exhibit increased ovarian estrogen production during the first year of life, analogous to the testosterone surge during the first 6 months of life in male infants (Bidlingmaier et al., 1987). Girls with TS presumably would lack this surge, secondary to their dysgenetic ovaries. This very early estrogen deficiency may affect later neurocognitive development.

The existing literature and our previous results support or suggest that (1) estrogen has significant effects on brain and behavior in animal studies, (2) absence or decrease in estrogen levels is related to some differences in cognitive function and psychological well-being, and (3) the neurophysiological mechanisms for the effects of estrogen on brain development are not fully known.

Animal studies have shown both structural (organizational) and activational effects of estrogen on subcortical nuclear regions such as the hypothalamic-preoptic area and forebrain regions that are related to behavior (Juraska, 1991; Matsumoto, 1991). Sex hormone alterations during the perinatal period and puberty influence cognitive function and behavior in animal models. Studies in monkeys demonstrated that learning ability can be altered by perinatal hormone manipulations (Bachevalier & Hagger, 1991). Nottebohm and Arnold (1976) have shown that in song birds, the level of androgen influences the development of specific anatomical brain structures that are necessary for song production in the male of the species. McEwen et al. (1987) have demonstrated specific morphological and chemical changes in neurons of the ventromedial nucleus of the hypothalamus in rats treated with estrogen, and these changes result in altered behavior.

Other support for sex hormone effects on behavior are the findings that spatial ability tends to lag at puberty in normal girls as compared to normal boys and male superiority in spatial ability tends to debut at the time of puberty (Waber, 1977). Additionally, the rate of pubertal development in girls influences the probable functional manifestation of hemispheric lateralization. Girls who experienced advanced puberty had increased verbal ability and diminished spatial ability in comparison to normal girls (Money & Meredith, 1967). Gender differences are reported for verbal learning, for which women have superior verbal recall and fluency (Kramer et al., 1988), and for spatial ability, an area in which men exhibit superiority over women (Linn & Retersen, 1985). The spatial and motoric abilities of adult women, as opposed to men, fluctuate in relation to their menstrual cycle (Ho et al., 1986; Hampson & Kimura, 1988; Sherwin, 1988; Hampson, 1990), suggesting biphasic estrogen dose effects on spatial ability. Hampson found that women had better spatial abilities in the lower estrogen phase of the menstrual cycle (Hampson, 1990). In contrast, motor speed and self-reported mood improved during the higher estrogen, preovulatory phase of the menstrual cycle. Other investigators have not found cognitive variations across the menstrual cycle or in relationship to estradiol levels (Gordon & Lee, 1993). Additional evidence in humans supports an estrogen dose effect on the brain. Warren & Brooks-Gonn (1989) noted transient behavioral changes in normal female adolescents that occur only in early puberty. They found that depression and poor impulse control were the greatest from early to middle puberty and improved by late puberty. Surgically menopausal women treated with estrogen replacement had improved memory and mood (Sherwin & Gelfand, 1985) as compared to such women in the untreated state. Estrogen replacement therapy may also be associated with improved verbal memory in postmenopausal women (Kampen & Sherwin, 1994) and improved attention, orientation, mood, and social interaction in some women with Alzheimer-type dementia (Fillit et al., 1986).

Nyborg argued that estrogen deficiency underlies at least part of the cognitive and behavioral differences in TS and that an optimal estrogen level is necessary for optimal spatial performance (Nielson & Nyborg, 1981). This conclusion is based not only on the striking absence of estrogen in TS but also on the improvement in spatial ability in TS subjects after short-term estrogen replacement. We currently are investigating the effects of continuous low-dose estrogen treatment of young girls with TS (age 8 or 12 years) in a randomized, double-blind, placebo-controlled study. We have not yet demonstrated positive or negative estrogen effects on spatial ability but plan to analyze these effects when the double-blind study is completed.

In the area of self-image, we recently examined the longitudinal effects of estrogen replacement in adolescent girls with TS, ages 12–16 years (table 11.4), who are followed up yearly in the ongoing growth and cognition study (Ross et al., 1996). Approximately 30% of these girls were included in the earlier cognitive analyses (see tables 11.1–11.3). These 12- to 16-year-old girls completed the Piers-Harris Children's Self-Concept Scale, and their parents completed the Child Behavior Checklist (Ross et al., 1996) when the girls were 12, just prior to their uniformly starting estrogen replacement therapy as part of the standard protocol. At that point, approximately 50% of the subjects were receiving very low-dose estrogen (25–50 ng/kg/day) or growth hormone (or both) for durations of 0.5 to 7.0 years, as part of the growth study evaluating the effect of growth hormone or estrogen on final adult height. All girls were started on estrogen (50–100 ng/kg/day) at age 12 and remained on this dose until age 14. The doses of estrogen then were doubled on a yearly basis until menses occurred. The effects of growth hormone on behavior in this population have not been analyzed owing to the ongoing requirement for the investigators to remain blinded to treatment effects. Growth hormone generally has not been found to affect cognitive function in girls with TS.

The Piers-Harris Self-Concept Scale is a self-reporting measure of self-concept. It consists of 80 statements that children rate as yes or no in accord with how they feel about themselves. Scoring provided a total overall score and scores on six subscales: behavior, popularity, intellectual and school

Table 11.4 Piers-Harris Children's Self-Concept Scale and Child Behavior Checklist (CBCL) T-score results

| | Estrogen-treated (yr) | | | | |
	Baseline	1 yr	2 yr	3 yr	P^a
Age	12.3 ± 0.2	13.4 ± 0.3	14.4 ± 0.3	15.4 ± 0.2	
n	25^b	31	31	25	
Piers					
Behavior	55 ± 9	58 ± 7	62 ± 6	59 ± 9	0.001
Intellect	55 ± 10	57 ± 8	59 ± 8	59 ± 9	0.003
Happy	53 ± 11	56 ± 9	60 ± 6	58 ± 6	0.007
Total	56 ± 12	59 ± 11	62 ± 9	61 ± 11	0.001
CBCL					
Behavior	54 ± 12	50 ± 12	49 ± 12	47 ± 12	0.003
Delinquent	55 ± 8	53 ± 5	52 ± 5	52 ± 5	0.005
Aggressive	57 ± 10	54 ± 7	53 ± 5	53 ± 5	0.002
Externalize	53 ± 12	50 ± 10	47 ± 10	47 ± 10	0.001
Attention problems	59 ± 9	56 ± 9	56 ± 7	55 ± 7	0.17
Social problems	62 ± 8	62 ± 13	60 ± 8	57 ± 7	0.03

[a] P value: repeated measures ANOVA.
[b] results were missing from six subjects at baseline and from six others at 3 years.

status, physical appearance, happiness, and anxiety. Higher scores indicate higher ability or more positive outcome. The Child Behavior Checklist was developed by Achenbach (1991) as a standardized measure of academic and social competency as well as of behavior problems in children ages 4 to 18. The checklist includes standard and percentile scores for 3 competency scales (activities, social, and school) and for 10 problem behavior areas. Internalizing, externalizing, and total behavior scales also are derived from the responses. The internalizing scales are believed to represent over-controlled symptoms, such as excessive worrying, whereas the externalizing scales are believed to represent undercontrolled or acting-out symptoms, such as aggressive behavior or lying. Lower scores indicate fewer problem behaviors.

Selected results are shown in table 11.4. Self-concept in the adolescent girls with TS improved significantly (by self-report and parental report) by age 16. No unblinding of the investigators was necessary because all the TS subjects are uniformly treated with low doses of estrogen after age 12. We previously reported a decline in self-image in untreated girls with TS syndrome between the ages of 9 and 12 that appears to reverse with estrogen treatment between the ages of 12 and 16 (Ross et al., 1996). We cannot demonstrate directly whether these improvements in self-image are secondary to direct estrogen effects on the brain, estrogen effects on inducing

Table 11.5 Cognitive abilities in 45, X subjects versus X chromosome parental origin

	Maternally derived X	Paternally derived X	P value
n	21	9	
Verbal IQ	103 ± 11	102 ± 14	0.83
Performance IQ	92 ± 11	95 ± 15	0.54

pubertal changes, growth hormone effects or to age effects that are independent of estrogen treatment. Growth hormone treatment is less likely to be influencing self-image because growth rates are typically waning in this age range. A non-age-dependent effect of estrogen on behavior is the most heuristic conclusion based on the positive effect of estrogen on mood in the higher-estrogen phase of the menstrual cycle (Hampson, 1990) and in estrogen-replaced, postmenopausal women (Sherwin & Gelfand, 1985).

GENETIC INFLUENCE ON THE NEUROCOGNITIVE PROFILE IN TURNER SYNDROME

One way to assess the role of genetic factors in the neurocognitive features of TS would be to identify genes that contribute to the phenotype. Physical and neurocognitive TS features could be due to one gene or to interactions among multiple genes. Phenotypic complexity does not necessarily imply that many genes are involved. Several possible explanations exist for the genetic effects of partial or complete monosomy X on cognitive development. First, in the case of imprinted genes, loss of one allele could result in the total absence of gene products. Second, deletions might unmask X-linked recessive mutations on the normal X chromosome. Finally, a reduced level of gene products could emanate from some X-linked genes.

Girls with 45, X TS retain either the maternal or the paternal X chromosome. If X-linked genes involved in cognitive development are imprinted, retention of the paternal rather than the maternal X would be expected to affect the neurocognitive outcome. We studied 30 nonmosaic 45, X subjects to determine whether imprinting affects cognitive abilities in TS girls. We measured VIQ and PIQ for each subject and, using restriction fragment–length polymorphism analysis (not shown), determined the parental origin of the single X chromosome. Table 11.5 shows the IQ results, grouped according to parental origin of the X chromosome. We found no apparent imprinting effects on VIQ or PIQ in our study of 30 45, X subjects. In other words, the TS neurocognitive phenotype is not the result of total absence of imprinted gene products.

The specific cognitive deficits associated with TS appear to be distinct from X-linked mental retardation. As mentioned previously, characteristic spatial or perceptual deficits are common in 45, X subjects, but diffuse mental retardation is unusual. Furthermore, neurocognitive deficits were demonstrated in a group of TS subjects even after excluding individuals with obvious mental retardation (VIQ < 70) (Ross et al., 1995). These data indicate that the neurocognitive phenotype of TS is not simply due to unmasking of X-linked recessive mental retardation mutations. It would be interesting to know whether distinct neurocognitive profiles also are associated with X-linked mental retardation, but the more global impairment in these syndromes makes performance of such studies difficult.

Given the pervasiveness and relative homogeneity of cognitive deficits in TS subjects, the most likely hypothesis for genetic effects of monosomy X on neurocognition is that the phenotype results from reduced dosage of as-yet-unidentified X-linked genes. Most X-linked genes show monoallelic expression in normal female individuals because of stochastic inactivation of one X chromosome during early development. The level of most X-linked gene products is presumably normal in 45, X TS patients because the single X chromosome is not inactivated. However, some genes escape X-inactivation (i.e., show biallelic expression in normal girls). The absence of one X chromosome in TS results in half-normal dosage of these genes that escape X-inactivation. Recent studies have shown that half-normal dosage of single genes is the culprit in several pleiotropic developmental disorders, including Greig polysyndactyly syndrome and Rubinstein-Taybi syndrome.

That the neurocognitive profile in TS represents a complex phenotype does not necessarily imply that many genes are responsible. Mutations in single genes can cause characteristic neurocognitive or social-behavioral phenotypes. Self-mutilation behavior in Lesch-Nyhan syndrome, an X-linked recessive disorder, is a well-known consequence of mutations in the hypoxanthine guanine phosphoribosyltransferase (HPRT) gene (Ernst et al., 1996). A mutation that inactivates the monoamine oxidase A gene has been linked in one kindred to disturbed regulation of impulsive aggression (Brunner et al., 1993). In both of these cases, loss of gene function is complete. More analogous to TS, the overall cognitive impairment with relatively spared verbal abilities seen in Williams syndrome appears to be due to half-normal dosage of one or a few genes in a small region of chromosome 7 (band 7q32) (Frangiskakis et al., 1996). It should be possible to localize genes responsible for TS cognitive deficits by comparing the phenotypes of subjects with different partial X deletions. However, expression of TS neurocognitive deficits varies within the population, even among nonmosaic 45, X subjects. Given the possibility that the TS cognitive phenotype is due to reduced dosage of X-linked genes, we would expect that girls who are genetically mosaic would be less severely affected than 45, X nonmosaic subjects. This has been confirmed by previous investigators (Rovet, 1991; Murphy et al., 1993, 1994; Temple & Carney, 1995) who noted less severe neurocognitive deficits and neuroanatomical abnormalities in women with mosaic TS as opposed to 45, X TS.

By comparing the neurocognitive profile of seven mosaic TS subjects (45, X/46, XX) with a group of 45, X subjects, we also investigated this

Table 11.6 Neurocognitive results from mosaic 45, X/46XX versus 45, X subjects

	45, X/46, XX	45, X	P value
n	7	66	
Age	11.1 ± 3.4	10.9 ± 2.6	0.85
SES	50 ± 14	50 ± 8	1.00
General intelligence			
VIQ	109 ± 15	101 ± 15	0.18
PIQ	98 ± 16	91 ± 13	0.19
FSIQ	107 ± 17	94 ± 11	0.06
Information	10.7 ± 2.7	9.8 ± 2.9	0.44
Similarities	12.3 ± 3.3	11.4 ± 3.4	0.51
Arithmetic	11.3 ± 3.6	9.1 ± 2.9	0.07
Vocabulary	12.0 ± 1.4	10.7 ± 3.3	0.31
Comprehension	12.7 ± 2.0	10.5 ± 2.9	0.06
Digit span	9.0 ± 2.7	7.4 ± 2.8	0.15
Picture completion	9.3 ± 2.8	8.2 ± 2.5	0.28
Picture arrangement	10.9 ± 2.5	10.2 ± 2.6	0.49
Block design	10.0 ± 3.9	9.0 ± 3.5	0.48
Object assembly	8.3 ± 3.0	8.0 ± 3.0	0.80
Coding	10.7 ± 1.9	8.3 ± 2.7	0.03
Academic skills and verbal memory			
Word list	12.5 ± 4.2	11.0 ± 2.3	0.14
Denman-immediate recall	24 ± 8	24 ± 8	0.99
Peabody	108 ± 11	114 ± 23	0.53
Wide-Range Achievement–Reading	59 ± 22	58 ± 18	0.90
Visuospatial/visuomotor			
Rey figure–copy	56 ± 17	46 ± 19	0.18
Rey figure–immediate recall	25 ± 16	23 ± 14	0.67
Judgment of Line Orientation	15 ± 10	15 ± 6	0.93
Motor-Visual Perception Test	33 ± 3	31 ± 4	0.25
Money Street Map, errors	10 ± 3	8 ± 3	0.02
Matching Familiar Figures	6.6 ± 3.7	6.0 ± 2.8	0.60
Beery Visual-Motor Integration	26 ± 9	21 ± 9	0.25
Test of Facial Recognition	44 ± 3	38 ± 6	0.03

SES, socioeconomic status; VIQ, verbal IQ; PIQ, performance IQ; FSIQ, full-scale IQ.

hypothesis (table 11.6). We chose to examine only those subjects with the combination of the 45, X and 46, XX lines, because the presence of other cell lines such as 47, XXX or 46, X, i(Xq) may introduce confounding effects of trisomy for all or part of the X. For example, girls with karyotype 47, XXX have been reported to have deficits in language comprehension and VIQ as compared to controls (Bender et al., 1993). We therefore chose a "homogeneous" mosaic group, with the understanding that the presence of detectable mosaicism implies considerable variation in phenotype. Our results (mean ± standard deviation) are shown in table 11.6.

The mosaic subjects in general had somewhat higher scores on many of the neurocognitive variables examined. However, only the results from the Money Street Map, the Test of Facial Recognition, and the coding subtest of the Wechsler Intelligence Scale for Children–Revised achieved statistical significance. Subjects may possess variable degrees of mosaicism in any body tissue, including the brain, accounting at least in part for the variable results. Interestingly, Murphy et al. (1994) noted a correlation between visuospatial ability and the percentage of lymphocytes in the karyotype having the 45, X result.

CONCLUSION

TS represents a unique model for evaluating the effects of the hormonal versus the genetic contribution to the neurocognitive and behavioral phenotype associated with the syndrome. TS subjects demonstrated evidence of right cerebral brain dysfunction and deficits generally involving nonverbal skills. This neuromaturational abnormality in TS may result from the X chromosome monosomy or from hormone deficiencies secondary to gonadal dysgenesis, or both. Early estrogen exposure from a functioning ovary early in infancy may affect these changes. Additionally, pubertal replacement of estrogen in adolescence may influence or ameliorate certain deficits.

Future studies will examine the role of estrogen replacement therapy on cognitive function and behavior in TS. In addition, our results and previous data from other investigators suggest X chromosome effects on brain maturation and development of cognition. It is possible that genes responsible for the neurocognitive profile in TS contribute to the variance in specific cognitive abilities among chromosomally normal individuals. The degree to which genetic effects of monosomy X are independent of ovarian failure in the neurocognitive development of girls with TS is also a subject for future investigation.

REFERENCES

Achenbach, T. M. (1991). *Manual for the Child Behavior Checklist/4–18 and 1991 Profile*. Burlington VT: University of Vermont, Department of Psychiatry.

Bachevalier, J., & Hagger, C. (1991). Sex differences in the development of learning abilities in primates. *Psychoneuroendocrinology, 16,* 177–188.

Bender, B. G., Linden, M. G., & Robinson, A. (1993). Neuropsychological impairment in 42 adolescents with sex chromosome abnormalities. *American Journal of Medical Genetics, 48,* 169–173.

Bender, B., Puck, M., Salbenblatt, J., & Robinson, A. (1984). Cognitive development of unselected girls with complete and partial X monosomy. *Pediatrics, 73,* 175–182.

Bidlingmaier, F., Strom, T. M., Dorr, H. G., Eisenmenger, W., & Knorr, D. (1987). Estrone and estradiol concentrations in human ovaries, testes, and adrenals during the first two years of life. *Journal of Clinical Endocrinology and Metabolism, 65,* 862–867.

Brunner, H. G., et al. (1993). Abnormal behavior associated with a point mutation in the structural gene for monoamine oxidase A. *Science, 262,* 578–580.

Clark, C., Klonoff, H., & Hayden, M. (1990). Regional cerebral glucose metabolism in Turner syndrome. *Canadian Journal of Neurological Sciences, 17,* 140–144.

Cowen, E. L., Pederson, A., Babigian, H., Izzo, L. D., & Trost, M. A. (1973). Long-term follow-up of early detected vulnerable children. *Journal of Consulting and Clinical Psychology, 41,* 438–446.

Downey, J., Elkin, E. J., Erhardt, A. A., Meyer Bahlburg, H., Bell, J., & Morishima, N. (1991). Cognitive ability and everyday functioning in women with Turner syndrome. *Journal of Learning Disabilities, 24,* 32–39.

Ernst, M., et al. (1996). Presynaptic dopaminergic deficits in Lesch-Nyhan diesase. *New England Journal of Medicine, 334,* 1568–1572.

Fillit, H., Weinrib, H., Cholst, I., Loine, V., McEwen, B., Amador, R., & Zabriskie, J. (1986). Observations in a preliminary open trial of estradiol therapy for senile dementia–Alzheimer's type. *Psychoneuroendocrinology, 11,* 337–345.

Frangiskakis, J. M., Ewart, A. D., Morris, C. A., Mervis, C. B., Bertrand, J., Robinson, B. F., Klein, B. P., Ensing, G. J., Everett, L. A., Green, E. D., Proschel, C., Gutowski, N. J., Noble, M., Atkinson, D. L., Odelberg, S. J., & Keating, M. T. (1996). LIM-kinase1 hemizygosity implicated in impaired visuospatial constructive cognition. *Cell, 86,* 59–69.

Gordon, H. W., & Lee, P. A. (1993). No difference in cognitive performance between phases of the menstrual cycle. *Psychoneuroendocrinology, 18,* 521–531.

Hampson, E. (1990). Estrogen-related variations in human spatial and articulatory-motor skills. *Psychoneuroendocrinology, 15,* 97–111.

Hampson, E., & Kimura, D. (1988). Reciprocal effects of hormonal fluctuations on human motor and perceptual-spatial skills. *Behavioral Neuroscience, 102,* 456–459.

Hassold, T. J. (1986). Chromosome abnormalities in human reproductive wastage. *Trends Genetics, 2,* 105–110.

Held, K. R., et al. (1992). Mosaicism in 45,X Turner syndrome: Does survival in early pregnancy depend on the presence of two sex chromosomes? *Human Genetics, 88,* 288–294.

Hier, D. B., & Crowley, W. F. (1982). Spatial ability in androgen-deficient men. *New England Journal of Medicine, 306,* 1202–1205.

Ho, H., Gilger, J. W., & Brink, T. M. (1986). Effect of menstrual cycle on spatial information processes. *Perceptual and Motor Skills, 63,* 743–751.

Hook, E. B., & Warburton, D. (1983). The distribution of chromosomal genotypes associated with Turner's syndrome: Livebirth prevalence rates and evidence for diminished fetal mortality and severity in genotypes associated with structural X abnormalities or mosaicism. *Human Genetics, 64,* 24–27.

Johnson, R., Jr., Rohrbaugh, J., & Ross, J. L. (1993). Altered brain development in Turner's syndrome: An event-related potential study. *Neurology, 43,* 801–808.

Juraska, J. M. (1991). Sex differences in "cognitive" regions of the rat brain. *Psychoneuroendocrinology, 16*(1), 105–119.

Kampen, D. L., & Sherwin, B. B. (1994). Estrogen use and verbal memory in healthy postmenopausal women. *Obstetrics and Gynecology, 83,* 979–983.

Kramer, J. H., Delis, D. C., & Daniel, M. (1988). Sex differences in verbal learning. *Journal of Clinical Psychology, 44,* 907–915.

Levandowski, L., Costenbader, V., & Richman R. (1985). Neuropsychological aspects of Turner syndrome. *International Journal of Clinical Psychology, 7*, 144–147.

Linn, M. C., & Petersen, A. I. (1985). Emergence and characterization of sex differences in spatial ability: A meta-analysis. *Child Development, 56*, 1479–1498.

Matsumoto, A. (1991). Synaptogenic action of sex steroids in developing and adult neuroendocrine brain. *Psychoneuroendocrinology, 16*(1–3), 25–40.

Matsumoto, A., Arai, Y., Urano, M., & Hyodo, S. (1991). Androgen regulates gap junction mRNA expression in androgen-sensitive motor neurons in the rat spinal cord. *Neuroscience Letters, 131*, 159–162.

McCauley, E., Kay, T., Ito, J., & Treder, R. (1987). The Turner syndrome: Cognitive deficits, affective discrimination, and behavior problems. *Child Development, 58*, 464–473.

McCauley, E., Ross, J. L., Kushner, H., & Cutler, G. B., Jr. (1995). Psychological adjustment in girls with Turner syndrome. *Journal of Developmental and Behavioral Pediatrics, 16*, 82–88.

McCauley, E., Sybert, V., & Ehrhardt, A. A. (1986). Psychosocial adjustment of adult women with Turner syndrome. *Clinical Genetics, 29*, 284–290.

McEwen, B. S., Jones, K. J., & Pfaff, D. W. (1987). Hormonal control of sexual behavior in the female rat: Molecular, cellular and neurochemical studies. *Biology of Reproduction, 36*, 37–45.

Money, J. (1973). Turner syndrome and parietal lobe functions. *Cortex, 9*, 313–326.

Money, J., & Meredith, T. (1967). Elevated verbal I. Q. and idiopathic precocious sexual maturation. *Pediatric Research, 1*, 59–65.

Murphy, D. G. M., Allen, G., Haxby, J. V., Largay, K. A., Daly, E., White, B. J., Powell, C. M., & Schapiro, M. B. (1994). The effects of sex steroids, and the X chromosome on female brain function: A study of the neuropsychology of adult Turner syndrome. *Neuropsychologica, 32*, 1309–1323.

Murphy, D. G. M., Decarli, C., Daly, E., Haxby, J. V., Allen, G., White, B. J., McIntosh, A. R., Powell, C. M., Horwitz, B., Rapoport, S. I., & Schapiro, M. B. (1993). X-chromosome effects on female brain: A magnetic resonance imaging study of Turner's syndrome. *Lancet, 342*, 197–2000.

Netley, C., & Rovet, J. (1982). Atypical hemispheric lateralization in Turner syndrome subjects. *Cortex, 18*, 377–384.

Nielson, J., & Nyborg, H. (1981). Sex hormone treatment and spatial ability in women with Turner's syndrome. In W. Schmid & J. Nielson (Ed.), *Human behavior and genetics* (pp. 167–181). Amsterdam: Elsevier.

Nottebohm, F., & Arnold, A. P. (1976). Sexual dimorphism in vocal control areas of the songbird brain. *Science, 94*, 211–213.

Nyborg, H. (1991). Sex hormones, brain development and spatial-perceptual strategies in women with Turner syndrome and in school girls. In B. Bender & D. Berch (Eds.), *Sex chromosome abnormalities and behavior: Psychological studies*, (pp. 100–128). Boulder, CO: Westview Press.

Pennington, B. F., Heaton, R. K., Karzmark, P., Pendleton, M. G., Lehman, R., & Shucard, D. W. (1985). The neuropsychological phenotype in Turner syndrome. *Cortex, 21*, 391–404.

Ratcliffe, S. G., Butler, G. E., & Jones, M. (1991). Edinburgh study of growth and development of children with sex chromosome abnormalities: IV. *Birth Defects Original Article Series, 26*(4), 1–44.

Reiss, A. L., Freund, L., Plotnick, L., Baumgardner, T., Green, K., Sozer, A. C., Reader, M., Boehm, C., & Denckla, M. B. (1993). The effects of X monosomy on brain development: Monozygotic twins discordant for Turner's syndrome. *Annals of Neurology, 34,* 95–107.

Reiss, A. L., Mazzocco, M. M. M., Greenlaw, R., Freund, L. S., & Ross, J. L. (1995). Neurodevelopmental effects of X monosomy: A volumetric imaging study, *Annals of Neurology, 38,* 731–738.

Reske-Nielson, E., Christiensen, A. L., & Nielson, J. (1982). A neuropathological and neuropsychological study of Turner syndrome. *Cortex, 18,* 181–190.

Robinson, A., Bender, B. G., Linden, M. G., & Salbenblatt, J. A. (1991). Sex chromosome aneuploidy: The Denver prospective study. *Birth Defects Original Article Series, 26(4),* 59–115.

Romans, S. M., Roeltgen, D. P., Kushner, H., & Ross, J. L. (1997) Executive function in females with Turner syndrome. *Developmental Neuropsychology, 13,* 23–40.

Ross, J. L., McCauley, E., Roeltgen, D., Kushner, H., & Cutler, G. B., Jr. (1996). Self-image in adolescent girls with Turner syndrome: Potential estrogen effects. *Journal of Clinical Endocrinology and Metabolism, 81,* 926–931.

Ross, J. L., Stefanatos, G., Roeltgen, D., Kushner, H., & Cutler, G. B., Jr. (1995). Ullrich-Turner syndrome: Neurodevelopmental changes from childhood through adolescence. *American Journal of Medical Genetics, 58,* 74–82.

Rovet, J. F. (1991). The cognitive and neuropsychological characteristics of females with Turner syndrome. In B. Bender & D. Berch (Eds.), *Sex chromosome abnormalities and behavior: Psychological studies* (pp. 39–77). Boulder, CO: Westview Press, 1991.

Rovet, J. (1993). The psychoeducational characteristics of children with Turner syndrome. *Journal of Learning Disabilities, 26,* 333–341.

Rovet, J. & Ireland, L. (1994). Behavioral phenotype in children with Turner syndrome. *Journal of Pediatric Psychology, 19,* 779–790.

Salbenblatt, J. A., Meyers, D. C., Bender, B. G., Linder, M. G., & Robinson, A. (1987). Gross and fine motor development in 45,X and 47,XXX girls. *Pediatrics, 84,* 678–682.

Sherwin, B. B. (1988). Estrogen and/or androgen replacement therapy and cognitive functioning in surgically menopausal women. *Psychoneuroendocrinology, 13,* 345–357.

Sherwin, B. B., & Gelfand, M. M. (1985). Sex steroids and affect in the surgical menopause: A double-blind crossover study. *Psychoneuroendocrinology, 10,* 325–335.

Stewart, D. A., Bailey, J. D., Netley, C. T., & Park, E. (1991). Growth, development, and behavioral outcome from mid-adolescence to adulthood in subjects with chromosome aneuploidy: The Toronto study. *Birth Defects Original Article Series, 2(4),* 131–188.

Swillen, A., Fryns, J. P., Kleczkowska, A., Massa, A., Vanderschueren-Lodeweyckx, M., & Van Den Berghe, H. (1993). Intelligence, behavior, and psychosocial development in Turner syndrome. *Genetic Counseling, 4,* 7–18.

Temple, C. M., & Carney, R. A. (1995). Patterns of spatial functioning in Turner syndrome. *Cortex, 31,* 109–118.

Tsuboi, T., Nielsen, J., & Nagayama, I. (1988). Turner syndrome: A qualitative and quantitative analysis of EEG background activity. *Human Genetics, 78,* 206–215.

Waber, D. (1979). Neuropsychological aspects of Turner syndrome. *Developmental Medicine and Child Neurology, 21,* 58–70.

Waber, D. P. (1977). Sex difference in mental abilities, hemispheric lateralization and rate of physical growth at adolescence. *Developmental Psychobiology, 13,* 29–38.

Warren, M. P., & Brooks-Gunn, J. (1989). Mood and behavior at adolescence: Evidence for hormonal factors. *Journal of Clinical Endocrinology and Metabolism, 69,* 77–83.

Williams, J., Richman, L., & Yarbrough, D. (1991). A comparison of memory and attention in Turner syndrome and learning disability. *Journal of Pediatric Psychology, 16,* 585–593.

Williams, J. K., Richman, C., & Yarbrough, D. B. (1992). Comparison of visual-spatial performance strategy training in children with Turner syndrome and learning disabilities. *Journal of Learning Disabilities, 25,* 658–664.

III Neurodevelopmental Disorders: Syndromes with Complex Genetic Etiologies

12 Conceptual and Methodological Issues in Dyslexia Research: A Lesson for Developmental Disorders

Jack M. Fletcher, Barbara R. Foorman,
Sally E. Shaywitz, and Bennett A. Shaywitz

The existence of children and adults who struggle to learn to read is without question. Depending on how reading disability is defined, estimates range from 5% to 17% of the school-age population (Shaywitz & Shaywitz, 1994). Whether reading disabilities represent a distinct disorder, syndrome, or a set of syndromes has been debated since the earliest observations of unexpected reading failure (Morgan, 1896). Much of this controversy reflects problems in defining and classifying children with unexpected reading failure. Here the vagueness and circularity of most definitions of reading disability have impeded attempts to identify potential biological and social correlates and the evaluation of approaches to the treatment of dyslexia (Fletcher & Morris, 1986).

This controversy is significant not only for dyslexia, but for other neurodevelopmental disorders (Fletcher, 1994). A cognitive neuroscience of developmental disorders is not possible without a careful approach to definition and, when necessary, classification. Without precise definitions, samples may be poorly defined and may be so heterogeneous that identification of neurobiological correlates will be obscured. This is exactly the case with dyslexia, wherein problems at the level of definition and classification have been known (and unknown) sources of controversy for decades. Hence, this chapter begins with a brief review of the history of attempts to define and classify dyslexia, which may provide an example for other neurodevelopmental disorders.

DEFINITION AND CLASSIFICATION OF DYSLEXIA

Commonly, dyslexia is viewed as a reading disability that occurs in children (and adults) who have normal intelligence and are free of sensory and neurological impairment (Critchley, 1970). This view often is operationalized as a discrepancy between scores on an intelligence test and a reading test. Interestingly, the nature of the reading deficit often is not specified, despite the fact that problems with the identification of single words in isolation always have been the pivotal or core deficit characterizing individuals with reading disabilities.

Initial Observations and Brief History

The initial observations of reading difficulties occurred more than 100 years ago, with simple descriptions of a disorder of "word blindness" (Hinschelwood, 1896; Morgan, 1896). That adults with brain injury lost their ability to identify visual representations of words was well-known at the time and commonly was viewed as a visual agnosia for words. However, Morgan (1896) and Hinschelwood (1896) reported cases of word blindness in the absence of brain injury that were less complete than in cases with brain injury (Doris, 1993). Hence, initial differentiations separated reading disorders that reflected a loss of reading ability (alexia) from a failure to develop reading ability (dyslexia). Subsequent attempts to define *dyslexia* simply eliminated other "known" causes (low intelligence, social deprivation, inadequate instruction, and emotional problems; Orton, 1925). These attempts were epitomized in the definition of dyslexia put forward by the World Federation of Neurology (Critchley, 1970, p. 11):

A disorder manifested by difficulties in learning to read despite conventional instruction, adequate intelligence, and socio-economic opportunity. It is dependent upon fundamental cognitive disabilities which are frequently of constitutional origin.

Isle of Wight Studies

This approach to definition received some support from the influential Isle of Wight studies in the late 1960s and early 1970s (Rutter & Yule, 1975; Rutter, 1978). These studies, conducted on an epidemiological sample of children on the Isle of Wight, addressed many issues in child development, including the validity of the concept of specific reading disability. As part of this study, children received the performance IQ scale of the Wechsler Intelligence Scale for Children (WISC) and measures of reading accuracy and rate. When the distribution of reading skills was plotted, it appeared bimodal, showing a "hump" in the lower end of the distribution and the expected central mode near the average of the distribution. This led to the hypothesis that two distinct subtypes of reading disability existed: *specific reading retardation*, representing children with reading levels well below expectations based on age and IQ score, and *general reading backwardness*, representing children who had reading levels below age-based expectations but whose reading levels were consistent with IQ expectations.

The hypothesis that these two groups represented separable disorders was supported by results showing that relative to children with general reading backwardness, children with specific reading retardation had higher IQ scores, a lower frequency of known and suspected neurological disorders, and poorer reading outcomes over time and were roughly equal in the proportion of male and female subjects. In contrast, more children with general reading backwardness were male than female, were mentally deficient, and had known or suspected brain disorders. Rutter and Yule (1975, p. 195) concluded:

Reading retardation is shown to differ significantly from reading backwardness in terms of sex ratio, neurological disorder, pattern of neurodevelopmental deficits and educational prognosis. It is concluded that the concept of specific reading retardation is valid ...

The Isle of Wight studies of reading disability were accepted widely, partly because, despite the authors' disclaimers, the results seemed to support the notion of dyslexia (i.e., specific reading retardation) set forth in the World Federation of Neurology definition. One of the important influences of the Isle of Wight studies was the implication that discrepancies between IQ and reading scores were a proxy or marker for dyslexia. Though the Isle of Wight studies were landmarks at the time of their completion, the studies of reading disabilities suffer from significant limitations.

The bimodality may be a product of a ceiling effect on the reading test (van der Wiesel & Zegers, 1985) and the failure to apply any common exclusionary criteria to children in the study (Fletcher et al., 1998). The latter issue is particularly critical because the general reading backwardness group included children with definite central nervous system (CNS) disorders (11.4%) and suspected CNS disorders (25.3%). In contrast, the specific reading retardation group included no children with a definite CNS disorder and 18.6% with a questionable CNS disorder. Many children in the general reading backwardness group had IQ scores below 70, so that the longer tail and hump in the reading score distribution may reflect the influence of CNS disorders on IQ test scores in a manner consistent with the two-factor theory of mental retardation (Zigler & Hodapp, 1986). Moreover, the reported neurodevelopmental differences between the two groups also can be explained by the presence of neurological disorders and lower IQ scores, which was noted by the investigators: "[T]he association with general reading backwardness was to be expected on the grounds of the below average intelligence of that group of children" (Rutter & Yule, 1975, p. 189).

Also noteworthy is that neither the bimodality of reading skills nor the presence of differences between discrepant and low-achieving readers has seen any form of systematic replication when exclusionary criteria have been applied. Several epidemiological investigations have failed to show bimodality, with the most recent study suggesting that "dyslexia occurs along a continuum that blends imperceptibly with normal reading ability ... the dyslexic children simply represent a lower portion of a continuum of reading capabilities" (Shaywitz et al., 1992, p. 148).

Other recent studies have addressed possible differences between children who meet IQ-discrepancy and low-achievement criteria. These studies generally failed to show differences between these two reading-disabled groups in cognitive profiles (Siegel, 1992; Fletcher et al., 1994; Stanovich & Siegel, 1994), heritability (Pennington et al., 1992), or long-term outcomes (Francis et al., 1996). As Stanovich and Siegel (1994, p. 48) stated:

[N]either the phenotypic nor the genotypic indicators of poor reading are correlated in a reliable way with IQ discrepancy. If there is a special group of children with reading disabilities who are behaviorally, cognitively, genetically, or neurologically different, it is becoming increasingly unlikely that they can be easily identified by using IQ discrepancy as a proxy for the genetic and neurological differences themselves. Thus, the basic assumption that underlies decades of classification in research and educational practice regarding reading disabilities is becoming increasingly untenable.

Alternative Definitions of Dyslexia

The results of these studies do not indicate that dyslexia does not exist, that dyslexia subtypes do not exist, or that dyslexia occurs in the absence of biological correlates. They do suggest that more traditional approaches to definition and classification, which view dyslexia as *more* than a disorder of reading, may impede the definition problem.

The traditional view of dyslexia as more than a disorder of reading contrasts with contemporary views of dyslexia that focus on the reading problem. These views, which have fueled current investigations of the cognitive and neurobiological correlates of dyslexia, use hypothetical models of the reading process and of the relationship of language and cognitive skills with reading to specify dependent variables (Vellutino, 1979; Wagner & Torgesen, 1987; Stanovich, 1988, 1991; Liberman et al., 1989; Castles & Coltheart, 1993). In addition to identifying a variety of correlates of reading disability, these investigations have focused dyslexia research on the core deficit, which involves the ability to decode single, isolated words.

This deficit is related closely to phonological processing skills. Nonetheless, dyslexia also is more than a disorder of word decoding. Children with dyslexia commonly (though variably) have neurological soft signs, problems in other academic areas (e.g., mathematics), attention deficit hyperactivity disorder (ADHD), and other sources of heterogeneity. This heterogeneity may have important implications for understanding potential biological correlates and individual differences within children with dyslexia, particularly response to treatment (Benton, 1975). However, this source of heterogeneity may not explain why children with dyslexia fail to develop effective reading skills. Here, more recent research that addresses the cognitive basis of the reading problem becomes critically important. Approaching the definition problem from this latter perspective allows dyslexia to be viewed as a disorder of single-word decoding skills. The problems in decoding can be associated reliably with language problems involving phonological processing. From this core, other correlates occur variably but are associated less reliably with the reading problem (Stanovich, 1988). Dyslexia then can be viewed simply as a variation on normal development consistent with a *dimensional* approach to definition (Ellis, 1984; Stanovich, 1988, 1991; Shaywitz et al., 1992). In other words, reading disability is simply the lower end of an undemarcated continuum of reading ability (Shaywitz, 1996). Identifying children with dyslexia could be based on establishing a cut-point on the dimension of reading disability, thus representing an *inclusionary* definition, with research proceeding to identify possible subtypes that account for individual differences. The "unexpectedness" occurs because the child is not mentally deficient and is underachieving relative to chronological age. Such an approach is reflected clearly in the research definition recently adopted by the Orton Dyslexia Society (Lyon, 1995a, p. 9):

Dyslexia is one of several distinct learning disabilities. It is a specific language-based disorder of constitutional origin characterized by difficulties in single word decoding, usually reflecting insufficient phonological processing abilities. These difficulties in single word decoding are often unexpected in relation to age and other cognitive and academic abilities; they are not the result of generalized developmental disability or sensory impairment. Dyslexia is manifest by variable difficulty with different forms of language, often including, in addition to problems reading, a conspicuous problem with acquiring proficiency in writing and spelling.

Problems with Dimensional Definitions

A dimensional approach simplifies approaches to definition but is not without problems. Most significant is the level of severity that represents a cut-point for identification of a child as disabled. Research on children with dyslexia has not been viewed as have been dimensional disorders in medicine (e.g., hypertension, obesity), wherein *treatment* at certain points on the continuum indicates the level of severity necessary to reduce adverse outcomes. Nonetheless, from a research perspective, little evidence corroborates that factors influencing poor reading are different from those influencing good reading. The key is for the researcher to measure appropriate reading skills and to demonstrate clearly a *replicable* cut-point (Fletcher et al., 1998).

The second set of concerns involves the use of exclusionary criteria. No empirical basis mandates excluding cases with brain injury, mental deficiency, emotional problems, social deprivation, and lack of opportunity. Although the cause may vary, reading problems most often reflect problems with decoding, which invariably reflect problems with phonological processing (Lyon, 1995b). In particular, no good basis calls for establishing the point on the continuum at which the cut-point for separating dyslexia and mental deficiency should occur. When this issue has been investigated empirically, lower-IQ children do not emerge as a separate subgroup unless IQ is used as a classification variable (Siegel, 1989, 1992; Fletcher et al., 1998). Again, for research purposes, exclusions make sense as long as the exclusionary criteria are not used to make strong causal inferences. Clearly, the cognitive factors that influence good and poor reading in children with brain injury and low IQ scores are similar to those that influence good and poor reading in neurologically normal children with average IQ scores (Siegel, 1989, 1992; Fletcher et al., 1995; Barnes & Dennis, 1996). The *cause* of the cognitive variations may vary but not the relationship of cognitive skills and reading.

The final issue involves the subset of children who fail to read at levels expected on the basis of their IQ but still read in the average range. Recent studies indicate that when these children are identified using regression-based criteria, this subgroup also is impaired in phonological awareness skills (Fletcher et al., 1998). Thus, because this group is not different from lower-IQ children with reading disorders, some investigators have proposed using both discrepancy and low-achievement definitions to identify cases (Shaywitz et al., 1992). More research is needed on this issue.

Definition

These examples render clear that dyslexia can be defined and demystified using dimensional criteria, particularly when the reading measure involves single-word decoding skills. In fact, such definitions have fueled recent investigations of genetic and neurobiological correlates and treatment approaches (Lyon, 1995a,b). This rapid progress occurs in part because definitions based on decoding identify children who are relatively homogeneous in terms of the reading problem but heterogeneous on other dimensions (Fletcher et al., 1998). The problem is not whether dyslexia exists or how to define it but the broadness of the definition and subsequent classification. These decisions will be facilitated by intervention studies that examine interactions of subtypes and outcome (Lyon, 1985) and begin to evaluate the level of severity necessary to support particular approaches to definition.

Several recent efforts have sought to broaden classification efforts in children with dyslexia and other forms of reading and learning disability (Fletcher et al., 1998; Stanovich et al., 1997), joining an older literature about these problems (Satz & Morris, 1981; Rourke, 1985; Fletcher & Morris, 1986; Morris, 1988; Hooper & Willis, 1989). (These studies are beyond the scope of this chapter). What is important is that one form of reading disability—dyslexia—can reliably be identified and defined. This form of reading disability accounts for up to 80% of cases of poor reading in children (Lerner, 1989; Lyon, 1995a). Indeed, across the age range, reading disability occurs primarily at the level of the single word and involves deficits in decoding skills (Bruck, 1992). The question is: What accounts not only for this core deficit but for variations around this core? At the cognitive level, an appropriate framework is the phonological core-variable differences model of Stanovich (1988, 1991) in which reading disability is viewed as consisting of an invariant, core deficit in phonological processing but with variability in the contribution of other cognitive skills. Good support is found for this model (Stanovich, 1988, 1991; Fletcher et al., 1994, 1998; Stanovich & Siegel, 1994).

At another level, certain factors influence these variations in cognitive ability. These factors are both biological and environmental. Much of the research on dyslexia has explored the relationship of cognitive and biological factors, but the contribution of social and environmental factors should not be discounted. A particularly difficult problem is the possibility, largely unexamined, that the phenotype associated with reading disability may not vary across potential causes. Hence, even in poor readers with a history of social deprivation, the initial problems reflect difficulties in learning decoding skills, and the cognitive correlates are similar to those in children who read poorly with no history of social deprivation.

This issue is addressed at the end of this chapter. In the next sections, four areas of investigation of the cognitive and neuropsychological factors related to dyslexia are discussed and are followed by a discussion of neurobiological factors in dyslexia. These four areas were selected for review because each area explicitly attempts to relate cognition to underlying neurobiological factors. This discussion is not a summary of the vast literature on dyslexia but a critical review of research findings and future directions.

COGNITIVE AND NEUROPSYCHOLOGICAL CORRELATES OF DYSLEXIA

Current approaches to evaluating the cognitive correlates of dyslexia are based on four frameworks: (1) traditional neuropsychology, (2) visual processes, (3) comparisons of adult alexia and developmental dyslexia, and (4) relationships of language and reading. Each of these frameworks makes an attempt to describe aspects of the phenotype of dyslexia and relate this phenotype to brain function.

Traditional Neuropsychological Framework

The neuropsychological framework is largely psychometric and has a long history in dyslexia research. It is based on the view that dyslexia is more than a reading problem. Studies from the neuropsychological framework clearly show that children with dyslexia have deficits in a variety of areas involving language, memory, spatial perception, motor skills, and associated deficits reflecting finger agnosia, right-left confusion, and soft neurological signs. This literature, reviewed by Satz and van Nostrand (1973), Rourke (1975), and Benton (1975), was based on the belief that understanding deficits presumably *unrelated* to the reading problem would provide evidence for the biological basis of dyslexia.

This belief has not been supported. Indeed, the lesson of the neuropsychological framework is important. These studies show clearly that comparisons of dyslexic and normal readers yield significant group differences on virtually every dimension studied. Effect sizes vary, but obtaining significant univariate differences depends mostly on sample size. The problems with this literature, including small, poorly defined samples, a focus on broad, factorially confounded dependent variables, and weak formulation of hypotheses, have been summarized (Benton, 1975; Doehring, 1978; Satz & Fletcher, 1980), with an emphasis on the need for larger, well-defined samples, the need to consider subtypes within dyslexic groups, and the importance of a multivariate approach. The sampling, definition, and measurement issues are obvious but continue to be slighted in many studies of dyslexia. The need for a multivariate conceptualization and for strong hypothesis formulation are less obvious but frequently are underemphasized.

The problem is still the common practice in research about dyslexia to take a univariate difference on a single dimension—given that comparisons on most dimensions will be significant—and to extrapolate this difference into a theory of dyslexia. This is the most important lesson from the neuropsychological framework: Univariate differences at a phenotypic level may not explain the entire phenotype, nor do such differences support identification of brain-based factors related to dyslexia. In particular, the notion that differences not clearly related to the core deficit in word reading are important not only lacks support but has been misleading; hence, the weak theoretical basis of many studies of dyslexia conducted from the neuropsychological framework.

The misleading nature of neuropsychological deficits based on such univariate analyses are most apparent on examination of some of the brain-based hypotheses about dyslexia generated from this framework. These hypotheses include variations of a maturational lag hypothesis (Satz & van Nostrand, 1973), incomplete cerebral dominance (Orton, 1925), and variations on parietal lobe hypotheses (Benton, 1975). In general, all these hypotheses are based on the visual inspection of performance patterns of children with dyslexia, often with extrapolations to the performance patterns of adults with brain injury. None of these hypotheses have proved viable, partly because of a focus on deficiencies that do not explain the core deficit in decoding and because extrapolations between adults with brain injury and children with dyslexia all too frequently are misleading. Certainly, mere similarities in phenotypic performance patterns do not confirm a similar brain basis in the absence of the capacity of the study independently to evaluate neurobiological variables (Fletcher & Taylor, 1984).

Possibly, the phenotypic variability exhibited by dyslexics may have implications for individual differences at the level of neurobiology or treatment. This question awaits additional evaluation. Most important are the *lessons* of the neuropsychological framework: Definition and sampling must be based on the core deficit, and a multivariate approach is essential for addressing phenotypic variability. This requires specification of dependent variables at an analytical and precise level to determine exactly those skills that account for variability across cases and in relationship to the core deficit. When samples are well defined and dependent variables are analytical and well specified, the possibility of relating neurobiological (and environmental) variables to the phenotype is enhanced.

Visual Processes

The lessons of the neuropsychological framework have not been learned by investigations of visual processes in children with reading disability. Older versions of these hypotheses, particularly those that focused on *visuospatial* skills (e.g., perceptual-motor skills), were criticized by Vellutino (1979) and generally have not been supported. Some children with dyslexia have spatial problems, but such difficulties do not account for significant variability in the core deficit in decoding. Studies of subtypes based on the neuropsychological framework identified groups impaired in spatial skills (Rourke, 1985; Hooper & Willis, 1989), but a recent study that also included a variety of analytical language measures clearly related to decoding skills did not identify subtypes exclusively impaired in spatial skills (Fletcher et al., 1998).

Transient Visual System Deficits

More recent studies have used models of the visual system to study children who are poor readers. The predominant set of studies is based on psychophysical distinctions between parallel sustained and transient channels in the visual system (Breitmeyer & Ganz, 1976). The sustained channel provides a longer-duration response to stimuli that are slowly moving with high frequency. The transient channel provides short, previsual responses to stimuli that have low spatial frequency and are moving rapidly. Sustained channel operations relate anatomically to the parvocellular visual pathway, whereas transient channel operations relate to the magnocellular pathway.

In reading (and other visual processes), these systems inhibit one another. Individuals with dyslexia have been hypothesized to have ineffective transient system inhibition that interferes with normal saccadic suppressions. This results in a persistence of the retinal image, resulting in a superimposition of successive visual inputs so that the words on a page seem jumbled (Lovegrove et al., 1986).

Some evidence supports this hypothesis (Lovegrove & Williams, 1993) and evidence also supports a broader range of vision defects in dyslexics (Stein, 1993). However, even studies that compare language- and visual-processing measures show that measures of language abilities—particularly phonological processing skills—account for most of the variability in reading skills in good and poor readers. To illustrate, Eden et al. (1995, p. 272) compared phonological- and visual-processing skills of children who were disabled and nondisabled readers, concluding as follows:

In addition to performing poorly on verbal tests, the children with reading disability were significantly worse than non-disabled children on many visual and eye-movement tasks ... These results provide further support for the hypothesis that reading disability may, to some extent, result from dysfunction of the visual and oculomotor systems.

Clearly, Eden et al. (1995) found between disabled and nondisabled readers differences that were statistically significant at conventional levels of alpha ($P < .05$). What they failed to report is that effect sizes clearly were much larger for the language tasks than for the visual tasks. Moreover, visual-processing tasks correlated "significantly" with reading ability, but the amount of variability explained by the visual tasks ranged from 4% to 15%, whereas correlations for language tasks ranged from 4% to 55%, and measures of phonological awareness accounted for 26% to 55% of the variability. A stepwise multiple regression analysis predicting reading skills entered a phonological awareness variable first, followed by verbal IQ, chronological age, and a dot localization measure. The latter entered into the regression model only after 63% of the variability between the first three variables had been explained and only incremented the model by 5%. As in other studies of visual processing, Eden et al. (1995) found "significant" differences that pale relative to the robustness of relationships of language and reading.

Methodological Issues

At this juncture, disputing whether individuals with reading disability have deficits in the visual system is less relevant than is the question of these deficits' meaning. However, addressing this question is difficult because of problems similar to those identified for the neuropsychological framework: definition, univariate conceptualization of the disorder, and weak hypothesis formulation.

The definition problem is significant. Regardless of one's beliefs about reading, language, and vision, the most common problem with reading in children who are poor readers occurs at the level of the single word. Groups of impaired readers should be identified on the basis of difficulties with single-word decoding. Possibly, other forms of reading disability exist, but the disorder identified currently and (to a lesser degree) historically as dyslexia represents a core deficit in the identification of single words in isolation (Doris, 1993).

Studies of visual processes often have failed to specify the definition used to form groups. Even when the definition is provided, recent studies use definitions that are known to be suspect on psychometric and empirical grounds, usually employing a "grades-below" criterion. For example, in discussing the definition problem, Willows et al. (1993, p. 267) stated:

[T]he term *reading disability* is defined by the conventional definition, which requires that subjects have normal general intellectual ability, educational opportunity, and social/emotional functioning but below normal reading achievement For children at or above the age of 8, a lag of 2 or more years below grade level in reading achievement is defined as a reading disability. For children who are below the age of 8, and therefore cannot be more than 2 years below grade level, an individual who is at least 1 year below age/grade at age 7 or at least 6 months below age/grade expectation at age 6 is designated as reading disabled.

The authors went on to note: [t]he operational definition of the group of readers is the key to the interpretation of the data (p. 267) and "... not all researchers have adopted an acceptable definition of reading disability" (p. 267). Furthermore, according to these authors, "There has been no systematic use of any other definition of reading disability in the disabled-normal reader literature examining visual processes" (p. 267).

These observations are cogent because definitions based on grades-below criteria were criticized widely 15 or more years prior to the appearance of these words (Angoff, 1971; Gaddes, 1976; Rutter, 1978; Reynolds, 1984). The primary problems reflect the unstandardized nature of grade- or age-based criteria and the increasing dispersion of such unstandardized metrics with age. The "number-of-years-below" criteria are arbitrary and fundamentally not meaningful in a cross-sectional study design wherein children vary in age. One could argue that such criteria, though imprecise, still will produce groups of good and poor readers. However, the effect of imprecise definitions is to introduce unmeasured sources of variability into the groups, increasing the possibility that good and poor readers will differ on multiple dimensions, so that univariate comparisons will be significant if the sample size provides sufficient power (Doehring, 1978; Fletcher & Morris, 1986; Siegel & Heaven, 1986). Compounding this problem is the common failure to specify how reading was measured to form the groups. Definitions based on comprehension skills commonly increase heterogeneity in the dependent variables. As Siegel and Heaven (1986) noted, many factors can produce low scores on measures of reading comprehension, few of which have to do with reading per se. Moreover, as the majority of children with reading disability have problems with decoding skills, not surprisingly, decoding ability is the best predictor of reading comprehension skills (Adams & Bruck, 1993; Lyon, 1995a).

Perhaps the most significant weakness of the visual hypotheses is the failure to explain the core single-word decoding deficit that characterizes dyslexia. The interaction of the transient and sustained channels is most apparent in the saccadic eye movements that occur in reading connected text. The transient system, which has been hypothesized to be deficient in children with reading disability, operates very early in the visual process, performing a spatial analysis of the stimulus to be processed. Problems with the transient system would be most apparent on dynamic visual-processing tasks, such as visible persistence, or in the perception of an object when the object is not physically present. However, the primary problem in children with dyslexia involves reading words in isolation, which is a *static* visual-processing task that does not significantly involve the transient visual system (Willows & LeCluyse, 1990). The difficulties that dyslexic people experience in reading connected text occur because they cannot decode isolated words, much less words in context. This deficiency is what any reasonable explanation of dyslexia must address, a deficiency presently not addressed by proponents of a visual-deficit hypothesis.

Interventions

Visual-deficit hypotheses have spawned a variety of interventions, including colored lenses to correct "scotopic sensitivity" (Blaskey et al., 1990; O'Connor et al., 1990; Robinson & Conway, 1990), monocular occlusion to correct unstable binocular control (Stein & Fowler, 1982), and the use of colored overlays to correct deficiencies in the transient system (Willows & LeCluyse, 1990).

Some evidence suggests that colored lenses lead to improvement in text reading in disabled readers (Blaskey et al., 1990; Robinson & Conway, 1990), but the evidence is mixed (O'Connor et al., 1990) and subject to multiple methodological problems (Parker, 1990; Solan, 1990). No evidence supports the ability of colored lenses to improve single-word decoding skills. Also, evidence suggests that treatment for unstable binocular control leads to improved reading in some children (Stein, 1993), but this evidence is fairly controversial (Bishop, 1989) .

The use of colored overlays also is associated with improvement in reading skills in some children (Willows & LeCluyse, 1990; Willows et al., 1992). However, the latter studies illustrate some of the problems with the approach to definition taken by these intervention studies. Poor reading was defined using a grades-below definition, based on what appear to be reading comprehension measures. No control for comorbid disorders, such as ADHD, was provided. In a recent study of the effect of colored overlays, Iovino (1995) defined groups using standardized tests of reading decoding skills and included groups of children with ADHD and no reading disability, mathematics and no reading disability, reading disability with and without mathematics disability, and normal controls. Single-word identification, reading comprehension, and reading rate were measured as outcome variables. The results revealed that blue transparencies led to a small (0.25 standard deviation) improvement in reading rate and comprehension in *all* groups, with no effect of any transparency (blue, red, clear) on single-word decoding. In short, the blue transparencies—which should have the most effect on the transient system—led to improved text reading, but this improvement occurred regardless of whether the child was dyslexic.

Visual-Processing Hypotheses

Like studies conducted from the traditional neuropsychological framework, the visual-processing hypotheses show group differences between disabled and nondisabled readers that are of questionable significance. Problems exist at the level of definition and sampling, specification of the dependent variables, and hypothesis formulation. Fundamental is the extent to which visual-processing hypotheses can explain the core deficit in dyslexia, which involves the decoding of words in isolation. Noteworthy is that phonological codes are activated very early in the word-recognition process (Rayner et al., 1995). Nonetheless, reading involves the visual system, and the investigation of visual processes is important, particularly if the research leads to new information on the neurobiology of dyslexia or on interventions. However, as Wolff and Melngailis (1996) recently observed, what tends to happen is that observations important to visual hypotheses do not stand up in more controlled investigations. This was the case with earlier observations of spatial deficits (Vellutino, 1979) and more recent studies of eye movements (Olsen & Fosberg, 1993), letter reversals and reading geometrically transformed text (Wolff & Melngailis, 1996), and even the efficacy of color overlays (Iovino, 1995). Some of these deficiencies in visual processing may be a *byproduct* of the decoding problem or of some presently unspecified comorbidity, such as ADHD.

Comparisons of Acquired and Developmental Reading Disability

Studies of acquired reading disorders due to brain injury have led to classification of the alexias based on patterns of reading and writing errors and on associated characteristics. This research was based on hypotheses about the nature of word-recognition processes, particularly those encapsulated in dual-route theory. This theory views word recognition in a lexicon as occurring through two routes: an indirect route mediated by phonological rules that relate graphemes to phonemes and a direct visual-orthographic route (Foorman, 1994b).

The dual-route theory provides an alternative to connectionist models that emphasize a single route, "bottom-up" process of constrained pattern recognition (Foorman, 1994a). Nonetheless, reading words in isolation also requires *orthographical* processes that involve awareness of spelling patterns and the representation of words in the alphabet. Orthographical processes include awareness of the spatial and sequential letter redundancies, which may involve visual processes. Proponents of a role for visual deficits in reading disability have explored the role of orthographical processes, viewing them as, for example, a "hypothetical print analyzer" (Seymour & Evans, 1993). A focus on orthographical processes has served other investigations of extralinguistic factors in reading disability (Bowers et al., 1994; Wolf et al., 1994) and represents an attempt to link some of the associated characteristics of reading disability with a core deficit in reading.

The findings from studies of alexia have been applied to non-brain-injured children with reading disability. Most striking are observations of individual cases with reading error patterns that appear to mimic error patterns in subtypes of adult alexia. For example, Castles and Coltheart (1993) separated dyslexics with specific deficits in either phonological or orthographical processes, referring to the former as *phonological dyslexics* and the latter as *surface dyslexics*. Phonological dyslexics show poorer reading of nonsense words than exception words; surface dyslexics show better nonsense-word reading than exception-word reading.

That children with phonological dyslexia can be reliably defined is clear. Such children emerge in virtually all the single-case studies and in larger studies conceptualized from the dual-route model. Whether surface dyslexics can be defined reliably is controversial (Stanovich et al., 1997). Murphy and Pollatsek (1994) did not obtain evidence supporting distinctions between phonological and surface dyslexics. However, Manis et al. (1996) and Stanovich et al. (1997) did obtain subtypes that supported this hypothesis. The support was apparent primarily in children younger than those used in Murphy and Pollatsek (1994) and only with normal readers who were matched on reading age with the disabled readers (i.e., comparisons of older poor readers and younger good readers).

Stanovich et al. (1997) reanalyzed the data from Castles and Coltheart (1993) and Manis et al. (1996), along with a data set of their own. The reanalysis of these two studies showed that most dyslexics had difficulties at both the phonological and orthographical level of the word, consistent with Foorman et al. (1998). When younger normal readers were matched on reading level to the older poor readers, children who had been identified as surface dyslexics on the basis of comparison to chronological-age-matched normal readers no longer showed evidence for surface dyslexia. In an analysis of a younger group of children with reading disabilities that included reading-level and chronological-age controls, Stanovich et al. (1997) also found that surface dyslexics largely were not apparent when reading-level controls were employed. Stanovich et al. (1997) suggested that phonological dyslexia was a distinct subtype, characterized by problems with both pseudowords and real words persistent across definitions and age. In contrast, surface dyslexia appeared to represent a subtype that was not stable across definition or age, representing a delay in the development of word recognition skills.

Independent of the distinction between phonological and surface dyslexia, the role of orthographical processes in dyslexia remains controversial. Stanovich et al. (1997) showed that disabled readers were poor in both phonological and orthographical processes, with phonological processes accounting for a much greater portion of the variability in reading skills. However, some studies using reading level match designs have implied that children with dyslexia compensate for these weaknesses in phonological processing through the orthographical route (Stanovich & Siegel, 1994) and actually may be superior orthographical processors (Siegel et al., 1995). In contrast, Foorman et al. (1998) showed that evidence of orthographical superiority most likely was an artifact of matching reading levels on grade equivalent scores (for all the problems already outlined regarding the use of "grades-below" criteria). The evidence for orthographical superiority disappeared when matching was conducted using interval-based metrics that measured reading ability on a scale that was constant across age range. In addition, the relationship between orthographical processing and decoding skills was nonlinear, with no evidence of a relationship at lower levels of decoding. As Stanovich et al. (1997) showed, disabled readers tend to do poorly on any type of word recognition task.

One of the factors underlying comparisons of adult alexics and developmental dyslexics was the hope that similarities in the error patterns would elucidate areas of the brain involved in dyslexia. According to this reasoning, because the adult alexics have known brain lesions, it may be possible to extrapolate to the brains of people with dyslexia. However, this type of "argument by analogy" does little more than suggest hypotheses. Similarities in error patterns may be mere homologies with no common origin (Fletcher & Taylor, 1984). Indeed, error patterns in children with reading disability are influenced significantly by the myriad interventions these children tend to receive.

Language and Reading

In contrast to the weak and inconsistent findings generated by the three previous paradigms, studies of children with dyslexia based on hypothesized relationships of specific language skills and reading provide robust findings concerning important aspects of the phenotype and provide potential neurobiological correlates. These studies are based on the view that reading is an outgrowth of the development of language. Although varied language skills have been evaluated, four general domains consistently emerge as important: phonological processing, rapid serial naming, verbal short-term memory, and lexical skills (Vellutino, 1987; Wagner & Torgesen, 1987; Liberman et al., 1989).

Phonological Processing Currently, a large body of research examines the language and cognitive correlates of good and poor reading. This research, which has emerged over the last 20 years, shows that language variables are the primary cognitive correlates of both good and poor reading. In particular, language variables that involve phonological processing are most significant (Wagner & Torgesen, 1987; Liberman et al., 1989). To learn to read, children must develop an awareness that words have an internal, sound-based structure (Liberman, 1973; Liberman et al., 1974; Adams, 1990). Learning to make the connection between speech and print so as to learn an alphabetical code for reading is essential for the development of decoding skills, which in turn represent the level at which most children who develop dyslexia struggle (Vellutino, 1979, 1987, 1991; Bradley & Bryant, 1983; Foorman et al., 1991; Adams & Bruck, 1993).

At this point, most investigations show and largely accept that phonological-processing skills account for much of the variability in reading skills in poor readers. At issue is whether other language (and cognitive) skills account for variability in decoding skills beyond what is explained by phonological-processing skills. One prominent view sees the phonological-processing deficits of dyslexia as a bottleneck that interferes with the development of other cognitive skills (Shankweiler & Crain, 1986). In this view, deficits in rapid serial naming and verbal short-term memory are manifestations of an underlying phonological deficit. Other investigations have shown that other measures account for variability in word recognition skills independently of phonological-processing abilities, particularly rapid serial naming (McBride-Chang, & Manis, 1996). In addition, orthographical measures account for variability in decoding skills (Wagner & Barker, 1994). The issue of untangling these relationships is addressed later in this chapter. At this juncture, clearly phonological-processing abilities are robustly related to good and poor reading.

Rapid Serial Naming   Along with problems with phonological processing, disabled readers also have difficulties with rapid serial naming skills (Denckla & Rudel, 1974; Katz & Shankweiler, 1985; Wolf et al., 1986; Wolf et al., 1994). The basis for these difficulties is unclear. Some have hypothesized that the problems with rapid serial naming are a manifestation of the weakness in phonological processing (Shankweiler & Crain, 1986; Wagner & Torgesen, 1987). In contrast, Wolf et al. (1994) have argued that these deficits often are related to a more general rate or automaticity factor that is independent of the phonological-processing problem. Support for this hypothesis has come from studies by Wolf et al. (1986, 1994) identifying poor readers who were impaired only in rapid serial naming but not in phonological-processing skills. However, it is important to note that these children are not impaired in *decoding* skills—only in *comprehension* skills. The intervention studies of Lovett et al. (1994) have separated children according to the rate and accuracy of reading versus problems with single-word decoding. Evidence also suggests that the problems that are identified on these measures of rapid serial naming may reflect more general rate-based difficulties outside the language system (Wolff, 1993).

The problem with these studies is that the samples are small. Few subjects who have deficits involving rapid serial naming but are not also phonologically impaired can be identified. These subjects are not classically dyslexic because the isolated rate deficits are not expected to produce single-word decoding deficits. Rather, the reading deficiencies have been related to orthographical processes that produce problems with the rate and automaticity of text reading (Bowers et al., 1994; Wolf et al., 1994). Finally, exactly what is measured by rapid serial naming and other rate-based measures is not clear. Possibly, rapid serial naming places a premium on phonological processing as well as on an automaticity factor, such that the measures are factorially confounded. A more analytical approach to the assessment of these skills may be necessary to determine the measurement characteristics of such tasks. This issue is addressed later.

Verbal Short-Term Memory   Verbal short-term memory deficits also have been identified frequently. Children with dyslexia often show difficulty in their ability to encode and retrieve verbally coded material, particularly if phonological structures are manipulated (Fletcher, 1985; Gathercole & Baddley, 1990; Brady, 1991; Torgesen, 1996). The memory problems are limited largely to the language domain (Shankweiler et al., 1979; Fletcher, 1985) and may be manifestations of the underlying deficits in phonology and language skills as opposed to specific problems with working memory and short-term memory (Shankweiler & Crain, 1986; Wagner et al., 1994).

Lexical Deficits   Finally, children with dyslexia commonly show both reductions in the size of vocabulary skills and problems on lexical retrieval tasks. Performance on measures of receptive vocabulary are good predictors of the development of reading skills (Satz & Fletcher, 1980; Vellutino et al., 1988). In addition, vocabulary deficits commonly are observed in older children who are poor readers. In that case, possibly the vocabulary difficulties are products of the reading difficulty, reflecting insufficient reading experience and lack of exposure to higher-level academics as opposed to a cause of the reading problem (Doehring, 1978; Vellutino et al., 1988).

Other Language Skills   Many other language skills also have been evaluated. Younger children with dyslexia do not appear to experience problems comprehending syntactical and grammatical structures (Fletcher et al., 1981; Shankweiler et al., 1995). However, such deficiencies may characterize older children but may be related more to problems in comprehension rather than in decoding skills (Fletcher, 1981). Tasks involving speed of articulation also have been implicated in reading disability (Olsen et al., 1985). Whether these tasks account for any variability in outcomes independent of phonological processing is unclear. Morphological deficits can be identified clearly (Shankweiler et al., 1995). Shankweiler and Crain (1986) and Liberman et al. (1989) suggested that the constellation of language-based deficits may reflect a coherent syndrome associated with reading disability. Deficits in phonological processing—clearly responsible for much of the variability in the core deficit in word decoding—would be expected to lead to problems with other aspects of language. If that be the case, this formulation may provide a coherent account of the variations in language skills observed in children with dyslexia.

Structural Modeling Studies   Studies of the language correlates of reading disability are characterized by increasingly improved approaches to issues involving definition and sampling. Although earlier studies were based on relatively small samples, now several large sample studies examine children with reading disabilities. Perhaps more importantly, several available studies address the language and cognitive correlates of dyslexia from a multivariate perspective, sometimes including sophisticated multivariate modeling techniques that permit the identification of *unique* underlying sources of variability in the relationships of cognitive skills in reading ability. Results from four of these studies are worthy of consideration: Fletcher et al. (1996); Katz et al., unpublished manuscript; McBride-Chang & Manis (1996); and Wagner et al. (1994).

The study by Fletcher et al. (1996) involved 378 children (ages 7.5–9.5 years). The sample included children recruited with a variety of deficits in reading, arithmetic, and attention, children who had IQ scores in the 60 to 79 range, and a group of normal children. From a large battery of cognitive and linguistic tests selected based on a hypothetical model of reading and cognitive skills, a confirmatory factor analysis was performed. The results of this analysis revealed that a model that included eight specific factors and a general factor best approximated the latent structure of the data. The eight latent variables included measures of phonological awareness, verbal short-term memory, rapid serial naming, lexical retrieval and vocabulary, speech production, visuospatial skills, nonverbal short-term memory, and visual attention. Each of the language factors was related also to a general language factor. The general language factor was accounted for primarily by measures involving vocabulary and verbal reasoning skills, such as the Peabody Picture Vocabulary Test-Revised, the Boston Naming Test, and verbal subtests of the WISC-Revised (WISC-R).

Figure 12.1 shows the cognitive profiles across these eight latent variables for children who are disabled in reading, reading and mathematics and only in mathematics, along with children with ADHD and no learning disability, children with IQ scores in the below-average–mentally deficient range, and normal children. Apparent from figure 12.1 is that children with reading disability and both reading and mathematics disability are not particularly different. Basically, the children with both reading and mathematics disability tend to have lower scores, but the shape of the profile is similar. Note that the low points in the profiles involve phonological awareness, rapid naming, and vocabulary and lexical skills for both groups. Other studies of the sample have not shown differences between those children who meet discrepancy and low-achievement definitions of reading disability (Fletcher et al., 1994) or between children with reading disability and with and without ADHD (Shaywitz et al., 1995). In general, regardless of comorbidity, measures of phonological processing, rapid serial naming, lexical and vocabulary skills, and verbal short-term memory explain the most variability in separating groups of good and poor readers, with measures of phonological awareness skills accounting for the largest amount of variability.

The contribution of these language domains to reading skills can be evaluated directly. A second confirmatory factor analysis took a battery of achievement tests administered to the sample and developed successive, hierarchical confirmatory factor models. The best model identified five different variables: real-word decoding, pseudoword decoding, spelling, reading comprehension, and mathematics (Fletcher et al., 1996). For each of the reading and spelling variables, a stepwise multiple regression was used to iden-

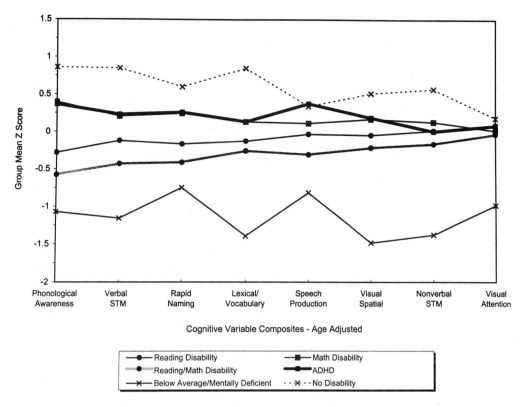

Figure 12.1 Profiles across eight cognitive constructs for children with reading disability (1); mathematics disability (2); reading and mathematics disability (3); attention deficit hyperactivity disorder (ADHD) and no learning disability (7); below average or mental deficiency (8); and no disability (9).

Table 12.1 Stepwise multiple regression predicting achievement construct skills with cognitive constructs

	Real Word Decoding (R^2)	Pseudoword Decoding (R^2)	Reading Comprehension (R^2)	Spelling (R^2)
Phonological awareness	.54	.60	.46	.49
Rapid naming	.59	.64	.59	.53
Lexical vocabulary skills	.62	.63	.54	
Verbal short-term memory				.56

tify those latent variables most closely related with the outcomes. These results are presented in table 12.1. As this table shows, measures of phonological awareness, rapid serial naming, and lexical and vocabulary skills were identified consistently as the best predictors of reading and spelling skills. Verbal short-term memory emerged as a significant predictor only if reading comprehension were involved but not for decoding. Phonological-awareness skills were the best single predictor in each analysis.

Katz et al. (unpublished manuscript) took the same dataset and developed a hypothetical model of language and reading skills. The model posited five determinants of real-word and pseudoword decoding: phonological awareness, automaticity (rapid serial naming), morphological awareness, lexical skills (indexed by vocabulary and verbal reasoning skills), and verbal short-term memory (working memory). Although the indicators of these constructs varied slightly relative to Fletcher et al. (1996), the latent variables were quite similar, with the addition of morphological awareness measures. The real-word and pseudoword decoding measures were viewed as mediators of outcomes involving reading comprehension and spelling. A listening comprehension measure also was included as a determinant of reading comprehension but not of decoding skills.

The results of this analysis showed that measures of phonological awareness accounted for most of the unique variance in the relationship of language skills and both real-word and pseudoword decoding. However, small paths were significant for morphological awareness and rapid serial naming with real-word decoding. In addition, listening comprehension had a significant influence on reading comprehension but not to the extent of decoding measures. Like the regression analyses, these results do not identify significant relationships between short-term memory skills and reading ability, suggesting that the problems experienced by children with dyslexia on measures of working memory and verbal short-term memory reflect their deficiencies in phonological processing. However, measures of rapid serial naming and morphological awareness accounted for small amounts of unique variance in decoding skills.

These findings are similar to another recent structural equation study in a smaller sample (McBride-Chang & Manis, 1996). This study showed that phonological awareness, rapid serial naming, and "verbal intelligence" (WISC-R Vocabulary and Similarities) all had significant relationships with real-word decoding that varied depending on reading skill. In poor readers, phonological awareness and rapid serial naming skills (but not verbal intelligence) were related uniquely to real-word decoding; in good readers, phonological awareness and verbal intelligence (but not rapid serial naming) were related to decoding skills.

The fourth study (Wagner et al., 1994) was longitudinal and developed a structural model relating test batteries administered in kindergarten, grade 1, and grade 2. This causal modeling study of 244 randomly selected children related five latent abilities (phonological analysis, phonological synthesis, phonological coding in working memory, isolated naming, and serial naming) to the development of decoding skills. The results revealed that these abilities develop at different rates and are remarkably stable over time. Models in which decoding skills exercised a causal influence on the development of phonological processing skills were not significant. Rather, phonological processing skills "caused" decoding skills. Neither serial nor isolated naming skills had a causal relationship with decoding skills. Markers of "verbal intelligence" (Stanford Binet Vocabulary) were not related to growth in either phonological processing or decoding skills. The relationship of rapid serial naming and decoding skills diminished over time. Letter-name knowledge in kindergarten mediated word-decoding skills influencing phonological-processing skills, but this influence was also independent of vocabulary size.

Conclusions

The structural modeling studies support the hypothesis that language skills can be fractionated into latent variables. These latent variables have differential relationships with academic skills. Katz et al. (unpublished manuscript) and McBride-Chang and Manis (1996) found that phonological awareness and rapid serial naming measures accounted for unique variance in relationship to word-decoding skills. Katz et al. (unpublished manuscript) and Wagner et al. (1994) found no unique relationship of lexical and vocabulary measures with word-decoding skills, whereas McBride-Chang and Manis (1996) found relationships of similar lexical and vocabulary measures—all involving verbal subtests of the WISC-R or Stanford Binet and measures, such as the Peabody Picture Vocabulary Test (Revised)—with word decoding *only* in good readers. The primary differences among the studies reflect the relationship of rapid serial naming to word decoding, which was not significant in Wagner et al. (1994). However the sample in Wagner et al. was a random sample and had relatively few disabled readers, whereas the samples in Katz et al. (unpublished manuscript) and McBride-Chang and Manis (1996) selected for disabled readers, who represented some 45% of both samples. McBride-Chang and Manis (1996) suggested that rapid-naming measures show considerable variability in disabled readers, a source of heterogeneity that clearly emerges in subtyping studies (Fletcher et al., 1998). None of these studies included orthographical measures, but Wagner and Barker (1994) completed a structural equation analysis and found relationships of both phonological and orthographical latent variables with word reading. Altogether, these studies show that measures of phonological-processing skills account for most of the variability in word reading abilities, with additional evidence for small but unique relationships of rapid serial naming, morphological awareness, and orthographical awareness.

NEUROBIOLOGICAL CORRELATES OF DYSLEXIA

Several approaches have been taken to the evaluation of the neurobiological correlates of dyslexia, including (1) the interpretation of performance patterns, (2) electrophysiological investigations, (3) autopsy studies, (4) structural neuroimaging studies, (5) functional neuroimaging investigations, and (6) genetic studies. Relative to the four models for research already reviewed, noteworthy is that most investigations have explored the visual process and language hypotheses. Reviews of each of these sets of studies are extensive (see chapter 13).

Performance Patterns

Approaches based on traditional neuropsychological studies of adults with alexia have generated hypotheses about the neurobiological basis of dyslexia related to extrapolations of performance patterns to individuals with brain injury. Because of the technology available at the time, this research (reviewed by Satz and van Nostrand, 1973; Benton, 1975; Rourke, 1975; and Coltheart, 1980) never included independent evaluations of the integrity of the brain-only extrapolations from performance patterns of adults and children. The limitations of these types of extrapolations were already described (Fletcher & Taylor, 1984), and these studies will not be reviewed further.

Electrophysiological Investigations

The older electrophysiological studies were reviewed by Hughes (1978), and more recent studies were reviewed by Dool et al. (1993). Clearly, many problems influence the evaluation of this research, particularly the tendency to study groups of children broadly defined as "learning disabled" and a large variety of nonspecific electrophysiological findings (Hughes, 1978).

More recent electrophysiological studies have used activation paradigms involving tones, clicks, and visual stimuli and stimuli sensitive to higher-order cognitive processes to study event-related potentials. These studies show differences between disabled and nondisabled readers in visual and auditory domains and in linguistic tasks. When the subject is defined clearly as reading-disabled, findings implicating a deficient left hemisphere are common. This is particularly true on tasks that manipulate phonological sensitivity and naming (Ackerman et al., 1994), but the deficiencies also occur on a variety of other language-based tasks, including semantic processing. Interestingly, responses to spatial stimuli or activations of the right hemisphere generally do not differentiate disabled and nondisabled readers.

Livingstone et al. (1991) and Lehmkuhle et al. (1993) evaluated evoked responses to stimuli eliciting responses of the transient visual system. In both studies, poor readers differed from good readers on visual evoked response measures in a manner consistent with deficient responsiveness of the magnocellular visual pathway. Lehmkule et al. (1993, p. 995) speculated that these deficiencies created "a timing disorder that precludes the rapid and smooth integration of detailed visual information necessary for efficient reading." These hypotheses are consistent with other studies that have observed rate-based deficiencies in poor readers (Wolff, 1993; Wolf et al., 1994). As we indicated these hypotheses await evaluation in better-defined samples, with some attempt to relate the findings to the core deficit in single-word decoding that characterizes dyslexia.

The electrophysiological studies are noteworthy in that consistent differences can be observed in subtypes of learning disability, particularly in relationship to ADHD (Harter et al., 1988; Ackerman et al., 1994) and reading versus arithmetical disability (Mattson et al., 1992; Miles & Stelmack, 1994). As children with ADHD also differ from comparison groups on electrophysiological measures, assessing the comorbidity of ADHD is critically important in any assessment of children with reading disability. As Dool et al. (1993) observed, electrophysiological research must include more precise definitions and assessments of possible subtypes. Definitions such as that used by Lehmkule et al. (1993, pp. 990–991)—"reading levels one to two years below their current grade levels, but with overall scores for mathematics and listening comprehension at or above grade level"—are not acceptable. Such an approach to subject selection, with an absence of an acceptable psychometric approach, no specification of how reading is measured, and no assessment of comorbidity of ADHD, increases the probability that the results are not specific to dyslexia. Moreover, one can only echo Dool et al. (1993) in calling "for theory-driven research" (pp. 395–396). Studies from Dykman's laboratory (Ackerman et al., 1994) provide excellent examples of the value of electrophysiological research when the samples are well defined and the activation paradigms theoretically are motivated by current hypotheses on the relationship of cognition and reading.

Autopsy Studies

The autopsy studies have been reviewed by Hynd and Semrud-Clikeman (1989) and Filipek (1995). Most of the interest has focused on studies of brains of adults with a history of dyslexia completed by Galaburda (1988), who found evidence of microdysgenesis and focal dysplasia in five of the seven brains analyzed. In addition, Galaburda (1988) found that the area of the planum temporale was symmetrical in all seven brains, whereas normal individuals usually have a larger left planum than right planum. Finally, Galaburda and Livingstone (1993) reported abnormalities of the magnocellular (but not parvocelluar) layers in five brains of dyslexics.

These autopsy studies have been controversial. Obviously, dyslexia is not fatal, so these cases are unusual. The sample is small, and the nature and severity of the dyslexia are unclear. Measuring the planum temporale is difficult (Galaburda, 1993). Perhaps what is more important than the nature of the abnormalities or their location is the evidence that these differences in the brains of dyslexics reflect early problems with neuronal migration that should lead to a host of abnormalities (Galaburda, 1988), which, in fact, the postmortem studies have demonstrated (Hynd & Semrud-Clikeman, 1989). However, prenatal or perinatal complications, which might relate to these disorders, are rare in children in dyslexia. It should not be surprising that electrophysiological and neuroimaging studies yield a variety of inconsistent findings or even that a variety of cognitive findings emerge. The tasks are to identify (1) correlates of the core deficit in word recognition, (2) how these correlates relate to brain function, and (3) how well these relationships predict individual differences among children with dyslexia.

Structural Neuroimaging Studies

Filipek (1995; see also chapter 13) summarized the 20 or so studies using cerebral tomography and magnetic resonance imaging (MRI) methods to quantitate brain areas in children and adults with reading disability. These studies vary widely in subjects, methods, and results, with little replication across studies. Clinical studies rarely are abnormal; even when abnormal, the findings are nonspecific. Consequently, more recent studies have attempted to measure the size of different brain regions. These studies have shown differences between disabled and nondisabled readers in hemispheric asymmetries, the corpus callosum, the temporal lobes, and the planum temporale. However, these differences are inconsistent and, as Filipek (1995, p. 567) concluded, "[N]o consistent morphologic correlates have been associated with developmental dyslexia in children and adults using *in vivo* imaging techniques." Filipek (1995, p. 567) noted the small sample sizes and variability in how well the subjects are described, observing, "Given the large variability in normal human neuroanatomy, larger homogeneous subject and control groups are needed." In contrast to this need is the amount of time required for precise morphological measurements from MRI and the numerous factors involved in MRI acquisition that influence measurements. This area has promise and likely will be enhanced by methods for more rapid acquisition and continued refinement of software and related methods essential for MRI morphometry.

Functional Neuroimaging Studies

Rumsey (1996) and Shaywitz et al. (1996) reviewed the functional neuroimaging studies. These studies largely analyze adults and are based on methods for measuring regional cerebral blood flow using xenon-inhalation techniques and brain metabolism using positron emission tomography. These studies produced a variety of findings implicating multiple cognitive processes and multiple areas of the brain, leading Rumsey (1996, p. 72) to hypothesize, "[S]evere, uncompensated dyslexia is associated with involvement of widely distributed neural circuits, affecting bilateral temporal and, possibly, other brain regions." At this point, although the temporal lobes are implicated, the results of these studies are discrepant, reflecting in part variations in samples and methods.

The foregoing studies are based on adults because of the risk of exposure of children to low levels of radiation. Hence, there is great interest in the development of functional magnetic resonance imaging (fMRI) methods because these paradigms are noninvasive, do not involve radiation, and can be used with children. A recent study (Eden et al., 1996) evaluated visual processing hypotheses using fMRI methods to evaluate brain metabolism is response to a motion sensitivity task. The subjects were six adults with reading disability and eight controls. Results revealed little activation within portions of the magnocellular visual system in response to the perception of subtle changes in motion. The authors concluded that the visual system abnormalities may be a marker for a deficiency in temporal processing that "may manifest itself as disorders of phonological awareness, rapid naming, rapid visual processing, or motion detection" (Eden et al., 1996, p. 69). Such hypotheses attest to the importance of relating results of all studies of dyslexia to the core deficit in decoding single words and phonological processing. Also entirely possible is that dyslexia is associated with a variety of cognitive and neurobiological phenomena that have little to do with the reading problem but have implications for the neurobiology of dyslexia and intervention.

Shaywitz et al. (1996) summarized fMRI studies on the basis of series of tasks that reliably activate different brain areas during reading. In addition to demonstrating gender differences in the activation of specific brain areas for phonological processing, the results suggest more frontal activations for phonological tasks and more temporal activations for semantic tasks. These developments will form the basis for a series of studies of adults and children with dyslexia.

Genetic Studies

Pennington (1995; see also chapter 13) reviewed the evidence for genetic factors in dyslexia. It has long been known that reading problems often are familial (Hallgren, 1950), with a risk in a child of a parent with dyslexia eight times higher than the general population (Pennington, 1995). Segregation studies indicate that dyslexia is genetically heterogeneous and reflect the operation of autosomal dominant transmission. Multiple genes likely are involved, with similar modes of transmission in dyslexic and nondyslexic families. Hence, the genetic basis for dyslexia represents susceptibility for a set of quantitative traits that interact with the environment in producing variations in reading skills. Linkage studies recently implicated a marker on chromosome 6 (Cardon et al., 1994), with additional evidence suggesting markers on chromosome 15 (see chapter 13). As Pennington (1995) noted, genetic studies represent an area that is developing rapidly and eventually may have significant implications for early intervention and prevention.

CONCLUSIONS: TOWARD A COMPREHENSIVE UNDERSTANDING OF DYSLEXIA

At this point, clearly the quality of research on dyslexia has improved over the last decade. In particular, major progress has been made in definition and sampling, along with the measurement of dependent variables. Strong hypotheses, particularly those relating language and reading skills, have been developed and tested, with robust findings. Defining samples with good specifications of phenotype has been critical in the identification of potential genetic variables that account for dyslexia, conceptualized as a core deficit in word decoding (Shaywitz, 1996). Although this conceptualization represents only one type of learning disability, this type is by far the largest subgroup, with most estimates suggesting that such cases involve both the majority of children with reading disability and children served in special education classes in the public schools (Lerner, 1989; Lyon, 1995b). Indeed, noteworthy is that attempts to subtype dyslexia on the basis of models of the relationship of word-recognition processes consistently identify one large subgroup, with little variability (Stanovich et al., 1997). In contrast, subtyping studies based on more general relationships of language and cognitive skills with reading identify more subtypes, largely because of variations in the relationship of rapid serial naming and verbal short-term memory with the core deficit in phonological processing (Fletcher et al., 1998). Such results clearly support the notion of dyslexia as a disorder of the language system with coherent variability around a phonological core (Shankweiler & Crain, 1986; Stanovich, 1988, 1991; Shaywitz, 1996).

The relationships of more general rate factors that influence automaticity and possible orthographical processing presently are not as well taken into account in children with dyslexia. Little evidence exists for subgroups impaired only in rate factors that have decoding difficulties, but clearly children with dyslexia experience problems in more than one aspect of the reading process. Even if they develop single-word decoding skills, many children may stumble in developing good text-reading skills because of basic problems automatizing these skills in a way that facilitates the reading of connected text. Such problems undoubtedly contribute to the comprehension problems observed in dyslexic children. However, as the structural equation studies show, decoding skills explain most of the variability in comprehension skills, and phonological-processing skills account for most of the variability in decoding skills in good and poor readers.

Other potential hypotheses involving dyslexia are somewhat limited because of problems at the level of definition and sampling and because of weak hypothesis formulation. At this point, any emerging theory attempting to explain dyslexia as defined in this chapter must account for the core deficit. In other words, any proposed deficiencies must account for the relationship of phonological processing and decoding in dyslexia. This is clearly the major weakness of the visual-processing hypotheses. Certainly possible is that the visual processes identified may be related to the rate and automaticity factors but do not appear to have a strong relationship with single-word decoding skills. Whether more general factors involving rate of temporal processing underlie the problems with phonological processing and decoding presently is nothing more than speculation. It is hoped that well-designed studies will provide rigorous tests of this hypothesis. What is important is not to study such variables in isolation of phonological processing. The history of dyslexia research shows that most studies find dyslexics to perform more poorly than do normal readers on many dependent variables. The issues are what aspects of dyslexia are explained, particularly in relationship to the core deficit, and the size of the group difference. Small to moderate effect sizes may be of limited use given the large effect sizes observed in the language domain.

This chapter has focused primarily on variables in the cognitive and biological domain. Clearly, such studies are only part of the picture. Most exclusionary definitions suggest that children who are socially deprived, victims of poor instruction, or have emotional problems should be excluded from definitions of dyslexia. However, little present evidence maintains that the phenotype of reading disability is different in children who are inadequately instructed, socially deprived, or emotionally disturbed relative to traditionally defined dyslexia. In addition, when children with brain injury have reading difficulties, the correlates appear to be similar (Fletcher et al., 1995; Barnes & Dennis, 1996). What is important to note is that definitions based on decoding skills and relationships of decoding skills and cognitive abilities do not establish causal relationships. Biological factors certainly are one cause of dyslexia, but other factors may lead to reading disabilities and are deserving of explanation, particularly as intervention studies emerge.

Figure 12.2 provides an assessment model useful for conceptualizing the relationship of the disability with cognitive and social factors, along with biological and environmental causes. In this figure, a particular outcome is identified as the manifest disability, which in children with dyslexia would represent the problems in decoding single words. Cognitive and social factors clearly are indicated as factors that interact to produce this disability. The cognitive factors are well-known; the social factors have been studied inadequately. These factors could involve inadequate instruction, poor self-esteem, and related factors that are undoubtedly important for outcome. The assessment model also identifies both biological and environmental causes of

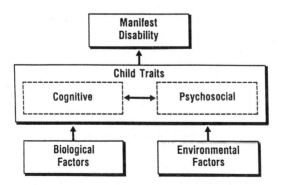

Figure 12.2 Measurement model underlying a comprehensive understanding of dyslexia.

these relationships between the manifest disability and child traits. Again, little research has been done on relationships of environmental causes.

These relationships will not be sorted out just by studying relationships of the manifest disability and the child's traits. Important for future investigations is to begin to flesh out the right side of this model. Such studies may have important implications for intervention studies, but also may be necessary to identify separately the various factors that influence the manifest disability. It is certainly convenient to conceptualize dyslexia as a biologically determined outcome, but in fact little evidence suggests specificity of the phenotype to a set of biological variables. In fact, multiple factors appear to produce similar outcomes at a phenotypic level. At this point, the important consideration is beginning to separate variability at the level of phenotype and relating this variability to both biological and environmental factors. Such an approach would provide a more comprehensive theory of reading disability and would help to move the field toward the ultimate outcome, which is the ability to intervene with poor readers.

ACKNOWLEDGMENTS

This study was supported in part by National Institute of Child Health and Human Development grants HD21888, HD25802, HD28172, and HD30995. Rita Taylor's assistance with manuscript preparation is gratefully acknowledged.

REFERENCES

Ackerman, P. T., Dykman, R., & Oglesby, D. M. (1994). EEG power spectra of children with dyslexia, slow learning, and normally reading children with ADHD during verbal processing. *Journal of Learning Disabilities, 10,* 619–630.

Adams, M. J. (1990). *Beginning to read.* Cambridge, MA: MIT Press.

Adams, M. J., & Bruck, M. (1993). Word recognition: The interface of education policies and scientific research. *Reading and Writing: An Interdisciplinary Journal, 5,* 113–139.

Angoff, W. M. (1971). Scales, norms, and equivalent scores. In R. L. Thorndike (Ed.), *Educational measurements* (2nd ed., pp. 508–600). Washington, DC: American Journal on Education.

Barnes, M. A., & Dennis, M. (1996). Reading comprehension deficits arise from diverse sources: Evidence from readers with and without developmental brain pathology. In C. Cornoldi & J. Oakhill (Eds.), *Reading comprehension difficulties: Processes and intervention.* Hillsdale, NJ: Erlbaum.

Benton, A. L. (1975). Developmental dyslexia: Neurological aspects. *Advances in Neurology, 7,* 2–5.

Bishop, D. V. M. (1989). Unstable vergence control and dyslexia—a critique. *British Journal of Ophthalmology, 73,* 223–245.

Blaskey, P., Scheiman, M., Parisi, M., Ciner, E. B., Gallaway, M., & Selznick, R. (1990). The effectiveness of Irlen filters for improving reading performance: A pilot study. *Journal of Learning Disabilities, 10,* 604–612.

Bowers, P., Golden, J., Kennedy, A., & Young, A. (1994). Limits upon orthographic knowledge due to processes indexed by naming speed. In V. W. Berninger (Ed.), *The varieties of orthographic knowledge* (Vol. 1, pp. 173–218). Dordrecht, The Netherlands: Kluwer.

Bradley, L., & Bryant, P. (1983). Categorizing sounds and learning to read: A causal connection. *Nature, 301,* 419–421.

Brady, S. (1991). The role of working memory in reading disability. In S. A. Brady & D. P. Shankweiler (Eds.), *Phonological processes in literacy: A tribute to Isabelle Y. Liberman* (pp. 129–151). Hillsdale, NJ: Erlbaum.

Breitmeyer, B. G., & Ganz, L. (1976). Implications of sustained and transient channels for theories of visual pattern matching, saccadic suppression, and information processing. *Psychological Review, 83,* 1–36.

Bruck, M. (1992). Persistence of dyslexics' phonological awareness deficits. *Developmental Psychology, 28,* 874–886.

Cardon, L. R., Smith, S. D., Fulker, D. W., Kimberling, B. S., Pennington, B. F., & DeFries, J. C. (1994). Quantitative trait locus for reading disability on chromosome 6. *Science, 226,* 276–279.

Castles, A., & Coltheart, M. (1993). Varieties of developmental dyslexia. *Cognition, 47,* 149–180.

Coltheart, M. (1981). Disorders of reading and their implications for models of reading. *Visible Language, 15,* 245–286.

Critchley, M. (1970). *The dyslexic child.* Springfield, IL: Charles C Thomas.

Denckla, M. B., & Rudel, R. G. (1974). Rapid "automatized" naming (R.A.N.): Dyslexia differentiated from other learning disabilities. *Cortex, 14,* 471–479.

Doehring, D. G. (1978). The tangled web of behavioral research on developmental dyslexia. In A. L. Benton & D. Pearl (Eds.), *Dyslexia: An appraisal of current knowledge* (pp. 123–138). New York: Oxford University Press.

Dool, C. B., Stelmack, R. M., & Rourke, B. P. (1993). Event-related potentials in children with learning disabilities. *Journal of Clinical Child Psychology, 22,* 387–398.

Doris, J. (1993). Defining learning disabilities: A history of the search for consensus. In G. R. Lyon, D. B. Gray, J. F. Kavanagh, & N. A. Krasnegor (Eds.), *Better understanding learning disabilities* (pp. 97–116). Baltimore: Paul H. Brookes.

Eden, G. F., Stern, J. F., Wood, M. H., & Wood, F. B. (1995). Verbal and visual problems in dyslexia. *Journal of Learning Disabilities, 28,* 272–290.

Eden, G. F., Van Meter, J. W., Rumsey, J. M., Maisog, J. M., Woods, R. P., & Zeffiro, T. A. (1996). Abnormal processing of visual notion in dyslexia revealed by functional brain imaging. *Nature, 382,* 66–69.

Ellis, A. W. (1984). The cognitive neuropsychology of developmental (and acquired) dyslexia: A critical survey. *Cognitive Neuropsychology, 2,* 169–205.

Filipek, P. A. (1995). Neurobiological correlates of developmental dyslexia: How do dyslexic's brains differ from those of normal readers? *Journal of Child Neurology, 10,* S61–S68.

Fletcher, J. M. (1981). Linguistic factors in reading acquisition: Evidence for developmental changes. In F. J. Pirozzolo & M. D. Wittrock (Eds.), *Neuropsychological and cognitive processes in reading* (pp. 274–294). New York: Academic.

Fletcher, J. M. (1985). Memory for verbal and nonverbal stimuli in learning disability subgroups: Analysis by selective reminding. *Journal of Experimental Child Psychology, 40,* 244–259.

Fletcher, J. M. (1994). Afterword: Brain-behavior relationships in children. In S. H. Broman & J. Grafman (Eds.), *Atypical cognitive deficits in developmental disorders: Implications for brain function* (pp. 297–326). Hillsdale, NJ: Erlbaum.

Fletcher, J. M., Brookshire, B., Bohan, T. P., Brandt, M., & Davidson, K. (1995). Early hydrocephalus. In B. P. Rourke (Ed.), *Nonverbal learning disabilities: Manifestations in neurologic disease, disorder, and dysfunction* (pp. 206–238). New York: Guilford.

Fletcher, J. M., Francis, D. J., Shaywitz, S. E., Lyon, G. R., Foorman, B. R., Stuebing, K. K., & Shaywitz, B. A. (1998). Intelligence testing and the discrepancy model for children with learning disabilities. *Learning Disabilities Research and Practice, 13*, 186–203.

Fletcher, J. M., Francis, D. J., Stuebing, K. K., Shaywitz, B. A., Shaywitz, S. E., Shankweiler, D. P., Katz, L., & Morris, R. (1996). Conceptual and methodological issues in construct definition. In G. R. Lyon (Ed.), *Attention, memory, and executive functions* (pp. 17–42). Baltimore: Paul H. Brookes.

Fletcher, J. M., & Morris, R. D. (1986). Classification of disabled learners: Beyond exclusionary definitions. In S. Ceci (Ed.), *Handbook of cognitive, social, and neuropsychological aspects of learning disabilities* (Vol. 1, pp. 55–80). Hillsdale, NJ: Erlbaum.

Fletcher, J. M., Satz, P., & Scholes, R. J. (1981). Developmental changes in the linguistic performance correlates of reading disabilities. *Brain and Language, 13*, 78–90.

Fletcher, J. M., Shaywitz, S. E., Shankweiler, D. P., Katz, L., Liberman, I. Y., Fowler, A., Francis, D. J., Stuebing, K. K., & Shaywitz, B. A. (1994). Cognitive profiles of reading disability: Comparisons of discrepancy and low achievement definitions. *Journal of Educational Psychology, 85*, 1–18.

Fletcher, J. M., & Taylor, H. G. (1984). Neuropsychological approaches to children: Towards a developmental neuropsychology. *Journal of Clinical Neuropsychology, 6*, 39–56.

Foorman, B. R. (1994a). The relevance of a connectionistic model of reading for "The Great Debate." *Educational Psychology Review, 6*, 25–47.

Foorman, B. R. (1994b). Phonological and orthographic processing: Separate but equal? In V. W. Berninger (Ed.), *The varieties of orthographic knowledge: I. Theoretical and developmental issues* (pp. 319–355). Dordrecht, The Netherlands: Kluwer.

Foorman, B. R., Francis, D. J., Fletcher, J. M., Schatschneider, C. & Mehta, P. (1998). The role of instruction in learning to read: Preventing reading failure in at-risk children. *Journal of Educational Psychology, 90*, 37–55.

Foorman, B. R., Francis, D. J., Novy, D. M., & Liberman, D. (1991). How letter-sound instruction mediates progress in first-grade reading and spelling. *Journal of Educational Psychology, 83*, 459–469.

Francis, D. J., Shaywitz, S. E., Stuebing, K. K., Shaywitz, B. A., & Fletcher, J. M. (1996). Developmental lag versus deficit models of reading disability: A longitudinal, individual growth curves analysis. *Journal of Educational Psychology, 88*, 3–17.

Gaddes, W. H. (1976). Prevalence estimates and the need for the definition of learning disabilities. In R. M. Knights, & D. J. Bakker (Eds.), *The neuropsychology of learning disorders: Theoretical approaches* (pp. 3–24). Baltimore: University Park Press.

Galaburda, A. M. (1988). The pathogenesis of childhood dyslexia. In F. Plum (Ed.), *Language communication and the brain* (pp. 127–138). New York: Raven.

Galaburda, A. M. (1993). The planum temporal. *Archives of Neurology, 50*, 457.

Galaburda, A. M., & Livingstone, M. (1993). Evidence for a magnocellular defect in developmental dyslexia. *Annals of the New York Academy of Sciences, 682*, 70–82.

Gathercole, S. E., & Baddeley, A. D. (1990). Phonological memory deficits in language disordered children: Is there a causal connection? *Journal of Memory and Language, 29,* 336–360.

Hallgren, B. (1950). Specific dyslexia (congenital word-blindness): A clinical and genetic study. *Acta Psychiatrica et Neurologica Scandanavica Supplementum, 65,* 1–287.

Harter, M. R., Diering, S., & Wood, F. B. (1988). Separate brain potential characteristics in children with reading disability and attention deficit disorder: Relevance-independent effects. *Brain and Cognition, 7,* 54–86.

Hinschelwood, J. (1896). A case of dyslexia: A peculiar form of word blindness. *Lancet, 101,* 1451–1454.

Hooper, S. R., & Willis, W. G. (1989). *Learning disability subtyping: Neuropsychological foundations, conceptual models, and issues, in clinical differentiation.* New York: Springer.

Hughes, J. R. (1978). Electroencephalographic and neurophysiological studies in dyslexia. In A. L. Benton & D. Pearl (Eds.), *Dyslexia: An appraisal of current knowledge* (pp. 205–240). New York: Oxford.

Hynd, G. W., & Semrud-Clikeman, M. (1989). Dyslexia and brain morphology. *Psychological Bulletin, 106,* 477–482.

Iovino, I. (1995). *Interventions for visual perceptual deficits in reading disabled and ADHD children: Are they really effective?* Unpublished doctoral dissertation, University of Houston, TX.

Katz, R. B., & Shankweiler, D. P. (1985). Receptive naming and the detection of word retrieval deficits in the beginning reader. *Cortex, 21,* 617–625.

Lehmkuhle, S., Garzia, R. P., Turner, L., Hash, T., & Baro, J. A. (1993). A defective visual pathway in children with reading disability. *New England Journal of Medicine, 328,* 989–996.

Lerner, J. W. (1989). Educational interventions in learning disabilities. *Journal of the American Academy of Child and Adolescent Psychiatry, 28,* 326–331.

Liberman, I. Y. (1973). Segmentation of the spoken word. *Bulletin of the Orton Society, 23,* 65–77.

Liberman, I. Y., Shankweiler, D. P., Fischer, F. W., & Carter, B. (1974). Explicit syllable and phoneme segmentation in the young child. *Journal of Experimental Child Psychology, 26,* 201–212.

Liberman, I. Y., Shankweiler, D. P., & Liberman, A. M. (1989). The alphabetic principle and learning to read. In D. P. Shankweiler & I. Y. Liberman (Eds.), *Phonology and reading disability: Solving the reading puzzle* (pp. 1–33) (IARLD Monograph Series). Ann Arbor: University of Michigan Press.

Livingstone, M. S., Rosen, G. D., Drislane, F., & Galaburda, A. M. (1991). Physiological and anatomical evidence for a magnocelluar defect in developmental dyslexia. *Proceedings of the National Academy of Sciences of the United States of America, 88,* 7943–7947.

Lovegrove, W., Martin, F., & Slaghuis, W. (1986). A theoretical and experimental case for a visual deficit in specific reading disability. *Cognitive Neuropsychology, 3,* 225–267.

Lovegrove, W. J., & Williams, M. C. (1993). Visual temporal processing deficits in specific reading disability. In D. M. Williams, R. S. Kruk, & E. Corcos (Eds.), *Visual processes in reading and reading disabilities* (pp. 311–330). Hillsdale, NJ: Erlbaum.

Lovett, M. W., Borden, S., DeLuca, T., Laceerenza, L., Benson, N., & Branckstone, D. (1994). Treating the core deficits of developmental dyslexia: Evidence of transfer of learning after phonologically- and strategy-based reading training programs. *Developmental Psychology, 30,* 805–822.

Lyon, G. R. (1985). Educational validation of learning disability subtypes. In B. P. Rourke (Ed.), *Neuropsychology of learning disabilities: Essentials of subtype analysis* (pp. 228–256). New York: Guilford.

Lyon, G. R. (1995a). Toward a definition of dyslexic. *Annals of Dyslexia, 45,* 3–27.

Lyon, G. R. (1995b). Research in learning initiatives disabilities: Contributions from scientists supported by the National Institute of Child Health and Human Development. *Journal of Child Neurology, 10,* 5120–5126.

Manis, F. R., Seidenberg, M. S., Doli, L. M., McBride-Chang, C., & Peterson, A. (1996). On the basis of two subtypes of developmental dyslexia. *Cognition, 58,* 157–195.

Mattson, A. J., Sheer, D. E., & Fletcher, J. M. (1992). Electrophysiological evidence of lateralized disturbances in children with learning disabilities. *Journal of Clinical and Experimental Neuropsychology, 14,* 707–716.

McBride-Chang, C., & Manis, F. R. (1996). Structural invariance in the associations of naming speed, phonological awareness, and verbal reasoning in good and poor readers: A test of the double deficit hypothesis. *Reading and Writing: An Interdisciplinary Journal, 8,* 323–339.

Miles, J. E., & Stelmack, R. M. (1994). Learning disability subtypes and the effects of auditory and visual priming on visual event-related potentials to words. *Journal of Clinical and Experimental Neuropsychology, 16,* 43–64.

Morgan, W. P. (1896). A case of congenital word blindness. *British Medical Journal, 2,* 1378.

Morris, R. D. (1988). Classification of learning disabilities: Old problems and new approaches. *Journal of Consulting and Clinical Psychology, 56,* 789–794.

Murphy, L., & Pollatsek, A. (1994). Developmental dyslexia: Heterogeneity without discrete subgroups. *Annals of Dyslexia, 44,* 120–146.

O'Connor, P. D., Sofo, F., Kendall, L., & Olsen, G. (1990). Reading disabilities and the effects of colored filters. *Journal of Learning Disability, 10,* 591–603.

Olsen, R. K., & Fosberg, H. (1993). Disabled and normal readers' eye movement in reading and nonreading tasks. In D. M. Williams, R. S. Kruk, & E. Corcos (Eds.), *Visual processes in reading and reading disabilities* (pp. 377–392). Hillsdale, NJ: Erlbaum.

Olsen, R. K., Lkiegl, R., Davidson, B. J., & Foltz, G. (1985). Individual and developmental differences in reading disability. In G. E. MacKinnon & T. G. Waller (Eds.), *Reading research: Advances in theory and practice* (Vol. 4, pp. 1–64). New York: Academic.

Orton, S. T. (1925). "Word-blindness" in school children. *Archives of Neurology and Psychiatry, 14,* 581–615.

Parker, R. M. (1990). Power, control, and validity in research. *Journal of Learning Disabilities, 10,* 613–620.

Pennington, B. F. (1995). Genetics of learning disabilities. *Journal of Child Neurology, 10,* 569–577.

Pennington, B. F., Gilger, J. W., Olson, R. K., & DeFries, J. C. (1992). External validity of age versus IQ discrepant definitions of reading disability: Lessons from a twin study. *Journal of Learning Disabilities, 25,* 639–654.

Rayner, K., Sereno, S. C., Lesch, M. F., & Pollatsek, A. (1995). Phonological codes are automatically activated during reading: Evidence for an eye movement priming paradigm. *Psychological Science, 6,* 26–31.

Reynolds, C. R. (1984). Critical measurement issues in learning disabilities. *Journal of Special Education, 18,* 451–476.

Robinson, G. L. W., & Conway, R. N. F. (1990). The effects of Irlen colored lenses on students specific reading skills and their perception of ability: A 12-month validity study. *Journal of Learning Disabilities, 10,* 588–596.

Rourke, B. P. (1975). Brain-behavior relationships in children with learning disabilities: A research programme. *American Psychologist, 30,* 911–920.

Rourke, B. P. (Ed.). (1985). *Neuropsychology of learning disabilities: Advances in subtype analysis.* New York: Guilford.

Rumsey, J. M. (1996). Neuroimaging in developmental dyslexia: A review and conceptualization. In G. R. Lyon & J. M. Rumsey (Eds.), *Neuroimaging* (pp. 57–78). Baltimore: Paul H. Brookes.

Rutter, M. (1978). Prevalence and types of dyslexia. In A. L. Benton & D. Pearl (Eds.), *Dyslexia: An appraisal of current knowledge* (pp. 3–28). New York: Oxford.

Rutter, M. (1989). Isle of Wight revisited: Twenty-five years of child psychiatric epidemiology. *Journal of the American Academy of Child and Adolescent Psychiatry, 29,* 633–653.

Rutter, M., & Yule, W. (1975). The concept of specific reading retardation. *Journal of Child Psychology and Psychiatry, 16,* 181–197.

Satz, P., & Fletcher, J. (1980). Minimal brain dysfunctions: An appraisal of research concepts and methods. In H. E. Rie & E. D. Rie (Eds.), *Handbook of minimal brain dysfunctions: A critical view* (pp. 669–714). New York: Wiley.

Satz, P., & Morris, R. (1981). Learning disability subtypes: A review. In F. J. Pirozzolo & M. C. Wittrock (Eds.), *Neuropsychological and cognitive processes in reading* (pp. 109–141). New York: Academic.

Satz, P., & van Nostrand, G. (1973). Developmental dyslexia: An evaluation of a theory. In P. Satz & J. Ross (Eds.), *The disabled learner: Early detection and intervention* (pp. 121–148). Rotterdam: Rotterdam University Press.

Seymour, P. H. K., & Evans, H. M. (1993). The visual (orthographic) processor and developmental dyslexia. In D. M. Willows, R. S. Kruk, & E. Corcos (Eds.), *Visual processes in reading and reading disabilities* (pp. 347–366). Hillsdale, NJ: Erlbaum.

Shankweiler, D. P., & Crain, S. (1986). Language mechanisms and reading disorder: A modular approach. *Cognition, 24,* 139–168.

Shankweiler, D. P., Crain, S., Katz, L., Fowler, A., Liberman, A., Brady, S., Thornton, R., Lundquist, E., Dreyer, L., Fletcher, J., Stuebing, K., Shaywitz, S., & Shaywitz, B. (1995). Cognitive profiles of reading-disabled children: Comparison of language skills in phonology, morphology, and syntax. *Psychological Science, 6,* 149–156.

Shankweiler, D. P., Liberman, I. Y., Mark, L. S., Fowler, C. A., & Fisher, F. (1979). The speech code and learning to read. *Journal of Experimental Psychology: Human Learning and Memory, 5,* 531–545.

Shaywitz, B., Fletcher, J., Holahan, J., & Shaywitz, S. (1992). Discrepancy compared to low achievement definitions of reading disability: Results from the Connecticut Longitudinal Study. *Journal of Learning Disabilities, 25,* 639–648.

Shaywitz, B. A., Fletcher, J. M., Holahan, J. M., Sadler, A., Marchione, K., Francis, D. J., Stuebing, K. K., Shankweiler, D. P., Katz, L., Liberman, I. Y., & Shaywitz, S. E. (1995). Cognitive profiles of reading disability: Interrelationships between reading disability and attention deficit-hyperactivity disorder. *Child Neuropsychology, 1,* 170–186.

Shaywitz, B. A., & Shaywitz, S. E. (1994). Learning disabilities and attention disorders. In K. Swaiman (Ed.), *Principles of pediatric neurology* (pp. 1119–1151). St. Louis: Mosby.

Shaywitz, S. E. (1996). Dyslexia. *Scientific American, 275,* 98–105.

Shaywitz, S. E., Escobar, M. D., Shaywitz, B. A., & Fletcher, J. M., & Makuch, R. (1992). Distribution and temporal stability of dyslexia in an epidemiological sample of 414 children followed longitudinally. *New England Journal of Medicine, 326,* 145–150.

Shaywitz, S. E., Shaywitz, B. A., Pugh, K. R., Skudlarski, P., Fulbright, R. K., Constable, R. T., Bronen, R. A., Fletcher, J. M., Liberman, A. M., Shankweiler, D. P., Katz, L., Lacadie, C., Marchoine, K. E., & Gore, J. C. (1996). The neurobiology of developmental dyslexia viewed through the lens of functional magnetic resonance imaging technology. In G. R. Lyon & J. M. Rumsey (Eds.), *Neuroimaging* (pp. 79–94). Baltimore: Paul H. Brookes.

Siegel, L. S. (1992). Dyslexic vs. poor readers: Is there a difference? *Journal of Learning Disabilities, 25,* 618–629.

Siegel, L. S., & Heaven, R. K. (1986). Categorization of learning disabilities. In S. S. Ceci (Ed.), *Handbook of cognitive, sound, and neuropsychological aspects of learning disabilities* (Vol. 1, pp. 95–121). Hillsdale, NJ: Erlbaum.

Siegel, L. S., Share, D., & Geva, E. (1995). Evidence for superior orthographic skills in dyslexics. *Psychological Science, 6,* 250–254.

Solan, H. A. (1990). An appraisal of the Irlen technique of correcting reading disorders using tinted overlays and tinted lenses. *Journal of Learning Disabilities, 10,* 621–623.

Stanovich, K. E. (1988). Explaining the differences between the dyslexic and the garden-variety poor reader: The phonological core variable difference model. *Journal of Learning Disabilities, 21,* 590–604.

Stanovich, K. E. (1991). Discrepancy definitions of reading disability: Has intelligence led us astray? *Reading Research Quarterly, 26,* 1–29.

Stanovich, K. E., & Siegel, L. S. (1994). Phenotypic performance profiles of children with reading disabilities: A regression-based test of the phonological-core variable difference model. *Journal of Educational Psychology, 86,* 24–53.

Stanovich, K. E., Siegel, L. S., & Gottardo, A. (1997). Converging evidence for phonological and surface subtypes of reading disability. *Journal of Education Psychology, 89,* 114–128.

Stein, J. F. (1993). Visuospatial perception in disabled readers. In D. M. Willows, R. S. Kruk, & E. Corcos (Eds.), *Visual processes in reading and reading disabilities* (pp. 331–346). Hillsdale, NJ: Erlbaum.

Stein, J. F., & Fowler, M. S. (1982). Diagnosis of dyslexia by means of a new indicator of eye dominance. *British Journal of Ophthalmology, 66,* 332–336.

Torgesen, J. K. (1996). A model of memory from an information processing perspective: The special case of phonological memory. In G. R. Lyon (Ed.), *Attention, memory, and executive function: Issues in conceptualization and measurement* (pp. 157–184). Baltimore: Paul H. Brookes.

Van der Wissell, A., & Zegers, F. E. (1985). Reading retardation revisited. *British Journal of Developmental Psychology, 3,* 3–9.

Vellutino, F. R. (1979). *Dyslexia: Theory and research.* Cambridge, MA: MIT Press.

Vellutino, F. R. (1987). Dyslexia. *Scientific American, 256,* 34–41.

Vellutino, F. R. (1991). Introduction to three studies on reading acquisition: Convergent findings on theoretical foundation of code-oriented versus whole language approaches to reading instruction. *Journal of Educational Psychology, 83,* 437–443.

Vellutino, F. R., Scanlon, D. M., & Tanzman, M. S. (1988). Lexical memory in poor and normal readers: Developmental differences in the use of category cues. *Canadian Journal of Psychology, 42,* 216–241.

Wagner, R. K., & Barker, T. A. (1994). The development of orthographic processing ability. In V. W. Berninger (Ed.), *The varieties of orthographic knowledge: I. Theoretical and developmental issues* (pp. 243–276). Dordrect, The Netherlands: Kluwer.

Wagner, R. K., & Torgesen, J. K. (1987). The nature of phonological processing and its causal role in the acquisition of reading skills. *Psychological Bulletin, 101,* 192–212.

Wagner, R. K., Torgesen, J. K., & Rachotte, C. A. (1994). Development of reading-related phonological processing abilities: New evidence of bidirectional causality from a latent variable longitudinal study. *Developmental Psychology, 30,* 73–78.

Williams, M. C., Littell, R. R., Reinoso, C., & Greve, K. (1994). Effect of wavelength on the performance of attention-disorder and normal children on the Wisconsin Card Sorting Test. *Neuropsychology, 8,* 187–193.

Willows, D. M., Kruk, R. S., & Corcos, E. (1993). Are there differences between disabled and normal readers in their processing of visual information? In D. M. Willows, R. S. Kruk, & E. Corcos (Eds.), *Visual processes in reading and reading disabilities* (pp. 265–287). Hillsdale, NJ: Erlbaum.

Willows, M. C., & LeCluyse, K. (1990). Perceptual consequences of a temporal processing deficit in reading disabled children. *Journal of the American Optometric Association, 61,* 111–121.

Willows, M. C., LeCluyse, K., & Rock-Faucheux, A. (1992). Effective intervention for reading disability. *Journal of the American Optometric Association, 63,* 411–417.

Wolf, M., Bally, H., & Morris, R. (1986). Automaticity, retrieval processes, and reading. A longitudinal study in average and impaired readers. *Child Development, 57,* 988–1000.

Wolf, M., Pfeil, C., Lotz, R., & Biddle, K. (1994). Towards a more universal understanding of the developmental dyslexias: The contribution of orthographic factors. In V. W. Berninger, *The varietes of orthographic knowledge* (Vol. 1, pp. 137–171). Dordrecht, The Netherlands: Kluwer.

Wolff, P. H. (1993). Impaired temporal resolution in developmental dyslexia. *Annals of the New York Academy of Sciences, 683,* 87–103.

Wolff, P. H., & Melngailis, I. (1996). Reversing letters and reading transformed text in dyslexia: A reassessment. *Reading and writing: An interdisciplinary journal, 8,* 317–355.

Zigler, E., & Hodapp, R. M. (1986). *Understanding mental retardation.* New York: Cambridge Univeristy Press.

13 Dyslexia as a Neurodevelopmental Disorder

Bruce F. Pennington

When I first entered training in clinical psychology nearly 25 years ago, some psychoanalytically trained supervisors encouraged their students to open a first session with a new patient, even a child, with the daunting question, "What brings you here?" This chapter attempts to address what an answer would look like for a child with reading disability, given our current state of knowledge.

The goals of this chapter are twofold: The first is to apply a fairly standard framework by which to review what is known about developmental dyslexia or reading disability. The second is to turn back on the framework itself and consider how our emerging understanding of dyslexia may challenge some of the implicit assumptions in this framework.

In this chapter, the framework is explained and applied to dyslexia. Then the limitations of the framework are examined as a way to draw out more general lessons for understanding neurodevelopmental disorders.

FRAMEWORK

In several publications (Pennington, 1991b; Pennington & Ozonoff, 1991; Pennington & Welsh, 1995), this author has developed a theoretical framework for analyzing developmental psychopathologies and has applied it to several disorders, including dyslexia, autism, attention deficit hyperactivity disorder (ADHD), and schizophrenia. Within this framework are four levels of analysis: etiology, brain mechanisms, neuropsychological mechanisms, and symptoms. The framework also specifies possible causal relations between levels of analysis. It divides symptoms into primary, secondary, correlated, and artifactual; each type of symptom is defined by different causal relations to underlying mechanisms at the three other levels of analysis.

A similar framework has been developed independently by Morton and Frith (1995) and has also been applied to dyslexia, autism, and ADHD. Within their model are three levels of analysis—biological, cognitive, and behavioral—so their biological level includes both etiology and brain mechanisms. Their last two levels of analysis are similar to the last two levels in the Pennington framework; however, the processes included in my neuropsychological level are broader than those included in Morton and Frith's cognitive level (1995). Their model likewise distinguishes different kinds of symptoms and considers possible causal relations between levels of analysis. An important function of their framework is to provide a theory-neutral, easily understood notation for diagramming theories and comparing them. Thus, although their framework is applied mainly to disorders whose cause appears to be biological, the framework can diagram theories in which the cause is completely nonbiological (i.e., due to the social environment). The same is true for my framework.

In each of our frameworks, and in our empirical work (largely because we are all cognitive developmentalists), our focus has been on disorders in which there appears to be a unitary, specific, underlying cognitive deficit. A working assumption that we all share is that an underlying cognitive deficit (or deficits) is the proximal cause of the pattern of symptoms observed in a given developmental psychopathology. In other words, we assume that the effects of biology on observable behavior (symptoms) often are mediated by underlying cognitive processes. In their account, Morton and Frith (1995) allow for a direct (i.e., not mediated by cognition) effect of brain mechanisms, and they give as examples of two motor symptoms—tics in Tourette syndrome and tremor in Parkinson disease. Of course, this implies that motor function is noncognitive. In the Pennington model, any observed behavior is mediated neuropsychologically. We also generally assume that whereas heterogeneity is likely in both etiologies and even brain mechanisms in a given disorder, homogeneity will be found at the cognitive level in disorders such as dyslexia and autism. Hence, the specific, underlying cognitive deficit in a given disorder will provide a powerful, parsimonious explanation of at least the core or primary signs and symptoms of the disorder, if not the correlated and secondary ones as well. Therefore, we give the cognitive level of analysis priority in a unified explanation of a disorder.

We also largely assume that the causal arrows are unidirectional; however, our frameworks are not restricted to depicting unidirectional causation. A sharply contrasting model used by many contemporary developmental psychopathologists is a transactional model in which the causal arrows are bidirectional (Sameroff & Chandler, 1975; Lewis, 1990). Both this and the previously discussed frameworks allow for transactions, but we doubt that a transactional model is the correct one for the disorders on which we have focused, such as dyslexia and autism.

Whether it is the right model for other developmental psychopathologies, such as childhood depression, is an interesting question. We have critiqued the adequacy of the transactional model as a comprehensive account of the etiology of developmental psychopathologies, using the perspective of behavior genetics (Pennington & Bennetto, 1993). Our main points were that a transaction is formally the same as what a behavior geneticist calls a *genotype-environment* (G-E) *correlation*. Quantitative genetic theory establishes that G-E correlations can account for, at most, half the variance in a given trait and that substantial main effects of both genotype and environment are needed for there to be G-E correlation. Hence, we argued that transactions cannot be the sole or even main causal mechanism in developmental psychopathologies.

Three important differences characterize our framework and that of Morton and Frith (1995). First, Morton and Frith (1995) use separate frameworks to model abnormal and normal development; we use the same framework for both. Second, they draw a sharp distinction between specific and general cognitive processes and disorders. A specific cognitive process is domain-specific, such as the phonological processes that are specific to speech or the visual recognition processes that are specific to faces. In Fodor's (1983) terminology, specific cognitive processes are "vertical faculties," whereas general cognitive processes, which operate across domains, are "horizontal faculties." Examples of general cognitive processes include aspects of memory and executive functions. Morton and Frith (1995, p. 5) maintain that features of a disorder "that can be accounted for as part of a general condition need not be accounted for within the causal theory for the specific condition." Of greatest interest for them is a specific disorder that occurs in a "pure form," without any other specific or general cognitive deficits. In contrast, because we assume interdependence among all cognitive processes, we doubt that there can be such a sharp separation between specific and general cognitive processes and, in any case, some theoretical account is needed of their relation. As will be discussed later, this author also has reservations about the concept of a "pure form" of a disorder and believes that some apparently specific disorders, such as autism, may be caused by a deficit in general cognitive processes. The third related difference concerns how modular the cognitive mechanisms are; this too will be discussed later in the chapter.

FRAMEWORK APPLIED TO DYSLEXIA

In this section, we review what is known about dyslexia at each of the four levels of analysis contained in the Pennington framework just discussed: (1) etiology, (2) brain mechanisms, (3) cognitive mechanisms, and (4) symptoms.

Etiology

In the last two decades, our understanding of the etiology of dyslexia has increased considerably due to advances in both behavioral and molecular genetics. For 50 years after dyslexia was first described by Kerr (1897) and Morgan (1896), evidence for recurrence in families was repeatedly documented in case reports, leading Hallgren (1950) to undertake a more formal genetic epidemiological study of a large sample of families. Besides conducting the first test of the mode of transmission, Hallgren's comprehensive monograph also documented several characteristics of dyslexia that have recently been rediscovered: The gender (male-female) ratio is nearly equal, being approximately 1.5 : 1 (Shaywitz et al., 1990; Wadsworth et al., 1992), and no significant association exists between dyslexia and non-right-handedness (Pennington et al. 1987). Hallgren (1950) also documented that dyslexia co-occurs with other language disorders; however, the degree and basis of this comorbidity has not yet been determined satisfactorily.

Although Hallgren and his predecessors provided considerable evidence that dyslexia is familial, modern twin studies ultimately demonstrated that this familial trait is substantially genetic and modern linkage studies have aided us in actually beginning to locate the genes involved. Unlike the situation in Hallgren's time, we now have very strong, converging evidence that dyslexia is both familial and heritable (see Pennington, 1994, for a review). We can also reject the hypotheses of classic, X-linked or simple recessive autosomal transmission, at least in the vast majority of cases. In addition, we have evidence that dyslexia is genetically heterogeneous (Smith et al., 1990). Perhaps most importantly, we have evidence that supports Hallgren's observation that what appears to be autosomal dominant transmission occurs in many dyslexic families. Hence, effects of major loci do appear to be acting in a dominant or additive fashion on the transmission of reading problems.

However, we can place several important constraints on Hallgren's hypothesis of a monohybrid, autosomal dominant gene influencing dyslexia. First, it is unlikely to be one gene because of the evidence for genetic heterogeneity. Second, it may not be a gene influencing dyslexia per se, as the familial nature of, heritability of, and transmission results for normal variations in reading skill are not clearly distinct from those for dyslexia (Gilger et al. 1994). If valid, the finding of a major locus effect on the transmission of normal reading skill, which acts to depress reading scores, suggests that the same loci may be involved in the transmission of both normal reading skill and dyslexia. Assuming that this were true, then dyslexics would have just more of the unfavorable alleles at these loci or more environmental risk factors, such that their reading scores would be pushed beyond the cutoff for dyslexia. In this case, the locus (or loci) is not necessarily a "disease" locus but is instead better conceptualized as a susceptibility locus. A susceptibility locus, unlike a disease locus, is neither necessary nor sufficient to produce the disorder in question. If a susceptibility locus influences a continuous (as opposed to categorical) trait, then it is called a *quantitative trait locus* (QTL). Complex behavioral traits are more likely to be influenced by several QTLs than by a single Mendelian locus.

Therefore, instead of a classic, autosomal dominant "disease" gene, which is rare in the population and which is, by itself, necessary and sufficient to produce the disorder of dyslexia, we may be dealing with several, more frequent QTLs that are involved in the transmission of both dyslexia and normal variations in reading skill. No one QTL is likely to be necessary to produce dyslexia. Whether one QTL has an effect sufficient to produce dyslexia is an open, empirical question that only linkage methods can answer.

Table 13.1 Multifactorial versus major locus transmission of normal and abnormal reading

	Major locus for normal	No major locus for normal
Major locus for abnormal	Quantitative trait loci	"Disease" locus
No major locus for abnormal	Reading disability environmental, polygenic	Reading disability not discrete

The concept of QTLs raises the question of whether dyslexia is a discrete disorder with a distinct etiology. Table 13.1 presents some of the possible answers: Most researchers have focused on the two possibilities in the right column; either there is a disease allele for dyslexia, or both dyslexia and normal variation in reading are multifactorial, with no major locus effects on either. In contrast, the answer that best fits the results reviewed here is an unexpected one—namely, that there are major locus effects on both normal variation and dyslexia. If these major loci are the same, then we would say that the etiology of dyslexia is not distinct from that of normal variation but, contrary to what might be expected, that both are due to a small number of discrete factors. Dyslexics would be distinct from normal readers only in their distribution of alleles and environmental risk factors (both biological and experimental), not in possessing a single necessary disease allele or a single necessary pathogenetic, environmental risk factor.

Nonetheless, if one (or more) of these alleles at different QTLs has a sizable effect and is moderately frequent in the population overall, then it will be more frequent among dyslexic individuals who have extreme reading scores. The concentration of deleterious alleles in a subset of the population would change the proportion of the phenotypic variance across the entire population that is due to genes (i.e., heritability, or h^2), resulting in higher observed heritabilities. DeFries and colleagues (Alarcon & DeFries, 1995; DeFries et al., 1997), in the Colorado Learning Disability Research Center twin sample, tested this possibility using multiple regression methods. They found that the h^2 for individual differences in reading was 0.82 in the dyslexic twin sample but 0.53 in the control twin sample, a difference that was significant when nonsignificant common environment terms were dropped from the model.

In summary, several hypotheses about the transmission of dyslexia can be rejected on the basis of available data reviewed in Pennington (1994): First, dyslexia is not an X-linked disorder, and little evidence of parental gender effects on transmission is available. There is converging evidence for gender differences in penetrance, which would produce the slight preponderance of male patients (male-female ratio, 1.5:1) that is observed. Second, simple polygenic or multifactorial transmission can be rejected because a major locus effect is seen in several samples. This major locus effect acts in an additive or dominant (but not in a recessive) fashion. Third, a monogenic hypothesis can be rejected because dyslexia is genetically heterogeneous.

Fourth, a necessary disease allele hypothesis can be rejected because evidence exists of a major locus effect on the transmission of normal variation in reading skill. A remaining hypothesis that fits the empirical data considered here is that a small number of QTLs underlie the transmission of both dyslexia and normal variations in reading skill.

Given the strong possibility that the major loci contributing to dyslexia are QTLs, and given the evidence for genetic heterogeneity, traditional linkage analysis (of large, extended, dyslexic families) is not the most appropriate method by which to identify these loci. Instead, a type of sibling-pair (sib-pair) linkage analysis is more appropriate. By selecting sibling pairs in which at least one sibling has an extreme score, one can perform linkage analyses that screen for genetic loci influencing extreme scores on a continuous measure (Fulker et al., 1991). We have used this and another sibling-pair linkage method (Smith et al., 1991) to begin to identify possible loci affecting dyslexia in the sibling pairs from the families in the linkage sample.

We have completed a replication test for the chromosome 6 results using new polymerase chain reaction markers in both the kindred and twin family reading study samples of sib pairs, analyzing the data with a new interval mapping technique (Cardon et al., 1994). Each sample gave significant evidence of a QTL located in a 2-centimorgan (2-cM) region of the interval between the D65105 and TNFB markers, which are situated in 6p21.332.

This finding recently was replicated by Grigorenko et al. (1997), who found a highly significant linkage between deficits in a phoneme awareness phenotype in dyslexic families and markers on essentially the same region of chromosome 6. They also found significant linkage in the same sample for a different phenotype, deficits in word recognition, and markers in the centromeric region of chromosome 15 initially linked to dyslexia by Smith et al. (1983). They argue for viewing these two phenotypes as separate components of reading, each with different genetic influences. Whether these are two separate reading phenotypes and whether the mapping between genes and component reading processes will be this precise is discussed in Pennington (1997).

These exciting findings eventually will allow us to address the degree of variance in reading scores for which these loci account and the frequency with which unaffected siblings have unfavorable alleles at these loci. If a similar sib-pair linkage study were conducted using probands selected for extremely high reading scores, we could determine whether different alleles at the same two loci influence exceptionally good reading. If so, we could conclude that the same QTLs are affecting reading scores across the entire distribution. If they are, then our speculation that the same genes are influencing normal and extreme individual differences in reading would be supported. If not, then we would have direct evidence that dyslexia is etiologically distinct. Once we have a better understanding of these genetic mechanisms, we also can conduct much more revealing studies of environmental factors, both risk factors and protective ones, which also undoubtedly operate in the transmission of both abnormal and normal reading skill. Most importantly, once these genes are identified clearly, we can begin to trace the dynamic, developmental pathway that runs from gene to brain to behavior.

Brain Mechanisms

Previous autopsy or magnetic resonance imaging (MRI) studies of brain structure in dyslexia have examined size differences in the planum temporale (Galaburda, 1988; Larsen et al., 1990; Hynd et al., 1991; Schultz et al., 1994), insula (Hynd et al., 1991), corpus callosum (Duara et al., 1991; Larsen et al., 1992; Hynd et al., 1995), and thalamus (Jernigan et al., 1991; Galaburda & Livingstone, 1993) although no finding for a given structure has been consistently replicated across studies. Moreover, the samples in these studies were small and usually highly selected, and both anatomical definitions and methods of image acquisition varied across studies (Filipek, 1995). One recent study (Schultz et al., 1994) found that group differences between dyslexics and controls were negligible, once one had accounted for gender, age, and IQ, although there are questions about the anatomical definitions used in that study (Filipek, 1995).

Of course, finding a brain difference in dyslexia in a cross-sectional study does not reveal the causal relation between the brain difference and dyslexia. The brain difference observed may merely be a correlate of the real brain cause of dyslexia or even a secondary effect of the behavioral phenotype itself, as it is known that environmental influences affect the size of brain structures. In a twin sample, we can go further and test competing causal models. Specifically, with large samples we can address the extent of genetic and environmental covariation between extreme brain and reading phenotypes. A null result for either genetic or environmental covariation would argue against that particular etiological pathway. However, a positive result, such as a finding of significant shared genetic influence on both a brain structure and dyslexia, still does not establish the causal relation between brain and dyslexia, again for the reasons just mentioned.

Using quantitative MRI analyses in a large sample of dyslexic and control twins, we have begun testing for differences in brain structure in dyslexia. Thus far, we have addressed whether there are genetic influences on size variations in brain structures.

A factor analysis of 14 structures composing the entire brain found two factors—a cortical and a subcortical factor—that accounted for 70.8% of the total variance. We examined genetic and environmental influences on these two factors by comparing intraclass correlations for monozygotic (MZ) ($N = 19$) pairs and dizygotic (DZ) ($N = 17$ pairs) pairs across the entire sample, both reading-disabled subjects (RD) and controls. If the MZ correlation is significant and significantly greater than the DZ correlation, then there is evidence for significant heritability, the magnitude of which can be roughly estimated by doubling the MZ − DZ difference [2(MZ − DZ)], with an upper bound being the value of the MZ correlation. The remaining variance $(1 - MZ)$ is unique to individuals and is explained by the combination of error and nonshared environmental influences (e^2). If the DZ correlation is significant, then the proportion of phenotypic variance accounted for by influences of the common or shared (shared by siblings in the same family) environment (c^2) is roughly estimated by the equation $2DZ - MZ$. The overall results were that we found significant h^2 for size variations in the subcortical factor but little evidence for shared environmental effects (c^2). The MZ correlation for the subcortical factor was .78 ($P < .001$), whereas the DZ correlation was essentially nil ($-.02$). The difference between these two correlations was significant (Fisher's $Z = 2.19$, $P < .05$), providing evidence of heritability. The estimates for h^2, bounded at 0.78, with 0.22 being the estimate for the combination of e^2 and error, and 0 being the estimate for c^2. In contrast, for the cortical factor, we found significant evidence for c^2 but not for h^2 at this point. The MZ correlation for the cortical factor was .80 ($P < .001$) and, for the DZ correlation, .61 ($P < .01$) yielding estimates of .42 for c^2, .20 for the combination of e^2 and error, and .38 for h^2, which is not significant with this sample size (Pennington et al., unpublished manuscript).

These results, if maintained in a larger sample, indicate different etiologies for individual differences in the size of cortex and subcortex. Subcortical structures, which develop earlier, appear to be more strongly genetically influenced, whereas the cortex, which develops later, appears to be under both genetic and environmental influences. Experience-dependent synaptogenesis, which varies across individuals, is known to be important in cortical development, whereas the environmental influence on subcortical structures may be mainly of the experience-expectant type, which varies little across individuals. Only environmental *differences* that cause individual *differences* will be detected in a behavioral genetic analysis.

These results are encouraging for the hypothesis that the brain mechanisms mediating the genetic influences on reading skill (which were discussed earlier) are structural, at least in part. To test this hypothesis further, we must determine whether brain structure differences in dyslexics differ from that of controls and whether genetic covariation exists between those structures and reading or reading-related skills (such as phoneme awareness). Positive results from both those additional tests would be consistent with the hypotheses that the QTLs discussed earlier alter brain structural development which, in turn, alters the development of reading skills.

The MRI results from earlier studies of dyslexia pose another potential difficulty for the framework. The brain changes observed are somewhat specific to reading but are distributed rather than localized. Either we need a computational account whereby distributed changes can lead to a fairly specific cognitive problem or we need to reconsider how specific the cognitive deficit in dyslexia really is.

Cognitive Mechanisms

Considerable evidence now supports the conclusion that the underlying cognitive deficit in dyslexia is in the phonological coding of written language and that this written language deficit is preceded and caused by a spoken language deficit in phoneme awareness and segmentation (Pennington, 1991a,b) Without exaggeration, one could say that this has become the standard or modal explanation of dyslexia at the cognitive level. Controversy arises around three issues:

1. Is the phonological skill that is impaired in dyslexia best described by a dual-process or a single-process account?

2. Can the deficit in phoneme awareness be reduced to a more fundamental deficit in either auditory or speech perception?

3. Are there visual processing deficits in addition to the well-documented phonological ones?

The third issue is beyond the scope of this chapter (but see chapter 12 for a critique of visual hypotheses of dyslexia); we briefly consider the first two issues here.

Following the standard dual-process account of both normal adult reading and of acquired dyslexias, at least two developmental analogs have been postulated: developmental phonological dyslexia and developmental surface dyslexia (Frith, 1985; Temple, 1985), due, respectively, to selective impairment in the phonological (or sublexical) and lexical routes for word pronunciation. Case studies have shown that relatively "pure" cases of developmental phonological dyslexia (Temple & Marshall, 1983) or developmental surface dyslexia (Coltheart et al., 1983) exist. However, the existence of pure cases does not prove the underlying theory, as the definition of a pure case involves a double circularity: First, different processing theories will identify different cases as "pure," so there is no theory-neutral way of defining pure cases. Second, the notion of a pure case itself presupposes some form of modularity (Van Orden et al., unpublished manuscript).

Moreover, among normally developing readers, particularly younger normal readers, Bryant and Impey (1986) have found many of the errors that supposedly are diagnostic of developmental surface dyslexia, casting doubt on its validity as a distinct developmental dyslexia syndrome. Hence, an epidemiological rather than a selective case study approach provides a better test of the separability of the hypothesized dual processes in normal and abnormal reading development.

Castles and Coltheart (1993) conducted such a study and found among 53 dyslexic children that 60% performed significantly below age level on both nonword and exception-word reading, whereas only approximately 20% were selectively impaired on either; hence, the pure subtypes are less frequent than the mixed subtype. Using a regression method, these investigators also found that impairment in nonword reading relative to exception-word reading was more common in their sample than was the reverse. Hence, this study indicates that, among developmental dyslexics, pure cases are rarer than mixed ones and the profile of phonological dyslexia is considerably more common than the profile of surface dyslexia. The predominance of mixed cases is problematic for dual-process theory. Because it postulates that the lexical and sublexical processes are separate, it must postulate separate alterations in the development of each in the predominant mixed type, whereas single-process models would find it easier to explain the predominance of the mixed type.

To address this and other issues, Manis et al. (1996) conducted a replication study and considered how one could account for the results from both studies by the connectionist framework developed by Seidenberg and McClelland (1989). In this framework, the development of visual word pronunciation is modeled by a three-layer neural network in which the input layer corresponds to graphemes, the output layer corresponds to phonemes, and the "hidden" or middle layer helps one to learn the complex, quasi-regular covariation between letters and sounds in English words. Through repeated training trials with feedback, the network gradually adjusts the weights on the connections between layers until it reaches near-optimal performance in generating the pronunciation of single printed words. Although the network does not contain any explicit pronunciation rules, it can generalize from its training corpus to new exemplars, including pronounceable nonwords. Because the correspondence between print and pronunciation in English is only quasi-regular, and the spelling of some words (e.g., *yacht*) is unlike that of any others, the network must strike a balance between encoding rulelike and word-specific information. If it goes too far in the rulelike direction, then it will mispronounce exception words on which it was trained: No network or human can pronounce exception words without training. On the other hand, if it goes too far in the word-specific direction, it will be unable to generalize and thus be poor at reading either new words or nonwords.

In their replication study, Manis et al. (1996) also found a similar predominance of the mixed subtype. In addition, like Bryant and Impey (1986), these investigators found that those subjects with a surface profile were similar to younger normal readers, whereas those with a phonological profile were not, suggesting that the former represents a general developmental delay in word recognition, whereas the latter represents a specific deficit in phonological processing. They argue that for the dual route to explain these two characteristics of the data, it must introduce additional assumptions, whereas the Seidenberg and McClelland (1989) model can explain these and other characteristics within a single-process model. Essentially, Seidenberg and McClelland explain the mixed and phonological types as arising from degraded phonological representations, which most often impair nonword reading, next most often impair exception-word reading, and least often impair regular-word reading. Depending on the degree of phonological degradation, either a mixed or more pure phonological subtype is observed. This is obviously a more parsimonious explanation than is provided by the dual-process account, which must explain impaired nonword and exception-word reading by dysfunction of separate processes rather than by degrees of dysfunction in the same underlying mechanism. To explain the rarer surface subtype and its similarity to younger normal readers, Seidenberg and McClelland (1989) postulate a different alteration in the model: A reduced number of hidden units. With fewer hidden units, the model can learn (albeit less efficiently) the rulelike regularities in the input (rendering it able to pronounce regular and nonwords) but lacks the resources to learn word-specific patterns (such as are found in exception words). This account explains not only why surface dyslexics are particularly bad at exception words but also why they rarely are completely normal with regular and nonwords; again, the single-process account is more parsimonious. In addition, because learning word-specific patterns requires more trials for even a normal network, the pattern of errors of this network should resemble that of a "younger" normal network, just as children with the surface profile resemble younger normal readers. (See also the reanalysis of these two studies by Stanovich et al. (1997), who found that the surface subtype disappeared when reading-level rather than chronological-level controls were used.)

This connectionist reinterpretation of subtypes of developmental dyslexia extends an earlier use of connectionist principles to critique the standard dual-process account of both mature reading and the acquired dyslexias (Seidenberg & McClelland, 1989; Van Orden et al., 1990, unpublished manuscript; Plaut, 1995; Plaut et al., 1996). One basic criticism mimics that discussed previously—namely, that single-process accounts exist that explain the relevant reading phenomena as well as do dual-process accounts, and the single-process accounts are preferable on the basis of parsimony. These accounts involve a connectionist or neural network mechanism that learns word pronunciation. Both frequency and regularity or consistency effects can be produced by the same mechanism, whereas each effect is due to separate processes in a dual-process account.

A second criticism is based on the empirical result that phonological mediation of mature reading is virtually ubiquitous and occurs very early in the time course of word recognition, neither of which is predicted by standard dual-process accounts, which holds that phonological mediation is optional and slow in mature word recognition. Perhaps most telling is the finding that virtually identical damage to a single interdependent network can, on different runs, produce an apparent double dissociation of the sort that has been taken as strong confirmation of the hypothesized dual processes (Plaut, 1995).

At a more general level, these connectionist results question the transparency of the mapping from the symptoms of dyslexia, whether acquired or developmental, to underlying processing mechanisms and hence their modularity and localizability. It is somewhat dismaying to relinquish these familiar theoretical notions and attempt to conceptualize dyslexia in terms of the dynamics of an interdependent network, but both recent neuroimaging and computational results are more consistent with the latter perspective.

Although attempts have been made to simulate developmental dyslexia in a connectionist network, thus far these have started with the task of learning to read. A realistic simulation needs to begin earlier in the developmental process, focusing initially on the development of phonological representations themselves and showing how a network can be altered in such a way that speech imitation is fairly normal but phoneme awareness is impaired. Then it needs to be shown that a network with immature phonological representations has trouble learning to read in the same ways as do individuals with dyslexia (which seems likely, given the arguments presented by Manis et al., 1996). In other words, we need a computational account of phonological development that will allow us to test the kinds of perturbations leading to the later developmental differences that characterize dyslexia and the kinds leading to other disturbances of speech and language development.

These considerations bring us to the second controversy mentioned earlier—namely, whether the deficit in phoneme awareness in dyslexia can be reduced to a more basic deficit in auditory or speech perception. This controversy has both a theoretical and an empirical aspect. On the theoretical side, the questions are whether there could be a deficit in phoneme awareness without a lower-level deficit in auditory or speech perception and identification of the developmental relations among the development of auditory perception, speech perception, and phoneme awareness. Suffice it to say that the answers to these questions are not well delineated in current theories. On the empirical side, the questions are whether the evidence for auditory or speech perception deficits in dyslexia meets the same stringent criteria that have established a deficit in phoneme awareness as the primary cognitive cause of dyslexia. Briefly, (1) very robust deficits in phoneme awareness exist in dyslexia samples, relative to both chronological-age and reading-age controls in cross-sectional studies; (2) deficits in phoneme awareness precede and predict later dyslexia; and (3) remediating phoneme awareness improves later reading outcome. Before we reduce the deficit in phoneme awareness to a deficit in either auditory or speech perception, we must have evidence that the replacement deficit meets these same empirical criteria and that it causes the phoneme awareness deficit in dyslexia.

We are completing a review of studies of auditory and speech perception in dyslexia (Markey et al., unpublished manuscript). Virtually all the studies are cross-sectional. The most important conclusion is that the evidence of deficits in dyslexia relative to reading-level controls in either auditory or speech perception is inconsistent. Therefore, at least at this point, the empirical criteria for reduction have not been met. Our review also considers how a deficit in phoneme awareness could arise without a more basic deficit in auditory or speech perception, using as a theoretical framework

Markey's (Markey, 1994; Markey et al., 1995) HABLAR model of speech development.

Logically, one can distinguish at least four competing hypotheses to account for reading deficits in dyslexia, some of which we can exclude using the evidence reviewed earlier. In the *learning deficit* hypothesis (similar to the connectionist account of surface dyslexia, explained earlier), dyslexics could have normal, segmental phonological representations and metalinguistic awareness of those representations (i.e., normal phoneme awareness) but have neural networks that learned the complex correspondence between graphemes and phonemes much more slowly, perhaps because of too few hidden units. However, the robust phoneme awareness deficit in dyslexia rejects this hypothesis. In the *metalinguistic* hypothesis, dyslexics would have normal underlying segmental phonological representations and normal learning resources but would lack metalinguistic awareness of the phonological representations; the representations would not be accessible to be mapped onto a new domain (printed letters). The existence of language deficits in future dyslexics before normal age of onset for phoneme awareness (Scarborough, 1990) threatens this hypothesis. In the *linguistic* or *segmental* hypothesis (Fowler, 1991; Walley, 1993), dyslexics have intact auditory perception but do not develop normal underlying phonological representations and therefore have problems with both phoneme awareness and learning the correspondence between graphemes and phonemes. The *segmental* hypothesis has been scarcely tested; that is an important task for future research. Finally, in the *auditory* hypothesis (discussed earlier), dyslexics have an impairment in nonspeech auditory perception that undermines the development of phonological representations.

In sum, considerable evidence supports a deficit in phoneme awareness as the cognitive cause of dyslexia. The proposal to reduce this deficit to a deficit in nonlingustic auditory perception is not strongly supported by current evidence. Whether this deficit in phoneme awareness can be reduced to a deficit in the development of underlying phonological representations (the linguistic or segmental hypothesis) remains to be tested. Theoretically, a deficit in phonological representations that is not caused by a more basic deficit in auditory perception appears possible, at least within one computational model of speech development. An important next task for computational modeling is simulation of the development of dyslexia beginning with the abnormal development of phonological representations. A more distant goal is to use the results from structural and functional neuroimaging studies of dyslexia to constrain these computational models.

Symptoms

As explained elsewhere (Pennington, 1991a), a primary underlying cognitive deficit in phoneme awareness or phoneme segmentation provides a good explanation for most of the constellation of symptoms found in dyslexia:

deficits in reading and spelling real and nonwords, visual and lexicalization errors in reading, dysphonetic errors in spelling, and problems in learning and retrieving rote verbal information. Of course, not all the causal links have been rigorously tested. In this section, we consider symptoms outside the linguistic domain, wherein the links between a phonological deficit and the symptom in question are less obvious. Specifically, we will focus on two psychosocial symptoms—ADHD and problems with self-esteem and mood—and one symptom in a very different domain—immune disorders. We hope to illustrate here the range of methods available for testing the causal relations between a developmental disorder and its symptoms.

Recently, we completed a series of studies that examined the psychosocial correlates of dyslexia across the life span (Boetsch et al., 1996; Boetsch & Pennington, unpublished manuscript), using both cross-sectional and longitudinal designs. The four cross-sectional studies examined the psychosocial functioning of children, adolescents, and adults with developmental dyslexia. One sample of nonreferred dyslexic and nondyslexic men and three different samples of dyslexic and normally achieving control children and adolescents were studied. The child samples included both clinic-referred and nonreferred populations and sibling and nonsibling control designs. Variables assessed included depressive and ADHD symptomatology, self-concept and, in the adult sample, socioeconomic status and other life adjustment variables.

We found that, across three samples, children and adolescents report lower global self-worth and lower perceived competence in scholastic domains, more depressive symptomatology, and (both by self-report and parental report) more ADHD symptomatology than do normal achievers. In contrast, adult dyslexic men, while also perceiving themselves as less intelligent than their peers, reporting more generalized psychological distress, and showing less social mobility, were nonetheless comparable to their peers in terms of global self-worth, depressive symptomatology, and other indices of adult adjustment and satisfaction. Results are discussed in terms of a developmental "niche-finding" model, in which the shift into adult life may foster more constructive experiences and internal processes.

The longitudinal study examined self-esteem and mood and ADHD symptoms in samples of children at high and low familial risk for dyslexia who were followed up for 3 years (from age 5 to 8), at which time the high-risk group was divided into those who were dyslexic and those who were not. There were too few low-risk dyslexia subjects to allow group comparisons. Fewer differences in self-esteem and mood were noted between high-risk children who became dyslexic and either high-risk or low-risk controls than were found in the cross-sectional studies, raising the possibility that these symptoms develop somewhat later in dyslexia (although differences in samples is a competing explanation). Moreover, the differences noted in self-esteem and mood arose only after the appearance of dyslexia symptoms, consistent with the hypothesis that dyslexia leads to secondary problems with self-esteem and mood.

In contrast, the pattern of results for symptoms of ADHD was strikingly different among the subjects. Both the high-risk dyslexics and the high-risk controls had significantly more ADHD symptoms than did low-risk controls, beginning at age 5 and at the three subsequent time points. This result is not consistent with there being a causal relation between dyslexia and ADHD in either direction; it indicates that having a dyslexic parent increases a child's risk for ADHD symptoms regardless of whether the child is dyslexic. One hypothesis that is consistent with these results is the cross-assortment hypothesis, which states that an individual with dyslexia is more likely to marry another individual with ADHD, leading to an increased risk for the occurrence of either or both disorders in the offspring. This hypothesis follows from the fact that there is substantial genetic influence on both dyslexia and ADHD. Hence, such marriages place the offspring at increased risk for both dyslexia and ADHD, without there necessarily being a common genetic etiology for dyslexia and ADHD.

Another set of methods for testing relations between a disorder and its symptoms (or comorbidities) includes behavioral genetic methods, particularly twin designs. In a series of studies, we have applied these to the observed comorbidity between dyslexia and ADHD.

Behavioral genetic methods provide a powerful means of testing hypotheses about the clinical basis of comorbidity. Comorbidity is just a specific case of phenotypic correlation. Bivariate extensions of the multiple regression models described earlier allow one to test for bivariate h^2 and bivariate h^2g (heritability of extreme scores at the tails of the distribution), which provide estimates of the degree to which a phenotypic correlation is due to shared genetic influences. A bivariate extension of the interval-mapping model described earlier provides a more direct test of shared genetic influence. In this project, we are using these and other methods to test hypotheses about the basis of comorbidities with reading disability.

Six competing hypotheses purport to explain the causal basis of the development of a comorbidity: (1) disorder A causes disorder B; (2) disorder B causes disorder A; (3) a third factor causes both disorders A and B in all cases (common etiology); (4) a third factor causes both disorders A and B in an etiological subtype, but the two disorders are otherwise etiologically independent; (5) there is cross-assortment between disorders A and B; and (6) no causal basis exists for the observed association; rather, it is an artifact of some kind. Possibilities 1 and 2 can be subdivided. In some cases, the first disorder could produce a complete copy of the second. In other cases, one disorder could produce only the symptoms of the second disorder but not the full syndrome. We call this latter possibility the *phenocopy hypothesis*, because only the symptoms of the secondary disorder would be present, but its "deeper" characteristics, such as a particular cognitive or brain deficit, would be lacking. This phenocopy hypothesis is particularly germane to the present project (and to the comorbidity of behaviorally defined disorders generally), because it is highly conceivable that reading disability could produce just the behavioral symptoms of ADHD (or cognitive deficit or dysthymia or vice versa), without producing the cognitive or brain deficits characteristic of these disorders.

For the comorbidity of reading disability and ADHD, hypotheses 3 (common etiology) and 6 (artifact) can be clearly rejected on the basis of previous studies (McGee & Share, 1988; Shaywitz & Shaywitz, 1988; Gilger et al., 1992a). One neuropsychological study (Pennington et al., 1993), lends support to the phenocopy hypothesis, but other neuropsychological studies of groups with reading disability, ADHD, and comorbid reading disability do not corroborate these findings (Dykman & Ackerman, 1991; Korkman & Pesonen, 1994; Narhi & Ahonen, 1995). Direct support for the cross-assortment hypothesis was provided by a cosegregation analysis (Faraone et al., 1993).

Results of direct tests of the etiological subtype hypothesis for reading disability and ADHD comorbidity using twin methods have been mixed, with one study failing to support this hypothesis (Gilger et al., 1992a) and two later ones providing support (Stevenson et al., 1993; Light et al., 1995).

In our current work, we are undertaking more definitive tests of these hypotheses by (1) separately ascertaining an ADHD twin sample, which will permit a *bidirectional* test of bivariate h^2g between reading disability and ADHD; (2) typing parents for history of both reading disability and ADHD, which provides a direct test of cross-assortment; (3) subdividing ADHD groups (and symptoms) into the categories *inattentive only*, *overactive or impulsive only*, and *combined*, as emerging evidence indicates that the comorbidity with reading disability is mainly found for the inattentive subtype; (4) continuing to compare the neuropsychological profiles for reading disability, ADHD, and reading disability plus ADHD groups; and (5) conducting an interval-mapping linkage study of the ADHD sample, testing for linkage both to the chromosome 6 markers already linked to reading disability and to candidate loci for ADHD, some of which have been preliminarily linked to ADHD [i.e., the dopamine transporter locus (Cook et al., 1995) and the D4 allele (Benjamin et al., 1996; Epstein et al., 1996)]. A linkage analysis provides the most direct test of the common etiology and etiological subtype hypotheses.

It is expected that the pattern of results across these converging methods will provide clearer answers about the causal basis of the comorbidity between reading disability and ADHD.

The final symptom to be considered is immune problems, originally proposed by Geschwind and Behan (1982) to be correlated with dyslexia. We have conducted three studies that examine the relation between dyslexia and immune problems (Pennington et al., 1987; Gilger et al., 1992b; Gilger & Pennington, 1995; Gilger et al., 1998). Although initially we found evidence for such an association, as we increased samples and sample sizes, the association disappeared. Moreover, the results of behavioral genetic tests in twins of a common genetic etiology for dyslexia and asthma or allergies, either in the entire sample or in a genetic subtype, were consistently null. The hypothesis of a common genetic etiology for dyslexia and immune problems was appealing, given the fact that the QTL identified on the short arm of chromosome 6 is in or near the human leukocytic antigen (HLA) region, which contains many genes for immune function (and dysfunction). We can now reject this hypothesis, at least in our linkage samples for the types of immune alterations we have measured.

In sum, behavioral genetic methods provide a powerful means of testing relations not only across but also within levels of analysis in the framework used here. We have illustrated how these and other methods have clarified relations at the symptom level. Clearly, both ADHD and problems in self-esteem and mood are symptoms in dyslexia, but each of these symptoms has different causal relations to dyslexia. Evidence presented here indicates that problems in self-esteem and mood are secondary to dyslexia, whereas ADHD symptoms are not, although further work still is needed to clarify the causal relation between dyslexia and ADHD. In contrast, we have rejected the hypothesis of an association between dyslexia and immune problems, at least in our two main samples that have been used for linkage studies.

LIMITATIONS OF THE FRAMEWORK

The foregoing review has summarized our progress toward reaching the long-term goal of an integrated neuroscientific explanation of dyslexia using a standard framework for such an explanation. Along the way, we have highlighted potential problems for this framework, raised either by empirical results from studies of dyslexia or by general theoretical considerations. In this section, we focus on these potential limitations.

Limitations raised by the empirical results include (1) the possibility that the genetic etiology appears more likely to be due to one or more QTLs rather than to a disease allele at a given locus; (2) the finding that the brain structures implicated in dyslexia are distributed rather than localized; and (3) the current lack of a computational model of phonological development. Because a QTL is, by definition, neither necessary nor sufficient to produce the condition in question, the etiology in any given dyslexiac individual would include other factors, some of which may be difficult to identify because their effect size is small. Identifying the QTLs involved will improve considerably our ability to identify individuals at risk, but it will not produce a perfectly accurate diagnostic test.

The finding that the brain differences in dyslexia are widespread is not surprising, given the fact that the developing brain is a highly interdependent system. A change in the thalamus, for instance, would be expected to have widespread effects on the neocortex, because the thalamus provides the main source of afferent input to the entire neocortex and because the specialization of neocortical areas depends critically on the type and timing of thalamic inputs. Therefore, if the etiologies for dyslexia are specific to thalamus, the thalamic changes will produce a cascade of changes in other parts of the brain. Similar arguments could be made for other structures. Because the developing brain is a self-organizing dynamic system, tracing back from the neurological phenotype to the causal sequence that produced it may prove to be very difficult, especially lacking a good animal model.

Finally, as was discussed earlier, some of the limitations intrinsic to the neurological level of analysis might be offset by experiments performed on computational models of phonological and reading development, but we currently lack those.

The standard framework implies that a discrete and specific cause will be found at each of the four levels of analysis and that a unidirectional causal path can be traced from etiology to brain to cognition to symptoms and among symptoms. The findings discussed earlier lead us to question how discrete and specific or, in other words, how localized, these causes will prove to be.

This brings us to limitations raised by general theoretical considerations, of which there are several. First, the nonlocalized changes found at some of the levels implies that the eventual behavioral changes will be a mix of both specific and general effects; an utterly "pure" case may be an impossible fiction! Second, the framework provides for unidirectional causation, but bidirectional causation clearly is possible between some levels in the framework; behavior may change brain, for instance. Therefore, it is conceivable that feedback loops might operate across some levels, allowing developmental transactions. Third, the framework gives priority to the cognitive level of analysis; there may be multiple etiologies or multiple brain mechanisms, but there is assumed convergence at the cognitive level; a single cognitive deficit explains a complex of symptoms. However, it could be that a single neurological change produces a complex of cognitive changes!

Finally, we have exposed some of the difficulties in testing causal paths between levels of analysis. At the genetic level, a strong theory (genes influence phenotypes, but phenotypes do not influence genes) permits strong tests of causality between the genetic level and the various phenotype levels, even though the overall method is only quasi-experimental (as we are not able randomly to assign genes to individuals). The lack of such a strong theory, and the inability to perform true experiments, limits the test of causality between brain and the two behavioral phenotype levels. Behavioral genetic tests of genetic covariation help somewhat with this problem but do not eliminate it, as discussed earlier. Of course, experiments are possible to test links between the cognitive and symptom levels (e.g., a longitudinal treatment study). Therefore, ironically, at least for dyslexia, the gene-mind problem is more tractable than the body-mind problem! (For neurodevelopmental disorders for which there is an animal model, such as Down syndrome, the situation is different.) Advances in genetics or neuroimaging alone will not ease this problem; we could know in complete detail how the etiologies of dyslexia change the structure and metabolism of the developing brain but still not know how these changes in brain cause the phonological deficit.

In summary, we are coming much closer to the goal of achieving an integrated, neuroscientific understanding of dyslexia due to fundamental advances in genetics, neuroimaging, and cognitive science. However, this work raises fundamental issues concerning both the relations between causal factors at these different levels of analysis and, more generally, the ways in which we conceptualize the mechanisms underlying both normal and abnormal cognitive development.

The study of neurodevelopmental disorders such as dyslexia is an important part of the emerging interdiscipline of developmental cognitive neuroscience. Whereas the lesion study has been the central approach in traditional neuropsychology, for several reasons a different approach is necessary in developmental cognitive neuroscience: An acquired lesion is rare in childhood, extrinsic to normal development, and essentially an irreproducible natural experiment. In contrast, genetic alterations in development are reasonably common, are intrinsic to the neurobiological mechanisms underlying cognitive and social development, and are reproducible, thus permitting group studies. At a deeper, theoretical level, the central ideas implicit in the lesion approach do not fit well with emerging findings in developmental neurobiology. The lesion approach assumes a relatively nonvariant, modular, species-typical cognitive architecture that can be dissected into independent cognitive components through the method of double dissociation. In contrast, brain development across the life span is turning out to be very plastic, both within and across individuals (Changeux, 1985; Edelman, 1987). Moreover, the neural architecture may well be better characterized by recurrent, connectionist networks, the activities of which are nonlinear and interdependent, than as a set of specialized, independent modules. Although the lesion approach has been extremely useful in giving us a "first-pass" mapping of structure-function relations, other methods (and metaphors) are needed to tell us how the self-organizing system of the brain puts itself together in both normal and abnormal development.

Simply put, genetic alterations in neurodevelopmental disorders such as the ones considered in this book alter or constrict the reaction range of brain development in a nonfocal way by changing the number, function, or connections between neurons; they do not "hard-wire" an aberrant circuit or ablate a normal one. All other things being equal, these early, distributed changes in brain development can alter the function of developing neural networks, thus affecting cognitive development and resulting behavior. However, an individual with a neurodevelopmental disorder does not have a static lesion; his or her neural network, and the resulting cognitive functions and behavior, still develop. Moreover, the principles that explain such development are the same as those that explain normal development.

Much of the work that has been performed to further our understanding different developmental psychopathologies has been implicitly guided by various assumptions in the lesion approach. Now is an appropriate time to examine critically those assumptions and to envision how this work would proceed under a different set of assumptions. Similar to neuropsychological studies of the effects of acquired lesions, research on the cognitive phenotype of neurodevelopmental disorders has used dissociations and double dissociations to provide a first pass-mapping of which cognitive processes appear to be impaired and intact in each disorder. Even this description is relative to our theory of specific and general cognitive processes and the relation between the two. Most importantly, what this descriptive account tells us about underlying cognitive mechanisms depends on answering more in-depth questions concerning the nature of those mechanisms.

ACKNOWLEDGMENTS

This research was supported by two National Institute of Child Health and Human Development Center grants—Learning Disability Research Center grant P50 HD27802 and a Mental Retardation Research Center (MRRC) grant P30 HD04024—and by two National Institute of Mental Health grants—K02 MH00419 (RSA) and R37 MH38820 (MERIT). Thanks go to Terry Goldhammer for help in recruiting and scheduling subjects.

REFERENCES

Alarcon, M., & DeFries, J. C. (1995). Quantitative trait locus for reading disability: An alternative test. *Behavior Genetics, 25,* 253.

Benjamin, J., Li, L., Patterson, C., Greenberg, B. D., Murphy, D. L., & Hamer, D. H. (1996). Population and familial association between the D4 dopamine receptor gene and measures of novelty seeking. *Nature Genetics, 12,* 81–84.

Boetsch, E. A., Green, P. A., & Pennington, B. F. (1996). Psychosocial correlates of dyslexia across the lifespan. *Development and Psychopathology, 8,* 539–562.

Bryant, P., & Impey, L. (1986). The similarity between normal readers and developmental and acquired dyslexics. *Cognition, 24,* 121–137.

Cardon, L. R., DeFries, J. C., Fulker, D. W., Kimberling, W. J., Pennington, B. F., & Smith, S. D. (1994). Quantitative trait locus for reading disability on chromosome 6. *Science, 265,* 276–279.

Castles, A., & Coltheart, M. C. (1993). Varieties of developmental dyslexia. *Cognition, 47,* 149–180.

Changeux, J. P. (1985). *Neuronal man.* New York: Oxford University Press.

Coltheart, M. C., Masterson, J., Byng, S. Prior, M., & Riddoch, J. (1983). Surface dyslexia. *Quarterly Journal of Experimental Psychology, 37A,* 469–495.

Cook, E. H., Stein, M. A., Krasowski, M. D., Cox, N. J., Olkon, D. M., Kieffer, J. E., & Leventhal, B. L. (1995). Association of attention deficit disorder and the dopamine transporter gene. *American Journal of Human Genetics, 56,* 993–998.

DeFries, J. C., Filipek, P. A., Fulker, D. W., Olson, R. K., Pennington, B. F., Smith, S. D., & Wise, B. W. (1997). Colorado Learning Disabilities Research Center. *Learning Disability Quarterly, 8,* 7–19.

Duara, R., Kushch, A., Gross-Glenn, K., et al. (1991). Neuroanatomic differences between dyslexic and normal readers on magnetic resonance imaging scans. *Archives of Neurology, 48,* 410–416.

Dykman, R. A., & Ackerman, P. T. (1991). Attention deficit disorder and specific reading disability: Separate but often overlapping disorders. *Journal of Learning Disabilities, 24,* 96–103.

Edelman, G. M. (1987). *Neural Darwinism.* New York: Basic Books.

Epstein, R. P., Novick, O., Umansky, R., Priel, B., Osher, Y., Blaine, D., Bennett, E. R., Nemanov, L., Katz, M., & Belmaker, R. H. (1996). Dopamine D4 receptor (D4DR) exon III polymorphism associated with the human personality trait of novelty seeking. *Nature Genetics, 12,* 78–80.

Faraone, S. V., Biederman, J., Kritcher, B., Keenan, K., et al. (1993). Evidence for the independent familial transmission of attention deficit hyperactivity disorder and learning disabilities: Results from a family genetic study. *American Journal of Psychiatry, 150,* 891–895.

Filipek, P. A. (1995). Neurobiological correlates of developmental dyslexia—what do we know about how dyslexic's brains differ from those of normal readers? *Journal of Child Neurology, 10,* S62–69.

Fodor, J. A. (1983). *The modularity of mind.* Cambridge, MA: MIT Press.

Fowler, A. (1991). How early phonological development might set the stage for phoneme awareness. In S. A. Brady & D. P. Shankweiler (Eds.), *Phonological processes in literacy: A tribute to Isabelle Y. Liberman* (pp. 97–117). Hillsdale, NJ: Erlbaum.

Frith, U. (1985). Beneath the surface of developmental dyslexia. In K. E. Patterson, J. C. Marshall, & M. Coltheart (Eds.), *Surface dyslexia: Neuropsychological and cognitive studies of phonological reading* (pp. 301–330). Hillsdale, NJ: Erlbaum.

Fulker, D. W., Cardon, L. R., DeFries, J. C., Kimberling, W. J., et al. (1991). Multiple regression analysis of sib-pair data on reading to detect quantitative trait loci. *Reading and Writing, 3,* 235–313.

Galaburda, A. M. (1988). The pathogenesis of childhood dyslexia. In F. Plum (Ed.), *Language, communication and the brain.* New York: Raven Press.

Galaburda, A. M., & Livingstone, M. (1993). Evidence for a magnocellular defect in developmental dyslexia. *Annals of the New York Academy of Science, 682,* 62–70.

Geschwind, N., & Behan, P. (1982). Left-handedness: Associations with immune disease, migraine, and developmental learning disorder. *Proceedings of the National Academy of Sciences of the United States of America, 79,* 5097–5100.

Gilger, J. W., Borecki, I., DeFries, J. C., & Pennington, B. F. (1994). Comingling and segregation analysis of reading performance in families of normal reading probands. *Behavior Genetics, 24,* 345–355.

Gilger, J. W., & Pennington, B. F. (1995). Why associations among traits do not necessarily indicate their common etiology: A comment on the Geschwind-Behan-Galaburda model. *Brain and Cognition, 27,* 89–93.

Gilger, J. W., Pennington, B. F., & DeFries, J. C. (1992a). A twin study of the etiology of comorbidity: Attention-deficit hyperactivity disorder and dyslexia. *Journal of the American Academy of Child and Adolescent Psychiatry, 31*(2), 343 348.

Gilger, J. W., Pennington, B. F., DeFries, J. C., Harbeck, R., Kotzin, B., Green, P., & Smith, S. (1998). A twin and family study of the association between immune system dysfunction and dyslexia using blood serum immunoassay and survey data. *Brain and Cognition, 36,* 310–333.

Gilger, J. W., Pennington, B. F., Green, P., Smith, S. M., & Smith, S. D. (1992b). Reading disability, immune disorders and non-right-handedness: Twin and family studies of their relations. *Neuropsychologia, 30,* 209–227.

Grigorenko, E. L., Wood, F. B., & Pauls, D. L. (1997). Susceptibility loci for distinct components of developmental dyslexia on chromosome 6 and 15. *American Journal of Human Genetics, 6,* 27.

Hallgren, B. (1950). Specific dyslexia (congenital word-blindness): A clinical and genetic study. *Acta Psychiatrica et Neurologica Scandinavica Supplementum, 65,* 1–287.

Hynd, G. W., Hall, J., Novey, E. S., et al. (1995). Dyslexia and corpus callosum morphology. *Archives of Neurology, 52,* 32–38.

Hynd, G. W., Semrud-Clikeman, M., Lorys, A. R., Novey, E. S., & Eliopulas, D. (1991). Brain morphology in developmental dyslexia and attention deficit disorder/hyperactivity. *Archives of Neurology, 47,* 919–926.

Jernigan, T. L., Hesselink, J. R., Stowell, E., & Tallal, P. (1991). Cerebral structure on magnetic resonance imaging in language- and learning-impaired children. *Archives of Neurology, 48,* 539–545.

Kerr, J. (1897). School hygiene, in its mental, moral, and physical aspects. Howard Medical Prize essay. *Journal of the Royal Statistical Society, 60,* 613–680.

Korkman, M., & Pesonen, A. (1994). A comparison of neuropsychological test profiles of children with attention deficit-hyperactivity disorder and/or learning disorder. *Journal of Learning Disabilities, 27,* 383–392.

Larsen, J. P., Høien, T., Lundberg, I., & Ödegaard, H. (1990). MRI evaluation of the size and symmetry of the planum temporale in adolescents with developmental dyslexia. *Brain and Language, 39,* 289–301.

Larsen, J. P., Høien, T., & Ödegaard, H. (1992). Magnetic resonance imaging of the corpus callosum in developmental dyslexia. *Cognitive Neuropsychology, 9,* 123–134.

Lewis, M. (1990). Models of developmental psychopathology. In M. Lewis and S. M. Miller (Eds.), *Handbook of developmental psychopathology.* New York: Plenum Press.

Light, J. G., Pennington, B. F., Gilger, J. W., & DeFries, J. C. (1995). Reading disability and hyperactivity disorder: Evidence for a common genetic etiology. *Developmental Neuropsychology, 11,* 323–335.

Manis, F. R., Seidenberg, M. S., Doi, L. M., McBride-Chang, C., & Petersen, A. (1996). On the bases of two subtypes of developmental dyslexia. *Cognition, 58,* 157–195.

Markey, K. L. (1994). *The sensorimotor foundations of phonology: A computational model of early childhood articulatory and phonetic development* (Tech. Rep. No. CU-CS-752-94) [doctoral dissertation]. Boulder, CO: University of Colorado, Department of Computer Science.

Markey, K. L., Menn, L., & Mozer, M. C. (1995). A developmental model of the sensorimotor foundations of phonology. *Proceedings of the Boston University Conference on Language Development, 19,* 367–378.

McGee, R., & Share, D. L. (1988). Attention deficit disorder-hyperactivity and academic failure: Which comes first and what should be treated? *Journal of the American Academy of Child and Adolescent Psychiatry, 27,* 318–325.

Morgan, W. (1896). A case of congenital word-blindness. *British Medical Journal, 2,* 1378.

Morton, J., & Frith, U. (1995). Causal modelling: A structural approach to developmental psychopathology. In D. Cicchetti and D. J. Cohen (Eds.), *Manual of developmental psychopathology* (Vol. 1). New York: John Wiley.

Narhi, V., & Ahonen, T. (1995). Reading disability with or without attention deficit hyperactivity disorder: Do attentional problems make a difference? *Developmental Neuropsychology, 11,* 337–349.

Pennington, B. F. (1991a). *Diagnosing learning disorders: A neuropsychological framework.* New York: Guilford Press.

Pennington, B. F. (1991b). Genetic and neurological influences on reading disability: An overview. *Reading and Writing, 3,* 191–201.

Pennington, B. F. (1994). Genetics of learning disabilities. *Journal of Child Neurology, 10(suppl.),* S69–S76.

Pennington, B. F. (1997). Using genetics to dissect cognition [invited editorial]. *American Journal of Human Genetics, 60,* 13–16.

Pennington, B. F., & Bennetto, L. (1993). Main effects or transactions in the neuropsychology of conduct disorder? Commentary on "the neuropsychology of conduct disorder." *Development and Psychopathology, 5,* 151–164.

Pennington, B. F., & Ozonoff, S. (1991). A neuroscientific perspective on continuity and discontinuity in developmental psychopathology. In D. Cicchetti (Ed.), *Rochester symposium on developmental psychopathology* (Vol. 3, pp. 117–159). New York: Cambridge University Press.

Pennington, B. F., & Welsh, M. C. (1995). Neuropsychology and developmental psychopathology. In D. Cicchetti and D. J. Cohen (Eds.), *Manual of developmental psychopathology* (Vol. 1, pp. 254–290). New York: John Wiley.

Pennington, B. F., Filipek, P., Kennedy, D. N., Lefly, D., Simon, J. H., Filley, C. M., Galaburda, A., & DeFries, J. C. (1998). *Brain morphometry in reading-disabled twins.* Manuscript submitted for publication.

Pennington, B. F., Groisser, D., & Welsh, M. C. (1993). Contrasting deficits in attention deficit hyperactivity disorder versus reading disability. *Developmental Psychology, 29,* 511–523.

Pennington, B. F., Smith, S. D., Kimberling, W. J., Green, P. A., & Haith, M. M. (1987). Left-handedness and immune disorders in familial dyslexics. *Archives of Neurology, 44,* 634–639.

Plaut, D. (1995). Double dissociation without modularity: Evidence from connectionist neuropsychology. *Journal of Clinical and Experimental Neuropsychology, 17,* 291–321.

Plaut, D., McClelland, J. L., Seidenberg, M. S., & Patterson, K. E. (1996). Visual word recognition: Are two routes really necessary? *Psychological Review, 103,* 56–115.

Sameroff, A., & Chandler, M. I. (1975). Reproductive risk and the continuum of caretaking causality. In F. D. Horowitz (Ed.), *Review of child development, Research* (Vol. 4). (pp. 64–93). Chicago, IL: University of Chicago Press.

Scarborough, H. S. (1990). Very early language deficits in dyslexic children. *Child Development, 61,* 1728–1743.

Schultz, R. T., Cho, N. K., Staib, L. H., et al. (1994). Brain morphology in normal and dyslexic children: The influence of sex and age. *Annals of Neurology, 35,* 732–742.

Seidenberg, M. S., & McClelland, J. L. (1989). A distributed developmental model of word recognition and naming. *Psychological Review, 96,* 447–452.

Shaywitz, S. E., & Shaywitz, B. E. (1988). Attention deficit disorder: Current perspectives. In J. F. Kavanaugh & T. J. Truss (Eds.), *Learning disabilities: Proceedings of the national conference.* Parkton, MD: York Press.

Shaywitz, S. E., Shaywitz, B. A., Fletcher, J. M., & Escobar, M. D. (1990). Prevalence of reading disability in boys and girls. Results of the Connecticut Longitudinal Study. *Journal of the American Medical Association, 264*(8), 998–1002.

Smith, S. D., Kimberling, W. J., Pennington, B. F., & Lubs, H. A. (1983). Specific reading disability: Identification of an inherited form through linkage analysis. *Science, 219,* 1345–1347.

Smith, S. D., Kimberling, W. J., & Pennington, B. F. (1991). Screening for multiple genes influencing dyslexia. *Reading and Writing, 3,* 285–298.

Smith, S. D., Pennington, B. F., Kimberling, W. J., & Ing, P. S. (1990). Familial dyslexia: Use of genetic linkage data to define subtypes. *Journal of the American Academy of Child and Adolescent Psychiatry, 29,* 204–213.

Stanovich, K. E., Siegel, L. S., & Gottardo, A. (1997). Converging evidence for phonological and surface subtypes of reading disability. *Journal of Education Psychology, 89,* 114–128.

Stevenson, J., Pennington, B. F., Gilger, J. W., DeFries, J. C., & Gillis, J. J. (1993). Hyperactivity and spelling disability: Testing for shared genetic aetiology. *Journal of Child Psychology and Psychiatry, 34,* 1137–1152.

Temple, C. M. (1985). Surface dyslexia and the development of reading. In K. E. Patterson, J. C. Marshall, & M. Coltheart (Eds.), *Surface dyslexia: Neuropsychological and cognitive studies of phonological reading* (pp. 261–288). Hillsdale, NJ: Erlbaum.

Temple, C. M., & Marshall, J. C. (1983). A case study of developmental phonological dyslexia. *British Journal of Psychology, 74,* 517–533.

Van Orden, G. C., Pennington, B. F., & Stone, G. O. (1990). Word identification reading and the promise of subsymbolic psycholinguistics. *Psychological Review, 97*(4), 488–522.

Wadsworth, S. J., DeFries, J. C., Stevenson, J., Gilger, J. W., et al. (1992). Gender ratios among reading-disabled children and their siblings as a function of parental impairment. *Journal of Child Psychology and Psychiatry, 33,* 1229–1239.

Walley, A. C. (1993). The role of vocabulary development in children's spoken word recognition and segmentation ability. *Developmental Review, 13,* 286–350.

14 Specific Grammatical Limitations in Children with Specific Language Impairment

Mabel L. Rice

CASE STUDY: CHILD WITH SPECIFIC LANGUAGE IMPAIRMENT

Jay is a rather ordinary little boy in general appearance and demeanor. He plays with other children in the usual ways, and his speech is quite clear. He was extraordinarily late in beginning to talk. His parents referred him for language intervention services because he was almost 3 years old before he began to talk, well beyond the age at which talking usually begins. His parents were concerned because his father had received speech and language therapy as a child. They are concerned, caring, and conscientious parents who sought out recommendations for enhancing Jay's language development.

In his clinical evaluation, Jay scored below age expectations on a standardized test of language acquisition, his utterances were shorter than expected for his age, and he showed poor performance on a test of receptive vocabulary. At the same time, audiological assessment showed his hearing to be within normal range and his nonverbal intelligence to be near normal levels for his age. His mother reported an uneventful birth history and early childhood development for Jay. The diagnosis was specific language impairment (SLI): receptive and expressive language development below age expectations without concomitant deficits of hearing, intelligence, or social-affective relationships. Jay was enrolled in a language intervention program for preschoolers offered by his local school district.

When Jay was almost 5 years old, he was enrolled in a longitudinal study of children with SLIs. The initial round of testing determined that Jay's morphological development showed a profile that proved to be characteristic of other children in the affected group. Some grammatical rules were evident, whereas others were not. On the unaffected side were rules governing plurals, the verbal inflection, -ing, and prepositions. Jay said these sentences clearly: (1) "Those guys got sore legs"; (2) "That baby's taking a nap"; and (3) "The babies sleep in this bed." In fact, in contexts wherein the adult grammar would require plural -s, as in sentence 1, Jay was accurate 96% of the time; for the verbal -ing, as in sentence 2, accuracy was 96%; for the prepositions *in* and *on*, as in sentence 3, accuracy was 100%. In these ways, Jay's grammar was very similar to that of unaffected, typically developing children. In other ways, however, Jay's grammar was very different from that of his age peers. This was evident in utterances involving grammatical tense marking. These utterances included the following [the asterisk indicating an ungrammatical utterance that was produced in contexts in which an adult would say the utterance following the virgule (/)]: (4) *"This thing drop/

this thing dropped"; (5) *"Dad sleep here/dad sleeps here"; (6) *"Her fine/she is fine"; and (7) *"He going to fall/he's going to fall". In contexts wherein the adult grammar would require -ed past, as in sentence 4, his accuracy was 27%; for -s third-person present, as in sentence 5, accuracy was 13%; for forms of BE[1] like those in sentences 6 and 7, his accuracy was 53%. These levels of grammatical performance are far below age expectations. Unaffected children at age $4\frac{1}{2}$ years are at 90% levels of accuracy, very near the adult grammar.

Jay's teachers (and even his parents) do not notice these details of his grammar. They notice instead that Jay is a somewhat withdrawn child. Although he seems to enjoy playing with other children, he hangs back somewhat from verbal conversations and is reluctant to assert his own wants and needs. He is not popular among his peers. When he goes to kindergarten, his teacher notices this apparent shyness and regards him as "socially immature." For this reason, she does not promote him to first grade with his age peers but instead recommends that he move to a "developmental first grade."

His reading readiness skills are limited, and he subsequently encounters difficulty with the transition to reading. If his academic outcome proceeds in a way similar to other children's with SLI, he likely will be a modest student who ultimately achieves a high-school degree and perhaps a semester or two of college. When matched for children of similar socioeconomic status and nonverbal intelligence levels, his final educational levels will be lower. Finally, also likely is that when he becomes a parent, one or more of his children will demonstrate a similar language acquisition profile.

The little boy Jay is representative of a group of children who have been the focus of study in the author's laboratory for some time. In all, we have detailed spontaneous language data on more than 100 such children, all of whom received the diagnosis of SLI, along with evidence from in excess of 100 unaffected control children. The children in this group meet the clinical profile of expressive and receptive language deficits. As described in the first two paragraphs of the case, youngsters such as Jay typically are referred for evaluation, during which they are given standardized tests of language acquisition and vocabulary development, supplemented by measures drawn from spontaneous speech, such as the mean length of utterance. In addition, measures of nonverbal intelligence are obtained, hearing is assessed, and parents are interviewed for information about other dimensions of development.

These diagnostic measures establish that Jay's profile of performance meets the definition of *language-impaired* relative to age expectations, and he further meets the exclusionary criteria invoked for SLI, (i.e., no known deficits of cognitive development, gross neuromotor development, or social-affective development and no hearing loss). In other words, no obvious associated conditions could account for the extreme delays in language acquisition. The causes of Jay's language impairment are unknown, although current scientific inquiry is bringing new advances in our understanding of the condition.

A long-standing issue in the study of children with SLI is whether the language delays can be thought of as the primary area of impairment or as symptoms secondary to limitations in more general perceptual or cognitive mechanisms. This issue links up with one of the fundamental issues in theories of children's language acquisition: the extent to which grammar emerges from dedicated cognitive mechanisms and processes or is intrinsic to more general perceptual and/or cognitive mechanisms. Do children with SLI have specific grammatical limitations or are any apparent language delays an epiphenomenon of faulty perceptual mechanisms or general learning processes?

The author would argue that the answer to these questions lies in careful consideration of the grammatical symptomatology associated with the condition of SLI. With regard to the closely related disorder of dyslexia, Lyon (1995) argued that specifying the key symptoms and characteristics of affected children is essential. That specificity is the objective of the work discussed in this chapter. A preview of some key findings is offered in paragraph three of the foregoing case study, showing that some but not all morphemes are likely to be affected (where *morphemes* refer to words and meaningful affixes, such as the *-ed* on *walked*). Because of the selective deficits, SLI should not be thought of as a general problem of grammatical acquisition. Most importantly, a close consideration of the pattern of affectedness proves to be enlightening: We can rule out some possible interpretations and can propose some new explanations. The account discussed here focuses on fundamental properties of clausal construction, to propose that children with SLI do not know that tense marking is obligatory in simple declarative sentences and in this way are very far behind their age peers and even behind younger unaffected children at similar language levels. Furthermore, this symptom is not apparent in children with Williams syndrome (see chapter 4) who are also delayed in emergence of their grammar relative to their age peers. Thus, we know that it is not always to be expected in cases of language delay.

Important as these advances are in understanding the grammatical symptoms, one would not want to create the impression that children with SLI realistically can be considered as otherwise unaffected children. Our experience (and that of other investigators) with these children is that grammatical limitations during the preschool years can be associated with, and perhaps lead to, other developmental and life span risks as well. The final paragraph of the case study description lays out some of the other risks, including relatively mild but nevertheless significant social differences and not-so-mild academic risks and genetic risks. Elsewhere, the author and others have reported on the social risks during the preschool and early school years (Hadley & Rice, 1991; Rice, 1993a,b; Rice et al., 1993; Gertner et al., 1994; Redmond et al., 1998) and have argued that the ways in which young children with SLI show social differences is remarkably similar to the ways in which young children learning English as a second language seem to be socially different. Therefore, we should suspect that the limited language competence is a causal factor and not the other way around. The academic risks for SLI are well documented (Aram et al., 1984; Catts, 1993; Watkins &

Rice, 1994). Emerging evidence also substantiates considerable genetic risk (Crago and Gopnik, 1994; Rice, 1996; Tomblin, 1996; chapter 15). Because this chapter explores in detail the grammatical deficits, these other dimensions are not addressed beyond this acknowledgment that they exist and should not be ignored in the full picture.

A final point is that Jay's profile is one of several possible profiles encountered in a clinically referred sample of children who meet the exclusionary criteria of SLI. Jay's language deficits are apparent in the receptive and expressive modalities, and his speech generally is clear (i.e., he is readily intelligible and does not omit sounds in single-word productions).

Why is this profile selected for study? Again, borrowing from the observations of Lyon (1995, p. 3) about studies of dyslexia, "It is crucial to study individuals who meet well-specified selection criteria." The receptive-expressive disorder is a well-specified selection criterion. Furthermore, this clinical profile characterizes preschool children who are least likely to "outgrow" their early language impairment (Rescorla & Schwartz, 1990; Thal et al., 1991), so it is likely to be a stable condition that can be studied to determine persistence over time. Because the focus of inquiry is on morphology, it should eliminate children who cannot pronounce the sounds that appear as surface morphemes, sounds such as the final -s in *two dogs* or *he runs*. Otherwise, it would not be possible to tell whether the difficulties lie in motor performance, in acoustic representations, or in underlying linguistic representations.

The initial sections of this chapter contain an overview of the grammatical property of finiteness and how it emerges in children's grammar. An optional infinitive stage is described. The following sections lay out evidence of an extended optional infinitive stage in children with SLI, drawing the conclusion that tense marking is a significant clinical marker in the grammars of affected children but that this symptom does not characterize the early grammars of children with Williams syndrome. This finding is taken as evidence that selective deficits of tense marking are not characteristic of all cases of language delay and probably originate in cognitive mechanisms selective to the grammar. In the next section, an auditory-processing account of SLI is examined, critiqued, and found to be unconvincing as an explanation of the grammatical deficits of children with this condition. The chapter concludes with a discussion of the implications for cognitive neuroscience and neurodevelopmental disorders.

THE SEARCH FOR A CLINICAL MARKER

The identification of a distinctive grammatical marker for SLI long has been sought and long has proved to be elusive. In a recent literature review, Leonard (1987) concluded that available evidence did not support a unique linguistic characteristic of this condition. Lahey et al. (1992) concluded that the range of normal variation is great in young children's early grammatical acquisition and that the reported deficits of children with SLI fall within the broad range of typical development. The standing question has been whether the grammar of children with this condition differs in interesting ways from the profile expected for younger levels of language acquisition. The null hypothesis has been that the grammar of affected children can be considered as a simple developmental delay within the broad range of normal variation for younger children. This can be regarded as an extended development theory of SLI. Within this view, the underlying grammar of children with SLI is undifferentiated from that of unaffected children; some unknown factor causes language acquisition to start slowly. Under some readings of an extended development theory, children should be expected to "outgrow" the early problem. Perhaps this is what happens in many children identified as late talkers who "catch up" with their age peers around school entry age (Rescorla & Schwartz, 1990; Thal et al., 1991).

For a long time, however, some have hinted that something more is at stake. Recognized for some time is that, in English, certain morphemes are more likely to lag behind, especially a small set of verbal affixes, such as third person singular -s in *she talks* (Lahey et al., 1992; Leonard et al., 1992; Rice & Oetting, 1993; Rice, 1994); regular past tense in *she talked* (Leonard, 1987; Bishop, 1994); and (although relatively neglected for some time) the forms of *to be* as in *she is talking* and *she is happy* (Ingram, 1972). To account for these observations, an existing group of theories can be considered loosely as extended development theory plus processing constraints. One group of explanations targets input processing mechanisms as faulty. Several versions of this view exist. One posits a deficit in auditory processing of rapidly changing speech, which leads to difficulty in discriminating between speech syllables (Tallal et al., 1996). A second view assumes that the underlying paradigm-building mechanisms of language are in place but that the problem is in the processing of surface forms of low phonetic salience (i.e., the small, unstressed parts of the input grammar). In effect, this view posits a filter in which grammatical information is selectively screened on input, such that the low salience parts get dropped from input and, therefore, cannot be considered by the paradigm-building mechanisms. This interpretation, known as a *surface account*, was put forth by Leonard et al. (1992) and recently was revised to a low phonetic substance interpretation (Leonard, 1996, 1998), which stipulates that relative morphophonemic duration determines the components likely to be dropped. Omissions are predicted to be morphophonemic material of shorter duration than neighboring material. Finally, an alternative version of a processing constraint is the production constraint explanation of Bishop (1994), in which observed surface omissions are attributed to constraints on the output side, such that as a child is formulating and producing an utterance, a ceiling of some sort influences available production resources. When this ceiling is exceeded, some parts of the utterance drop out. What the processing models, collectively, have in common is the expectation that the underlying grammar of SLI is basically intact, and does not differ in interesting ways from younger, normally developing children. Differences are attributable to processing breakdowns.

Important recent breakthroughs bring a new theoretical perspective and provide strong evidence that certain grammatical functions lag far behind in the language acquisition of children such as Jay. Also corroborated is that the grammar of SLI is in interesting ways like younger children's grammars but that, at the same time, the affected grammar is unlike younger grammars in the persistence of a specific grammatical difference over a long period. This account is the extended optional infinitive account (described later). The extended optional infinitive model can be viewed as a highly enriched version of the extended development theory, which assumes highly explicit models of the adult and child grammars, models that allow for specification of affected parts of the grammar. The theoretical import of the extended optional infinitive account is that the observed findings do not yield readily to processing accounts of linguistic limitations.

THE GRAMMATICAL PROPERTY OF FINITENESS

Contemporary theories of linguistic structure and language acquisition focus on the grammatical property of finiteness (cf. Chomsky, 1993, 1995). Finiteness is marked on verbs, which can appear in finite or nonfinite forms. Finite forms are those marked for tense and grammatical agreement. Each declarative clause must have a finite form to be grammatical. Consider the following sentences (asterisk indicates that the sentence is ungrammatical):

(1) a. Patsy *walks*.
     b. *Patsy walk.

(2) a. Yesterday Patsy walked home after work.
     b. *Yesterday Patsy walk home after work.

(3) a. Patsy is walking.
     b. *Patsy walking.

(4) a. Patsy is happy.
     b. *Patsy happy.

(5) a. Patsy did not work today/Does Patsy work today?
     b. *Patsy not work today/*Patsy work today?

In examples 1 to 5, the *a* examples are grammatical, whereas the *b* examples are not. The reason they are ungrammatical is that they are missing finiteness markings, which in English can be seen in the use of -*s* as a verbal affix with third-person singular present-tense subjects (where both tense and subject-verb agreement are operative); in the use of -*ed* to mark past tense (irrespective of subject personhood, so that grammatical tense is evident but subject-verb agreement is not); in the use of *BE* forms (which includes the surface forms of *is, am, are, was, were*, so that tense and subject-verb agreement are evident) as auxiliary verbs (as in example 3a) or as main verbs (as in example 4a); and in the use of *DO* forms (which includes the surface forms of *do, does,* and *did,* thus showing tense and agreement, as in example 5a). Notice that although these different surface forms share the grammatical property of finiteness marking, they do not share speech properties. Some are affixes (i.e., *-s, -ed*) and some are free-standing morphemes (i.e., *BE* and *DO,* although *BE* can appear as a contracted form attached as an affix, which is possible for examples 3a and 4a, and *DO* can appear as a stem carrying a contracted form of *not,* as in example 5a and b). The point to notice here is that perceptual properties do not define this set of grammatical forms.

Next consider that in English, finiteness marking may or may not appear on a surface form. This does not mean that finiteness marking does not exist but only that it is not apparent on the surface. This is illustrated in examples 6, 7, and 8 that follow. In example 6a, we see that the third-person singular present-tense *-s* does not appear for plural subjects and, in example 6b, for first person singular subjects. This shows that bare stems of lexical verbs can appear in finiteness-carrying syntactical positions.

(6) a. They walk.
　　 b. I walk.

In example 7a we see that not all bare stem verbs are in finiteness-carrying contexts. In example 7a, *walk* cannot carry finiteness marking, as is evident in example 7b.

(7) a. Patsy likes to walk.
　　 b. *Patsy likes to walks.

In example 8a, we see that nonfinite verb positions do not necessarily require the infinitival *to* evident in example 7a. We know this bare stem *walk* is not finite because, as illustrated in example 8b, it becomes ungrammatical if overt finiteness is applied.

(8) a. Patsy made him walk.
　　 b. *Patsy made him walks.

Examples 6 to 8 show that children learning English must know the syntactic contexts that allow finiteness marking and those that do not. They cannot follow a simple strategy of "find the verb and attach an affix." If they do, it will be apparent in misapplications of overt morphemes. The main point here is that morphological marking of finiteness is related intrinsically to knowledge of the configurational structures of sentences (i.e., the syntax). Hence, the term *morphosyntax.*

Finally, consider that in English, small, unstressed grammatical morphemes share surface properties with the finiteness markers described, but these morphemes do not mark finiteness. For example, plural *-s* (as in example 9) is very similar to the *-s* affix for third-person singular present tense.

(9) Clocks tell time.

Note also that the -s affix is phonetically very similar to sounds that appear within word boundaries, such as the final sound of the words *fox* or *box*. A child learning English early on knows that the final sound of *fox* is linguistically different from the plural affix of *clocks*, and (as I will show) different from the affix of -s in *walks*. Keep in mind, however, that for children with problems in pronouncing the -s sound, it can be omitted in words as well as morphological affixes. In such cases, determining which level of linguistic representation is involved may not be possible.

Other plausible comparison morphemes are the prepositions *in* and *on*, as in examples 10a and b following, and the verbal -*ing* of examples 3a and b previously, which is thought to mark progressive aspect.

(10) a. Patsy is in the office
      b. The phone is on the desk.

Each of these, like the morphemes, third-person -s, -ed, BE, and DO, are small, unstressed parts of sentences. So, if small, unstressed parts of the surface grammar are vulnerable to processing constraints, plural -s, *in*, *on*, and -*ing* should be omitted as should the finiteness marking morphemes.

A final, important observation is that the finiteness markers are *obligatory* parts of each main declarative clause, whereas the acoustically similar morphemes for prepositions, plurals, and progressive aspect are not. Sentences without plurals are not ungrammatical; sentences without small words (e.g., the prepositions *in* and *on*) are not ungrammatical; sentences without the progressive aspect marker -*ing* are not ungrammatical. Many of the sentences that appear in the text of this chapter do not have one of these morphemes. On the other hand, literally every sentence in this text has a finiteness marker. In this fundamental sense in the adult grammar, finiteness is obligatory and must be carried in the mental representation of underlying sentence structures. Finiteness is part of "deep syntactic processes that interact with morphology to produce surface inflectional patterns" (Wexler, 1994, p. 319). (Currently, an extensive literature analyzes the formal linguistic properties of finiteness and sentence representations. See Pollock, 1989; Rizzi, 1990; Chomsky, 1993, 1995; and Haegeman, 1994, for discussion and references.)

CHILDREN'S ACQUISITION OF FINITENESS: AN OPTIONAL INFINITIVE STAGE

A recent and rather surprising discovery is that young, normally developing children for some time use nonfinite (infinitival) forms and finite forms of verbs in grammatical contexts wherein verbs are required. Wexler (1994, 1996) called this the *optional infinitive stage*, because infinitives were optional in finite contexts. In a given sample of young children's utterances, children sometimes used infinitival forms and sometimes used finite forms of the main verb; in many of the languages studied, the infinitival form clearly differs from the finite form. This period has now been attested across many languages, including Danish, Faroese, French, German, Icelandic, Norwegian, and Swedish.

Among the current areas of investigation, interest focuses on how to characterize this period in terms of what children know and do not know about clause structure early on, and in terms of why some languages and not others show this period of language acquisition. (For reviews, see Bottari et al., 1996; Clahsen et al., 1994; Guasti, 1994; Lust et al., 1994; Rizzi, 1994; Wexler, 1994, 1996; Haegeman, 1995; Rice & Wexler, 1995, 1996a; Schutze et al., 1995.)

Wexler (1994, 1996) worked out predictions for English. He argued that even though the many bare stems of English verbs reduce the number of contexts in which finiteness marking is clear, nevertheless some clear grammatical contexts would evince an apparent optional infinitive grammar. In particular, he predicted the following: For the third-person -s and -ed markings on lexical verbs, bare stems may be used optionally where inflected forms are required, and auxiliary and main verb uses of BE may be omitted, as can auxiliary (but not main verb) DO. The predicted errors are those illustrated in the asterisk-marked sentences in examples 1 to 5 previously.

A further, and very important, prediction is that when children do use a finite form in a given utterance—even when they are optionally dropping these forms from other utterances—they nevertheless know that the form used must agree with the subject of the sentence (i.e., subject-verb agreement must be evident) and that finiteness marking can appear only in the positions within the clause in which it is allowed (i.e., errors such as those in examples 7b and 8b should not appear). This is a strong prediction that says that children who do not know that tense is obligatory nevertheless know the structural configuration of a sentence (i.e., where finiteness can appear) and that the choice of a finiteness form is correlated with the subject of the sentence. In other words, grammatical morphology is intricately bound to knowledge of clausal structure (i.e., the syntax), and even young children know this.

To summarize; The optional infinitive account offers a view of normative language acquisition in which child grammars show a developmental delay in the obligatory use of tense marking. At the same time, children know about the relationship of morphology and syntax and the obligatory properties of subject-verb agreement. In this framework, children do not acquire morphemes one at a time independently of what they know about word order and other properties of a sentence. Inflectional patterns and underlying syntax are associated closely, and morphemes are understood in terms of grammatical function.

AN EXTENDED OPTIONAL INFINITIVE PERIOD FOR CHILDREN WITH SLI

In this section are reported findings from a series of studies investigating a possible extended optional infinitive stage in children such as Jay. These studies were carried out in the author's laboratory, in collaboration with Ken Wexler. Detailed reports appear elsewhere (Rice & Wexler, 1995, 1996a,b,c; Rice et al., 1995; Rice et al., unpublished manuscript). Summarized here are some key findings.

The findings are both cross-sectional and longitudinal. The basic design includes an affected group of children who were identified in the year prior to school entry (when their mean age is near 60 months) and who meet the inclusionary and exclusionary criteria described in the case study. This group is compared to two control groups of unaffected children, one matched for chronological age (henceforth termed the *5N group* because their mean age is right at 60 months at the time of first measurement), the other group of children at equivalent levels of language acquisition, as indexed by mean length of utterance. The members of this group are 2 years younger than those in the affected and age control groups at initial testing, with a mean age of some 36 months, so they are termed the *3N group*. In the cross-sectional studies, the three groups of children were compared when all three groups were preschoolers. A group of 37 children with SLI participated in the cross-sectional study reported here, 45 5N children, and 40 children in the 3N group.

In a longitudinal study, 20 children in each of the three groups (N = 60) were followed for subsequent testing over a period of 4 years, for a total of seven data points, with testing at 6-month intervals. Collapsed over the three groups of children, the developmental interval observed encompassed ages 2. 5 to 9 years.

Important methodological refinements in these studies are the exclusion from the affected group of those children who failed a screening for single-word pronunciation of the target sounds (final *s, z, t, d*) and specification of both receptive and expressive impairments. In these two ways, the sample of affected children is specified more fully than it is in many comparison studies reported in the literature. The full battery of assessments given and criteria for inclusion in the affected group are reported in table 14.1. A further methodological refinement is an a priori plan for measuring target morphemes in elicitation probes and in detailed analyses of spontaneous utterances. Thus, the available evidence for morphological use is more extensive than that in many other studies.

Accuracy of SLI Children in Tense Marking Morphemes

A very robust picture emerges on comparison of the performance of the SLI group to that of the two normal control groups on the set of morphemes thought to mark tense (Rice & Wexler, 1996b). This set includes *-s* third-person singular present, *-ed* past, *BE*, and *DO*. For each of these morphemes, the SLI group mean is lower than that of either of the comparison groups, with means statistically significantly lower than that of younger 3N group

Table 14.1 Assessment for the children diagnosed as specific language impaired

Instrument	Criterion
Peabody Picture Vocabulary Test–Revised (Dunn & Dunn, 1981)	In clinical range
Mean length of utterance in spontaneous speech sample	In clinical range
Test of language development–primary speaker language quotient (TOLD2-P; Newcomer & Hammill, 1988)	In clinical range
Goldman Fristoe Test of Articulation (Goldman & Fristoe, 1986)	Exclude for multiple and severe articulation errors
Phonological screening for final −s, −z, −t, and −d in single-syllable words	80% Accuracy required
Columbia Mental Maturity Scale (Burgemeister et al., 1972)	Within or above normal range
Audiological assessment	Within normal range on pure tones

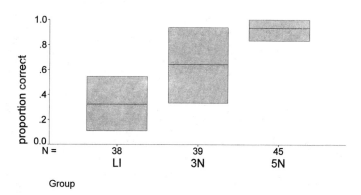

Figure 14.1 Distribution of children's performance on third-person −s within groups.

and much, much lower than that of the 5N age-matched group, who are essentially at adult levels of use of the morphemes.

A representative example of the findings can be seen in figure 14.1. This boxplot depicts the performance of the three groups on -s third-person singular present in an experimental probe. In this task, children are shown a picture of a person doing something (e.g., a doctor seeing a patient), and the children are asked to tell what the doctor does (e.g., "He makes people get well"). The variable is the percentage of correct uses of third-person -s. The mean values for the groups are as follows: SLI, 23%; 3N, 44%; 5N, 92%. The figure shows for each group the median score (indicated by the line in the middle of the box for each group) and the deviation from the median (indicated by the width of the box, which extends from the twenty-fifth percentile to the seventy-fifth percentile, a box that includes half the children in the group).

Several findings are clear. One is that the affected group is considerably less accurate than is the younger group of children at equivalent levels of utterance length, and the affected group is virtually nonoverlapping with their age peers. Their age peers, in the year before kindergarten, know that finiteness marking is obligatory, whereas the affected children are very likely to drop the third-person -s. The younger 3N group members also show optionality in their use of third-person -s, using it (on average) 44% of the time.

This pattern of results is evident for each of the morphemes in the tense-marking group (i.e., third-person -s, -ed, BE as either copula or auxiliary, and DO). Furthermore, this difference appears irrespective of task differences (i.e., it appears in spontaneous samples and in experimentally elicited probes as well).

In this domain of the grammar, the conclusion is clear: The affected children do in fact differ from unaffected children. By age 5, unaffected children are performing virtually as adults in this part of their grammar; they know that finiteness marking is required in clauses, and they insert the appropriate morphemes. The variance from one child to another is very small, within a narrow range at the uppermost levels of performance consistency. Younger unaffected children do not know that finiteness marking is obligatory, and they sometimes drop these markers in their utterances. What is strikingly true of the children in the affected group is that their rate of finiteness dropping is even greater than that of younger children and that it is far from the performance levels of their age peers.

A clinically relevant way to compare the affected children with their age peers is to evaluate the identification rates for individual children. This analysis yields levels of sensitivity and specificity, wherein sensitivity is the rate of identification of true cases (i.e., children in the affected group) and specificity is the rate of identification of true noncases (i.e., children in the control group). For this purpose, we calculated a composite score, collapsing across the different measures of tense marking morphemes (TNS). As can be seen in figure 14.2, if the cut-off is set at 80% correct, 97% (30 of 31) of the true cases are identified correctly, and 97% (36 of 37) of the true noncases are identified. These are very high levels of specificity and selectivity, indicating accurate classification of the children according to diagnostic categories.

Several important conclusions can be drawn. Tense marking is a robust clinical marker for young children who have SLI and meet the clinical profile studied here. Performance in this domain is low for affected children and high for unaffected age peers, a pattern desirable for an effective diagnostic marker. Furthermore, this grammatical difference exceeds the grammatical delay associated with younger children at equivalent utterance lengths, suggesting that the problem is more than a simple delay of early language skills.

Comparison of Preschool SLI Children and Normal Controls in Non-Tense Marking Morphemes

Perhaps the morphological difficulties of children with SLI should not be thought of as specific to tense marking but instead as representing a general-

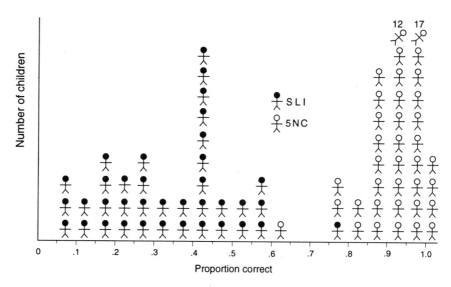

Figure 14.2 Distribution of individual children's performance on a composite tense marking score: SLI and age-matched controls.

ized problem with acquisition of grammatical morphemes. This would be one possible interpretation of an extended development theory view. Another possible alternative view is that morphemes with similar surface characteristics, such as the -s of plurals, will be affected, showing that it is surface properties, not underlying grammatical properties, that account for the dropping of surface morphemes, a prediction most clearly put forth by Leonard (Leonard et al., 1992; Leonard, 1996). An earlier investigation by Rice and Oetting (1993) reported that third-person singular -s (but not plurals) were affected (see Oetting & Rice, 1993, for further evidence of what children with SLI know about plural marking). The cross-sectional study reported here renders possible examination of the non-tense-marking morphemes in spontaneous utterances (i.e., plural -s, progressive -ing, and the prepositions *in* and *on*), and a comparison of them to the tense-marking set of morphemes, third person -s, -ed, and BE. DO appears so infrequently in spontaneous utterances of young children that it was not included in the spontaneous analyses.

The findings are illustrated in figure 14.3, which reports the findings for plural -s. Obviously, the group performances are much more similar for the non-tense morphemes than they are for the tense-marking morphemes, even when the comparison involves the -s morphemes, which are highly similar acoustically for plurals and third-person singular present tense. Children with SLI are very similar to those in their comparison groups for their use of regular plural affixes. Mean accuracy levels are as follows: SLI, 88%; 3N, 97%; 5N, 97%.

In a separate study carried out by Rice and Oetting (1993), the affected children appeared likely to drop plural affixes in only one particular context:

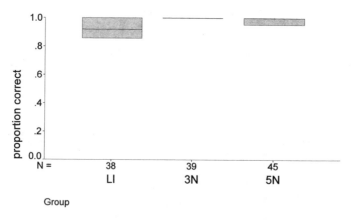

Figure 14.3 Distribution of children's performance on plural −s within groups.

that in which a plural noun is preceded by a numerical quantifier, such as *two cats*, which those authors suggested may be indicative of the way children represent number marking in semantic items, such as *two*. Whatever the reasons for the occasional dropping of regular plurals, obviously plural -s does not show the strong optionality apparent with tense marking for either the children with SLI or the younger unaffected children. Furthermore, this finding holds for progressive -*ing* and the prepositions *in* and *on* as well. This leads to the following conclusion: By age 5, children's performance on plurals, prepositions, and progressives is not likely to differentiate affected from unaffected children. A further implication is that a generalized measure of morpheme performance, summarized across morphemes, is not likely to reveal affectedness, a point that will come up again in subsequent discussions.

An important part of the analyses carried out in the studies summarized here is detailed investigation of the records for possible errors. The extended optional infinitive account predicts that errors of application and form choice will not appear (see Rice et al., 1995; Rice & Wexler, 1996c; and Wexler, 1996, for detailed discussions of these predictions). Children's attempts to apply affixes or to insert finiteness marking in non-finiteness-carrying sentence positions (as in the errors illustrated in examples 7b and 8b), would suggest that they do not know the underlying sentence configurations. The extended optional infinitive account posits that the children do know where finiteness markers can appear in sentences. An alternative possibility is that, because of faulty input-processing mechanisms, they are confused as to the possible location of an affix. Presumably because they do not hear or process the incoming information, under this explanation they would have to make some guesses as to where a morpheme may appear.

The evidence shows that children with SLI and the control children seldom make errors of misapplication. For the affected children, the error rate is 1% to 2%; for the control groups, it is 0.5%. The conclusion is that application of the tense-marking morphemes is highly constrained by syntactical knowledge.

Another possible kind of error can be seen in the use of BE and DO. Children could be confused about which form of BE goes with which subject, in which case they would make errors such as illustrated in example 11:

(11)   a.   *I is happy.
        b.   *She am happy.
        c.   *They is happy.

The extended optional infinitive account predicts that children will know subject-verb agreement (i.e., that they will know that if a form of BE is in the surface structure, it will be the form specified by the person and number features carried by the subject). Even affected children who drop BE forms frequently will know this; the evidence strongly supports this prediction. The group means for correct form choice are as follows: SLI, 89%; 3N, 91%; 5N, 94%. Clearly, although the affected children do not know that BE must appear in such utterances as those in examples 3a and 4a, at the same time they know a lot about the underlying paradigm of forms assigned to subject person and number and about the need to choose the form of BE that is required for subject-verb agreement. That is to say, the paradigm is available, and their choice of forms is governed by the paradigm. As will be argued further, the robustness of the paradigm would be rather mysterious if we assume that the children have faulty input-processing mechanisms.

Persistence of Tense-Marking Deficits in SLI Children

Findings from other laboratories have reported that past-tense marking is not mastered fully by individuals who have SLI and are elementary school age or older (Bishop, 1994; Marchman & Weismer, 1994; Tomblin, 1994; Ullman & Gopnik, 1994; King et al., 1995; Oetting et al., 1995). What have been unknown are the developmental trajectory in this part of the grammar and the way in which multiple morphemes change over time. The extended optional infinitive framework generates the prediction that the set of morphemes that mark grammatical tense should cohere over time and should show—both as a set and individually—protracted slower development for affected children.

As we followed the children in the longitudinal study, we were impressed with how long the extended optional infinitive stage persists. This is evident is growth curve data shown in figure 14.4, which illustrates the development of children's performance on the experimental probe task for the -s third-person singular present-tense affix. In this figure, the 3N group is shown in the dotted line to the left, over the time from 3 to 5 years, when this group overlaps with the first round of data available for the 5N group, which is shown in the uppermost dashed line on the right, from 5 to 7 years (when

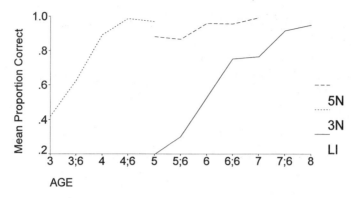

Figure 14.4 Third person −s probe data: growth curves per group.

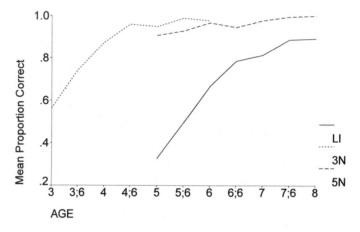

Figure 14.5 Composite tense: growth curves per group.

data collection ended for this variable because of ceiling effects of performance). The SLI group is the solid line on the right side, far below the 5N comparison group, for ages 5 to 8. What is striking in these data is the fact that the affected children's low performance on third-person -s persists throughout this time of measurement.

Growth curve statistical analyses (Rice et al., unpublished manuscript) yielded the following conclusions. First, similar patterns of growth were evident for each of the morphemes in the tense-marking set. For this reason, the findings can be summarized as a composite tense measure, collapsed across the individual measures, as is shown in figure 14.5. Clearly, the younger 3N group achieves mastery in less time than does the SLI group. The time from 36 to 48 months in unaffected children is the period in which they rapidly adjust the optionality of tense marking to the fully obligatory status expected of the adult grammar, and this is fully achieved prior to school entry. On the other hand, for the sample of affected children, as a group their mean performance levels lag far behind those of the unaffected children. Even though they are 8 years old at the last time of measurement, they do not consistently insert tense marking in obligatory contexts.

Although the rates of acquisition differ for the affected children, in other and important ways they are similar to those of their younger controls. For both groups of children, much of the growth curve shows steady change over time (i.e., linear components) and times of uneven acceleration (i.e., nonlinear components), and the overall patterns of change look highly similar. Thus, the underlying mechanisms for change probably are very much alike.

What accounts for the observed patterns of change? To explore this question, we examined four different predictors measured at the first time of data collection (Rice et al., unpublished manuscript): the children's nonverbal intelligence performance and their performance on a picture vocabulary test; their mean length of utterance (as a simple index of general language growth); and their mother's educational level (as a simple indicator of the richness of maternal input in the home). The outcomes showed that the only significant predictor was the child's initial mean length of utterance. Thus, children whose mothers are better educated are not necessarily more likely to show faster acquisition of these morphemes, nor do children with higher vocabulary levels or nonverbal intelligence scores have an advantage. In fact, even when the mean length of utterance is included in the predictor set, only 1% of the variance in grammatical growth is explained. This means that the change over time in this set of morphemes is driven by factors outside the domain of nonverbal intelligence, vocabulary size, mother's education, or length of sentences. Thus, although the exact mechanisms driving the emergence of this part of the grammar are unknown, they seem to be similar for affected and younger unaffected children and not part of a general trajectory of growth in other cognitive and linguistic domains.

Evidence of Extended Optional Infinitive Stage in Williams Syndrome Children

Perhaps an extended optional infinitive stage is characteristic of any condition in which language delay is apparent. This would be interesting to know because, if this is true, it would suggest that tense marking is one symptom of children whose language emerges late and follows a slow trajectory of acquisition. Perhaps this symptom may emerge anytime in the presence of risk for language development, which could be intellectual limitations, hearing loss, or differences in the integrity of the nervous system.

Children with Williams syndrome present interesting comparison profiles. These children are known to have significant intellectual limitations and to have a late appearance of language. By adolescence and young adulthood, however, their grammatical abilities are strong relative to their general cognitive abilities. Possibly, given their early language delay, children with Williams syndrome also show tense as a clinical marker.

Table 14.2 Group descriptors for the comparison of children with specific language impairment (SLI), children with Williams syndrome (WMS), and unaffected children (N)

| | Group | | | |
	SLI	3N	5N	WMS
Mean length of utterance	3.48	3.57	4.53	3.35
Intelligence testing	96	109	106	60
Chronological age (in months)	58	36	60	91
Third-person −s spontaneous	35%	61%	88%	83%
−ed Past spontaneous	22%	48%	92%	85%
BE spontaneous	47%	70%	96%	91%

In a recent study (Rice et al., unpublished manuscript), we examined a sample of children who had a diagnosis of Williams syndrome and whose language development was at a general level equivalent to the children with SLI in the cross-sectional Rice and Wexler sample (1996b). We identified Williams syndrome children whose mean length of utterances were equivalent to the children with SLI. This allowed for comparison of the Williams syndrome children, the children with SLI, the 3N group, and the 5N group. As shown in table 14.2, the first three groups were at equivalent mean length of utterance levels. The groups varied in cognitive performance, with the children in the SLI and normal control groups within normative range and the children in the Williams syndrome group in the range of intellectual deficits. Also, the groups varied in chronological age, with the Williams children older than those in the other three groups.

The findings show that the children with Williams syndrome do not have selective difficulty with tense marking, as reported in table 14.2. In their spontaneous samples, their mean percentage of use in obligatory contexts for third-person -s was 83%; for -ed, it was 85%; for BE, it was 91%. In this part of their grammar, their performance exceeds that of those in the SLI group and that of the younger 3N children at equivalent language levels (and pairwise comparisons carried out with t-tests yielded statistically significant differences: $P < .05$). This suggests that tense marking is not a concomitant by-product of the utterance expansions measured by mean length of utterance but instead is to some degree independent of utterance length. This is not surprising within the extended optional infinitive framework because finiteness marking is not defined in terms of utterance length.

Finally, the children with Williams syndrome perform at levels of accuracy that do not differ from those in the 5N group. Essentially, the Williams syndrome children with the much lower cognitive abilities are functioning very near adult levels on tense marking. The conclusion is that children with Williams syndrome know that tense marking is obligatory at a time in which their general language development is comparable to that of children who have SLI and do not know that tense marking is obligatory. Whatever the source of the early language delay of children with Williams syndrome, it does not seem to show the same grammatical properties as does the early language delay of children with SLI.

Considered as a collection of findings, the evidence strongly points in the direction of grammatical tense as a clinical marker for SLI. This symptom is proving to be highly informative. It shows a selective difference in affected children's grammar relative to the adult grammar, not unlike what is seen in younger unaffected children. Morphemes unrelated to tense appear not to be affected, at least not beyond the delays attributable to the initially slow emergence of language, a pattern of findings that points away from a general problem of morphological acquisition. For the affected children, this part of the grammar can remain unadultlike for a very protracted period. Change over time shows similar patterns across tense-marking morphemes and shows similar trajectories for affected and unaffected children, although the affected children trail behind the younger controls to a significant degree. Finally, change in this domain seems to be driven by relatively specific factors, independent of general intelligence, vocabulary development, or environmental differences linked to mother's education.

Elsewhere, Rice and Wexler propose that an extended optional infinitive stage is a strong candidate as a phenotype for an inherited language disorder, a phenotype involving a slowly maturing linguistic system (Rice & Wexler, 1996c; Rice, 1997; see Gilger, 1996; Tomblin, 1996; and chapter 15 for relevant reviews of genetic bases of language impairments). The possibility of a genetic contribution to an extended optional infinitive stage is supported by a recent study (Rice et al., 1997), which shows that, for the children in the study summarized here (Rice and Wexler, 1996b), the reported occurrence of speech and language impairments in the family members of these children is higher than that in the families of the control children. For example, for the affected children, the rate of reported positive histories for fathers is 29%, compared to 9% for those in controls; for brothers, 26% versus 3%; for sisters, 29% versus 4%. Thus, seemingly, an extended optional infinitive stage very likely could run in families (or at the very least, families with a child with this symptom are also very likely to have other individuals with speech-language impairments).

A final and important characteristic of this symptom is that it appears in a generally very robust grammatical system. That is to say, children who have SLI and show an extended optional infinitive stage know a great deal about the adult grammar, and much of this knowledge is apparent in the sentences they generate. Their general language acquisition mechanisms are very, very robust, probably in much the same way as are those seen in unaffected children. In this regard, the extended optional infinitive account is similar to the position of other scholars who assume that the underlying grammatical competence is intact (Bishop, 1994; Leonard, 1996). What is distinctive about the extended optional infinitive account is the conclusion that tense marking is a selective area of the grammar not fully specified for children with SLI.

The new findings with the Williams syndrome children support the possibility that tense as a clinical marker may be selective for children with SLI, the import of which is discussed later.

RELATION OF AUDITORY PROCESSING DEFICITS TO EXTENDED OPTIONAL INFINITIVE STAGE

A very different view of the language impairments of children with SLI has been put forth by Tallal et al., (1996): an auditory processing deficit account of language impairments. Because the auditory processing deficit account is a strong version of a perspective referred to earlier as extended development theory plus processing constraints and because this view is important in current scientific forums, it is worth close consideration. More importantly (for the purposes of this chapter), a critical examination of the auditory-processing deficit account in terms of the findings of the extended optional infinitive account will help to clarify the ways in which a grammatical approach to SLI can contribute to our understanding of the phenomenon.

According to the auditory-processing deficit account of Tallal et al. (1996), the surface grammatical symptoms of language impairment arise because a certain kind of

"basic temporal processing deficit may disrupt the normal sharpening of neurally represented phonetic prototypes for the native language in L[anguage] L[earning] I[mpaired] children, resulting in a cascade of negative effects on subsequent receptive and expressive language development (p. 82).

... the symptomology of L[anguage] L[earning] I[mpaired] children may reflect primarily bottom-up processing constraints rather than a defect in linguistic competence per se. (p. 83)

The auditory processing deficits, some claim, cause affected children to have difficulty in differentiating between syllables such as [ba] and [da]. Such a problem is thought to extend to the contrast between uninflected and inflected words, such as *pack* and *packed*, wherein the interpretation is that affected children cannot perceive these two as unique words (i.e., that they literally perceive *pack* and *packed* as the same; see Travis, 1996).

Although this account has much appeal, it is unconvincing as an account of language acquisition or language impairment of the form demonstrated earlier in this chapter. Other scholars have challenged this interpretation of auditory temporal perception deficits (Studdert-Kennedy & Mody, 1995) and have questioned whether an auditory processing deficit of the kind proposed by Tallal could account for children's language impairments (Leonard, 1987). We take up the argument by assuming that the auditory-processing deficit account is true, projecting some predictions for observed morphology (keep in mind that the advocates for auditory-processing deficit account have not specified such morphological predictions) and evaluating the extent to which the predictions concur with foregoing evidence for the observed grammatical deficits of children with SLI.

What are the predictions of an auditory-processing deficit account? To simplify matters, the predictions examined here are limited to the English language, even though English provides a greatly reduced set of relevant evidence and the challenges to the auditory-processing deficit account become greater if evidence from other languages is brought to bear. If children literally do not hear the difference between *pack* and *packed*, what are the plausible consequences? If they have "bottom-up processing constraints" of this sort, how can they arrive at a "language competence?"

We propose the following predictions generated by the auditory-processing deficit account. First, *children will be likely to omit surface morphology*. As we can see from the evidence already presented this prediction would capture some (but not all) of the evidence. It would account for why children drop tense-marking morphemes but not for why they do not drop all morphemes with similar surface properties. In short, this prediction overpredicts morpheme dropping to include both morphemes that are not dropped (e.g., plural *-s* and prepositions and *-ing*) and those that are. A way would have to be found to constrain the application of the "bottom-up processor" such that it allows some morphological information to be processed but screens out other instances even when the surface acoustic properties are similar.

Also, *children will be likely to make errors of application when they do attempt to insert morphemes*. If the input is filtered or masked in a way to lead a child to confuse *pack* versus *packed*, how is a child to know that the affix can appear in some contexts but not in others? For instance, in examples 7b and 8b, we see that affixes cannot be attached to every occurrence of the lexical verb. What would block such errors from occurring? We can see from the evidence that these errors are very unlikely. Thus, this prediction also is overly broad, predicting errors that do not appear. A related possible error does not appear. Children, even those with SLI, do not seem to apply third-person *-s* when they mean *-ed* (i.e., no evidence corroborates that children confuse present and past tense affixes). How could they sort this out if they were getting faulty information about the third-person *-s* and *-ed*? If children heard *walk*, *walks*, and *walked* as interchangeable, how would they ever determine when the *-s* is required rather than the *-ed*? Again, the prediction is overly broad and predicts errors that do not happen.

Further, *children will be likely to confuse the surface forms required for subject-verb agreement*. Consider the third-person *-s* of *walks*. In children's speech, this morpheme appears with third-person singular subjects, as in "He walks," and only rarely (at best) is applied to subjects that are not third-person singular, such as "I walks," a generalization that holds both for children with SLI and for unaffected children. What would block this application to subjects other than third-person singular? Consider the forms of *BE*. Children who have limited or filtered input processing of *BE* might be expected sometimes to hear the *'s* in sentences such as example 3a when pronounced as "Patsy's walking" and sometimes not to hear them. So, they would be expected to drop the contracted form more frequently than an uncontracted form, such as appears in such sentences as "She is?" That, however, is not the case. Detailed analyses reported by Cleave and Rice (1997) clearly, show that *BE* in the contracted context is more likely to appear in the sentences than in the uncontracted context. Now, let us go further and examine how children who may not detect the appearance of a form of *BE* will be able clearly to separate *is, am, are* and to pair them with the subjects with which they appear. The problem is: How could children build a paradigm for subject-verb agreement and tense marking? One would expect considerable confusion of form choice as children were trying to sort out whether *'s* can go with both *I* and *he*. If children cannot consistently hear the final sounds for *I'm* and *he's*, how are they to know that *'m* is restricted to *I*?

Additionally, *children will learn morphemes one at a time, without knowing the common functions of a diverse set of surface forms.* Presumably, children who sometimes hear morphemes and sometimes do not will experience difficulty in noticing that third person *-s* appears in the same syntactical contexts as does *-ed*, and that if *BE* appears, *DO* cannot. Finiteness markers follow distributional rules such that they can appear in certain places in the syntax, but only one of the small set of finiteness markers can appear at a time, and if one is present, it blocks the appearance of others. If children cannot consistently detect the presence of these forms, how will they come to know their syntactical functions? How will they come to know the small set of morphemes that shares the grammatical function of finiteness marking and the fact that it does not include, for example, *in* or *ing*? Again, how will they come to know that if one appears, another is blocked? As with the other predictions, this prediction falsely expects children to make such errors as "*He is does running" or "*He is makes paper" or "*I is makes paper" and so forth. Such errors do not appear.

Finally, *children will not know the deep syntactical processes that interact with morphology to produce inflectional patterns.* Children know that a set of morphemes shares the property of finiteness marking, as is evident in their use of third-person *-s, -ed, BE* and *DO* and in the near-perfect avoidance of errors in their application. Evidence also suggests that they know the syntactical processes that interact with morphology. For example, in English, children must learn that *DO* is inserted when the lexical verb cannot raise (i.e., move to the left in the sentence). This happens when *not* appears, as in example 12a following:

(12) a. Patsy does not fly.
      b. *Patsy flies not.
      c. *Patsy does not flies.

This is a property of English unlike that of many other languages, such as French, where the lexical verb can raise. As indicated in example 12b, this option is not grammatical in English. Children must know that *DO* is inserted. Furthermore, they must know that when *DO* is inserted, finiteness marking shifts to the *DO*. As illustrated in example 12c, the lexical verb cannot carry the affix if auxiliary *DO* is inserted. If children cannot hear the difference between *fly* and *flies* or between *do* and *does*, how are they ever to sort out the relationships with *DO* and negation? Yet young children (and children with SLI) do in fact generate sentences that show that they know these relationships.

The conclusion to be drawn is clear: An auditory-processing deficit account predicts omissions that do not occur and errors that do not happen; presents a piecemeal approach to grammar instead of the finely tuned distributional regularities that are evident in the use of finiteness marking; and results in an impoverished sentence formulation process instead of the complex inter-related morphosyntax that is evident. Understanding how children with an auditory-processing deficit of this sort could arrive at a coherent form of the adult grammar is difficult.

IMPLICATIONS FOR COGNITIVE NEUROSCIENCE AND NEURODEVELOPMENTAL DISORDERS

The focus of this chapter has been a careful analysis of the grammatical symptomatology of a well-specified clinical group of children having a diagnosis of SLI. What is revealed is a group of grammatical characteristics shown to occur in an extended optional infinitive stage of development. At the core of the extended optional infinitive model, according to the theoretical framework, is an incomplete knowledge of the obligatory property of tense marking. In this chapter and elsewhere, we argued that these findings point clearly toward a specific grammatical limitation. Alternative accounts that put the source of limitation outside the grammar, such as the aforementioned auditory-processing deficit account, do not provide a satisfactory account of what is known and not known by children with SLI, in part because such accounts tend to overpredict errors and omissions. The grammatical limitations evident in the extended optional infinitive grammar are highly constrained, in terms of linguistic function, and at the same time are generalized across different surface forms. The most parsimonious account of these patterns, we argue, is one that recognizes the grammatical properties and processes involved.

What implications do these conclusions present to cognitive neuroscience and the study of neurodevelopmental disorders? As noted earlier, a long-standing issue is the relationship between language acquisition and more general cognitive processes, such as those measured by nonverbal intelligence testing. Because the intellectual development of children with SLI meets normative expectations, we assume that general intellectual limitations do not contribute to the extended optional infinitive stage. This assumption is certainly not universally held; Johnston (1994), among others, argued that children with SLI show differences from control children in a variety of cognitive tasks. Johnston also acknowledged the limitations of this viewpoint. Paramount among them is that the nature of the underlying deficits is unknown, as is the way in which those deficits would account for the surface symptomology of language impairment.

The previously reported natural experiment comparison of the sample of children having SLI with the sample of children with Williams syndrome brings new evidence not obtainable in experimental manipulations nor in clinical versus normative control comparisons. In this comparison, the two clinical groups yield complementary profiles regarding cognitive and morphosyntactic competencies. The Williams syndrome children are surprisingly consistent in tense marking, almost at adult grammar levels, even though their intellectual competencies are far below those of their comparison group of children with SLI. On the other hand, the children with SLI are surprisingly inconsistent in tense marking, given their intellectual competencies and their chronological age. At the very least, the performance of the two clinical groups indicates that the relationship between general intellectual development of the sort measured by intelligence tests and children's morphosyntactical development is not a direct, positive association. Children can have strong morphosyntax with limited intellectual ability; an extended optional infinitive stage is evident in children who have normative levels of intellectual development. What is suggested is that an extended optional infinitive stage is not caused by an intellectual factor missing in the children with SLI but evident in the Williams syndrome children. Instead, tense marking seemingly can be either strong or weak, at either midrange or lowrange of intellectual aptitude. Note that this conclusion also is congruent with the result of the growth curve analyses reported earlier, which showed no predictive effect for nonverbal intelligence for either the children with SLI or the younger control children.

Further group comparisons of the natural experiment sort could further clarify the extent to which the grammatical symptomology of SLI (i.e., the extended optional infinitive stage) appears in other groups of children known to have a late emergence of language and subsequent language impairment. For example, it would be interesting to know whether children whose primary impairments are social-affective disorders also would manifest an extended optional infinitive stage. Such a comparison would help to clarify the relationship between fundamental social-affective development and grammatical development.

The natural experiment comparisons have proved to be a very informative scientific strategy for sorting out the role of factors inherently confounded in nature; see the comparisons of individuals with Down syndrome and individuals with Williams syndrome in chapter 4; comparisons of autistic children and children with Williams syndrome (Tager-Flusberg, 1995) and comparisons of autistic children with deaf children (Gale et al., 1995). However, to date the group of children with SLI seldom have entered into such comparisons. The implication put forward here is that such comparisons could be very productive in sorting out the extent to which grammatical limitations, such as the extended optional infinitive stage, are symptomatic of SLI alone or can be found in other clinical conditions as well. Perhaps morphosyntax can run, to an interesting degree, either ahead of or behind general intellectual developments or can run (to an equally interesting degree) either ahead of or behind other markers of general linguistic development (e.g., the mean length of utterance) as suggested by the growth curve analysis of the children with SLI and by the comparison to the children with Williams syndrome. Strategic comparisons across selected clinical populations would be crucially significant in determining the ways in which morphosyntax is represented in the mind and its associated neural and cortical pathways.

Another major implication derives from the fact that careful specification of the grammatical symptomatology of SLI is essential for evaluating possible etiological factors. As described, when children drop grammatical forms, it could be because they have problems with speech and pronunciation or because they do not realize that grammatical forms must appear in the surface structure of clauses. Sorting out which level of performance is involved requires at the very least, checking to see whether the first level of speech pronunciation could be implicated. If the method of characterizing a given sample of children is not clear, an investigator could arrive at erroneous conclusions about causal factors.

For example, auditory-processing deficits may (or may not) account for one symptom but not the other. Neuromotor deficits, for example, may be related to speech (i.e., motor) performance but not to higher-order morphosyntactical representations. The phonological processing deficits known to be associated with dyslexia, for example, may be related to one kind of speech or language symptom but not to others (Catts, 1993; Lyon, 1995; Gilger, 1996; Lefly & Pennington, 1996; Smith et al., 1996; see chapters 12 and 13). The point to make here is that the standards of contemporary inquiry require careful specification of language symptomatology. In fact, careful specification is essential for evaluation of potential clinical markers for subject identification, for evaluation of possible concomitant conditions or factors, and for investigation of etiological contributions. As we move into sophisticated studies of neural and cortical processing associated with language disorders, the establishment of a clear sense of the pertinent dimensions of language is imperative. Just as we would not confuse a motor balance problem with epilepsy, we should not confuse speech production with morphology or confuse grammatical affixes with morphosyntax.

One conclusion to be drawn from the evidence and arguments presented here is that behavioral scientists who want to understand conditions of language impairment can profit from considering the insights of contemporary linguistics. Global characterizations of language aptitude are not as illuminating as are carefully specified distinctions, and such distinctions are to be found in the current models and descriptions of the human linguistic capacity and the essential features of a given language. If we are to move to a stage of inquiry in which we can meaningfully compare linguistic performance with genetic material and brain functioning, precision is essential in all three areas of inquiry.

To return to the case study of Jay, the child with SLI: It is fitting to note that though the symptoms of grammatical impairments can be fairly specified and unobvious to a casual observer, at the same time affected individuals face pervasive and long-standing consequences that in all probability play out over their entire lifetime. Accurate description of the phenotype is an important first step toward the ultimate goals of determination of the etiology of the condition, the way it is manifest in the cortical cognitive structures and functions, and the provision of effective intervention. Because language impairments are evident in many syndromic conditions, advances in our understanding of SLI may hold the key to a better understanding of other developmental impairments. If, as many scholars suspect, children with SLI go on to comprise much of the group of children later given diagnoses of dyslexic, study of the linguistic underpinnings of SLI ultimately may yield information relevant to reading aptitude as well. Studies of these highly related disorders in a comparative manner surely will add to our understanding of neurodevelopmental disorders in general and of the ways in which cognitive abilities and impairments are manifest over the course of child development.

ACKNOWLEDGMENT

This study was supported by National Institute of Deafness and Communicative Disorders award R01 DC01803 to Mabel L. Rice and Kenneth Wexler. I thank Patsy Woods for assistance with text preparation and Esther Lerner for assistance with preparation of the figures. Special appreciation is extended to Makoto Kariyasu for preparation of figure 14.2.

NOTE

1. In this chapter, the term *BE* stands for all uses of the verb *to be* in auxiliary or main verb (copula) contexts. This would include *is* in "He is running" and "He is happy;" *am* in "I am running" and "I am happy;" and *are* in "They are running" and "They are happy."

REFERENCES

Aram, D. M., Ekelman, B. L., & Nation, J. E. (1984). Preschoolers with language disorders: 10 years later. *Journal of Speech and Hearing Research, 27*, 232–244.

Bishop, D. V. M. (1994). Grammatical errors in specific language impairment: Competence or performance limitations? *Applied Psycholinguistics, 15*, 507–550.

Bottari, P., Cipriani, P., & Chilosi, A. M. (1996). Root infinitives in Italian SLI children. In A. Stringfellow, D. Cahana-Amitay, E. Hughes, & A. Zukowski (Eds.), *Proceedings of the twentieth annual Boston University conference on language development* (Vol. 2). Somerville, MA: Cascadilla Press.

Burgemeister, B. B., Blum, L. H., & Lorge, I. (1972). *Columbia mental maturity scale*. San Antonio, TX: Psychological Corporation.

Catts, H. (1993). The relationship between speech-language impairments and reading disabilities. *Journal of Speech and Hearing Research, 36*, 948–958.

Chomsky, N. (1993). A minimalist program for linguistic theory. In K. Hale & S. J. Keyser (Eds.), *The view from building 20: Essays in linguistics in honor of Sylvain Bromberger* (pp. 1–52). Cambridge, MA: MIT Press.

Chomsky, N. (1995). *Minimalism*. Cambridge: MIT Press.

Clahsen, H., Penke, M., & Parodi, T. (1994). Functional categories in early child German. *Language Acquisition, 3*, 395–430.

Cleave, P. L., & Rice, M. L. (1997). An examination of the morpheme BE in children with specific language impairment: The role of contractibility and grammatical form class. *Journal of Speech, Language, and Hearing Research, 40*, 480–492.

Crago, M., & Gopnik, M. (1994). From families to phenotypes: Theoretical and clinical implications of research into the genetic basis of specific language impairment. In R. V. Watkins & M. L. Rice (Eds.). *Specific language impairments in children* (pp. 35–51). Baltimore: Paul H. Brookes.

Gale, E., de Villiers, P. A., de Villiers, J. G., & Pyle, J. (1995, November). *Language and theory of mind in oral deaf children*. Paper presented at the Boston University Conference on Child Language, Boston, MA.

Gertner, B. L., Rice, M. L., & Hadley, P. A. (1994). The influence of communicative competence on peer preferences in a preschool classroom. *Journal of Speech and Hearing Research, 37*. 913–923.

Gilger, J. W. (1996). How can behavioral genetic research help us understand language development and disorders? In M. L. Rice (Ed.), *Toward a genetics of language* (pp. 77–110). Mahwah, NJ: Erlbaum.

Guasti, M. T. (1994). Verb syntax in Italian child grammar: Finite and nonfinite verbs. *Language Acquisition, 3*, 1–40.

Hadley, P. A., & Rice, M. L. (1991). Conversational responsiveness of speech and language impaired preschoolers. *Journal of Speech and Hearing Research, 34*, 1308–1317.

Haegeman, L. (1994). *Introduction to government and binding theory* (2nd ed.). Cambridge, MA: Blackwell.

Haegeman, L. (1995). Root infinitives, tense, and truncated structures in Dutch. *Language Acquisition, 4*, 205–255.

Ingram, D. (1972). The acquisition of the English verbal auxiliary and copula in normal and linguistically deviant children. *Papers and Reports in Child Language Development, 4*, 79–92.

Johnston, J. R. (1994). Cognitive abilities of children with language impairment. In R. V. Watkins & M. L. Rice (Eds.), *Specific language impairments in children* (pp. 107–122). Baltimore: Brookes Publishing.

King, G., Schelletter, C., Sinka, I., Fletcher, P, & Ingham, R. (1995). Are English-speaking SLI children with morpho-syntactic deficits impaired in their use of locative-contact and causative alternating verbs? *University of Reading Working Papers in Linguistics, 2*, 45–66.

Lahey, M., Liebergott, J., Chesnick, M., Menyuk, P., & Adams, J. (1992). Variability in children's use of grammatical morphemes. *Applied Psycholinguistics, 13*, 373–398.

Lefly, D. L., & Pennington, B. F. (1996). Longitudinal study of children at high family risk for dyslexia: The first two years. In M. L. Rice (Ed.), *Toward a genetics of language* (pp. 49–75). Mahwah, NJ: Erlbaum.

Leonard, L. B. (1987). Is specific language impairment a useful construct? In S. Rosenberg (Ed.), *Advances in applied psycholinguistics: Vol. 1. Disorders of first language development* (pp. 1–39). New York: Cambridge University Press.

Leonard, L. B. (1996). Characterizing specific language impairment: A crosslinguistic perspective. In M. L. Rice (Ed.), *Toward a genetics of language* (pp. 243–256). Mahwah, NJ: Erlbaum.

Leonard, L. B. (1998). *Children with specific language impairment.* Cambridge, MA: MIT Press.

Leonard, L. B., Bortolini, U., Caselli, M. C., McGregor, K. K., & Sabbadini, L (1992). Morphological deficits in children with specific language impairment: The status of features in the underlying grammar. *Language Acquisition, 2,* 151–179.

Lust, B., Suner, M., & Whitman, J. (1994). *Syntactic theory and first language acquisition: Crosslinguistic perspectives: Vol. 1. Heads, projections, and learnability.* Hillsdale, NJ: Erlbaum.

Lyon, G. R. (1995). Toward a definition of dyslexia. *Annals of Dyslexia, 45,* 3–27.

Marchman, V. A., Weismer, S. E. (1994, June). *Patterns of productivity in children with SLI and NL: A Study of the English past tense.* Poster presented at the Society for Research in Child Language Disorders, University of Wisconsin, Madison, WI.

Newcomer, P. L., & Hammill, D. D. (1988). *Test of language development 2–primary.* Austin, TX: Pro-Ed.

Oetting, J., Horohov, J. E., & Costanza, A. L. (1995, June). *Influences of stem and root characteristics on past tense marking: Evaluation of children with SLI.* Poster presented at the annual meeting of the Symposium on Research in Child Language Disorders, Madison, WI.

Pollock, J. (1989). Verb movement, universal grammar, and the structure of IP. *Linguistic Inquiry, 20,* 365–424.

Redmond, S. M., & Rice, M. L. (1998). The socioemotional behaviors of children with specific language impairment: Social adaptation or social deviance? *Journal of Speech, Language, and Hearing Research, 41,* 688–700.

Rescorla, L., & Schwartz, E. (1990). Outcome of toddlers with expressive language delay. *Applied Psycholinguistics, 11,* 393–407.

Rice, M. L. (1993a). "Don't talk to him; He's weird" A social consequences account of language and social interactions. In A. P. Kaiser & D. B. Gray (Eds.), *Enhancing children's communication: Research foundations for intervention* (pp. 139–158). Baltimore: Brookes.

Rice, M. L. (1993b). Social consequences of specific language impairment. In H. Grimm & H. Skowronek (Eds.), *Language acquisition problems and reading disorders: Aspects of diagnosis and intervention* (pp. 111–128). New York: de Gruyter.

Rice, M. L. (1994). Grammatical categories of children with specific language impairments. In R. V. Watkins & M. L. Rice (Eds.), *Specific language impairments in children* (pp. 69–88). Baltimore: Brookes.

Rice, M. L. (1997). Specific language impairments: In search of diagnostic markers and genetic contributions. *Mental Retardation and Developmental Disabilities Research Reviews, 3,* 330–357.

Rice, M. L., Hadley, P. A., & Alexander, A. L. (1993). Social biases toward children with speech and language impairments: A correlative causal model of language limitations. *Applied Psycholinguistics, 14,* 445–471.

Rice, M. L., & Oetting, J. B. (1993). Morphological deficits of children with SLI: Evaluation of number marking and agreement. *Journal of Speech and Hearing Research, 36,* 1249–1257.

Rice, M. L., Haney, K. R., & Wexler, K. (1998). Family histories of children with extended optional infinitives. *Journal of Speech, Language, and Hearing Research, 41,* 419–432.

Rice, M. L., & Wexler, K. (1995). Extended optional infinitive (EOI) account of specific language impairment. In D. MacLaughlin & S. McEwen (Eds.), *Proceedings of the nineteenth annual Boston University conference on language development* (Vol. 2, pp. 451–462). Somerville, MA: Cascadilla Press.

Rice, M. L., & Wexler, K. (1996a). Tense over time: The persistence of optional infinitives in English in children with SLI. In A. Stringfellow, D. Cahana-Amitay, E. Hughes, & A. Zukowski (Eds.), *Proceedings of the twentieth annual Boston University conference on language development* (Vol. 2, pp. 610–621). Somerville, MA: Cascadilla Press.

Rice, M. L., & Wexler, K. (1996b). Toward tense as a clinical marker of specific language impairment in English-speaking children. *Journal of Speech and Hearing Research, 29,* 1239–1257.

Rice, M. L., & Wexler, K. (1996c). A phenotype of specific language impairment: Extended optional infinitives. In M. L. Rice (Ed.), *Toward a genetics of language* (pp. 215–237). Mahwah, NJ: Erlbaum.

Rice, M. L., Wexler, K, & Cleave, P. (1995). Specific language impairment and a period of Extended Optional Infinitive. *Journal of Speech and Hearing Research, 38,* 850–863.

Rizzi, L. (1990). *Relativized minimality.* Cambridge, MA: MIT Press.

Rizzi, L. (1994). Some notes on linguistic theory and language development: The case of root infinitives. *Language Acquisition, 3,* 371–394.

Schutze, C. T., Ganger, J. B., & Broihier, K. (Eds). (1995). Papers on language processing and acquisition. *MIT Working Papers in Linguistics, 26.*

Smith, S. D., Pennington, B. F., & DeFries, J. C. (1996). Linkage analysis with complex behavioral traits. In M. L. Rice (Ed.), *Toward a genetics of language* (pp. 29–44). Mahwah, NJ: Erlbaum.

Studdert-Kennedy, M., & Mody, M. (1995). Auditory temporal perception deficits in the reading-impaired: A critical review of the evidence. *Psychonomic Bulletin & Review, 2,* 508–514.

Tager-Flusberg, H. (1995, March). *Language and the acquisition of a theory of mind: Evidence from autism and Williams Syndrome.* Paper presented at the Society for Research in Child Development Conference, Indianapolis, IN.

Tallal, P., Miller, S. L., Bedi, G., Byma, G., Wang, X., Nagarajan, S. S., Schreiner, C., Jenkins, W. M., & Merzenick, M. M. (1996). Language comprehension in language-learning impaired children improved with acoustically modified speech. *Science, 271,* 81–84.

Thal, D., Tobias, S., & Morrison, D. (1991). Language and gesture in late talkers: A one-year follow-up. *Journal of Speech and Language Research, 23,* 604–612.

Tomblin, B. (1994, February). *Family and twin studies of language impairment. Inherited speech and language disorders: In search of a phenotype.* Session conducted at the AAAS Annual Meeting, San Francisco, CA.

Tomblin, J. B. (1996). Genetic and environmental contributions to the risk for specific language impairment. In M. L. Rice (Ed.), *Toward a genetics of language* (pp. 191–210). Mahwah, NJ: Erlbaum.

Travis, J. (1996). Let the games begin. *Science News, 149,* 104–106.

Ullman, M., & Gopnik, M. (1994). The production of inflectional morphology in hereditary specific language impairment. *McGill Working Papers, 10,* 1–38.

Watkins, R. V., & Rice, M. L. (Eds.) (1994). *Specific language impairments in children.* Baltimore: Brookes.

Wexler, K. (1994). Optional infinitives. In D. Lightfoot & N. Hornstein (Eds.), *Verb movement* (pp. 305–350). New York: Cambridge University Press.

Wexler, K. (1996). The development of inflection in a biologically based theory of language acquisition. In M. L. Rice (Ed.), *Toward a genetics of language* (pp. 113–144). Mahwah, NJ: Erlbaum.

15 Language Patterns and Etiology in Children with Specific Language Impairment

J. Bruce Tomblin and Xuyang Zhang

Among children with developmental forms of spoken language impairment are those who have normal hearing and no signs of other developmental impairments such as mental retardation, autism, or cerebral palsy and who have been provided with ordinary rearing experiences. These children present specific language impairment (SLI). They are common in the case loads of speech-language clinicians and are found in disproportionate numbers of programs for children with academic and behavioral disorders (Stark & Tallal, 1988; Beitchman et al., 1989; Bishop & Adams, 1990; Catts 1991).

Descriptions of children with SLI can be found in the literature as early as 1872 (Myklebust, 1971). Until very recently, this form of developmental language impairment was named *congenital, childhood*, or *developmental aphasia*. Benton (1964) provided a broad definition of developmental aphasia that continues to incorporate the principal aspects of this syndrome. He noted (Benton, 1964, p. 41) that

We use the term [developmental aphasia] to designate the condition in which a child shows a relatively specific failure of the normal growth of language functions. The failure can manifest itself either in a disability in speaking with near normal speech understanding or in a disability in both understanding and expression of speech. The disability is called a "specific" one because it cannot readily be ascribed to those factors which often provide the general setting in which failure of language development is usually observed, namely deafness, mental deficiency, motor disability or severe personality disorder.

The sensory, motor, and cognitive conditions mentioned in Benton's definition have been termed *exclusionary conditions*. Although the clinical construct described by Benton has persisted, in recent years within the United States, the term *specific language impairment* has replaced the term *developmental aphasia* to avoid the neurogenic implications of the term *aphasia* and its confusion with acquired language impairment.

Since 1964, besides the trend toward the use of the term SLI, changes also have taken place in the specific ways in which the construct has been defined. Most of the variation has focused on the manner in which one accounts for nonverbal IQ in the definition. Researchers and clinicians began to use the child's nonverbal IQ or mental age, instead of chronological age, as the standard on which to base language development expectations. This was motivated in part by theories assigning a strong cognitive role in language development and by changes in the diagnoses of learning disability and dyslexia, which also emphasized a discrepancy between achievement and potential. Also, normal nonverbal IQ (IQ > 84) replaced the exclusionary criterion of an absence of mental retardation (Stark & Tallal, 1981): Thus, rather than an absence of mental retardation, the child with SLI was required to show clearly normal levels of nonverbal intellectual development. The other exclusionary conditions continued to be employed as a part of the diagnosis of SLI. Much of the work that will be reported in this study uses a diagnostic standard for SLI that requires the child to have language skills of less than −1 standard deviation (SD) (on the basis of chronological age expectation) and to have a nonverbal IQ in excess of 85 without the other exclusionary conditions.

The diagnostic entity of developmental aphasia and, now, SLI is a durable notion, thus, giving it some validity. However, unlike many syndromic forms of developmental disorders discussed within this book, children with SLI present no dysmorphic features, known organ function differences, or chromosomal or genetic markers that allow us to make a diagnosis that is independent of language. On the surface, children with SLI seem just like other typically developing children except for their poor language achievement. This leads us to the question that this chapter will address, which has been a topic of concern for several years: Are children with SLI a different group of language learners who have a distinctive form of linguistic behavior and a unique etiology, as described by Clahsen (1989) and Gopnik and Crago (1991)? Or are these children most likely to be the tail end of the distribution of normal language learners, as proposed by Leonard (1987)? For those familiar with the literature on dyslexia, this question will sound familiar, as this question was posed recently with respect to specific reading impairment (Shaywitz et al., 1992b; Stanovich, 1993). A considerable amount of research bears on this topic. Rather than reviewing this literature, we plan to use this chapter to add to this discussion our voices and the data we have obtained, specifically with respect to the patterns of performance on a set of typical diagnostic language measures and the genetic basis of SLI.

PATTERNS OF LANGUAGE PERFORMANCE

Is there a profile of language and nonlanguage performance that is distinctive for children with SLI? This issue is very similar to one addressed on the topic of dyslexia in chapter 12. During the past 4 years, we have been conducting an epidemiological study of SLI in a large sample of kindergarten children living in Iowa. From this study, we have examined the language and nonverbal intellectual status of 1992 children who were selected from a larger sample of 7272 kindergarten children. Half the children we selected for diagnosis had passed a language screening test (Tomblin et al., 1996) and

Table 15.1 Diagnostic measures obtained during diagnostic phase of study

Test of Oral Language Development—Primary: 2 (TOLD-P:2; Newcomer & Hammill, 1988)
    Picture vocabulary
    Oral vocabulary
    Grammatical understanding
    Sentence imitation
    Grammatical completion
    Word articulation

Narrative comprehension and expression (Culatta et al., 1983)

Wechsler Preschool and Primary Scale of Intelligence—Revised (WPPSI—R; Wechsler, 1989)
    Picture identification
    Block design

Pure-tone hearing screening

Table 15.2 Language subtests used to compute five composite scores and total composite scores for language diagnosis

	Receptive	Expressive	
Vocabulary	TOLD-P:2 picture identification	TOLD-P:2 oral vocabulary	*Vocabulary composite*
Grammar	TOLD-P:2 grammatical understanding	TOLD-P:2 grammatic completion & sentence imitation	*Grammar composite*
Narrative	Cullata et al. (1983) narrative comprehension	Cullata et al. (1983) narrative expression	*Narrative composite*
	Comprehension composite	*Expression composite*	*Total composite*

TOLD-P:2 = Test of Oral Language Development—Primary: 2 (Newcomer & Hammill, 1988).

half had failed. Those children for whom English was not their first language were excluded from this study. Table 15.1 provides a list of some tests administered to these children, which provide the data for our analyses. For diagnostic purposes, the language measures were combined to form five composite scores reflecting three domains of language function and two modalities of language use, as shown in table 15.2. Children were considered to be language-impaired if two or more of these composite scores fell below −1.25 SD for children of their age. A child was determined to be specifically language-impaired if there was a language impairment present in association with a nonverbal IQ greater than 87 and no exclusionary conditions were present. When this diagnostic system was employed with these children, three groups were formed: those with SLI, those who have SLI and both poor language and poor nonverbal status (general delay), and those who have normal language status. Figure 15.1 shows the mean composite language scores, along with composite performance IQ based on the block design and picture completion tasks of the Wechsler Intelligence Scale for

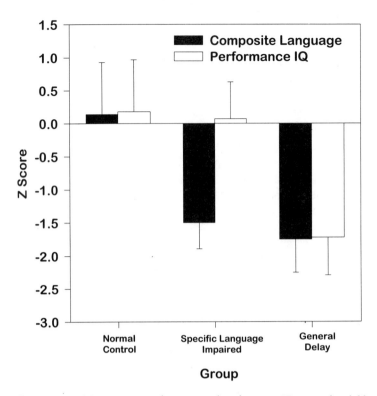

Figure 15.1 Mean composite language and performance IQ scores for children with specific language impairment, normal language development, and children with general delay.

Children–Revised (Wechsler, 1989) for each of these three groups. As expected, these profiles differ. The children with SLI had nonverbal skills that were similar to the normal language learners but had overall language skills substantially lower than the normal learners. Further, the language skills of the specifically language-impaired group were close to, though slightly better than, those of the children who had general developmental delays. These results, of course, are not surprising, because our criteria for diagnosis imposed these differences on the sample of children. Therefore, it is unreasonable to claim that because there are three distinctive profiles, there are three different groups of language users.

We can now turn to the question of whether there is a distinctive linguistic profile that distinguishes the children with SLI from either the normal language users or the children with general delay. During the past 20 years, many researchers have reported that children with SLI present an interesting deficit of grammatical morphology. This was first noted by Johnston and Schery (1976), was further confirmed by many authors (Khan & James, 1983; Johnston & Kamhi, 1984; Leonard et al., 1988; Bliss, 1989), and is the focus of Rice's recent work described in chapter 14. Do we find that there are certain areas of language that are more vulnerable than others for children with SLI? On the basis of the literature just cited, we could expect that the domain

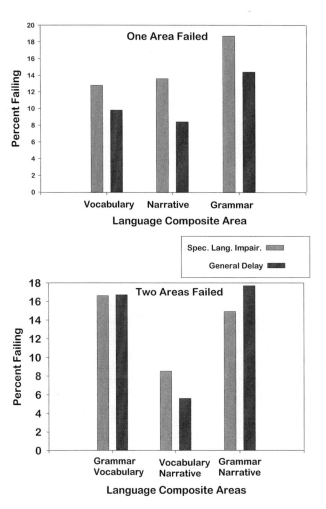

Figure 15.2 Rates of failure in three different areas of language for children with specific language impairment and children with general delay. (*Top panel*) Rates of failure in each of the three areas for two groups of language-impaired children. (*Bottom panel*) Rates of failure in each group wherein failure encompassed two areas of language.

of grammatical performance might be the most vulnerable for children with SLI and that these children would be more likely to fail this aspect of language than would the other two groups of children. Figure 15.2 displays the patterns of failure for these three domains for the two groups of language-impaired children. Children could fail in one area, two areas, or all three. For those children who failed in only one area, for both groups, grammatical performance was clearly more challenging than vocabulary or narration. Likewise, for those children who failed two subtests, they also were most likely to fail the grammatical area plus either vocabulary or narration. The pattern of failure in which narration and vocabulary were failed and grammatical performance was spared was the least likely to occur. These data

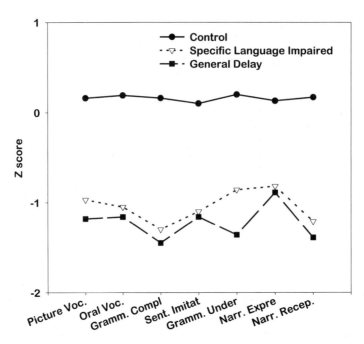

Figure 15.3 Mean scores for measures of picture vocabulary, oral vocabulary, grammatical completion, sentence imitation, grammatical understanding, narrative expression, and narrative comprehension (reception) for children with specific language impairment, general delay, and normal language development.

support the contention that grammatical performance in children with SLI is weaker than other aspects of language achievement and may support those theories of SLI that claim a grammatical deficit as a cardinal sign of such impairment (as noted in chapter 14). We also see, however, that the same pattern occurs among children with general delay. Thus, grammar may be more challenging to both groups of children with limited language development skills.

An alternate way of examining the language profiles of these children is to inspect the mean scores for each language subtest administered in the protocol. This provides for a way to compare the two language-impaired groups with the normal controls. Furthermore, by examining each subtest, we can determine whether the modality (reception versus expression) of the language task influenced the profile. Figure 15.3 presents the mean scores in z-score units for the three groups of language users across the seven language tests given to these children. These data show that the control group had a very flat profile; these children showed no signs that the grammatical tests were particularly challenging. In contrast to the normal controls, the children in the two language-impaired groups show more variability across the subtests. The poorest performance for each group occurred on the grammatical closure subtest, which requires that the child complete a sentence with a word that involves grammatical marking such as plurality (*dresses*), possession (*boy's*), or tense (*threw*). Tasks involving receptive vocabulary, sentence comprehension, and narrative recall were relative strengths for the children with SLI. The presence of a strength in vocabulary and a relative weakness in grammar, particularly morphology, has been found in several other studies (Aram et al., 1984; Stark et al., 1984; Johnston et al., 1998). These data suggest, however, that this disassociation between grammatical development and lexical development is not unique to children with SLI but may be a general property of being less skilled at language development. Dale and Cole (1991) have presented evidence that children who are precocious language learners show the opposite profile, with grammatical development exceeding lexical development. These data also remind us that children with SLI suffer from difficulties in most aspects of language and thus, vocabulary and narratives also are problematic for these children and, in fact, are only slightly better than grammatical performance. This point sometimes is lost, as some (Gopnik, 1990) have argued that SLI is marked by a very specific deficit in grammar with preservation of vocabulary. The data emphasize that theoretical accounts—whether genetic, neurological, psychological, or linguistic—that aim to explain SLI as it currently is diagnosed must explain more than a grammatical deficit.

These are the first data to compare children with SLI to a general-delay group of children of the same chronological age and a very similar language level. They show that the children with general delay closely parallel the specifically language-impaired group except that the children with general delay were worse in each area of language and noticeably poorer on the test involving comprehension of sentences (grammatical understanding). Many comparisons have been made between the language skills of children with SLI and younger normal children who are matched for language level (see Johnston, 1988, for a review). These studies show that, in most respects, the character and developmental sequence of language development of children with SLI are very similar to those of younger normal children. Thus, the character of SLI can be captured more by the notion of an inefficient learning process than by the notion of a qualitatively different learning process. This suggests that our current diagnostic methods and standards for SLI do not result in a group of children whose profiles of language achievement are unique. As will be noted later, this does not eliminate the possibility that such children exist; rather, it indicates merely that our traditional diagnostic methods do not result in such a group.

Alternate Subtypes of Language Learners

One might conclude from the foregoing data that the process of language acquisition is highly constrained and that the ways that children can vary with respect to the development of language are few. Thus, the dimensionality of language impairment is limited predominantly to the rate of acquisition. Before we can reach this conclusion, however, we must recognize that we have made comparisons only of the language of groups formed a priori from differential patterns of verbal and nonverbal achievement. Possibly, there exist distinct groups of children (with respect to their language performance) that are not revealed by the current diagnostic scheme. To explore whether alternate subgroups of language users occur within the set of 1933 children who received the diagnostic battery, we submitted to a cluster analysis the scores of these children obtained from the language tests, nonverbal intelligence test, and articulation test. A cluster analysis was used first to precluster the children into 70 preliminary clusters based on the subjects' performance on the set of language, nonverbal IQ, and articulation tests.

After this analysis was completed, a mean for each variable of each of the 70 preliminary clusters was computed. A second cluster analysis then was performed on this reduced set. The second analysis yielded seven main clusters that accounted for all but 20 of the children. In the top panel of figure 15.4, the mean test score profiles for each of the seven clusters are displayed. The predominant feature of the plots of these data is a layered pattern across the language tests and the nonverbal intelligence test, which suggests that these clusters of children differ primarily with regard to the level of language achievement rather than to substantial qualitative differences. This layered pattern is disrupted at the far right of the figure, where speech sound production skills are represented by the articulation test. Performance among the tasks involving vocabulary, grammar, and narration hung together, whereas performance in speech sound production was independent of these other three aspects of spoken language. These results should not be too surprising, as other research employing factor analysis of children's performance on subtests of the Test of Oral Language Development—Primary: 2 (TOLD-P:2) and other language and cognitive measures also have shown solutions wherein one factor accounted for the lexical and grammatical aspects of language and the second factor comprised phonological skill (Newcomer & Hammill, 1988; Beitchman et al., 1989). Currently, it is unclear whether this phonological skill pertains to sound representations or the motor abilities to execute these representations. However, these results suggest that cognitive systems subserving the speech sound skills of these children differ from those serving grammar, word meaning, and narration. Further, it appears that these latter systems of grammar, word meaning, and narration share with nonverbal cognitive skills the same pool of etiological factors. One might also hypothesize that this common set of etiological factors influences the status of children at all levels of development: That is, what makes poor language learners different from average learners also influences the differences between average and superior learners.

The clusters shown in figure 15.4 are discouraging to those of us who claim to be studying SLI, as most of these clusters do not display evidence of any special group of poor language learners. However, one cluster (C7),

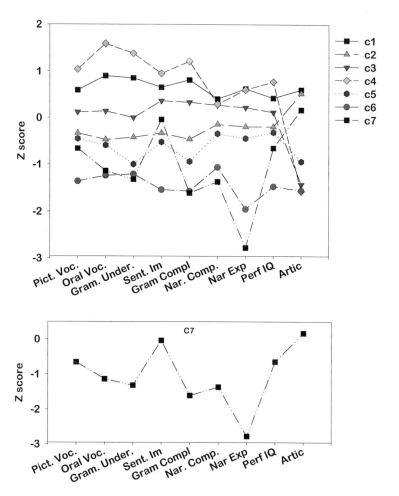

Figure 15.4 (*Top panel*) Mean scores for measures of picture vocabulary, oral vocabulary, grammatical understanding, sentence imitation, grammatical completion, narrative comprehension, narrative expression, performance IQ, and articulation for seven groups of children formed by cluster analysis. (*Bottom panel*) Cluster 7 (C7) scores.

consisting of 22 children, stands out as a possible group of children who are very different language users. This cluster is shown separately in the lower panel of figure 15.4. This unusual group of children presents very poor narrative comprehension and grammatical completion scores (a measure of expressive use of grammar) but displays normal levels of sentence comprehension and performance IQ and low but probably adequate levels of receptive vocabulary and speech sound production. Thus, unlike the other groups of children, the children in this group exhibit considerable variability in language achievement in association with normal nonverbal cognitive abilities. Therefore, these children provide some evidence for the existence of a group of children who may be considered to have some form of SLI.

Implications of Profiles

In our assessments discussed thus far, we were concerned with whether our current diagnostic scheme for SLI yielded a group of language learners who were unique as compared to other children, as evidenced by their standardized test performance. The data suggest that these children were challenged relatively more by grammatical morphology than by other areas of language but that this pattern is not unique to children with SLI and can be found among those children with general delays in language and nonverbal development. Thus, children with SLI, as diagnosed using typical standards, do not appear to be a uniquely different group of language users. Further, the cluster analysis suggested that most of the individual differences in language performance were in a single dimension concerning overall language proficiency and that only when speech sound production skill was included did groups with distinctive patterns emerge.

Hence, that a different system for interpreting these test scores would provide distinctively different diagnostic groups is unlikely. These results can mean one of two things. Possibly, our language tests are not measuring the areas of language development that will reveal the important differences among children who are poor language learners. The test measures used in this work, and most other clinical measures of language, are not constructed around linguistic models that make principled claims concerning separate linguistic modules. Thus, these tests are not the best measures for showing subtle distinctions in patterns of language development that may reveal a separate group of language learners. Rice and her colleagues are working on an approach that reflects the use of such a linguistically principled approach (see chapter 14).

An alternative interpretation of our results is that children with SLI are not distinctly different from other children who have poor language skills but rather represent a group of children who are at the lower end of the normal distribution. Thus, any account of the behavior or etiology of specifically language-impaired children is an extension of an account of the individual differences in language acquisition of children in general. This is not a new claim. As we noted earlier, Leonard (1991) has made this claim based on his review of the research and his own work. Leonard (1991, p. 68) concluded that "these [SLI] children may be different solely because they fall at the very low end of the normal distribution in ability." Likewise regarding the distinctiveness of children with SLI, Bishop (1994) contrasted in twins the pattern of concordance for language impairment under two diagnostic systems, one using a performance IQ discrepancy and one without such a discrepancy. The concordance rate was better under the system that did not require a discrepancy. Bishop (1994, p. 108) concluded that "there is no fundamental difference between children with language impairment who have a large discrepancy between IQ and verbal functions, and those who do not."

The absence of a distinctive quality of learning difficulty is not unique to SLI. In recent years, researchers studying dyslexia have expressed very similar concerns as noted in chapter 12 and by Stanovich (1993). Shaywitz et al. (1992b, p. 646) stated, "Reading disability is distributed along a continuum that blends imperceptibly with normal reading ability." However appealing is an account of SLI that characterizes it as a distinctive syndrome of unique language-learning difficulty with an associated unique etiological base, we must face the likelihood that this account is not true, at least for the majority of the children currently identified. If this hypothesis about the indistinctiveness of SLI is true, one might conclude that there is no value in asking about its etiology. We focus on this issue in the next section.

GENETICS AND SLI

Etiological accounts of SLI, like most disorders of complex behaviors, can be generated at several different levels that may be viewed as proximal or distal to the actual behavior of interest. Most of the research on the etiology of SLI has focused on sensory or cognitive explanations. These range from studies emphasizing basic perceptual processes, such as Tallal's deficit in temporal processing (Tallal & Stark, 1981), to deficits in general representational symbolic systems (Terrell et al., 1984), to deficits in general-purpose information-processing systems (Johnston, 1991; Kail, 1994). Some workers also have examined hypotheses concerned with differences in basic brain structure, revealing some evidence of anatomical volumetric differences in certain cortical and subcortical areas (Plante et al., 1991). Along with this mix of etiologically directed research during the last 10 years has been work examining the hypothesis that SLI has, at least in part, a genetic basis.

The belief that genes play a significant role in the etiology of SLI has both theoretical and empirical support. At a theoretical level, for several decades those who have adopted nativist positions about language development have argued that the capacity to acquire language must depend on a uniquely human genetic endowment. This position has been strengthened during the last two decades by advancements in a linguistic theory often called *universal grammar* (Chomsky, 1980). This theory posits that there are universal constraints on the form of human languages, that the origin of these constraints resides in special neural systems dedicated to language functions (including language acquisition), and that these neural systems are genetically determined. This strong form of linguistic nativism is not embraced by all those who study language acquisition. Many psychologists believe that language acquisition is accomplished by more general-purpose cognitive systems and, therefore, genes whose expression lead to linguistically dedicated neural systems are very unlikely to exist (Bates et al., 1991). Even these individuals, however, do not reject the plausibility that the capacity to acquire language is at least partly heritable and under some genetic influence

(O'Grady, 1987). Few researchers question that the capacity to acquire language is nearly universal in humans and that successful language acquisition requires very little of children's caregivers other than the provision of some basic exposure to language. Most would agree, therefore, that the child brings a considerable amount to the language acquisition process. The primary point of the debate, with respect to genes and language acquisition, pertains mainly to the kind of endowment for language acquisition that genes provide to the child. Is this genetic endowment related to a specific language learning and representational system, or is it associated with cognitive systems that provide the support to acquire complex knowledge structures, one of which is language?

Given that contemporary theories of language acquisition require or, at the very least, accept a role for genetics, then a genetic contribution to the etiology of SLI is a reasonable hypothesis. In fact, the belief that some forms of developmental speech and language impairments are heritable is not entirely new. Ingram (1959) noted that specific disorders of speech and language presented a familial character suggesting a genetic etiology. Systematic studies directed toward genetic hypotheses, however, are much more recent. Much of this recent work has shown that there is a familial aggregation for reported histories of specific language or learning impairments (Neils & Aram, 1986; Tallal et al., 1989; Tomblin, 1989; Beitchman et al., 1992). The phenotype used in most of these studies included speech, language, and reading problems but, in the Tomblin (1989), study the phenotype was limited to specific language and speech sound disorders. Only one study (Whitehurst et al., 1991) has reported no statistically significant elevation in the rate of language impairment among the family members of children with language impairment as compared with control families, but the former group of children were, in fact, late talkers, many of whom did not have persistent language impairments. Thus, among children with developmental speech and language impairments that persist into school age, considerable evidence points to a familial character to these communication problems.

A common feature of the studies just cited was that the status of many family members was established by historical report. Furthermore, the diagnostic entity under study was not SLI but rather speech, language, and (often) reading impairment or learning problems, with no evidence of exclusionary conditions or requirement of a normal nonverbal IQ. Thus, that SLI itself is familial, in contrast to the associated conditions such as reading impairment, is uncertain. Also, regarding these studies, Whitehurst et al. (1991) have noted that the reported positive histories in the families of the affected probands could have been biased by the inclusion of a child with a diagnosed speech problem. Recently, we examined the rate of SLI in 45 families of children in whom SLI was diagnosed, wherein the diagnostic criteria required that the child have a composite language score 1 SD below age expectation and a performance IQ in excess of 80, no other exclusionary conditions being applicable. The same standard was applied to the proband's

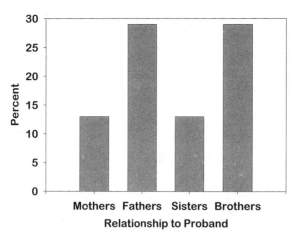

Figure 15.5 Rates of specific language impairment among first-degree relatives of children with specific language impairment who served as probands in these families.

siblings. The parents also were assessed diagnostically, using a language assessment protocol developed by us to identify adults with SLI (Tomblin et al., 1992). Figure 15.5 displays the results of this study. Even with a phenotype that is clearly more representative of SLI and using a diagnostic method that employs direct examination of the family members, strong evidence exists that SLI runs in families and that the male relatives of the affected probands are at more risk than are the female relatives. Though we do not have a control sample in this study, the prevalence rate of this phenotype among children is approximately 7% and is even lower for female subjects. These data then lead additional support to the view that SLI does run in families.

Evidence of familial aggregation of a trait or disease establishes the plausibility of a genetic explanation for the condition but is inadequate proof of a genetic etiology. Stronger evidence for a genetic etiology comes from the classical twin design wherein, if the trait is genetic, it is predicted that monozygotic twins will be more similar for the trait than are dizygotic twins. When the phenotype is a dichotomous condition (affected, unaffected), this similarity is measured as concordance that represents the proportion of twins for each zygosity who share the phenotypic state. When the phenotype can be quantified, estimates of heritability can be computed. Heritability is an estimate of the proportion of the phenotypic variance *in a population* associated with genotypic variance in that population. Heritability does not express the size of genetic influence for a trait in each case, nor can we generalize levels of heritability from one population to another. Finding high heritabilities for a phenotype in a population provides evidence that genes can contribute in an important way to the phenotype, but such a finding does not mean that this genetic effect is always great or cannot become greater. Genes and environment, particularly nutrition, influence stature. In countries in which the population is well fed, stature is more heritable than in those countries in which large numbers of people suffer malnutrition. Similarly, the heritability of speech and language impairment estimated in a population in which the children are receiving adequate linguistic input will be higher than that in a population where adequate linguistic input may not be the norm.

A few recent twin studies of specific speech and language disorders have been reported. Lewis and Thompson (1992) conducted a twin study of speech and language problems using a questionnaire. Parents of twins were contacted by telephone and were asked questions regarding the twins' communication status and the communication abilities of other family members. Although most of these twins (80%) had articulation difficulties, 12% had language difficulties. The authors found concordance rates of .86 for the monozygotic twins and .48 for the dizygotic twins; the expected greater rate of concordance among monozygotic twins than dizygotic twins supported a genetic contribution to this trait. Tomblin (1996) reported the results of a twin study involving 33 monozygotic twins and 14 dizygotic twins in which at least one of the pair presented with SLI. Concordance rates of .69 for the monozygotic twins and .40 for the dizygotic twins were obtained. Similar results were reported recently by Bishop et al., (1994), who examined the concordance of several phenotypes of articulation and language impairment in 63 monozygotic and 27 dizygotic twins who were administered a diagnostic battery. Using the diagnostic standard for SLI found in DSM-III-R, which requires a discrepancy between language and performance IQ, these authors reported a concordance of .70 and .46 for the monozygotic and dizygotic twins, respectively. When a broader phenotype was used that considered co-twins as affected if they showed evidence of any form of language impairment, including a positive history, the authors found even higher concordance rates. Thus, in all studies, a substantial difference is noted in the diagnostic concordance for speech and language impairments (including SLI) between monozygotic and dizygotic twins. Because monozygotic twins share all their genes and dizygotic twins share only 50% of their genes, this differential rate of concordance is associated with different rates of gene sharing, a fact that provides stronger evidence that SLI is genetically influenced.

The twin method provides a valuable means of examining for a genetic contribution to a familial trait. However, it has limitations. First, twins are a unique type of familial relationship and, although they provide a convenient natural experiment in which gene sharing is systematically varied, twinning also presents special challenges to language acquisition. For instance, twins are slower to develop language skills (Hay et al., 1987; Tomasello et al., 1989), possibly because of the high rate of prematurity or because of their special communicative circumstances in which they often compete with each other for the attention of the caregiver. Thus, what we learn from twin studies of language impairment must be cautiously generalized to the population at large.

Another limitation of the twin design is that, although it provides for a test of the degree to which genes contribute to a trait, the twin design does not provide information concerning the nature of this genetic contribution to the trait. A heritable trait may be caused by a single gene (monogenic), many genes (polygenic), or a single primary gene along with several other less influential genes and, possibly, environmental factors (mixed model). Also, other properties of the genetic contribution exist, such as dominance, which is the nonadditive effect of alleles at the same locus to the trait. The twin study design does not provide a means of estimating these properties of genetic transmission.

Other methods are available to identify the presence and role of genetic factors in a wide range of phenotypes, including complex behavior disorders in more typical populations. These methods provide much more information about the particular genetic mechanism involved in the phenotype.

One of these methods, segregation analysis, is a model-fitting approach that obtains parameter values for different genetic models based on phenotypic measures of the family members. The parameters relate to such things as phenotypic means and variances for persons of different genotypes and gene transmission probabilities. Different models of gene transmission contain different value constraints for these parameters. Thus, segregation analysis tests the degree to which a pattern of familial resemblance for a phenotype measured in a set of families (pedigrees) fits the expectations generated from mathematical models of different gene transmission. When a particular type of transmission is tested within segregation analysis, the null hypothesis for the relevant parameters is what is tested. Thus, if one wants to prove that a parent-to-offspring transmission of the trait exists, the null hypothesis to be tested is that there is no transmission. Rejection of the null hypothesis provides support for parent-to-child transmission.

Very few segregation analyses have been performed on families of children with specific speech and language impairment. Lewis et al., (1993) performed a segregation analysis on the pedigrees of 45 families who were selected through a proband in whom there was a preschool speech and language disorder. The phenotype being studied was a dichotomous phenotype reflecting the presence or absence of speech and language impairment, reflected primarily by a history of speech therapy. The researchers could reject models of no transmission, but they could not distinguish between a major locus model (that is, a mode of transmission involving a single gene) and one involving multiple gene and environmental factors (multifactorial model).

We have submitted the pedigrees of all nuclear and selected extended family members who participated in our family study involving direct diagnosis of family members. The phenotype being explored in this analysis was a quantitative value representing likelihood of SLI on the basis of a dis-

Table 15.3 Results of segregation analysis of 58 families of specific language impairment probands using the regressive model C of Statistical Analysis for Genetic Epidemiology

Model	Chi-square	Degrees of freedom	Rejection
Dominance	0.01	1	Not rejected
No transmission	17.17	2	Rejected
No major effect	19.33	5	Rejected
No polygenic effect	3.07	1	Not rejected
Mendelian transmission	9.51	3	Rejected

criminant analysis, and affected individuals were required to be free of exclusionary conditions. Because a discrepancy between nonverbal IQ and language was not required, this phenotype might more properly be called *developmental language impairment*, as suggested by Bishop (1994). This analysis involved pedigrees from 58 families, each selected because of a proband with SLI.

The results of this segregation analysis are shown in table 15.3. We could reject the null hypothesis that there was no transmission of the trait from parents to offspring. Thus, children resembled their parents. We could also reject the hypothesis that there was no major locus. This no-major-locus hypothesis predicted that the liability for the condition came from many independent causal factors. The rejection of this hypothesis showed that at least part of the transmitted liability for our phenotype of developmental language impairment was transmitted in a unitary fashion, as though there were a single transmitted etiological entity, such as a single gene. Thus, individuals in the family could be characterized according to a limited set of etiological types that had a discontinuous character, such as that of a genotype. We cannot claim that these types are genetic but, if they were, they could be represented as genotypes for a particular gene locus such as *AA*, *Aa*, and *aa*.

In this segregation analysis, the hypothesis concerning dominance also was supported, and those family members who were of mixed types (*Aa*) had a phenotype similar to that of family members whose type was homogeneous (*AA*). Thus, the distribution of the trait within the studied families took on a bimodal character. The hypothesis of no polygenic transmission was not rejected, the chi-square value obtaining a significance level close to .05. This hypothesis referred to a prediction that the liability was passed from parent to offspring only through a major-locus effect. Failing to reject the hypothesis of no polygenic transmission complemented the major-locus results. This suggests that whatever was the familial aspect of the etiology for SLI, it did not consist of numerous independent sources. The null hypothesis of Mendelian transmission was rejected. This hypothesis predicted that the offspring of matings between *AA* individuals would always be *AA*; among matings of *Aa* individuals, this phenotype would occur 50% of the time and, for *aa* individuals, it would never happen. If we had rejected this hypothesis, we would have concluded that the type entity identified by the major locus was likely to be a gene.

At this time, we cannot conclude that this single locus is genetic or that any of this transmissible liability is genetic. Our results provide further confirmation that a transmissible etiology is passed from parent to offspring, and it may not be in the form of many sources, as would occur in a polygenic trait. The segregation analysis does not provide evidence that this transmissible etiology is (or is not) genetic, although we do have separate evidence from twin work that suggests that it could be. This failure of the segregation analysis to provide clear-cut answers is common with respect to complex traits. The procedure of segregation analysis involves fitting parameter estimates to theoretical models for genetic etiology and, in the process, is very sensitive to distortions of the distributional characteristics of the phenotype. For SLI, measuring the same language or cognitive skills across the age groups studied in these families is not possible, nor is it possible to interpret the scores in the same fashion. Thus, the phenotypic measures obtained for different generations (grandparent, parent, child) may vary systematically and may violate assumptions such as multivariate normality and thus lead to inconclusive results. Fortunately, new approaches are now available (discussed later) that allow us to examine for genetic factors without the requirement for transgenerational phenotypic data.

DIRECTIONS IN THE STUDY OF THE ETIOLOGY OF SLI

In the first part of this chapter, evidence from our research and others' was provided to dispute the notion that children with SLI are a unique group of language learners. They do not appear to be different from younger normal children or agemates who have poor language skills and low nonverbal skills. Thus, from the phenotypic evidence, we might predict that the etiological factors that cause children to present SLI are no different from those factors that cause general delay or variation in normal levels of language achievement. The research to date concerning the familiality of SLI supports a hypothesis that complex genetic factors are important contributors to the variance in language achievement of children with SLI. Most likely, multiple factors, including multiple genes, contribute to this performance deficit. In light of our findings regarding the linguistic patterns of children with SLI, it also is unlikely that these multiple genes are unique to SLI; instead, they probably contribute to the variance in language achievement of many children.

Conditions with complex genetic etiologies are likely to be common but, until recently, such disorders were intractable to molecular genetic study. This situation is changing very rapidly, and now studying the genetic basis of complex behavior disorders is considered possible. Recently, Plomin et al.

(1994b) proposed two models for representing the etiology of complex human behavior. In one model, the complexity of the disorder is formed by the aggregation of several relatively simple diseases into one complex form. For each subtype, a single gene is the primary etiological agent and thus there is one gene for one disorder (OGOD), and the complexity is formed by the aggregation of these distinguishable subtypes. The single etiological agent here will serve as a necessary, though possibly insufficient, condition for the subtype of the disease. Plomin's group (1994b) uses Alzheimer disease as an example of such an OGOD model, because the disease subtypes (e.g., early onset, late onset) have different genetic etiologies. If a disorder such as SLI forms an OGOD type of complexity, the challenge is to find subtypes that have plausible etiological differences. As was noted earlier, few attempts have been made at subtyping developmental language impairments in general, but several of these have focused on children with SLI. The only robust distinction among subtypes involves the presence or absence of speech sound disorders and the presence and absence of language disorders; little clear evidence exists of subtypes based on language characteristics. All these attempts to identify subtypes have focused on the language and cognitive behaviors of affected children. Possibly, subtypes of SLI may be revealed in other ways, such as in patterns of comorbidities (e.g., attention deficit disorder, reading impairment).

We also may have to consider the possibility that the complexity of the etiology of SLI may not fit the OGOD model. As an alternative to the OGOD form of etiological complexity, Plomin et al. (1994b) provides a multigene model called a *quantitative trait loci* (QTL) model (also see chapter 13). Although Plomin restricts his etiological agents to genes, "loci" can simply be considered to be any etiological source influencing the trait of interest. In the QTL model, etiological complexity comes from the contribution of multiple additive and interchangeable etiological agents, each of which contributes to the variance of the trait, though none are necessary or sufficient for the disorder. In fact, these QTLs may not be uniquely associated with levels of function that are considered as disordered but rather may contribute to the language trait variance in the population at large. Here, etiological complexity cannot be resolved by identifying subtypes of the disorder, as the etiological complexity will be found at the level of the individual.

Plomin et al. (1994b) are not the only ones to discuss the notion of a construct such as QTLs. Others have distinguished between disease genes that are necessary and sufficient for a disease and liability genes that are genetic variants that increase one's risk for a disorder or disease. The difference between QTLs and liability genes mainly relates to whether the trait of interest is considered binary or is a quantitative trait. Thus, liability genes and QTLs are similar. The data concerning the patterns of language deficits in SLI support a QTL view of SLI, at least for most affected children. Possibly, the group we labeled as C7 represent a different group, in which the pattern of language deficits would be resolved according to an OGOD approach. The segregation analysis we performed suggests that risk for SLI is bunched among relatives of children with SLI. Thus, some carry one kind of etiological type (e.g., *AA or Aa*), whereas others are of another form (*aa*). The fact that these types are not transmitted in a Mendelian fashion may suggest that these types are more complex bundles of several risk factors or liability factors for SLI. Some, or perhaps all, these factors are genes that contribute to the variance in language skills of children. Because our analysis did not support a polygenic model, it appears that the number of such factors is small.

As few as 3 years ago, if we had concluded that a clinical condition had a genetic etiology that fit the QTL model, we would have effectively eliminated any possibility of learning about the specific genes involved in the disorder. This was true because the molecular genetic methods for identifying genetic loci required that the gene contribute to most of the trait variance, and this occurred only in Mendelian traits. High-density maps of anonymous DNA markers of the human genome (such as microsatellite-based short tandem repeat polymorphisms), increases in the number of known loci of genes themselves, and advances in the technology for DNA analysis have made possible the use of molecular genetic strategies to search for QTLs. Plomin et al. (1994a) have reported one such locus associated with variation in IQ. We believe that identification of at least the primary genetic factors associated with SLI is possible. We further believe that these genetic factors very likely contribute to the individual differences in language of children at all levels.

Research into the nature of SLI began under the assumption that affected children suffered language learning problems because of brain damage. Thus, these children were believed to be truly neurologically and linguistically abnormal. Increasingly, we are finding that the behavior and underlying causal systems of most children with SLI are far more similar to the normal and poor learner than we originally believed. This does not mean, however, that we cannot or need not understand the basis of their poor performance. Whether these children are at the low end of a normal distribution or are discretely different does not change the fact that they face substantial challenges in our society because of their limitations in language development. Further, it should be no more difficult or less interesting to understand the etiology of the low end of achievement than to develop an explanation for individual differences within the normal range.

ACKNOWLEDGMENT

Portions of this chapter were supported by contract NIH-DC-19-90 and research grant 5 R01 DC 00612-06, both from the National Institute on Deafness and Other Communication Disorders, National Institutes of Health. Also, some results reported in this chapter were obtained by using the program package Statistical Analysis for Genetic Epidemiology (S.A.G.E.), which is supported by a US Public Health Service Resource Grant (1 P41 RR03655) from the National Center for Research Resources.

REFERENCES

Aram, D., Ekelman, B., & Nation, J. (1984). Preschoolers with language disorders: 10 years later. *Journal of Speech and Hearing Research, 27*, 232–244.

Bates, E., Thal, D., & Marchman, V. (1991). Symbols and syntax: A Darwinian approach to language development. In N. A. Krasnegor, D. M. Rumbaugh, R. I. Schiefelbusch, & M. Studer-Kennedy (Eds.), *Biological and behavioral determinants of language development*. Hillsdale, NJ: Erlbaum.

Beitchman, J. H., Hood, J., & Inglis, A. (1992). Familial transmission of speech and language impairment: A preliminary investigation. *Canadian Journal of Psychiatry–Revue Canadienne De Psychiatrie, 37*, 151–156.

Beitchman, J. H., Hood, J., Rochon, J., et al. (1989). Empirical classification of speech/language impairment in children: I. Identification of speech/language categories. *Journal of the American Academy of Child and Adolescent Psychiatry, 28*, 112–117.

Benton, A. (1964). Developmental aphasia and brain damage. *Cortex, 1*, 40–52.

Bishop, D. V. M. (1994). Is specific language impairment a valid diagnostic category? Genetic and psycholinguistic evidence. *Philosophical Transactions of the Royal Society of London: B. Biological Sciences, 346*, 106–111.

Bishop, D. & Adams, C. (1990). A prospective study of the relationship between specific language impairment, phonological disorders and reading retardation. *Journal of Child Psychology and Psychiatry, 31*, 1027–1050.

Bishop, D. V. M., North, T., & Donlan, C. (1994). Genetic basis of specific language impairment: Evidence from a twin study. *Developmental Medicine and Child Neurology, 37*, 56–71.

Bliss, L. (1989). Selected syntactic usage by language-impaired children. *Journal of Communication Disorders, 22*, 277–289.

Catts, H. (1991). Early identification on dyslexia: Evidence from a follow-up study of speech-language impaired children. *Annals of Dyslexia, 41*, 163–175.

Chomsky, N. (1980). *Rules and representation*. New York: Columbia University Press.

Clahsen, H. (1989). The grammatical characterization of developmental dysphasia. *Linguistics, 27*, 897–920.

Culatta, B., Page, J., & Ellis, J. (1983). Story retelling as a communicative performance screening tool. *Language Speech and Hearing Services in Schools, 14*, 66–74.

Gopnik, M. (1990). Feature blindness: A case study. *Language Acquisition, 1*, 139–164.

Gopnik, M. & Crago, M. (1991). Familial aggregation of a developmental language disorder. *Cognition, 39*, 1–50.

Hay, D. A., Prior, M., Collett, S., & Williams, M. (1987). Speech and language development in preschool twins. *Acta Geneticae Medicae et Gemellologiae Twin Research, 36*, 213–223.

Ingram, T. T. S. (1959). Specific developmental disorders of speech in childhood. *Brain, 82*, 450–454.

Johnston, J. (1988). Specific language impairment in the child. In N. Lass, L. McReynolds, J. Northern, & D. Yoder (Eds.), *Handbook of speech-language pathology and audiology* (pp. 686–715). Philadelphia: B. C. Decker.

Johnston, J. (1991). Questions about cognition in children with specific language impairment. In J. Miller (Ed.), *Research on child language disorders*, (pp. 299–307). Austin, TX: Pro-Ed.

Johnston, J., & Kamhi, A. (1984). Syntactic and semantic aspects of the utterances of language-impaired children: The same can be less. *Merrill-Palmer Quarterly, 30*, 66–85.

Johnston, J., & Schery, T. K. (1976). The use of grammatical morphemes by children with communication disorders. In D. M. Morehead & A. E. Morehead (Eds.), *Normal and deficient child language*, (pp. 239–258). Baltimore, MD: University Park Press.

Kail, R. (1994). A method for studying the generalized slowing hypothesis in children with specific language impairment. *Journal of Speech and Hearing Research, 37*, 418–421.

Khan, L., & James, S. (1983). Grammatical morpheme development in three language disordered children. *Journal of Childhood Communication Disorders, 6*, 85–100.

Leonard, L. (1991). Specific language impairment as a clinical category. *Language, Speech, and Hearing Services in Schools, 22*, 66–68.

Leonard, L. B. (1987). Is specific language impairment a useful construct? In S. Rosenberg (Ed.), *Advances in applied psycholinguistics* (Vol. 1, pp. 1–39). New York: Cambridge University Press.

Leonard, L. B., Sabbadini, L., Volterra, V., & Leonard, J. S. (1988). Some influences on the grammar of English- and Italian-speaking children with specific language impairment. *Applied Psycholinguistics, 9*, 39–57.

Lewis, B. A., Cox, N. J., & Byard, P. J. (1993). Segregation analysis of speech and language disorders. *Behavior Genetics, 23*, 291–297.

Lewis, B. A., & Thompson, L. A. (1992). A study of developmental speech and language disorders in twins. *Journal of Speech and Hearing Research, 35*, 1086–1094.

Myklebust, H. (1971). Childhood aphasia: An evolving concept. In L. E. Travis (Ed.), *Handbook of speech pathology and audiology* (pp. 1181–1202). New York: Appleton-Century-Crofts.

Neils, J., & Aram, D. M. (1986). Family history of children with developmental language disorders. *Perceptual and Motor Skills, 63*, 655–658.

Newcomer, P., & Hammill, D. (1988). *Test of language development: 2. Primary*. Austin, TX: ProEd.

O'Grady, W. (1987). *Principles of grammar learning*. Chicago: University of Chicago Press.

Plante, E., Swisher, L., Vance, R., & Rapcsak, S. (1991). MRI findings in boys with specific language impairment. *Brain and Language, 41*, 52–66.

Plomin, R., McClearn, G. E., Smith, D. L., Vignetti, S., Chorney, M. J., Venditti, C. P., Kasarda, S., Thompson, L. A., Detterman, D. K., Daniels, J., Owen, M., & McGuffin, P. (1994a). DNA markers associated with high versus low IQ: The IQ quantitative trait loci (QTL) project. *Behavior Genetics, 24*, 107–118.

Plomin, R., Owen, M., & McGuffin, P. (1994b). The genetic basis of complex human behaviors. *Science, 264*, 1733–1739.

Shaywitz, B., Escobar, M., Shaywitz, B., Fletcher, J., & Makuch, R. (1992a). Evidence that dyslexia may represent the lower tail of a normal distribution of reading ability. *New England Journal of Medicine, 326*, 146–150.

Shaywitz, B., Fletcher, J., Holahan, J., & Shaywitz, S. (1992b). Discrepancy compared to low achievement definitions of reading disability: Results from the Conneticut Longitudinal Study. *Journal of Learning Disabilities, 25*, 639–648.

Stanovich, K. (1993). A model for studies of reading disability. *Developmental Review, 13*, 225–245.

Stark, R., Bernstein, L., Condino, R., Bender, M., Tallal, P., & Catts, H. (1984). Four-year followup study of language impaired children. *Annals of Dyslexia, 34*, 49–68.

Stark, R. E., & Tallal, P. (1988). *Language, speech, and reading disorders in children: Neuropsychological studies.* San Diego: College Hill.

Stark, R. E., & Tallal, P. (1981). Selection of children with specific language deficits. *Journal of Speech and Hearing Disorders, 46*, 114–122.

Tallal, P., Ross, R., & Curtiss, S. (1989). Familial aggregation in specific language impairment. *Journal of Speech and Hearing Research, 54*, 167–173.

Tallal, P., & Stark, R. (1981). Speech acoustic cue discrimination abilities of normally developing and language impaired children. *Journal of Speech and Hearing Research, 69*, 569–574.

Terrell, B., Schwartz, R., Prelock, P., & Messick, C. (1984). Symbolic play in normal and language-impaired children. *Journal of Speech and Hearing Research, 27*, 424–429.

Tomasello, M., Mannle, S., & Barton, M. (1989). The development of communicative competence in twins. *Revue Internationale de Psychologie Sociate, 2, 49–59.*

Tomblin, J. B. (1989). Familial concentration of developmental language impairment. *Journal of Speech and Hearing Disorders, 54*, 287–295.

Tomblin, J. B. (1996). Genetic and environmental contributions to the risk for specific language impairment. In M. Rice (Ed.), *Toward a genetics of language,* (pp. 191–210). Hillsdale, NJ: Erlbaum.

Tomblin, J. B., Freese, P. R., & Records, N. L. (1992). Diagnosing specific language impairment in adults for the purpose of pedigree analysis. *Journal of Speech and Hearing Research, 35*, 832–843.

Tomblin, J. B., Records, N., & Zhang, X. (1996). A system for the diagnosis of specific language impairment in kindergarten children. *Journal of Speech and Hearing Research, 39*, 1284–1294.

Wechsler, D. (1989). *WPPSI-R manual: Wechsler Preschool and Primary Scale of Intelligence–Revised.* New York: Psychological Corporation.

Whitehurst, G. J., Arnold, D. S., Smith, M., et al. (1991). Family history in developmental expressive language delay. *Journal of Speech and Hearing Research, 34*, 1150–1157.

16 Autism: Clinical Features and Neurobiological Observations

Margaret L. Bauman

Since its first description in 1943 (Kanner, 1943), autism has intrigued clinicians and scientists alike, largely because of its association with significant disturbances in cognition and behavior in the absence of obvious physical and brain dysmorphology. For many years, parenting and environmental factors were believed to be to blame for the social aloofness, obsessive need for sameness, perseverative and stereotypic behaviors, and impaired language that characterize this disorder. However, with the advent of improved neurobiological technology and with the awareness of the high incidence of seizures (Deykin & MacMahon, 1979) and abnormal electroencephalograms (Small, 1975) within the autistic population, evidence for a neurological basis for the disorder began to mount.

In any consideration of the clinical deficits exhibited by autistic children, disturbances in language development are usually the first concern and are the symptom that most frequently brings the child to the attention of a physician (Rapin, 1991). Initially, some autistic children may appear deaf, failing to respond to being called by their name or to follow simple commands. Rapin and Allen (1987) have suggested that many (if not most) autistic children have impaired comprehension of language and that some may exhibit a verbal-auditory agnosia or word-deafness (Rapin et al., 1977).

In the majority of autistic children, expressive language also is significantly delayed, and a significant proportion of these fail to develop any meaningful communication skills (Rutter, 1978). Approximately one-fifth of autistic children appear to develop language at the appropriate time, some of which development can seem to be precocious and associated with an exceptional vocabulary. However, these skills undergo regression, usually between 12 and 18 months of age, following which language development in these children is similar to that of autistic children whose verbal output was delayed from the beginning (Kurita, 1985).

Those children who eventually do develop language display a wide variation in the quantity and quality of communication patterns exhibited. Frequently, little spontaneous language is exhibited, and expressive output is obtained with the assistance of verbal or physical prompts. Some children will demonstrate rote patterns of counting, reciting the alphabet, or repeating scripts they have acquired from television, videotapes, books, or parents with little understanding of their meaning. Echolalia may be present, and children perseveratively may repeat a word or the last several words of a sentence just heard. For those children who become fluent speakers, abnormalities of prosody or the melody and intonation of speech may substantially impair communicative intent. Their verbal output may have a sing-song or monotone quality, and they may have difficulty in modulating the volume of their voice. Some highly verbal autistic children may speak pedantically to others, particularly on a favorite topic, with little appreciation of the interest of the listener. Many of these children can appear to have little need of a conversational partner, and social language often is impaired. Typically, they have difficulty in maintaining a topic of conversation, particularly if it is a topic which they themselves have not chosen. They have difficulty with conversational turn taking, do not easily establish or use eye contact during communication, and typically interpret poorly the body language, tone of voice, or facial expression of others (Rapin, 1991).

Nonverbal communication also is impaired in autistic children. They rarely use a pointing response, nor do they exhibit joint attention. Rather than gesture, autistic children will lead the hand of an adult to a desired object or obtain the object themselves (Minshew & Payton, 1988).

Though it is now acknowledged that autistic individuals exhibit a wide range of intellectual abilities, estimates suggest that approximately 75% function within the retarded range [Diagnostic and Statistical Manual of Mental Disorders (fourth edition) (DSM-IV)]. Regardless of the level of function, the profile of cognitive development tends to be uneven (DSM-IV). Many are very concrete, and even very intelligent autistic individuals may experience difficulty with concept formation, reasoning, abstract thought, and insight (Rapin, 1991). Typically, autistic children tend to have better nonverbal than verbal skills and tend to be better visual learners than auditory learners (Rapin, 1991). They tend to have an exceptional memory for details and tend to overgeneralize rules. In contrast, autistic individuals often have difficulty with the processing of information related to the integration and generalization of concepts and the development of abstract thought (Minshew & Payton, 1988). Some autistic persons have shown superior skills for a narrow range of abilities, such as calendars, calculations, music, drawing, and rote verbal tasks, despite otherwise impaired cognitive abilities (Rapin, 1991).

During early childhood, the majority of autistic children demonstrate significant deficits in imaginary or symbolic play. In the high-functioning adult, this deficit may contribute to the inability to develop generic notions in regard to abstract concepts, such as justice, beauty, or jealousy (Grandin, 1995).

Along with language and cognitive impairments, social deficits are one of the most striking clinical manifestations of autism. During infancy, autistic children may be extremely passive babies requiring little attention, or they may be very irritable, difficult to feed, have irregular sleep patterns, and resist cuddling. As young children, they appear to be socially aloof, seemingly unaware of the presence or feelings of others. Alternatively, some autistic children can be overly and inappropriately affectionate, even with strangers. They can become excessively attached to and clingy with one parent and tolerate separation poorly. Autistic children do not know how to make friends or to engage others in their activities or play. They tend to be rigid and do not easily learn socially appropriate behavior, such as initial greetings. Some basic social skills can be taught, but only rarely do they become automatic and used with total ease. The extent to which socialization abilities are related to or interdigitate with either language or cognitive functioning remains unknown.

Nearly all autistic children appear to have difficulty with the regulation of attention (Dawson & Lew, 1989). Many are easily distractible and hyperactive, rarely giving any task or toy more than momentary interest. Alternatively, others may become hyperfocused and "lock into" a task of particular interest to them, such as the computer, lining up objects, or twirling string. In this case, shifting or transitioning their attention to another activity often is difficult and leads to disruptive behavior (Kinsbourne, 1991).

Although autistic children initially were believed to be motorically normal, more careful observation has found that many demonstrate a generalized hypotonia with hyperextensibility of some of the joints. Posture tends to be poor. Though most of these children meet their developmental gross motor milestones on time, a significant proportion walk late. Gait patterns may lack fluidity, and bilateral motor coordination for such skills as skipping and cutting with scissors may be executed poorly. Some children walk on their toes, but whether this practice is related to a dysfunctional motor pattern or to excessive sensitivity on the bottoms of the feet (or both) is unclear. Refined fine motor skills, such as buttoning, controlling a pencil, or tying shoes, often are exceedingly difficult and (in some cases) are never achieved. In addition, a deficit may be possible in the ability to imitate motor movements and automatically to execute skilled motor tasks or to perform these tasks in a demand situation, suggesting the presence of motor dyspraxia in these children (Rapin, 1991). Poorly executed oral motor movements can be associated with drooling, poor articulation (resulting in reduced intelligibility), and difficulty in chewing. Repetitive and stereotypical motor movements are seen in approximately one-third of autistic children. Although the disorder frequently is termed "self-stimulatory" behavior, its etiology and functional significance remains a matter of debate.

Many autistic children appear to have difficulty in modulating the input of sensory information. Some appear to be particularly sensitive to auditory stimuli, such as mechanical noises, school bells, a baby's cry, or the subtle noises made by fluorescent lighting. Some are particularly sensitive to light touch, such as tags in their shirts, seams in their socks, haircuts, and new unwashed clothing that is perceived as scratchy. Alternatively, these same children may appear impervious to pain, failing to cry even when severely hurt. Some seek comfort from the sensation of pressure and may be found contentedly curled up between two mattresses in their bedroom. Occasionally, some autistic children also appear to be excessively sensitive to odors and others to food textures, which may result in restricted dietary intake.

NEUROPHYSIOLOGICAL STUDIES

Given the variety and complexity of symptoms with which the autistic child presents, some benefit derives from considering possible brain mechanisms that may underlie some of the clinical features of the disorder. Some of the earliest studies that attempted to address this question were neurophysiological investigations that demonstrated abnormal auditory-nerve and brainstem-evoked responses (Student & Schmer, 1978; Tanguay et al., 1982) and rapid eye movement sleep patterns (Tanguay et al., 1976). However, in retrospect, these abnormalities were found to be related primarily to the heterogeneity of the study population and to methodological factors. Subsequent investigations on well-documented autistic subjects have failed to confirm the original reports (Rumsey et al., 1984; Courchesne et al., 1985a).

P300 and negative component (Nc) have been the most common event-related potentials (ERPs) studied in autism. P300s are believed to originate from the modality-nonspecific association cortex in the parietal lobes and are thought to be dependent on the intact connectivity between this cortical region and the hippocampus and limbic cortex (Wood et al., 1984). Nc is believed to originate from the frontal cortex. ERPs are of cortical origin and depend on the brain's intrinsic processing of sensory information, not on the stimulus.

Small or absent auditory P300s and visual P400s have been recorded in autistic subjects who were required to detect random missing stimuli from a regular series of auditory or visual stimuli (Novick et al., 1979). Because the subjects were able to detect the missing stimuli, the authors suggested that the attenuated ERPs were related to a disturbance in information storage secondary to a dysfunction in the circuitry connecting the inferior parietal cortex with the entorhinal cortex and hippocampus, not to motivational or attentional factors. Further, cross-modulation studies involving both auditory and visual stimuli have suggested an impairment in information processing (Novick et al., 1979). This hypothesis was revised in 1980 when the same authors reported significantly smaller auditory P200 and P300 potentials in autistic subjects in response to pitch changes and deleted stimuli (Novick et al., 1980). It was noted that the depression in the late potentials occurred during tasks that required direct sequential comparison of auditory stimuli and was not limited to conditions in which a temporal interval must be registered. Based on these findings, the authors hypothesized that the abnormalities were not related to a dysfunction in information storage as previously proposed but to a disturbance in the processing of auditory information and that the abnormality most likely was located in the parietal association cortex. Subsequently, Courchesne et al. (1985b) noted the absence of Nc to novel visual or auditory stimuli in autistic subjects, despite normal task performance and sustained attention, suggesting abnormalities involving the frontal cortex. Thus, evidence appears to point to neurophysiological abnormalities in the parietal and frontal association cortices in autism; they have been hypothesized to be related to inefficient cortical auditory processing or to dysfunctional cortical handling of selective attention (Minshew, 1991).

POSITRON EMISSION TOMOGRAPHY AND FUNCTIONAL IMAGING STUDIES

Relatively few positron emission tomographic (PET) studies have been reported in autism. In 1985, Rumsey et al. noted increased 2-fluoro-2-deoxy-D-glucose uptake throughout the cerebral cortex, hippocampus, thalamus, and basal ganglia in a series of adult high-functioning male autistic subjects. However, substantial overlap occurred in the data between the control and autistic groups in this study. When these data later were subjected to correlation analysis, reduced frontal-parietal intercorrelations were found in the autistic individuals and were hypothesized to be related to an imbalance in mutually inhibitory neuronal circuits associated with attention (Horwitz et al., 1988). Two additional studies have failed to show any statistically significant differences between the autistic and control subjects (De Volder et al., 1987; Herold et al., 1988). More recently, Chugani et al. (1996) studied serotonin synthesis with PET in 10 normal adults in comparison with 4 adult autistic subjects. The results of this study demonstrated significantly higher serotonin synthesis in normal female subjects as compared to male subjects and increased serotonin synthesis in the autistic subjects in comparison with that in controls. These preliminary findings are intriguing and warrant further investigation.

Using (31)P nuclear magnetic resonance spectroscopy, Minshew et al. (1994) reported a decrease in phosphocreatine and adenosine triphosphate levels, borderline decreased phosphomonoesters, and increased phosphodiesters in the dorsal prefrontal cortex in a group of high-functioning autistic adolescents and young adults, suggesting neuronal membrane alteration and altered energy metabolism in the frontal cortex. The authors hypothesize that these preliminary findings may be reflective of inefficient information processing in autism.

IN VIVO NEUROANATOMY

The first imaging study to suggest a neuroanatomical basis for autism was a pneumoencephalographic study performed on 18 children who presented with retarded language development and autistic behavior (Hauser et al., 1975). Enlargement of the left temporal horn was noted in 15 cases, with some subjects showing enlargement of both temporal horns or mild enlargement of the lateral ventricles, more pronounced on the left. On the basis of these observations, the authors suggested that abnormalities involving the medial temporal lobe structures might play a role in the symptomatology of autism.

The introduction of computed tomography (CT) in the mid-1970s resulted in numerous attempts further to define brain abnormalities in autism. In 1979, Hier et al. reported a reversal of the normal left-right parietal-occipital asymmetry in 57% of the autistic subjects who were studied in comparison with mentally retarded and neurological control groups. On the basis of these findings, the failure of normal language development in autism was speculated possibly to be related to the morphological inferiority of the left hemisphere. However, subsequent CT studies failed to replicate these initial findings (Damasio et al., 1980; Tsai et al., 1983; Rumsey et al., 1988). Further CT studies focused on observations of ventricular size (Jacobson et al., 1988; Rumsey et al., 1988) without documentation of consistent abnormalities.

With the emergence of magnetic resonance imaging (MRI) technology, in vivo morphometrical studies of the brain have focused on the analysis of specific brain regions. The major focus of these studies has been on the cerebellum (following the initial reports of Courchesne et al. in 1987 and 1988) and on a remeasurement of the same cases in 1989 (Murakami et al., 1989), indicating a selective hypoplasia of lobules VI and VII of the vermis on midsaggital images in autistic subjects. However, five well-designed subsequent studies have failed to replicate these findings (Ritvo & Garber, 1988; Holttum et al., 1992; Filipek et al., 1992; Kleiman et al., 1992; Piven et al., 1992). In 1994, Courchesne et al. reanalyzed data from previously published MRI vermal measurements in 78 autistic subjects. Although the majority of the patients were found to demonstrate hypoplasia of lobule VI and VII as originally reported, a small subgroup was noted to have hyperplasia of these same lobules. The authors concluded that, because of the presence of both vermal hypoplasia and hyperplasia and the averaging of these measurements, cerebellar midline abnormalities were not detected in several of the previously reported series. However, given that only a single midsaggital section was measured, they did not address the possibility that the shape and total volume of the cerebellum, age, intelligence quotient, and other factors unrelated to autism may be significant variables. Further studies involving large numbers of carefully matched subjects will be needed before the significance of cerebellar findings on MRI can be resolved.

Other areas of the brain also have been studied by MRI in autism, including the brainstem and more recently the parietal lobe and corpus callosum (Gaffney et al., 1988; Filipek et al., 1992; Piven et al., 1992). So far, the findings in these studies have been inconsistent, and their significance at this time is uncertain.

HISTOANATOMICAL OBSERVATIONS OF THE BRAIN

Relatively few neuropathological studies have been reported in autism. In large part, this has been due to the limited availability of postmortem material for study and to the fact that, in most cases, the brains appear to be grossly normal, giving few clues to the location and nature of the neuropathology that underlies this disorder. On the basis of the clinical features of autism, and extrapolating from observations derived from clinical and animal research, a variety of candidate sites of abnormality have been hypothesized. These have included the basal ganglia (Vilensky et al., 1981), the thalamus (Coleman, 1979), the vestibular system (Ornitz & Ritvo, 1968), and structures of the medial temporal lobe (Boucher & Warrington, 1976; Delong, 1978; Damasio & Maurer, 1978; Maurer & Damasio, 1982). Despite these considerations, early neuropathological studies failed to determine any consistent morphological abnormalities (Aarkrog, 1968; Darby, 1976; Williams et al., 1980; Coleman et al., 1985).

Using the technique of whole-brain serial section (Yakovlev, 1970), the brains of nine well-documented autistic patients have been systematically studied in comparison with identically processed age- and sex-matched control material (Bauman & Kemper, 1995). All cases studied to date have shown no abnormalities of external brain structure or myelin. With the exception of the anterior cingulate gyrus, microscopical analysis of multiple cortical regions in all the autistic brains also have shown no abnormality of cortical lamination, neuronal size or number, or cellular migration consistent with the findings of Coleman et al. (1985). In addition, a systematic survey of the basal ganglia, thalamus, hypothalamus, and basal forebrain failed to delineate any differences from the controls.

Areas of the forebrain that were found to be abnormal were confined to the hippocampus, subiculum, entorhinal cortex, amygdala, mammillary body, anterior cingulate cortex, and septum. These structures are known to be related to each other by interconnecting circuits and make up a major portion of the limbic system of the brain. In comparison with controls, these areas showed reduced neuronal cell size and increased cell-packing density (number of neurons per unit volume), which appeared to be equal bilaterally. Using the rapid Golgi technique, pyramidal neurons of areas CA1 and CA4 of the hippocampus showed reduced complexity and extent of dendritic arbors (Raymond et al., 1996). In the amygdala, small cell size and increased cell-packing density was most pronounced medially in the cortical, medial, and central nuclei, whereas the lateral nucleus appeared to be comparable to controls. The exception to this profile was observed in the brain of a 12-year-old autistic boy with a history of serious behavioral disturbances but with documented average intelligence. In this case, the findings of small cell size and increased cell-packing density was less robust in the hippocampal complex, compared with that of more severely impaired subjects, but the entire amygdala was diffusely abnormal.

In the septum, reduced cell size and increased cell-packing density were similarly observed in the medial septal nucleus in all cases. However, a different pattern of abnormality was found in the nucleus of the vertical limb of the diagonal band of Broca (NDB). Compared with controls, unusually large but otherwise normal-appearing neurons, present in adequate numbers, were found in all the autistic patients younger than age 12. In contrast, these same neurons were noted to be small and markedly fewer in all the autistic patients older than age 22.

Outside of the forebrain, additional abnormalities in the autistic brains have been limited to the cerebellum and related inferior olive. In all cases, a marked reduction in the number of Purkinje cells was observed throughout the cerebellar hemispheres, most dramatically in the posterolateral neocerebellar cortex and adjacent archicerebellar cortex, with sparing of the vermis (Arin et al., 1991; Bauman & Kemper, 1996). Abnormalities also have been found in the globose, emboliform, and fastigial nuclei located in the roof of the cerebellum which, like the findings in the septum, appear to differ with age. Small pale neurons that are reduced in number are seen in these nuclei in all the autistic patients older than age 22. However, in all the younger autistic subjects, these same neurons and those of the dentate nucleus are enlarged and present in adequate numbers (Bauman & Kemper, 1994).

No evidence of atrophy or cell loss was found in the principal inferior olivary nucleus of the brainstem in any of the autistic brains, areas known to be related to the abnormal regions of the cerebellum (Holmes and Stewart, 1908). Because of this close relationship, neuronal cell loss and atrophy of the inferior olive invariably have been noted in human neuropathology after the perinatal and postnatal loss of Purkinje cells (Norman, 1940; Greenfield, 1954). In the three oldest cases, the olivary neurons were small and pale but exhibited no evidence of cell loss. In all the younger subjects, these same neurons were enlarged but otherwise normal-appearing.

IMPLICATIONS OF LIMBIC SYSTEM ABNORMALITIES FOR AUTISM

Microscopical analysis of the brain in autism has shown abnormalities that have been confined consistently to the limbic system, the cerebellum, and the related inferior olive. The findings of decreased neuronal cell size and increased cell-packing density that characterize the limbic system are consistent with a pattern of developmental curtailment involving this circuitry. This concept is supported further by the presence of decreased complexity and extent of dendritic arbors observed in the pyramidal cells of the hippocampus.

Given its extensive network of interrelated circuits and widespread connections to other parts of the brain, abnormalities of the limbic system could disrupt significantly the function of the limbic and sensory association neocortex and the reticulate core of the brain. Lesions in experimental animals involving the structures of the medial temporal lobe have shown pronounced effects on emotion, behavior, motivation, and learning, many of which effects resemble the clinical features of autism. Purposeless hyperactivity, severe impairment in social relatedness, hyperexploratory behavior, and the inability to remember or recognize the significance of visually or manually examined objects have been observed in monkeys after bilateral surgical ablations of the medial temporal lobe (Kluver & Bucy, 1939). Similar behaviors have been noted after comparable neurosurgical lesions in humans (Terzian & Delle-Ore, 1955).

Selective lesions involving specific medial temporal lobe structures, introduced experimentally in adult animals, have provided further insight into the function of each of these individual regions. In the rat, bilateral ablations of the hippocampus produced hyperactive animals with stereotypical motor behavior and unusual responses to novel stimuli (Roberts et al., 1962; Kimble, 1963). Similar surgical lesions in monkeys, confined to the amygdala, resulted in animals who exhibited loss of fear of normally aversive stimuli, compulsive indiscriminate examination of objects, and withdrawal from formerly socially rewarding situations (Mishkin & Aggleton, 1981). Further, these same animals showed a reduced ability to attach meaning to new environments based on past experience, resulting in poor adaptability to novel situations. When ablations were confined to the most medially located amygdalar structures (the central, medial, and cortical nuclei), the influence of familiarization on learning was reduced significantly (Vergnes, 1981). Further evidence for the importance of the amygdala for learning has been supplied by Murray and Mishkin (1985). In these studies, monkeys experienced a severe impairment of cross-modal associative memory after bilateral ablations of the amygdala. These animals failed to recognize visually an object that had been examined previously by taste or touch. These observations suggest that one of the major functions of the amygdala may be the integration and generalization of information that is processed by multiple sensory systems in the brain, a skill that is typically difficult for autistic individuals.

In 1991, Squire and Zola-Morgan reconsidered the hypothesized relationship of medial temporal lobe structures to memory. They noted that the severe memory loss previously attributed to bilateral combined lesions of the amygdala and hippocampus was the result of inadvertent surgical damage to the cortical regions adjacent to the amygdala, not to the inclusion of the amygdala, as previously believed (Mishkin, 1978). Thus, it appears that structures involved in the medial temporal lobe memory system include the hippocampal formation and related entorhinal, perirhinal, and parahippcampal cortices and that the amygdala is not a component of this system.

Studies in human and nonhuman primates have suggested the presence of at least two memory systems: representational or associative memory and procedural or habit memory (Mishkin & Appenzeller, 1987; Murray, 1990; Squire & Zola-Morgan, 1991). Representational memory is believed to involve all sensory modalities and mediates the processing of facts, experiences, and events and the integration and generalization of information that leads to higher-order cognition and learning. In contrast, habit memory is involved in skill learning and automatic connections between stimulus and response. The two systems are believed to be anatomically separate, representational memory depending on the hippocampus, amygdala and areas related to them, whereas the anatomical substrate for habit memory is believed to reside in the striatum and neocortex of the cerebral hemispheres. Neuropathological studies of the brain in autism have shown no abnormalities of the striatum and, with the exception of the anterior cingulate cortex, the neocortex likewise is unremarkable. In contrast, the hippocampal complex, amygdala, entorhinal cortex, septum, and medial mammillary body have shown significant abnormalities. Thus, the substrate for representational memory appears to be selectively abnormal in the autistic brain, whereas the structures responsible for habit memory appear to be spared.

Though the effect of an early disturbance to the limbic system structures is unknown, likely curtailment of development and prenatally acquired lesions in these regions could disrupt or distort the acquisition and interpretation of information. Such a disturbance in the processing of information could lead to the disordered cognition, social interaction, and language characteristic of the autistic child. In contrast, the preservation of the habit memory system could account for the need for sameness and preoccupation with a narrow range of interests and activities and for the outstanding memory for rote information observed in some autistic individuals.

Studies have suggested that these two neural systems mature at different times in both human and nonhuman primates, the habit system being functional early in life, though the representational system develops later in childhood (Bachevalier & Mishkin, 1991, Overman et al, 1992). Given this pattern of cognitive maturation, possibly a developmentally dysfunctional neuronal circuitry involving the limbic system would have little impact during the first 1 to 2 years of life. However, with development, the effect of this dysfunctional circuitry gradually may become evident, leading to what appears to be social, language, and cognitive deterioration, features frequently reported as part of the early history of childhood autism.

IMPLICATIONS OF CEREBELLAR ABNORMALITIES

Areas of abnormality outside the forebrain in autism have been confined to the cerebellum and related inferior olive. Marked reduction in the number and size of Purkinje cells has been noted, primarily in the posterior and inferior regions of the hemispheres, with sparing of the vermis and without the presence of significant gliosis. The absence of glial hyperplasia suggests that the lesions have been acquired early in development. Animal studies have shown a progressively decreasing glial response after cerebellar lesions at increasingly early ages (Brodal, 1940).

The preservation of the neurons of the inferior olive further support an early origin for the cerebellar abnormalities. Retrograde loss of olivary neurons regularly occurs after cerebellar lesions in immature postnatal and adult animals (Brodal, 1940) and neonatal (Norman, 1940) and adult humans (Holmes & Stewart, 1908; Greenfield, 1954), presumably because of the close relationship of the olivary climbing-fiber axons to the Purkinje cell dendrites (Eccles et al., 1967).

In the fetal monkey, prior to establishing their definitive relationship with the Purkinje cells dendrites, the olivary climbing fibers have been shown to synapse in a transitory zone beneath the Purkinje cells called the *lamina desiccans* (Rakic, 1971). In the human fetus, this zone is no longer present after 30 to 32 weeks' gestation (Rakic & Sidman, 1970). Therefore, in the absence of retrograde cell loss in the olive in the presence of a marked reduction in the number of Purkinje cells, likely the cerebellar cortical lesions seen in autism have their onset at or before this time.

The relationship of the cerebellar findings to the clinical features of autism is unclear. Dysfunction of the cerebellum beginning before birth may be associated with few if any neurological symptoms (Norman, 1940; Adams et al., 1984). Studies in adult animals have demonstrated both a pathway between the fastigial nucleus of the cerebellum and the amygdala and septal nuclei of the limbic system and a reciprocal connection between this nucleus and the hippocampus, suggesting that the cerebellum may play a role in the regulation of emotion and higher cortical thought (Heath & Harper, 1974; Heath et al., 1978). The cerebellum also has been implicated in the regulation of affective behavior (Berman et al., 1974) and in functional psychiatric disorders (Heath et al., 1979).

More recently, studies in animals and humans have suggested a role for the cerebellum in cognition, including mental imagery and anticipatory planning (Leiner et al., 1987) and in some aspects of language processing (Peterson et al., 1989). Further, the cerebellum has been implicated in the control of voluntary shift of selective attention between one sensory modality and another, for example, shifting between auditory and visual attention (Akshoomoff & Courchesne, 1992; Courchesne et al., 1994). Also, the cerebellum has been suggested to play a possible role in cognitive planning, a function independent of memory and most significant in novel situations (Grafman et al., 1992). More recently, studies in monkeys have established that the dorsolateral prefrontal cortex, believed to be involved in spatial working memory, is the target of output from the dentate nucleus of the cerebellum (Middleton & Strick, 1994). This relationship to the prefrontal cortex suggests that the cerebellum may be involved in the planning and timing of future behavior. Thus, a growing body of evidence suggests that the cerebellum is important in the regulation of the speed, consistency, and appropriateness of mental and cognitive processes and in the control of motor and sensory information and activity (Schmahmann, 1991). Therefore likely the anatomical abnormalities observed in the cerebellum in autism contribute to many of the atypical behaviors and disordered information-processing characteristic of the syndrome. However, the precise functional significance of these abnormalities, their relationship to the findings observed in the limbic system, and their impact on the specific features of autism remain to be elucidated.

CONCLUSION

Although science has made significant advances in our understanding of autism, particularly within the last 15 years, numerous challenges remain. Most now accept that autism is a disorder of neurological development probably occurring or beginning before birth. The most obvious anatomical abnormalities of the brain appear to be selective and appear to be confined to the limbic system and to the cerebellum and related inferior olive. Although now genetics appears possibly to play a significant etiological role, the pathogenic mechanisms for the disorder remain unknown. Future research undoubtedly will be directed toward elucidating the genetic profile associated with autism, thereby offering opportunities for prenatal and more precise and earlier postnatal diagnosis. Equally important will be the pursuit of in vivo functional imaging studies and neurochemical analysis of autopsy material, with a particular emphasis on the parts of the brain identified as being abnormal. Autism also is a disorder that offers the clinical investigator an unusual opportunity to study multiple aspects of atypical cognition, emotion, social awareness, language, and behavior from a developmental perspective, and likely, science ultimately may have a better understanding of normal development as the result of these present and future research efforts.

REFERENCES

Aarkrog, T. (1968). Organic factors in infantile psychoses and borderline psychoses: Retrospective study of 45 cases subjected to pneumoencephalography. *Danish Medical Bulletin, 15,* 283–288.

Adams, J. H., Corselis, J. A. N., & Duchen, L. W. (1984). *Greenfield's neuropathology.* New York: Wiley.

Akshoomoff, N. A., & Courchesne, E. (1992). A new role for the cerebellum in cognitive operations. *Behavioral Neuroscience, 106,* 731–738.

Arin, D. M., Bauman, M. L., & Kemper, T. L. (1991). The distribution of Purkinje cell loss in the cerebellum in autism [abstract]. *Neurology, 41,* 307.

Bachevalier, J., & Mishkin, M. (1991). Effects of neonatal lesions of the amygdaloid complex or hippocampal formation on the development of visual recognition memory. *Society Neuroscience Abstract, 17,* 338.

Bauman, M. L., & Kemper, T. L. (1994). Neuroanatomic observations of the brain in autism. In M. L. Bauman & T. L. Kemper (Eds.), *The neurobiology of autism* (pp. 119–145). Baltimore: Johns Hopkins University Press.

Bauman, M. L., & Kemper, T. L. (1995). Neuroanatomical observations of the brain in autism. In J. Panksepp (Ed.), *Advances in biological psychiatry* (pp. 1–26). New York: JAI Press.

Bauman, M. L., & Kemper, T. L. (1996). Observations on the Purkinje cells in the cerebellar vermis in autism [abstract]. *Journal of Neuropathology and Experimental Neurology, 55,* 613.

Berman, A. J., Berman, D., & Prescott, J. W. (1974). The effect of cerebellar lesions on emotional behavior in the rhesus monkey. In I. S. Cooper, M. Riklan, & R. S. Snyder (Eds.), *The cerebellum, epilepsy and behavior* (pp. 227–284). New York: Plenum.

Boucher, J., & Warrington, E. K. (1976). Memory deficits in early infantile autism: Some similarities to the amnestic syndrome. *British Journal of Psychology, 67*, 73–87.

Brodal, A. (1940). Modification of the Gudden method for study of cerebral localization. *Archives of Neurology and Psychiatry, 43*, 46–58.

Chugani, D. C., Muzil, O., Chakraborty, P., et al. (1996). Brain serotonin synthesis measured with 11C alpha methyl-tryptophan positron emission tomography in normal and autistic subjects [abstract]. *Annals of Neurology, 40*, 296.

Coleman, M. (1979). Studies of autistic syndromes. In R. Katzman (Ed.), *Congenital and acquired cognitive disorders* (pp. 265–303). New York: Raven.

Coleman, P. D., Romano, J., Lapham, L., et al. (1985). Cell counts in cerebral cortex in an autistic patient. *Journal of Autism and Developmental Disorders, 15*, 245–255.

Courchesne, E., Courchesne, R. Y., Hicks, G., et al. (1985a). Functioning of the brain stem auditory pathway in non-retarded autistic individuals. *Electroencephalography and Clinical Neurophysiology, 51*, 491–501.

Courchesne, E., Hesselink, J. R., Jernigan, T. L., et al. (1987). Abnormal neuroanatomy in a non-retarded person with autism. *Archives of Neurology, 44*, 335–341.

Courchesne, E., Lincoln, A. J., Kilman, B. A., et al. (1985b). Event-related brain potential correlates of the processing of novel visual and auditory information in autism. *Journal of Autism and Developmental Disorders, 15*, 55–76.

Courchesne, E., Townsend, J., & Saitoh, O. (1994). The brain in infantile autism. *Neurology, 44*, 214–228.

Courchesne, E., Yeung-Courchesne, R., Press, G. A., et al. (1988). Hypoplasia of cerebellar vermal lobules VI and VII in autism. *New England Journal of Medicine, 318*, 1349–1354.

Darby, J. H. (1976). Neuropathological aspects of psychosis in childhood. *Journal of Autism and Childhood Schizophrenia, 6*, 339–352.

Dawson, G., & Lew, A. (1989). Arousal, attention, and socioemotional impairments of individuals with autism. In G. Dawson (Ed.), *Autism: Nature, diagnosis and treatment* (pp. 49–74). New York: Guilford.

Delong, G. R. (1978). A neuropsychological interpretation of infantile autism. In M. Rutter & E. Schopler (Eds.), *Autism*. New York: Plenum.

Damasio, A. R., & Maurer, R. G. (1978). A neurological model for childhood autism. *Archives of Neurology, 35*, 777–786.

Damasio, H., Maurer, R. G., Damasio, A. R., et al. (1980). Computerized tomographic scan findings in patients with autistic behavior. *Archives of Neurology, 37*, 504–510.

De Volder, A., Bol, A., Michel, C., et al. (1987). Brain glucose metabolism in children with the autistic syndrome: Positron tomography analysis. *Brain Development, 9*, 581–587.

Deykin, E. Y., & MacMahon, B. (1979). The incidence of seizures among children with autistic symptoms. *American Journal of Psychiatry, 136*, 1312–1313.

Diagnostic and Statistical Manual of Mental Disorders (4th ed.). (1994). Washington, DC: American Psychiatric Association.

Eccles, J. C., Ito, M., & Szentagothai, J. (1967). *The cerebellum as a neural machine*. New York: Springer.

Filipek, P. A., Richelme, C., Kennedy, D. N., et al. (1992). Morphometric analysis of the brain in developmental language disorders and autism [abstract]. *Annals of Neurology, 32*, 475.

Gaffney, G. R., Kuperman, S., Tsai, L. Y., et al. (1988). Morphological evidence of brainstem involvement in infantile autism. *Biological Psychiatry, 24*, 578–586.

Grafman, J., Litvan, I., Massaquoi, S., et al. (1992). Cognitive planning deficit in patients with cerebellar atrophy. *Neurology, 42*, 1493–1496.

Grandin, T. (1995, November). *Autism: A personal perspective.* Paper presented at Current Trends in Autism, Boston, MA.

Greenfield, J. G. (1954). *The Spino-cerebellar degenerations.* Springfield, IL: Charles C Thomas.

Hauser, S. L., Delong, G. R., & Rosman, N. P. (1975). Pneumographic findings in the infantile autism syndrome. A correlation with temporal lobe disease. *Brain, 98*, 667–688.

Heath, R. G., Dempsey, C. W., Fontana, C. J., et al. (1978). Cerebellar stimulation: Effects on septal region, hippocampus and amygdala of cats and rats. *Biological Psychiatry. 113*, 501–529.

Heath, R. G., Franklin, D. E., & Shraberg, D. (1979). Gross pathology of the cerebellum in patients diagnosed and treated as functional psychiatric disorders. *Journal of Nervous and Mental Disorders, 167*, 585–592.

Heath, R. G., & Harper, J. W. (1974). Ascending projections of the cerebellar fastigial nucleus to the hippocampus, amygdala and other temporal lobe sites: Evoked potential and other histologic studies in monkeys and cats. *Experimental Neurology, 45*, 268–287.

Herold, S., Frackowiak, R. S. J., LeCouteur, A., et al. (1988). Cerebral blood flow and metabolism of oxygen and glucose in young autistic adults. *Psychological Medicine 18*, 823–831.

Hier, D. B., LeMay, M., & Rosenberger, P. B. (1979). Autism and unfavorable left-right asymmetries of the brain. *Journal of Autism and Developmemtal Disorders, 9*, 153–159.

Holmes, G., & Stewart, T. G. (1908). On the connection of the inferior olives with the cerebellum in man. *Brain, 31*, 125–137.

Holttum, J. R., Minshew, N. J., Sanders, R. S., et al. (1992). Magnetic resonance imaging of the posterior fossa in autism. *Biological Psychiatry, 32*, 1091–1101.

Horwitz, B., Rumsey, J. M., Grady, C., et al. (1988). The cerebral metabolic landscape in autism: Intercorrelations of regional glucose utilization. *Archives of Neurology, 45*, 749–755.

Jacobson, R., Lecouteur, A., Howlin, P., et al. (1988). Selective subcortical abnormalities in autism. *Psychological Medicine, 18*, 39–48.

Kanner, L. (1943). Autistic disturbances of affective contact. *Nervous Child, 2*, 217–250.

Kimble, D. P. (1963). The effects of bilateral hippocampal lesions in rats. *Journal of Physiological Psychology, 56*, 273–283.

Kinsbourne, M. (1991). Overfocussing: An apparent subtype of attention deficit-hyperactivity disorder. *Pediatric and Adolescent Medicine, 1*, 18–35.

Kleiman, M. D., Neff, S., & Rosman, N. P. (1992). The brain in infantile autism. *Neurology, 42*, 753–760.

Kluver, H., & Bucy, P. (1939). Preliminary analysis of functions of the temporal lobes in monkeys. *Archives of Neurology and Psychiatry, 42*, 979–1000.

Kurita, H. (1985). Infantile autism with speech loss before the age of thirty months. *Journal of Child Psychiatry, 24*(2), 191–196.

Leiner, H. C., Leiner, A. L., & Dow, R. S. (1987). Cerebellar learning loops in apes and humans. *Italian Journal of Neurological Science, 8,* 425–436.

Maurer, R. G., & Demasio, A. R. (1982). Childhood autism from the point of view of behavioral neurology. *Journal of Autism and Developmental Disorders, 12,* 195–205.

Middleton, F. A., & Strick, P. L. (1994). Anatomical evidence for cerebellar and basal ganglia involvement in higher cognitive function. *Science, 266,* 458–461.

Minshew, N. J. (1991). Indices of neural function in autism: Clinical and biologic implications. *Pediatrics, 87* (suppl.), 774–780.

Minshew, N. J. (1994). In vivo brain chemistry of autism: 31P magnetic resonance spectroscopy studies. In M. L. Bauman & T. L. Kemper (Eds.), *The neurobiology of autism* (pp. 86–101). Baltimore: Johns Hopkins University Press.

Minshew, N. J., & Payton, J. B. (1988). New perspectives in autism: I. The clinical spectrum of autism. *Current Problems in Pediatrics, 18*(10), 567–610.

Mishkin, M. (1978). Memory in monkeys severely impaired by combined but not separate removal of amygdala and hippocampus. *Nature, 273,* 297–298.

Mishkin, M., & Aggleton, J. P. (1981). Multiple functional contributors of the amygdala in the monkey from the amygdaloid complex. In Y. Ben-Ari, (Ed.), *The amygdaloid complex. INSERM symposium* no. 20 (pp. 409–419). Amsterdam: Elsevier–North Holland.

Mishkin, M., & Appenzeller, T. (1987). The anatomy of memory. *Scientific American, 256,* 80–89.

Murakami, J. W., Courchesne, E., Press, G. A., et al. (1989). Reduced cerebellar hemisphere size and its relationship to vermal hypoplasia in autism. *Archives of Neurology, 46,* 689–694.

Murray, E. A. (1990). Representational memory in non-human primates. In R. P. Kesner & D. S. Olton (Eds.), *Neurobiology of comparative cognition* (pp. 127–155). Hillsdale, NJ: Erlbaum.

Murray, E. A., & Mishkin, M. (1985). Amygdaloidectomy impairs crossmodal association in monkeys. *Science, 228,* 604–606.

Norman, R. M. (1940). Cerebellar atrophy associated with etat marbre of the basal ganglia. *Journal of Neurology and Psychiatry, 3,* 311–318.

Novick, B., Kurtzberg, D., and Vaughan, H. G. (1979). An electrophysiologic indication of defective information storage in childhood autism. *Psychiatry Research, 1,* 101–108.

Ornitz, E. M., & Ritvo, E. R. (1968). Neurophysiologic mechanisms underlying perceptual inconstancy in autistic and schizophrenic children. *Archives of General Psychiatry, 19,* 22–27.

Overman, W., Bachevalier, J., Turner, M., et al. (1992). Object recognition versus object discrimination: Comparison between human infants and infant monkeys. *Behavioral Neuroscience, 106,* 15–29.

Peterson, S. F., Fox, P. T., Posner, M. I., et al. (1989). Positron emission tomographic studies in the processing of single words. *Journal of Cognitive Neuroscience, 1,* 153–170.

Piven, J., Nehme, E., Simon, J., et al. (1992). Magnetic resonance imaging in autism: Measurement of the cerebellum, pons and fourth ventricle. *Biological Psychiatry, 31,* 491–504.

Rakic, P. (1971). Neuron-glia relationship during granule cell migration in developing cerebellar cortex: A Golgi and electron microscopic study in macacus rhesus. *Journal of Comparative Neurology, 141,* 282–312.

Rakic, P., & Sidman, R. L. (1970). Histogenesis of the cortical layers in the human cerebellum particularly the lamina dissecans. *Journal of Comparative Neurology, 139,* 473–500.

Rapin, I. (1991). Autistic children: diagnosis and clinical features. *Pediatrics, 87* (suppl), 751–760.

Rapin, I., & Allen, D. A. (1987). Developmental dysphasia and autism in preschool children: Characteristics and subtypes. In *Proceedings of the first international symposium on specific speech and language disorders in children* (pp. 20–35). London, England: Association of All Speech Impaired Children.

Rapin, I., Mattis, S., Rowan, A. J., et al. (1977). Verbal auditory agnosia in children. *Developmental Medicine and Child Neurology, 19*, 192–207.

Raymond, G., Bauman, M. L., & Kemper, T. L. (1996). Hippocampus in autism: A Golgi analysis. *Acta Neuropathologica, 91*, 117–119.

Ritvo, E. R., & Garber, J. H. (1988). Cerebellar hypoplasia and autism [abstract]. *New England Journal of Medicine, 319*, 1152.

Roberts, W. W., Dember, W. N., & Brodwick, H. (1962). Alteration and exploration in rats with hippocampal lesions. *Journal of Comparative Psychiatry, 55*, 695–700.

Rumsey, J. M., Creasey, H., Stepanek, J. S., et al. (1988). Hemispheric asymmetries, fourth ventricular size and cerebellar morphology in autism. *Journal of Autism and Developmental Disorders, 18*, 127–137.

Rumsey, J. M., Duara, R., Grady, C., et al. (1985). Brain metabolism in autism. *Archives of General Psychiatry, 42*, 448–455.

Rumsey, J. M., Grimes, A. M., Pikus, A. M., et al. (1984). Auditory brainstem responses in pervasive developmental disorders. *Biological Psychiatry, 19*, 1403–1417.

Rutter, M. (1978). Diagnosis and definition of childhood autism. In M. Rutter & E. Schopler (Eds.), *Autism: A reappraisal of concepts and treatment* (pp. 1–25). New York: Plenum.

Schmahmann, J. D. (1991). An emerging concept. The cerebellar contribution to higher function. *Archives of Neurology, 48*, 1178–1187.

Small, J. G. (1975). EEG and neurophysiologic studies of early infantile autism. *Biological Psychiatry, 10*(4), 385–397.

Squire, L. R., & Zola-Morgan, S. (1991). The medial temporal lobe memory system. *Science, 253*, 1380–1386.

Student, M., & Schmer, H. (1978). Evidence from auditory nerve and brainstem evoked responses for an organic lesion in children with autistic traits. *Journal of Autism and Childhood Schizophrenia, 8*, 13–20.

Tanguay, P. E., Edwards, R. M., Buchwald, J., Schwofel, J., & Allen, V. (1982). Auditory brain stem evoked responses in autistic children. *Archives of General Psychiatry, 38*, 174–180.

Tanguay, P. E., Ornitz, E. M., Forsythe, A. B., & Ritvo, E. R. (1976). Rapid eye movement (REM) activity in normal and autistic children during REM sleep. *Journal of Autism and Childhood Schizophrenia, 6*, 275–288.

Terzian, H. & Delle-Ore, G. (1955). Syndrome of Kluver and Bucy reproduced in man by bilateral removal of the temporal lobes. *Neurology, 3*, 373–380.

Tsai, L. Y., Jacoby, O. G., & Stewart, M. A. (1983). Morphological cerebral asymmetries in autistic children. *Biological Psychiatry, 18*, 317–327.

Vergnes, M. (1981). Effect of prior familiarization with mice on elicitation of mouse killing in rats: Role of the amygdala. In Y. Ben-Ari (Ed.), *The amygdaloid complex. INSERM symposium no. 20* (pp. 293–304). Amsterdam: Elsevier–North Holland.

Vilensky, J. A., Demasio, A. R., & Maurer, R. G. (1981). Gait disturbances in patients with autistic behavior. *Archives of Neurology, 38*, 646–649.

Williams, R. S., Hauser, S. L., Purpura, D. P., et al. (1980). Autism and mental retardation. *Archives of Neurology, 37,* 749–753.

Wood, C. C., McCarthy, G., Squires, N. K., et al. (1984). Anatomical and physiological substrates of event related potentials: Two case studies. *Annals of the New York Academy of Science, 425,* 681–721.

Yakovlev, P. I. (1970). Whole brain serial sections. In C. G. Tedeschi (Ed.), *Neuropathology: Methods and diagnosis* (pp. 371–378). Boston: Little, Brown.

17 The Extreme Male-Brain Theory of Autism

Simon Baron-Cohen

Autism is regarded widely to be the most severe of the childhood psychiatric conditions (Rutter, 1983; Frith, 1989; Baron-Cohen, 1995). It is diagnosed on the basis of abnormal social development, abnormal communicative development, and the presence of narrow, restricted interests and repetitive activity, along with limited imaginative ability [Diagnostic and Statistical Manual of Mental Disorders (fourth edition) (DSM-IV), 1994]. Such children fail to become social, instead remaining on the periphery of any social group and becoming absorbed in repetitive interests and activities, such as collecting unusual objects or facts. Their isolation is a tragedy for their families, who work tirelessly to attempt to engage with and socialize their child, mostly with very limited results.

This chapter begins with a summary of psychological findings from studies of autism. A brief review of genetic evidence appears next, as a bridge into the next section, wherein a recent notion is introduced: the "male brain." Evidence for biologically based psychological gender differences is presented, and the "male brain" is defined. Finally, this notion is related to autism, summarizing the author's new theory (Baron-Cohen & Hammer, 1997a) that autism is an extreme form of the male brain. This theory makes a number of predictions possible, and the current evidence relevant to these predictions is presented.

PSYCHOLOGICAL THEORIES OF AUTISM

In this section, evidence for three psychological theories is reviewed: the mindblindness theory, the central coherence theory, and the executive dysfunction theory.

The Mindblindness Theory

Our early theory of autism suggested that the social and communicative abnormalities in this syndrome could be the result of an impairment in the development of a "theory of mind,"or the capacity for "mind-reading." This is defined as the ability to attribute mental states to oneself and others and to make sense of and predict behavior on the basis of mental states. This is held to be important to autism simply because it is arguably the main way in which the normal individual succeeds in understanding and participating in social relationships and communication.

Wimmer and Perner (1983) devised an elegant paradigm to test when normally developing children show evidence of possessing a theory of mind—specifically, when they are aware of another person's beliefs. The child was given a short story with the simplest of plots. The story involves one character's not being present when an object is moved and therefore not *knowing* that the object is in a new location. The child being tested is asked where the character *thinks* the object is. Wimmer and Perner called this the *false belief test*, because it focuses on the subject's ability to infer a story character's mistaken belief about a situation. These authors found that normal 4-year-olds correctly infer that the character thinks the object is where the character last left it, rather than where it actually is. This is impressive evidence for normal children's ability to distinguish between their own knowledge (about reality) and someone else's false belief (about reality).

When this test was given to a sample of children with autism and mild degrees of mental retardation, a large majority of them "failed" this test by indicating that the character thinks the object is where it actually is (Baron-Cohen et al., 1985). That is, they appeared to disregard the critical fact that, by virtue of being *absent* during the critical scene, the character's mental state necessarily would be different from the child's mental state. In contrast, a control group of children with Down syndrome and moderate degrees of mental retardation passed this test as easily as did the normal children. The implication was that the ability to infer mental states may be an aspect of social intelligence that is relatively independent of general intelligence (Cosmides, 1989) and that children with autism might be impaired specifically in the development of a theory of mind.

Of course, simply failing one test would not necessarily mean that children with autism lacked awareness of the mind. Many reasons might account for failure on such a test. (Interestingly, control questions in the original procedure ruled out memory or language difficulties or inattention as possible causes of failure.) The conclusion that children with autism are indeed impaired in this domain only becomes possible because of the convergence of results from widely differing experimental paradigms. These are reviewed in detail in an edited volume (Baron-Cohen et al., 1993) and for that reason are summarized only briefly here.

Results from Studies of Mind-Reading in Autistic Children[1] The majority of children with autism are at chance on tests of the mental-physical distinction (Baron-Cohen, 1989a). That is, they do not show a clear understanding of how physical objects differ from *thoughts* about objects. For example, when asked which can be touched, a biscuit, or a thought (about a biscuit), young, normal, 3-year-olds rapidly identify the former, whereas most autistic children respond at chance levels.

They also have an appropriate understanding of the functions of the brain but have a poor understanding of the functions of the mind (Baron-Cohen, 1989a). They recognize that the brain's physical function is to make you move and do things, but they do not spontaneously mention the mind's mental function (in thinking, dreaming, wishing, deceiving, etc.). Again, contrast this with normal 3-year-old children who do spontaneously use such mental-state terms in their descriptions of what the mind is for (Wellman & Estes, 1986).

Most children with autism also fail to make the appearance-reality distinction (Baron-Cohen, 1989a), meaning that in their description of misleading objects (like a red candle in the shape of an apple), they do not distinguish between what the object *looks* like and what they *know* it really is. For example, the normal 4-year-old child will say of an ambiguous object— when asked what it looks like, and what it really is—that "It *looks* like an apple, but *really* it's a candle made of wax" (Flavell et al., 1986). In contrast, autistic children tend to refer to just one aspect of the object (e.g., saying "It looks like an apple, and it really is an apple").

Most children with autism fail a range of first-order false belief tasks of the kind just described (Baron-Cohen et al., 1985, 1986; Perner et al., 1989; Reed & Petersen, 1990; Leekam & Perner, 1991; Swettenham, 1996); they show deficits in thinking about someone else's different beliefs.

They also fail tests assessing their understanding of the principle that "seeing leads to knowing" (Leslie & Frith, 1988; Baron-Cohen & Goodhart, 1994). For example, when presented with two dolls, one of whom touches a box and the other of whom *looks inside* the box, and when asked "Which one *knows* what's inside the box?" they are at chance in their response. In contrast, normal children of 3 to 4 years of age correctly judge that the one who looked knows what is in the box.

Whereas normally developing children are rather good at picking out mental-state words (e.g., *think, know,* and *imagine*) in a word list that contains both mental-state and non-mental-state words, most autistic children are at chance (Baron-Cohen et al., 1994). In contrast, they have no difficulty in picking out words describing physical states.

Also, most children with autism do not *produce* the same range of mental-state words in their spontaneous speech (Baron-Cohen et al., 1986; Tager-Flusberg, 1992). Thus, from perhaps 18 to 36 months of age, normally developing children spontaneously use such words as *think, know, pretend, imagine, wish, hope,* and the like and use such terms appropriately (Wellman, 1990). In contrast, such words occur less frequently and often are even absent in the spontaneous speech of children with autism.

Such children also are impaired in the production of spontaneous pretend play (Wing et al., 1977; Baron-Cohen, 1987; Lewis & Boucher, 1988). Pretend play is relevant here simply because it involves understanding the mental state of *pretending*. The normal child of even age 2 effortlessly distinguishes between someone's acting veridically and "just pretending" (Leslie, 1987). Sometimes mommy actually is eating (putting a real spoon with real food into her mouth), whereas at other times, mommy is just pretending to eat (holding a pen to her lips and making funny slurping noises between her smiles).

Young normal children rapidly make sense of such behavior, presumably because they can represent the latter case as being driven by the mental state of "pretending." They also spontaneously generate examples of pretense themselves and do not show any confusion as they switch back and forth between pretense (the mental world), and reality (the physical world). In contrast, most children with autism produce little pretense and often appear confused about the intent of pretense and whether someone is pretending.

Though they can understand simple causes of emotion (such as reactions to *physical* situations), the majority of children with autism have difficulty in understanding more *mentalistic* causes of emotion (such as beliefs; Baron-Cohen, 1991a; Baron-Cohen et al., 1993). For example, they can understand that if Jane *actually* falls over and cuts her knee, she will feel sad and that if John *actually* gets a present, he will feel happy. However, they are poor at understanding that if John *thinks* he's getting a present (even if in reality he is not), he will still feel happy. In contrast, normal 4-year-old children comprehend such belief-based emotions.

Most children with autism also fail to recognize the eye region of the face as indicating that a person is *thinking* and what a person might *want* (Baron-Cohen & Cross, 1992; Baron-Cohen et al., 1995). Children and adults without autism use gaze to infer both of these mental states.

For example, when presented with pairs of photos such as those in figure 17.1, normal 3- to 4-year-olds easily identify the person looking upward and away as the one who is thinking. Children with autism are less sure of this. When shown a display such as the one in figure 17.2, normal 4-year-olds identify the candy that Charlie is looking at as the one he wants. Autistic children mostly fail to intuit that gaze can be an indicator of what a person might want.

In addition, many children with autism fail to make the accidental-intentional distinction (Phillips, 1993); they are poor at distinguishing whether someone "meant" to do something or whether something simply happened accidentally.

They also seem unable to deceive (Baron-Cohen, 1992; Sodian & Frith, 1992), a result that would be expected if one were unaware that people's beliefs can differ and therefore can be manipulated. In contrast, normal children of age 4 begin to be fairly adept at lying, thus revealing their awareness of the mental lives of others.

Most children with autism also have disproportionate difficulty on tests of understanding metaphor, sarcasm, and irony, all statements that cannot be decoded literally but are meaningful only by reference to the speaker's *inten-*

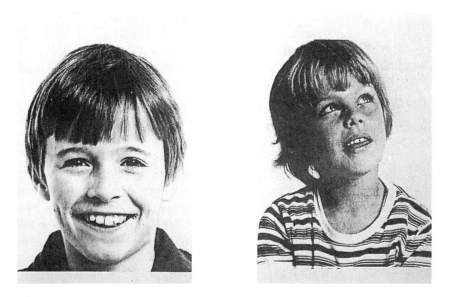

Figure 17.1 Which one is thinking? (Reproduced from Baron-Cohen & Cross, 1992, with permission.)

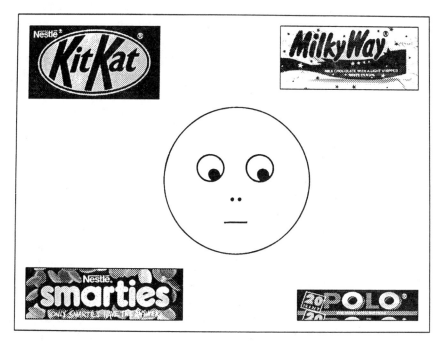

Figure 17.2 Which candy does Charlie want? (Reproduced from Baron-Cohen et al., 1995, with permission.)

tion (Happe, 1994). An example would be understanding "The drinks are on the house," a statement that one adult with autism (and above-average IQ) could interpret only literally. This suggests that children with autism are aware of the physical (the actual words uttered) but are relatively unaware of the mental states (the intentions) behind them.

Indeed, most children with autism fail to produce most aspects of pragmatics in their speech (see review in Baron-Cohen, 1988, and Tager-Flusberg, 1993) and fail to recognize violations of pragmatic rules, such as the Gricean Maxims of conversational cooperation (Surian et al., 1996). For example, one Gricean Maxim of conversation is "Be relevant." If someone replies to a question with an irrelevant answer, normal young children are very sensitive to this pragmatic failure, but most children with autism are not. As many pragmatic rules involve tailoring one's speech to what the listener expects or needs to know or might be interested in, this can be seen as linked intrinsically to a sensitivity of another person's mental states.

Crucially, most children with autism are unimpaired at understanding how physical representations (such as drawings, photos, maps, and models) work, even though they cannot understand mental representations (such as beliefs; Leekam & Perner, 1991; Charman & Baron-Cohen, 1992, 1995; Leslie & Thaiss, 1992). To the extent that both types of task require understanding of representation, this suggests something special about understanding mental representations that causes problems in autism.

Autistic children also are unimpaired in logical reasoning (i.e., about the physical world), even though they have difficulty in psychological reasoning (i.e., about the mental world; Scott & Baron-Cohen, 1996).

This long list of experiments provides strong evidence that children with autism lack the normal understanding of mental states. For this reason, autism can be conceptualized as involving degrees of *mindblindness* (Baron-Cohen, 1990, 1995).

Importantly, a small minority of children or adults with autism pass first-order false-belief tests. (First-order tests involve inferring what one person thinks.) However, these individuals often fail second-order false-belief tests (Baron-Cohen, 1989b): tests of understanding what one character thinks another character thinks. Such second-order reasoning usually is understood by normal children of age 5 to 6, and yet these tests are failed by autistic individuals with a mental age above this level.

Therefore, we can interpret these results in terms of a specific developmental delay in mind-reading at a number of different points (Baron-Cohen, 1991b). Some autistic individuals who are very high-functioning (in terms of IQ and language level) and usually are adults may pass even second-order tests (Ozonoff et al., 1991; Bowler, 1992; Happe, 1993). Those who can pass second-order tests correspondingly also pass the appropriate tests of understanding figurative language (Happe, 1993). However, their deficit shows up on tests of adult mind-reading (Baron-Cohen et al., 1997).

Thus, being able as an adult to pass a test designed for a 6-year-old may mask persisting mind-reading deficits by ceiling effects.

In summary, an impairment seems apparent in the development of a theory of mind in the majority of cases with autism. This finding has the potential to explain the social, communicative, and imaginative abnormalities that are diagnostic of the condition, because being able to reflect on one's own mental states (and those of others) would appear to be essential in all these domains. This deficit has been found to correlate with real-life social skills, as measured by a modified version of the Vineland Adaptive Behavior Scale (Frith et al., 1994).

The Brain Basis of Theory of Mind   One possibility arising from these studies is the presence of a particular part of the brain that in the normal case is responsible for our mind-reading ability and specifically is impaired in autism. If this view is correct, the assumption is that this may be for genetic reasons, as autism appears to be strongly heritable (see chapter 18). The idea that the development of our theory of mind is under genetic control in the normal case is consistent with evidence from cross-cultural studies: Normally developing children from markedly different cultures seem to pass tests of mind-reading at roughly the same ages (Avis & Harris, 1991).

Exactly which parts of the brain might be involved in this is not yet clear, though candidate regions include right orbitofrontal cortex, which is active when subjects are thinking about mental-state terms during functional imaging using single-photon emission computed tomography SPECT (Baron-Cohen et al., 1994) and left medial frontal cortex, which is active when subjects are drawing inferences about thoughts while being scanned with positron emission tomography (Fletcher et al., 1995; Goel et al., 1995). Other candidate regions include the superior temporal sulcus and the amygdala (for reasons explained later). These regions may form parts of a neural circuit supporting theory-of-mind processing (Baron-Cohen & Ring, 1994).

Developmental Origins of Theory of Mind   In an influential article, Leslie (1987) proposed that in the normal case, the developmental origins of mind-reading lie in the capacity for pretense and that in the case of children with autism, the developmental origins of their mindblindness lies in their inability to pretend. In Leslie's model, pretense was the "crucible" for theory of mind, as both involved the same computational complexity. Thus (according to Leslie), to understand that someone else might *think* "This banana is real" or might *pretend* "This banana is real," the child would need to be able to represent the agent's mental attitude toward the proposition, because the only difference between these two states of affairs *is* the person's mental attitude. One idea, then, is that mind-reading is first evident from perhaps 18 to 24 months of age in the normal toddler's emerging pretend play.

However, some evidence suggests that this ability might have even earlier developmental origins. Soon after the first demonstrations of mindblindness in autism, Sigman et al. (1986) also reported severe deficits in *joint attention* in children with autism. Joint attention refers to those behaviors produced by the child and involving monitoring or directing the target of attention of another person, so as to coordinate the child's own attention with that of somebody else (Bruner, 1983). Such behaviors include the pointing gesture, gaze monitoring, and showing gestures, most of which are absent in most children with autism.

This discovery was important because joint attention behaviors are normally well developed by age 14 months (Scaife & Bruner, 1975; Butterworth, 1991), so their absence in autism signifies a very early occurring deficit. This was important also because the traditional mind-reading skills already discussed are mostly those one would expect to see in a 3- to 4-year old normal child. Deficits in these areas cannot, therefore, be the developmentally earliest signs of autism, because we know that autism is present from at least the second year of life (Rutter, 1978), if not earlier.

Implicit in the idea of joint attention deficits in autism was the notion that these might relate to a failure to appreciate other people's point of view (Sigman et al., 1986). Bretherton et al. (1981) also had suggested that joint attention should be understood as an "implicit theory of mind"—or an implicit awareness of the mental. Baron-Cohen (1989c,d; 1991c) explicitly argued that the joint attention and mind-reading deficits in autism were no coincidence and proposed that joint attention was a *precursor* to the development of mind-reading. In that study (Baron-Cohen, 1989c), young children with autism (under age 5) were shown to produce one form of the pointing gesture (imperative pointing, or pointing to request) while failing to produce another form of pointing (declarative pointing, or pointing to share interest).

This dissociation was interpreted in terms of the declarative form of pointing alone being an indicator of the child monitoring another person's mental state (in this case, the mental state of "interest" or "attention"). More recent laboratory studies have confirmed the lack of spontaneous gaze monitoring (Leekam et al., 1997; Phillips et al., 1992; Phillips et al., 1995). Early diagnosis studies also have borne this out (Baron-Cohen et al., 1992; Baron-Cohen et al., 1996). The demonstration of a joint attention deficit in autism and the role that the superior temporal sulcus in the monkey brain plays in the monitoring of gaze direction (Perrett et al., 1985) has led to the idea that the superior temporal sulcus may be involved in the development of mind-reading (Baron-Cohen, 1994, 1995; Baron-Cohen & Ring, 1994). Brothers (1990) also reviewed evidence suggesting that the amygdala contains cells sensitive to gaze and facial expressions of mental states.

Though now considerable evidence supports the theory of mind deficit in autism, clearly this is not the only cognitive deficit in autism. Two others have emerged as important in the last 5 years. First, children with autism fail tests of "executive function." Secondly, they also fail tests of "central coherence." This is important, because though the theory of mind deficits may account for aspects of the social, communicative, and imaginative abnormalities, other symptoms (such as their repetitive behavior and unusual perception) are not explained easily by this cognitive deficit.

Central Coherence and Autism

The second cognitive deficit in autism that we review is in what Frith (1989) calls "central coherence." Defining this notion is slippery. The essence of it is the normal drive to integrate information into a context, or "Gestalt." Frith argued that the superior ability on the embedded figures test seen in autism (Shah & Frith, 1983) and on an unsegmented version of the block design subtest in the Wechsler Intelligence Scale for Children and the Wechsler Adult Intelligence Scale (Shah & Frith, 1993) arises because of a relative immunity to context effects in autism. Happe (1997) also reported a failure by autistic people to use context in reading, such that homophones are mispronounced. For example, "There was a *tear* in her eye" might be misread as "There was a *tear* in her dress." A recent study has shown that children with autism are equally good at judging the identity of familiar faces in photographs, whether they are given the entire face or just part of the face. Nonautistic controls show a "global advantage" on such a test, performing significantly better when given the entire face, not just the parts of the face (Campbell et al., 1995). The central coherence account of autism is attractive in having the potential to explain the nonholistic, piecemeal perceptual style characteristic of autism and the unusual cognitive profile seen in this condition (including the islets of ability).

A strong version of the central coherence account cannot be correct, however, because children with autism perform in line with their mental age on a range of tasks that would seem to involve integration across context. These include (1) transitive inference tests (A > B, and B > C, therefore A?C; Scott & Baron-Cohen, 1996); (2) analogical reasoning tests (A is to B as C is to?; Scott & Baron-Cohen, 1996); and (3) counterfactual syllogistic reasoning tests (e.g., all cats bark; Rex is a cat; therefore Rex?; Scott et al., 1995).

Finally, Happe (1997) reported that some very high-functioning people with autism who pass second-order theory-of-mind tasks nevertheless fail tasks of central coherence, such as the homophone task mentioned earlier. This dissociation implies that theory of mind and central coherence may be relatively independent processes (Frith & Happe, 1994). Whether both deficits in autism in fact reduce to a more basic deficit is still the subject of controversy. In sum, a weak form of central coherence theory seems likely to be correct, disabling individuals with autism from making full use of context. Whether this can account for islets of ability in autism (and even in savant syndrome) remains to be investigated in detail.

Executive Function and Autism

Regarding this third and final area of psychological studies, claims have been made of impairments in autism. Executive function is the postulated mechanism that enables a normal person to shift attention flexibly, inhibit prepotent responses, generate goal-directed behavior, and solve problems in a planful, strategic way (see Shallice, 1988; Baddeley, 1991). The basic idea, developed by Norman and Shallice (1980), is that without a "central executive" (or a *supervisory attentional system,* as it is also called), actions are controlled by the environment, such that an organism simply responds to cues that elicit behavior. Without a supervisory attentional system, action schemas or motor programs "contend" among themselves for execution. This contention takes place in a system known as the *contention scheduling system.* Shallice's notion is that the contention scheduling system is broadly a basal ganglia function, whereas the supervisory attentional system is basically a frontal lobe function. The supervisory attentional system allows inhibition of routine actions. The claim that this is a frontal function derives from the evidence that patients with frontal lobe damage fail tests of this (or executive) function.

Tests of executive function include (1) the Wisconsin Card Sorting Test (Milner, 1964), in which the subject has to shift card-sorting strategies flexibly; (2) the Tower of Hanoi (and its modified version, the Tower of London; Shallice, 1982), in which the subject has to solve problems by planning before acting; (3) the verbal fluency test (or FAS test; see Perret, 1974), in which the subject has to generate novel examples of words beginning with a given letter, in a fixed time period; and (4) the detour-reaching test (Diamond, 1991), in which the subject has to inhibit reaching directly for a visible goal and instead has to take a detour route to the goal.

Patients with frontal lobe damage fail on these tasks (reviewed in Shallice, 1988), as do people with autism (Rumsey & Hamberger, 1988; Prior & Hoffman, 1990; Ozonoff et al., 1991; Hughes & Russell, 1993; Hughes et al., 1994). This has led to the conclusion that children with autism might have frontal lobe damage. One suggestion arising from this finding is that they might fail theory of mind tests listed earlier because they cannot "disengage from the salience of reality" (Hughes & Russell, 1993).

Little doubt remains that in autism an executive dysfunction is likely to be a sign of frontal pathology. However, an important note is that executive dysfunction occurs in a large number of clinical disorders, and in this respect, it is not specific to autism. Thus, all the following eight patient groups show impairments on different tests of executive function:

• Schizophrenia (Frith, 1992; Elliot et al., 1995)

• Treated patients with phenylketonuria (Pennington et al., 1985; Welsh et al., 1990; Diamond, 1994)

• Obsessive-compulsive disorder (Head et al., 1989; Zelinski et al., 1991; Christensen et al., 1992)

- Gilles de la Tourette syndrome (Bornstein, 1990, 1991; Baron-Cohen & Robertson, 1995)

- Attention deficit with hyperactivity disorder (Chelune et al., 1986; Gorenstein et al., 1989; Loge et al., 1990; Grodzinsky & Diamond, 1992)

- Parkinson disease (Downes et al., 1989)

- Frontal lobe syndrome (Owen et al., 1991)

- Children and adults with mental handicap (Borys et al., 1982)

Studies demonstrating executive dysfunction across different populations suggest the absence of any specific mapping between psychiatric classification and the concept of what Baddeley and Wilson (1988) call a *dysexecutive syndrome* (Baron-Cohen & Moriarty, 1995). That all these conditions involve an executive impairment and yet do not lead to autism strongly suggests that, by itself, an impairment in executive function cannot explain autism. Note that examples of patients or disorders that show a double dissociation between executive function and theory of mind would be the strongest test of the independence of these processes.[2]

Possibly, as presently construed, the concept of executive function is too broad a level of analysis. The model suggests that this has several component processes (generativity, attention shifting, disengaging, etc.), and possibly specificity of deficit will be more apparent at this more fine-grain level of analysis. One example of a component process hypothesis is that in autism resides a deficit in "disengaging from the salience of reality." However, this cannot be correct in its strong form because, in a number of studies, subjects have to perform just such a task, and yet children with autism *pass* such tests as the following:

- Visual perspective taking (Hobson, 1984; Baron-Cohen, 1989c, 1991b; Tan & Harris, 1991): In these tasks, a child has to infer what others can see from their spatial position, even if that differs from what the child currently sees.

- False photograph tests (Leekam & Perner, 1991; Leslie & Thaiss, 1992; Swettenham et al., 1996): In these tasks, a child has to infer where something will be in an outdated photograph of reality, when they know that reality has been changed such that the object is actually in a new position.

- False map tests (Leekam & Perner, 1991; Leslie & Thaiss, 1992): These tasks test the same ability as that in the false photograph task but use a map rather than a photograph.

- False drawing tests (Charman & Baron-Cohen, 1992): These tasks also test the same ability as that in the false photograph task but use a drawing rather than a photograph.

- False model tests (Charman & Baron-Cohen, 1995): These tasks test the same ability as that in the false photograph task but use a model rather than a photograph.

• Intellectual realism tests in drawing (Charman & Baron-Cohen, 1993): In these tasks, a subject is asked to draw an object that is partially occluded (e.g., drawing a coffee mug in which the handle is out of view).

Children with autism show "intellectual realism" at the same mental age as that in nonautistic children (i.e., below a mental age of perhaps 6 years) in that they include the occluded object even though it is out of view. For example, they draw the handle of the coffee mug, even when it is not visible. (It is not until after a mental age MA of nearly 6 years has been achieved that subjects—with or without autism—show "visual realism," drawing only what they see, not what they know about.) This task is relevant in that if children with autism were "prisoners" of reality, they should show precocious visual realism, which they do not.

For these reasons, the executive function hypothesis remains in need of considerable clarification. In addition, theory of mind probably is not reducible to executive function. Executive function deficits in autism may instead co-occur with theory of mind deficits because of their shared frontal origin in the brain. Despite these provisos, the executive hypothesis of autism is important, as an attraction of the account is its potential to explain the perseverative, repetitive behaviors in this condition, behaviors not explained by the theory of mind hypothesis. Perseveration and repetitive behaviors are symptomatic of frontal lobe syndrome, in which executive dysfunction also is seen (Shallice, 1988). On this view, the two cognitive deficits may be separately responsible for different types of abnormal behavior.

GENETICS AND AUTISM

Chapter 18 provides a thorough review of the genetics of autism, to which the interested reader is referred. However, as a bridge between the psychological evidence already reviewed and the new model of autism discussed later, the key evidence for genetic factors in autism is briefly summarized.

Autism and Asperger syndrome appear to be strongly heritable according to heritability evidence. First, family studies have shown that first-degree relatives of people with autism have a raised risk of autism, compared to population baseline levels (Folstein & Rutter, 1988). For example, though estimates of autism in the general population range from 1 in 2500 to 1 in 1000 (Wing et al., 1977), the sibling risk rate in families with an autistic child is 3%. Therefore, this is significantly higher than the population baseline rate. Such family data could imply an environmental or hereditary cause. However, twin studies implicate a genetic etiology more persuasively. The concordance rate for autism among monozygotic (MZ) twins is as high as 60%, whereas the concordance rate among dizygotic (DZ) twins is no higher than the sibling risk rate (Folstein & Rutter, 1988; Bolton & Rutter, 1990). Steffenberg et al. (1989) found an even stronger difference between MZ and

DZ concordance rates (91% versus 0%). Though such twin studies are not watertight evidence for hereditary factors, they strongly suggest it.

Autism also is predominantly a male condition. If one takes the population of autism as a whole (75% of whom not only have autism but also have mental handicap), the male-female ratio is 4:1; (Rutter, 1978). If one takes just the "pure" cases of autism (also sometimes designated as having Asperger syndrome) whose IQs are in the normal range, the male-female ratio is even more dramatic: 9:1 (Wing, 1981).[3] Without doubt, then, autism and Asperger syndrome bear a strong relationship to being male. Precisely what this relationship is has received little research attention. The following discussion outlines a model to explain the connection between autism and being male.

THE MALE-BRAIN THEORY OF AUTISM

Our new model of brain development may have considerable relevance for our understanding of autism (Baron-Cohen & Hammer, 1997a). The model depends on the possibility of a "male brain" (defined psychometrically). The relevant background for this notion comes from the long history of research into gender differences in cognition.

Differences in Male and Female Cognition

Some of the key findings (for reviews, see Buffery & Gray, 1972; McGee, 1979; Halpern, 1992; Kimura, 1992; Geary, 1996) are that (as a group) women are superior to men in the following areas:

• Language tasks (e.g., the verbal fluency task calling for listing as many words as possible, beginning with the letter *L*. Female subjects also show a faster rate of language development and a lower risk for specific language impairment. (See Hyde and Linn, 1988, regarding gender differences in language, and Bishop, 1990, regarding language disorder.)

• Tests of social judgment (Argyle & Cooke, 1976; Hall, 1977; Halpern, 1992)

• Measures of empathy and cooperation (Hutt, 1972)

• Rapid identification of matching items (also known as *perceptual speed*; Kimura, 1992)

• Ideational fluency (e.g., list as many things as possible of the same color; Kimura, 1992)

• Fine-motor coordination (e.g., placing pegs in pegboard holes; Kimura, 1992)

• Mathematical calculation tests (Kimura, 1992)

• Pretend play in childhood (Hutt, 1972)

In contrast, men (as a group) are superior to women in the following areas:

• Mathematical reasoning, especially geometry and mathematical word problems (Johnson, 1984; Mills et al., 1993; Steinkamp et al., 1985; Marshall & Smith, 1987; Lummis & Stevenson, 1990; Stevenson et al., 1990). Benbow and Stanley (1980, 1983), for example, reported that at high-level mathematics, the male-female ratio is 13:1.

• The embedded figures task (i.e., finding a part within a whole; Witkin et al., 1971).

• The mental rotation task (i.e., imagining how an object will look when it is rotated or how a sheet of paper will look when it is folded; Masters et al., Sanders, 1993; Kalichman, 1989).

• Some (but not all)[4] spatial skills: mostly Euclidean geometrical navigation (Witelson, 1976; Linn & Petersen, 1985; Gilger & Ho, 1989; Law et al., 1993; Voyer et al., 1995). Spatial superiority in male individuals is found even in childhood (Kerns & Berenbaum, 1991).

• Target-directed motor skills, such as guiding or intercepting projectiles, irrespective of the amount of practice (Buffery & Gray, 1972; Kimura, 1992).

Prenatal Determination of Male and Female Brain

After conception, the embryo undergoes cell differentiation. In a male embryo, the XY genotype controls the growth of testes; at approximately 8 weeks' gestational age, the testes are not only formed but release bursts of testosterone. Testosterone frequently has been proposed to have a causal effect on subsequent fetal brain development,[5] such that by birth, clear gender differences are evident. In rats, the "masculinizing" effects are confined to a critical or sensitive period of testosterone release, around gestational day 17 and postnatal days 8 to 10 (Rhees et al., 1990). At birth, human female babies attend for longer to social stimuli, such as faces and voices, whereas male babies will attend for longer to nonsocial, spatial stimuli, such as mobiles (Goodenough, 1957; McGuiness & Pribam, 1979; Eibl-Ebelsfeldt, 1989). Levels of prenatal testosterone (as assessed during amniocentesis) predict spatial ability at follow-up at age 7 (Grimshaw et al., 1995).[6] One suggestion is that the release of testosterone at this stage of fetal life may determine aspects of brain development, leading to either the male or female brain type.

Defining the Male and Female Brain

Aforementioned evidence points to the notion that during fetal life, endocrine factors shape the brain as either "the male-brain type" or vice versa, more developed in terms of "folk psychology" and less developed in terms of "folk physics" (Moir and Jessel, 1989, in their popular book, for shorthand call this *the female-brain type*).

Table 17.1 Summary of the brain types

Brain type	Cognitive profile
The cognitively balanced brain	Folk physics = folk psychology
The normal female brain	Folk physics < folk psychology
The normal male brain	Folk physics > folk psychology
Asperger syndrome	Folk physics >> folk psychology
Autism	Folk physics >>> folk psychology

Folk psychology is broadly "mind reading," and folk physics is broadly understanding physical objects (and this includes mechanical, constructional, mathematical, and spatial skills; Pinker, 1998). In our model, we operationally define the male-brain type as individuals whose folk physics skills are in advance of their social folk psychology skills. That is, they show a folk physics > folk psychology discrepancy. This is regardless of one's chromosomal gender. Similarly, we define the female-brain type as individuals whose folk psychology skills are in advance of their spatial, folk physics skills[7] (i.e., they show a folk psychology > folk physics discrepancy). Again, this is regardless of one's gender. Clearly, this suggests that yet other people might have neither the male- nor the female-brain type, because their folk psychology skills are roughly equal to their folk physics skills. We call this third possibility the *cognitively balanced brain type*. Autism and Asperger syndrome arguably are extreme forms of the male-brain type; the folk physics > folk psychology discrepancy is even larger than in the normal male-brain type. These types of brain are summarized in table 17.1.

Neural Substrates of the Male and Female Brain

Precisely which structures distinguish these two brain types is still controversial (see Fitch and Dennenberg, 1996, for a review). Kimura (1992) reviewed evidence for differences in cerebral lateralization. In particular, she reviewed evidence that at birth, the right hemisphere cortex in the human male fetus is thicker than the left is. Some reports also show that the corpus callosum is larger in female subjects (De Lacoste-Utamsing & Holloway, 1982), though reports are conflicting (Wittelson, 1989, 1991; Dennenberg et al., 1991; Habib et al., 1991). Hines (1990) reviewed 13 studies and concluded that the female corpus callosum is larger and that this might cause the female superiority in verbal fluency (as a function of better interhemispheric transfer of information).

Finally, evidence suggests that aspects of folk physics, such as spatial ability, are affected by hormonal changes. For example, exposure to androgens prenatally increases spatial performance in female humans and females of other species (Resnick et al., 1986; Hines & Green, 1991; Halpern, 1992), and castration of the rat decreases spatial ability (Williams et al., 1990). The neuroendocrine evidence may be consistent with the notion that a male or female brain type is a function of the levels of circulating male or female hormones during critical periods of neural development.[8]

Any consideration of neurocognitive gender differences should also investigate the voluminous literature on cerebral lateralization. Geschwind and Galaburda's (1987) well-known model assumes the presence of a "standard dominance pattern" (strong left hemisphere dominance for language and handedness and strong right hemisphere dominance for such nonlinguistic functions as visuospatial abilities). Their model predicted that elevated fetal testosterone levels push lateralization away from this standard pattern and toward an "anomalous" pattern. Their model has been criticized on many grounds (see Bryden et al., 1994, for peer commentary regarding their review), but certainly, important connections have been demonstrated between lateralization, gender, and handedness.

In the normal population, 95% of right-handed people have language lateralized to the left hemisphere (as assessed by dichotic listening tasks) and only very rarely to the right (approximately 5% of cases). In left-handed people, lateralization of language to the right hemisphere is more common (some 25%). In his extensive review, Bryden (1988) concluded that left-handers show reduced language-laterality effects (i.e., they show a smaller difference in how quickly they respond to stimuli presented to their right or left ear or visual field, relative to right-handers). Thus, he found 82% of right-handers (but only 62% of left handers) show a right-ear advantage in dichotic listening (verbal) tasks. Male subjects have a rate of left-handedness much higher than that in female subjects (Halpern, 1992). Thus, when Bryden analyzed the same data by gender, he found that 81% of male (but only 74% of female) subjects showed a right-ear advantage. He concluded that, in general, female subjects have a more bilateral organization of cognitive abilities than do male subjects. Hines (1990) expressed the same idea differently: The degree of left-hemisphere dominance is greater in male than in female subjects.

Regarding the link between lateralization and folk physics, Benbow (1986) reported an elevated incidence of that left-handedness in children gifted mathematically. Hassler and Gupta (1993) also found that left-handers score higher on a measure of musical talent and (replicating the earlier work) show reduced right-ear advantage. In addition, Cranberg and Albert (1988) reported an elevated incidence of non-right-handedness in high-level male chess players. Rosenblatt and Winner (1988) found a very high rate of left-handedness and ambidexterity in children with exceptional drawing ability. Kimura and D'Amico (1989) found that non-right-handed university science students have higher spatial ability than that in right-handed controls. Sanders et al., (1982) found in their family study that left-handed men score higher than do right-handed men on spatial tasks (though left-handed women scored lower than did right-handed women). Indeed, elevated rates of left-handedness occur in those working in the visuospatial arts (Peterson, 1979;

Mebert & Michel, 1980), in architecture, and in engineering (Petersen & Lansky, 1974)—all aspects of folk physics.[9] Direction of handedness appears to be strongly familial (McManus, 1985).

The foregoing review therefore suggests that the male-brain type (as defined earlier) is likely to involve complex gender-by-laterality interactions. Halpern (1992) summarized some of the evidence for this. Right-handed male subjects perform better on spatial tests but worse on verbal tests, relative to left-handed male subjects. Right-handed female subjects perform worse on spatial tests but better on verbal tests, relative to left-handed female subjects. This evidence points to the importance of these two variables but does not yet enable us to draw final conclusions about the brain basis of these different brain types.

EVIDENCE FROM AUTISM FOR THE EXTREME MALE-BRAIN THEORY

Some of the evidence from autism relevant to the extreme male-brain theory of autism is listed. As will be seen, this evidence is largely consistent with the theory, though at least one piece of evidence raises problems for it.

Consistency with the Male-Brain Theory

Certain evidence from autism is consistent with the male-brain theory. For example, normal male subjects are superior in spatial tasks as compared to normal female subjects, and people with autism or Asperger syndrome are even better on spatial tasks, such as the embedded figures test (Jolliffe & Baron-Cohen, 1997). A strong male bias exists in the gender ratio of autism or Asperger syndrome. Also, normal male subjects are slower to develop language than are normal female subjects, and autistic children are even more delayed in language development (Rutter, 1978).

Normal male individuals develop socially more slowly than do normal female individuals, and autistic people are even more delayed in social development (Baron-Cohen et al., in press). Additionally, normal female subjects are superior to male subjects in mind-reading tasks, and people with autism or Asperger syndrome are severely impaired in mind-reading (Baron-Cohen et al., 1996).

Parents of children with autism or Asperger syndrome (who can be assumed to share the genotype of their child) also show superior spatial abilities and relative deficits in mind-reading (i.e., a marked male-brain pattern; Baron-Cohen & Hammer, 1997b). Normal male persons have a smaller corpus callosum than that in normal female persons, and in people with autism or Asperger syndrome they are even smaller (Egaas et al., 1994).

Left-handedness is more common among male subjects, and people with autism or Asperger syndrome show an elevated incidence of left-handedness. Fein et al. (1984) found an 18% incidence of left-handedness in autism. Satz et al. (1985) and Soper et al. (1986) found a very similar picture: In their autistic sample, 22% were left-handed.[10]

In the normal population, the male brain is heavier than is the female brain, and people with autism have brains even heavier than those in normal male subjects. (Piren et al., 1995). In the normal population, more male persons are found in mathematical, mechanical, and spatial occupations than are female persons. Parents of children with autism or Asperger syndrome are disproportionately represented in such occupations (Baron-Cohen et al., 1997). All these occupations require good folk physics, though not necessarily requiring equally developed folk psychological skills.

Inconsistencies with the Male-Brain Theory

Some evidence from autism raises inconsistencies with the male-brain theory. Because males are more strongly lateralized than are females, people with autism should show strong lateralization. Studies looking at lateralization in autism using dichotic listening tasks and evoked auditory potentials reveal abnormalities but in the direction opposite to those predicted by the theory. Thus, Prior and Bradshaw (1979) found that children with autism show no clear right-ear advantage in dichotic listening tasks, and Dawson et al. (1986) found that autistic children did not show the asymmetry of evoked response to auditory speech, unlike that of normal controls. The most recent relevant study is a SPECT neuroimaging investigation of autism reporting a lack of normal hemispheric asymmetry (Chiron et al., 1995). Satz et al. (1985) concluded that children with autism are less strongly lateralized, as compared to normal children. This is not consistent with the extreme male-brain theory of autism. However, this may have arisen because these studies looked at lateralization of language in children with autism plus significant language delay. Interesting future studies might look for lateralization of spatial abilities, in cases of "pure" autism or Asperger syndrome to test the extreme male-brain theory further.

CONCLUSIONS: THE CONTINUUM OF MALE- AND FEMALE-BRAIN TYPES

An important assumption of the aforementioned model is that all individuals fall on a continuum as regards male- and female-brain types. As stated earlier, we have referred to some individuals as *cognitively balanced*, being equally good at folk physics and folk psychology. They show no discrepancy. Other individuals are better at folk physics than at folk psychology; this corresponds to the male-brain type. People with the male-brain type might show this discrepancy just marginally (the normal male-brain type); slightly more than this (a touch of Asperger syndrome); or markedly still (frank Asperger syndrome); or in an extreme way (classic autism). Such a model encompasses Wing's (1988) important notion of an autistic continuum blurring into the normal population.[11] The work reviewed here constitutes preliminary but suggestive evidence for the notion of male- and female-brain types defined in psychometrical ways. The foregoing psychological studies are consistent also with the claim that autism (including Asperger syndrome) is an extreme form of the male brain. Currently, the neurobiological basis of such a model remains unclear.

ACKNOWLEDGMENTS

I am grateful for support from the Medical Research Council (UK), the Wellcome Trust, and the Gatsby Foundation during the preparation of this work. Parts of this chapter are reprinted from Baron-Cohen and Hammer (1997a) and Baron-Cohen and Swettenham (1997), with permission.

NOTES

1. In the following list of studies, all the tests mentioned are at the level of a normal 4-year-old child.

2. A further confounding variable is that many tests of theory of mind involve some attention shifting and that many tests of executive function involve accounting for one's mental states, such as one's plans and thoughts.

3. Such individuals are described as having either "high-functioning autism" or "Asperger syndrome" (after Hans Asperger, 1944, who first described such a group of children). A difference may exist between these two conditions (Ozonoff et al., 1991) but, for the present purposes, we consider them as one group.

4. Kimura (1992), for example, reported that men are not superior to women in measures of recall of landmarks from a route.

5. Perhaps the best known formulation of the testosterone model is that of Geschwind and Galaburda (1987). Their model is far-ranging, including predictions that testosterone in fetal life will affect immune status, cerebral lateralization, handedness, risk for neurodevelopmental disorder, and many other factors. Evidence for it is mixed. See Bryden et al. (1994) for a critical review, and see the commentaries on their target article for full debate. For more recent review of the role of both male and female sex hormones in development, see Grimshaw et al., (1995) and Fitch and Dennenberg (1996).

6. In the Grimshaw et al. (1995) study, an association was found only between prenatal testosterone and spatial ability in girls, not in boys. The authors of that study interpret this finding in the context of the claim by Gouchie and Kimura (1991) that high levels of prenatal testosterone might have a *curvilinear* relationship with spatial ability.

7. This model should not be used to reinforce traditional occupational and economic inequalities between the genders. A detailed reading of the model should lead the reader to draw conclusions based on individuals' brain type rather than on their gender.

8. Precisely when these critical periods occur is left open here, though these likely occur during fetal and early infant stages of development

9. See Martino and Winner (1995) for a recent study of this area.

10. It should be noted though that anomalous handedness is present also in children with general developmental delay (irrespective of whether they have autism; see Bishop, 1990). What

remains to be seen, then, is whether the anomalous handedness in autism is specific to this condition or is secondary to general developmental delay present in two-thirds of children with autism.

11. It is tempting to surmise that children with Williams syndrome might have an extreme form of the *female* brain type, (Karmiloff-Smith et al., 1995).

REFERENCES

Argyle, M., & Cook, M. (1976). *Gaze and Mutual Gaze*. Cambridge: Cambridge University Press.

Asperger, H. (1944). Die "Autistischen Psychopathen" im Kindesalter. *Archiv fur Psychiatrie und Nervenkrankheiten, 117,* 76–136.

Avis, J., & Harris, P. (1991). Belief-desire reasoning among Baka children: Evidence for a universal conception of mind. *Child Development, 62,* 460–467.

Baddeley, A. (1991). *Human memory: Theory and practice*. Hillsdale, NJ: Erlbaum.

Baddeley, A., & Wilson, B. (1988). Frontal amnesia and the dysexecutive syndrome. *Brain and Cognition, 7,* 212–230.

Baron-Cohen, S. (1987). Autism and symbolic play. *British Journal of Developmental Psychology, 5,* 139–148.

Baron-Cohen, S. (1988). Social and pragmatic deficits in autism: Cognitive or affective? *Journal of Autism and Developmental Disorders, 18,* 379–402.

Baron-Cohen, S. (1989a). Are autistic children behaviorists? An examination of their mental-physical and appearance-reality distinctions. *Journal of Autism and Developmental Disorders, 19,* 579–600.

Baron-Cohen, S. (1989b). The autistic child's theory of mind: A case of specific developmental delay. *Journal of Child Psychology and Psychiatry, 30,* 285–298.

Baron-Cohen, S. (1989c). Perceptual role-taking and protodeclarative pointing in autism. *British Journal of Developmental Psychology, 7,* 113–127.

Baron-Cohen, S. (1989d). Joint attention deficits in autism: Towards a cognitive analysis. *Development and Psychopathology, 1,* 185–189.

Baron-Cohen, S. (1990). Autism: A specific cognitive disorder of "mind-blindness." *International Review of Psychiatry, 2,* 79–88.

Baron-Cohen, S. (1991a). Do people with autism understand what causes emotion? *Child Development, 62,* 385–395.

Baron-Cohen, S. (1991b). The development of a theory of mind in autism: Deviance and delay? *Psychiatric Clinics of North America, 14,* 33–51.

Baron-Cohen, S. (1991c). Precursors to a theory of mind: Understanding attention in others. In A. Whiten (Ed.), *Natural theories of mind*. Oxford: Basil Blackwell.

Baron-Cohen, S. (1992). Out of sight or out of mind: Another look at deception in autism. *Journal of Child Psychology and Psychiatry, 33,* 1141–1155.

Baron-Cohen, S. (1994). How to build a baby that can read minds: Cognitive mechanisms in mindreading. *Cahiers de Psychologie Cognitive/Current Psychology of Cognition, 13(5),* 513–552.

Baron-Cohen, S. (1995). *Mindblindness: An essay on autism and theory of mind*. Boston: MIT Press.

Baron-Cohen, S., Allen, J., & Gillberg, C., (1992). Can autism be detected at 18 months? The needle, the haystack, and the CHAT. *British Journal of Psychiatry, 161,* 839–843.

Baron-Cohen, S., Campbell, R., Karmiloff-Smith, A., Grant, J., & Walker, J. (1995). Are children with autism blind to the mentalistic significance of the eyes? *British Journal of Developmental Psychology, 13,* 379–398.

Baron-Cohen, S., Cox, A., Baird, G., Swettenham, J., Drew, A., Nightingale, N., & Charman, T. (1996a). Psychological markers of autism at 18 months of age in a large population. *British Journal of Psychiatry, 168,* 158–163.

Baron-Cohen, S., & Cross, P. (1992). Reading the eyes: Evidence for the role of perception in the development of a theory of mind. *Mind and Language, 6,* 173–186.

Baron-Cohen, S., & Goodhart, F. (1994). The "seeing leads to knowing" deficit in autism: The Pratt and Bryant probe. *British Journal of Developmental Psychology, 12,* 397–402.

Baron-Cohen, S., Jolliffe, T., Mortimore, C., & Robertson, M. (1997). Another advanced test of theory of mind: Evidence from very high functioning adults with autism or Asperger syndrome. *Journal of Child Psychology and Psychiatry, 38,* 813–822.

Baron-Cohen, S., & Hammer J. (1997a). Is autism an extreme form of the male brain? *Advances in Infancy Research, 11,* 193–217.

Baron-Cohen, S., & Hammer, J. (1997b). Parents of children with Asperger Syndrome: What is the cognitive phenotype? *Journal of Cognitive Neuroscience, 9,* 548–554.

Baron-Cohen, S., Leslie, A. M., & Frith, U. (1985). Does the autistic child have a "theory of mind"? *Cognition, 21,* 37–46.

Baron-Cohen, S., Leslie, A. M., & Frith, U. (1986). Mechanical, behavioral and intentional understanding of picture stories in autistic children. *British Journal of Developmental Psychology, 4,* 113–125.

Baron-Cohen, S., & Moriarty, J. (1995). Developmental dysexecutive syndrome: Does it exist? A neuropsychological perspective. In M. Robertson & V. Eapen (Eds.), *Movement and allied disorders in childhood.* New York: Wiley.

Baron-Cohen, S., O'Riordan, M., Stone, V., Jones, R., & Plaisted, K. (in press). Recognition of faux pas by normally developing children and children with Asperger syndrome or high functioning autism. *Journal of Autism and Developmental Disorders.*

Baron-Cohen, S., & Ring, H. (1994). A model of the mindreading system: Neuropsychological and neurobiological perspectives. In P. Mitchell, & C. Lewis (Eds.), *Origins of an understanding of mind.* Hillsdale, NJ: Erlbaum.

Baron-Cohen, S., Ring, H., Moriarty, J., Shmitz, P., Costa, D., & Ell, P. (1994). Recognition of mental state terms: A clinical study of autism, and a functional neuroimaging study of normal adults. *British Journal of Psychiatry, 165,* 640–649.

Baron-Cohen, S., & Robertson, M. (1995). Children with either autism, Gilles de la Tourette Syndrome, or both: Mapping cognition to specific syndromes. *Neurocase, 1,* 101–104.

Baron-Cohen, S., Spitz, A., & Cross, P. (1993). Can children with autism recognize surprise? *Cognition and Emotion, 7,* 507–516.

Baron-Cohen, S., Tager-Flusberg, H., and Cohen, D. J. (Eds.) (1993). *Understanding other minds: Perspectives from autism.* Oxford: Oxford University Press.

Baron-Cohen, S., Wheelwright, S., Bolton, P., Stott, C., & Goodyer, I. (1997). Is there a link between engineering and autism? *Autism, 1,* 101–109.

Benbow, C., & Stanley, J. (1980). Sex differences in mathematical ability: Fact or artifact? *Science, 210,* 1262–1264.

Benbow, C., & Stanley, J. (1983). Sex differences in mathematical reasoning ability: More facts. *Science, 222,* 1029–1031.

Bishop, D. (1990). *Handedness and developmental disorder.* Oxford: Blackwell.

Bolton, P., & Rutter, M. (1990). Genetic influences in autism. *International Review of Psychiatry, 2,* 67–80.

Bornstein, R. (1990). Neuropsychological performance in children with Tourette syndrome. *Psychiatry Research, 33,* 73–81.

Bornstein, R. (1991). Neuropsychological correlates of obsessive characteristics in Tourette syndrome. *Journal of Neuropsychiatry and Clinical Neurosciences, 3,* 157–162.

Borys, S., Spitz, H., & Dorans, B. (1982). Tower of Hanoi performance of retarded young adults and nonretarded children as a function of solution length and goal state. *Journal of Experimental Psychology, 33,* 87–110.

Bowler, D. M. (1992). Theory of mind in Asperger syndrome. *Journal of Child Psychology and Psychiatry, 33,* 877–893.

Bretherton, I., McNew, S., & Beeghly-Smith, M. (1981). Early person knowledge as expressed in gestural and verbal communication: When do infants acquire a "theory of mind"? In M. Lamb & L. Sharrod (Eds.), *Infant social cognition.* (pp. 333–374) Hillsdale, NJ: Erlbaum.

Brothers, L. (1990). The social brain: A project for integrating primate behavior and neurophysiology in a new domain. *Concepts in Neuroscience, 1,* 27–51.

Bruner, J. (1983). *Child's talk: Learning to use language.* Oxford: Oxford University Press.

Bryden, M. (1988). An overview of the dichotic listening procedure and its relation to cerebral organization. In K. Hugdahl (Ed.), *Handbook of dichotic listening.* Chichester, UK: Wiley.

Bryden, M., McManus, I. C., & Bulman-Fleming, M. (1994). Evaluating the empirical support for the Geschwind-Behan-Galaburda model of cerebral lateralization. *Brain and Cognition, 26,* 103–167.

Buffery, A., & Gray, J. (1972). Sex differences in the development of spatial and linguistic skills. In C. Ounsted & D. Taylor (Eds.), *Gender differences: Their ontogeny and significance.* London: Churchill Livingstone.

Butterworth, G. (1991). The ontogeny and phylogeny of joint visual attention. In A. Whiten (Ed.) *Natural theories of mind.* Oxford: Basil Blackwell.

Campbell, R., Baron-Cohen, S., & Walker, J. (1995). *Do people with autism show a whole face advantage in recognition of familiar faces and their parts? A test of central coherence theory.* Unpublished manuscript, Goldsmith's College, University of London.

Charman, T., and Baron-Cohen, S. (1992). Understanding beliefs and drawings: A further test of the metarepresentation theory of autism. *Journal of Child Psychology and Psychiatry, 33,* 1105–1112.

Charman, T., & Baron-Cohen, S. (1993). Drawing development in autism: The intellectual to visual realism shift. *British Journal of Developmental Psychology, 11,* 171–185.

Charman, T., & Baron-Cohen, S. (1995). Understanding models, photos, and beliefs: A test of the modularity thesis of metarepresentation. *Cognitive Development, 10,* 287–298.

Chelune, G., Ferguson, W., Koon, R., & Dickey, T. (1986). Frontal lobe disinhibition in attention deficit disorder. *Child Psychiatry and Human Development, 16,* 221–234.

Chiron, C., Leboyer, M., Leon, F., Jambaque, I., Nuttin, N., & Syrota, A. (1995). SPECT study of the brain in childhood autism: Evidence for a lack of normal hemispheril asymmetry. *Developmental Medicine and Childhood Neurology, 37,* 849–861.

Christensen, K., Kim, S., Dysken, M., & Hoover, K. (1992). Neuropsychological performance in obsessive compulsive disorder. *Biological Psychiatry, 31*, 4–18.

Cosmides, L. (1989). The logic of social exchange: Has natural selection shaped how humans reason? Studies with the Wason selection task. *Cognition, 31*, 187–276.

Cranberg, L., & Albert, M. (1988). The chess mind. In L. Obler & D. Fein (Eds.), *The exceptional brain: Neuropsychology of talent and special abilities* (pp. 69–83). New York: Guilford.

Dawson, G., Finley, C., Phillips, S., & Galpert, L. (1986). Hemispheric specialization and the language abilities of autistic children. *Child Development, 57*, 1440–1453.

De Lacoste-Utamsing, C., & Holloway, R. (1982). Sexual differences in the human corpus callosum. *Science, 216*, 1431–1432.

Denenberg, V., Kertesz, A., & Cowell, P. (1991). A factor analysis of the human's corpus callosum. *Brain Research, 548*, 126–132.

Diamond, A. (1991). Neuropsychological insights into the meaning of object concept development. In S. Carey & R. Gelman (Eds.), *The epigenesis of mind: Essays on biology and knowledge.* Hillsdale, NJ: Erlbaum.

Diamond, A. (1994). Phenylaline levels of 6–10 mg/dl may not be as benign as once thought. *Acta Paediatrica, 83*, 89–91.

Downes, J., Roberts, A., Sahakian, B., Evenden, J., Morris, R., & Robbins, T. (1989). Impaired extra-dimensional shift performance in medicated and unmedicated Parkinson's disease: Evidence for a specific attentional dysfunction. *Neuropsychologia, 27*, 1329–1343.

Egaas, B., Courchesne, E., & Saitoh, O. (1995). Reduced size of the corpus callosum in autism. *Archives of Neurology, 52*, 794–801.

Eibl-Eibesfeldt, I. (1989). *Human ethology.* New York: Aldine de Gruyter.

Elliot, R., McKenna, P., Robbins, T., & Sahakian, B. (1995). Neuropsychological evidence for frontostriatal dysfunction in schizophrenia. *Psychological Medicine, 25*, 619–630.

Elliot, R., & Sahakian, B. (1995). The neuropsychology of schizophrenia: Relations with clinical and neurobiological dimensions. *Psychological Medicine, 25*, 581–594.

Fein, D., Humes, M., Kaplan, E., Lucci, D., & Waterhouse, L. (1988). The question of left-hemisphere dysfunction in infantile autism. *Psychological Bulletin, 95*, 258–281.

Fitch, R., & Denenberg, V. (1996). A role for ovarian hormones in sexual differentiation of the brain. *Psychology.*

Flavell, J. H., Green, F. L., & Flavell, E. R. (1986). Development of knowledge about the appearance-reality distinction. *Monographs of the Society for Research in Child Development, 51.*

Fletcher, P., Happe, F., Frith, U., Baker, S., Dolan, R., Frackowiak, R., & Frith, C. (1995). Other minds in the brain: A functional imaging study of "theory of mind" in story comprehension. *Cognition, 57*, 109–128.

Folstein, S., & Rutter, M. (1988). Autism: Familial aggregation and genetic implications. *Journal of Autism and Developmental Disorders, 18*, 3–30.

Frith, U. (1989). *Autism: Explaining the enigma.* Oxford: Basil Blackwell.

Frith, U., and Happe, F. (1994). Autism: Beyond "theory of mind." *Cognition, 50*, 115–132.

Frith, U., Happe, F., & Siddons, F. (1994). Autism and theory of mind in everyday life. *Social Development, 3*, 108–124.

Geary, D. (1996). Sexual selection and sex differences in mathematical abilities. *Behavior and Brain Sciences, 19*, 229–284.

Geschwind, N., & Galaburda, A. (1987). *Cerebral lateralization*. Cambridge, MA: MIT Press.

Gilger, J., & Ho, H. (1989). Gender differences in adult spatial information processing: Their relationship to pubertal timing, adolescent activities, and sex-typing of personality. *Cognitive Development, 4*, 197–214.

Goel, V., Grafman, J., Sadato, N., & Hallett, M. (1995). Modelling other minds. *Neuroreport, 6*, 1741–1746.

Goodenough, E. (1957). Interest in persons as an aspect of sex differences in the early years. *Genetic Psychology Monographs, 55*, 287–323.

Gorenstein, E., Mammato, C., & Sandy, J. (1989). Performance of inattentive-overactive children on selected measures of prefrontal type. *Journal of Clinical Psychology, 45*, 619–632.

Gouchie, C., & Kimura, D. (1991). The relationship between testosterone level and cognitive ability patterns. *Psychoneuroendocrinology, 16*, 323–334.

Grimshaw, G., Sitarenios, G., & Finegan, J. (1995). Mental rotation at 7 years: Relations with prenatal testosterone levels and spatial play experiences. *Brain and Cognition, 29*, 85–100.

Grodzinsky, G., & Diamond, A. (1992). Frontal lobe functioning in boys with attention deficit hyperactivity disorder. *Developmental Neuropsychology, 8*, 427–445.

Habib, M., Gayraud, D., Olivia, A., Regis, J., Salamon, G., & Khalil, R. (1991). Effects of handedness and sex on the morphology of the corpus callosum: A study with brain magnetic resonance imaging. *Brain and Cognition, 16*, 41–61.

Hall, J. (1977). Gender effects in decoding non-verbal cues. *Psychological Bulletin, 85*, 845–857.

Halpern, D. (1992). *Sex differences in cognitive ability* (2nd ed.). Hillsdale, NJ: Erlbaum.

Hassler, M., & Gupta, D. (1993). Functional brain organization, handedness and immune vulnerability in musicians and non-musicians. *Neuropsychologia, 31*, 655–660.

Happe, F. (1993). Communicative competence and theory of mind in autism: A test of relevance theory. *Cognition, 48*, 101–119.

Happe, F. (1994). An advanced test of theory of mind: Understanding of story characters' thoughts and feelings by able autistic, mentally handicapped, and normal children and adults. *Journal of Autism and Developmental Disorders, 24*, 129–154.

Happe, F. (1997). Central coherence and theory of mind in autism. Reading homographs in context. *British Journal of Developmental Psychology, 15*, 1–12.

Head, D., Bolton, D., & Hymas, N. (1989). Deficit in cognitive shifting ability in patients with obsessive-compulsive disorder. *Biological Psychiatry, 25*, 929–937.

Hines, M. (1990). Gonadal hormones and human cognitive development. In J. Balthazart (Ed.), *Hormones, brain and behavior in vertebrates: I. Sexual differentiation, neuroanatomical aspects, neurotransmitters, and neuropeptides*. Basel: Karger.

Hines, M., & Green, R. (1991). Human hormonal and neural correlates of sex-typed behaviors. *Review of Psychiatry, 10*, 536–555.

Hobson, R. P. (1984). Early childhood autism and the question of egocentrism. *Journal of Autism and Developmental Disorders, 14*, 85–104.

Hughes, C., & Russell, J. (1993). Autistic children's difficulty with mental disengagement from an object: Its implications for theories of autism. *Developmental Psychology, 29*, 498–510.

Hughes, C., Russell, J., & Robbins, T. (1994). Specific planning deficit in autism: Evidence of a central executive dysfunction. *Neuropsychologia, 33*, 477–492.

Hutt, C. (1972). Neuroendocrinal behavior and intellectual aspects of sexual differentiation in human development. In C. Ounsted & D. Taylor (Eds.), *Gender differences: Their ontogeny and significance*. Edinburgh: Churchill Livingstone.

Hyde, J., & Linn, M. (1988). Gender differences in verbal ability: A meta-analysis. *Psychological Bulletin, 104*, 53–69.

Johnson, E. (1984). Sex differences in problem-solving. *Journal of Educational Psychology, 76*, 1359–1371.

Jolliffe, T., & Baron-Cohen, S. (1997). Are people with autism and Asperger syndrome faster than normal on the embedded figures test? *Journal of Child Psychology and Psychiatry, 38*, 527–534.

Kalichman, S. (1989). The effects of stimulus context on paper and pencil spatial task performance. *Journal of General Psychology, 116*, 133–139.

Karmiloff-Smith, A., Klima, E., Bellugi, U., Grant, J., & Baron-Cohen, S. (1995). Is there a social module? Language, face-processing and theory of mind in subjects with William's syndrome and autism. *Journal of Cognitive Neuroscience, 7*, 196–208.

Kerns, K., & Berenbaum, S. (1991). Sex differences in spatial ability in childhood. Behavior Genetics, *21*, 383–396.

Kimura, D. (1992). Sex differences in the brain. *Scientific American, September*, 119–125.

Kimura, D., & D'Amico, C. (1989). Evidence for subgroups of adextrals based on speech lateralization and cognitive patterns. *Neuropsychologia, 27*, 977–986.

Law, D., Pellegrino, J., & Hunt, E. (1993). Comparing the tortoise and the hare: Gender differences and experiences in dynamic spatial reasoning tasks. *Psychological Science, 4*, 35–40.

Leekam, S., Baron-Cohen, S., Brown, S., Perrett, D., & Milders, M., (1997). Eye-direction detection: A dissociation between geometric and joint-attention skills in autism. *British Journal of Developmental Psychology, 15*, 77–95.

Leekam, S., & Perner, J. (1991). Does the autistic child have a metarepresentational deficit? *Cognition, 40*, 203–218.

Leslie, A. M. (1987). Pretence and representation: The origins of "theory of mind." *Psychological Review, 94*, 412–426.

Leslie, A. M., & Frith, U. (1988). Autistic children's understanding of seeing, knowing, and believing. *British Journal of Developmental Psychology, 6*, 315–324.

Leslie, A. M., & Thaiss, L. (1992). Domain specificity in conceptual development: Evidence from autism. *Cognition, 43*, 225–251.

Lewis, V., & Boucher, J. (1988). Spontaneous, instructed and elicited play in relatively able autistic children. *British Journal of Developmental Psychology, 6*, 325–339.

Linn, M., & Petersen, A. (1985). Emergence and characterization of sex differences in spatial ability: A meta-analysis. *Child Development, 56*, 1479–1498.

Loge, D., Staton, D., & Beatty, W. (1990). Performance of children with ADHD on tests sensitive to frontal lobe dysfunction. *Journal of the American Academy of Child and Adolescent Psychiatry, 29*, 540–545.

Lummis, M., & Stevenson, H. (1990). Gender differences in beliefs and achievement: A cross-cultural study. *Developmental Psychology, 26*, 254–263.

Martino, G., & Winner, E. (1995). Talents and disorders: Relationships among handedness, sex, and college major. *Brain and Cognition, 29*, 66–84.

Marshall, S., & Smith, J. (1987). Sex differences in learning mathematics: A longitudinal study with item and error analyses. *Journal of Educational Psychology, 79*, 372–383.

Masters, M., & Sanders, B. (1993). Is the gender difference in mental rotation disappearing? *Behavior Genetics, 23*, 337–341.

McGee, M. (1979). Human spatial abilities: Psychometric studies and environmental, genetic, hormonal, and neurological influences. *Psychological Bulletin, 86*, 889–918.

McGuinness, D., & Pribam, K. (1979). The origins of sensory bias in the development of gender differences in perception and cognition. In M. Bortner (Ed.), *Cognitive growth and development: Essays in memory of Herbert Birch*. New York: Brunner/Mazel.

McManus, I. C. (1985). Handedness, language dominance, and aphasia: A genetic model. *Psychological Medicine*, Monograph Supplement 8.

Mebert, C., & Michel, G. (1980). Handedness in artists. In L. Herron, (Ed.), *Neuropsychology of left-handedness*. New York: Academic.

Mills, C., Ablard, K., & Stumpf, H. (1993). Gender differences in academically talented young students' mathematical reasoning: Patterns across age and subskills. *Journal of Educational Psychology, 85*, 340–346.

Milner, B. (1964). Some effects of frontal lobectomy in man. In J. Warren & K. Akert (Eds.), *The frontal granular cortex and behavior*. New York: McGraw-Hill.

Moir, A., & Jessel, D. (1989). *Brainsex*. London: Mandarin Press.

Norman, D., & Shallice, T. (1980). Attention to action: Willed and automatic control of behavior. In R. Davidson G. Schwartz & D. Shapiro (Eds.), *Consciousness and self-regulation: Vol 4*. New York: Plenum.

Owen, A., Roberts, A., Polkey, C., Sahakian, B., & Robbins, T. (1991). Extradimensional versus intradimensional set shifting performance following frontal lobe excisions, temporal lobe excisions, or amygdalo-hippocampectomy in man. *Neuropsychologia, 10*, 99–106.

Ozonoff, S., Pennington, B., & Rogers, S. (1991). Executive function deficits in high-functioning autistic children: Relationship to theory of mind. *Journal of Child Psychology and Psychiatry, 32*, 1081–1106.

Ozonoff, S., Rogers, S., & Pennington, B. (1991). Asperger's syndrome: Evidence of an empirical distinction from high-functioning autism. *Journal of Child Psychiatry and Psychology, 32*, 1107–1122.

Pennington, B., van Doorninck, W., McCabe, L., & McCabe, E. (1985). Neurological deficits in early treated phenylketonurics. *American Journal of Mental Deficiency, 89*, 467–474.

Perner, J., Frith, U., Leslie, A. M., & Leekam, S. (1989). Exploration of the autistic child's theory of mind: Knowledge, belief, and communication. *Child Development, 60*, 689–700.

Perret, E. (1974). The left frontal lobe of man and the suppression of habitual responses in verbal categorical behavior. *Neuropsychologia, 16*, 527–537.

Perrett, D., Smith, P., Potter, D., Mistlin, A., Head, A., Milner, A., & Jeeves, M. (1985). Visual cells in the temporal cortex sensitive to face view and gaze direction. *Proceedings of the Royal Society of London, B223*, 293–317.

Peterson, J. (1979). Left-handedness: Difference between student artists and scientists. *Perceptual and Motor Skills, 48*, 961–962.

Peterson, J., & Lansky, L. (1974). Left-handedness among architects: Some facts and speculations. *Perceptual and Motor Skills, 38*, 547–550.

Phillips, W. (1993). *Understanding intention and desire by children with autism*. Unpublished doctoral dissertation, Institute of Psychiatry, University of London.

Phillips, W., Baron-Cohen, S., & Rutter, M. (1992). The role of eye-contact in the detection of goals: Evidence from normal toddlers, and children with autism or mental handicap. *Development and Psychopathology, 4,* 375–383.

Phillips, W., Gomez, J-C., Baron-Cohen, S., Riviere, A., & Laa, V. (1995). Treating people as objects, agents, or subjects: How young children with and without autism make requests. *Journal of Child Psychology and Psychiatry, 36,* 1383–1398.

Pinker, S. (1998). *How the mind works*. New York: Norton.

Piren, J., Arndt, S., Bailey, J., Havercamp, S., Andeason, N., & Palmer, P. (1995). An MRI study of brain size in autism. *American Journal of Psychiatry, 152,* 1145–1149.

Prior, M., & Bradshaw, J. (1979). Hemispheric functioning in autistic children. *Cortex, 15,* 73–81.

Prior, M., & Hoffman, W. (1990). Neuropsychological testing of autistic children through exploration with frontal lobe tests. *Journal of Autism and Developmental Disorders, 20,* 581–590.

Reed, T., & Peterson, C. (1990). A comparative study of autistic subjects' performance at two levels of visual and cognitive perspective taking. *Journal of Autism and Developmental Disorders, 20,* 555–568.

Resnick, S., Berenbaum, S., Gottesman, I., & Bouchard, T., Jr. (1986). Early hormonal influences on cognitive functioning in congenital adrenal hyperplasia. *Developmental Psychology, 22,* 191–198.

Rhees, R., Shyrne, J., & Gorski, R. (1990). Onset of the hormone-sensitive perinatal period for sexual differentation of the sexually dimorphic nucleus of the preoptic area. *Journal of Neurobiology, 21,* 781–786.

Rosenblatt, E., & Winner, E. (1988). Is superior visual memory a component of superior drawing ability? In L. Obler & D. Fein (Eds.), *The exceptional brain: Neuropsychology of talent and special abilities*. New York: Guilford Press.

Rumsey, J., & Hamburger, S. (1988). Neuropsychological findings in high functioning men with infantile autism, residual state. *Journal of Clinical and Experimental Neuropsychology, 10,* 201–221.

Rutter, M. (1978). Diagnosis and definition. In M. Rutter & E. Schopler (Eds.), *Autism: A reappraisal of concepts and treatment*. New York: Plenum Press.

Rutter, M. (1983). Cognitive deficits in the pathogenesis of autism. *Journal of Child Psychology and Psychiatry, 24,* 513–531.

Satz, P., Soper, H., Orsini, D., Henry, R., & Zvi, J. (1985). Handedness subtypes in autism. *Psychiatric Annals, 15,* 447–451.

Scaife, M., & Bruner, J. (1975). The capacity for joint visual attention in the infant. *Nature, 253,* 265–266.

Scott, F., & Baron-Cohen, S. (1996). Logical, analogical, and psychological reasoning in autism: A test of the Cosmides theory. *Development and Psychopathology, 8,* 235–246.

Shah, A., & Frith, U. (1983). An islet of ability in autism: A research note. *Journal of Child Psychology and Psychiatry, 24,* 613–620.

Shah, A., & Frith, U. (1993). Why do autistic individuals show superior performance on the block design test? *Journal of Child Psychology and Psychiatry, 34,* 1351–1364.

Shallice, T. (1982). Specific impairments of planning. *Philosophical Transactions of the Royal Society of London, B298,* 199–209.

Shallice, T. (1988). *From neuropsychology to mental structure*. Cambridge, UK: Cambridge University Press.

Sigman, M., Mundy, P., Ungerer, J., & Sherman, T. (1986). Social interactions of autistic, mentally retarded, and normal children and their caregivers. *Journal of Child Psychology and Psychiatry, 27*, 647–656.

Sodian, B., & Frith, U. (1992). Deception and sabotage in autistic, retarded, and normal children. *Journal of Child Psychology and Psychiatry, 33*, 591–606.

Soper, H., Satz, P., Orsini, D., Henry, R., Zvi, J., & Schulman, M. (1986). Handedness patterns in autism suggests subtypes. *Journal of Autism and Developmental Disorders, 16*, 155–167.

Steffenberg, S., Gillberg, C., Hellgren, L., Andersson, L., Gillberg, C., Jakobsson, G., & Bohman, M. (1989). A twin study of autism in Denmark, Finland, Iceland, Norway, and Sweden. *Journal of Child Psychology and Psychiatry, 30*, 405–416.

Steinkamp, M., Harnisch, D., Walberg, H., & Tsai, S. (1985). Cross national gender differences in mathematics attitude and achievement among 13 year olds. *Journal of Mathematical Behavior, 4*, 259–277.

Stevenson, H., Lee, S., Chen, C., Lummis, M., Stigler, J., Fan, L., & Ge, F. (1990). Mathematics achievement of children in China and the United States. *Child Development, 61*, 1053–1066.

Surian, L., Baron-Cohen, S., & Van der Lely, H. (1996). Are children with autism deaf to Gricean Maxims? *Cognitive Neuropsychiatry, 1*, 55–72.

Swettenham, J. (1996). Can children be taught to understand false belief using computers? *Journal of Child Psychology and Psychiatry, 37*, 157–166.

Swettenham, J., Baron-Cohen, S., Gomez, J-C., & Walsh, S. (1996). What's inside a person's head? Conceiving of the mind as a camera helps children with autism develop an alternative to a theory of mind. *Cognitive Neurospychiatry, 1*, 73–88.

Tager-Flusberg, H. (1992). Autistic children's talk about psychological states: Deficits in the early acquisition of a theory of mind. *Child Development, 63*, 161–172.

Tager-Flusberg, H. (1993). What language reveals about the understanding of minds in children with autism. In S. Baron-Cohen, H. Tager-Flusberg, & D. J. Cohen (Eds.), *Understanding other minds: Perspectives from autism*. Oxford: Oxford University Press.

Tan, J., & Harris, P. (1991). Autistic children understand seeing and wanting. *Development and Psychopathology, 3*, 163–174.

Voyer, D., Voyer, S., & Bryden, M. (1995). Magnitude of sex differences in spatial abilities: A meta-analysis and consideration of critical variables. *Psychological Bulletin, 117*, 250–270.

Wellman, H. (1990). *Children's theories of mind*. Cambridge, MA: MIT Press Bradford Books.

Wellman, H., & Estes, D. (1986). Early understanding of mental entities: A reexamination of childhood realism. *Child Development, 57*, 910–923.

Welsh, M., Pennington, B., Ozonoff, S., Rouse, B., & McCabe, E. (1990). Neuropsychology of early-treated phenylketonuria: Specific executive function deficits. *Child Development, 61*, 1679–1713.

Williams, C., Barnett, A., & Meck, W. (1990). Organizational effects of early gonadal secretions on sexual differentiation in spatial memory. *Behavioral Neuroscience, 104*, 84–97.

Wimmer, H., & Perner, J. (1983). Beliefs about beliefs: Representation and constraining function of wrong beliefs in young children's understanding of deception. *Cognition, 13*, 103–128.

Wing, L. (1981). Asperger syndrome: A clinical account. *Psychological Medicine, 11,* 115–130.

Wing, L. (1988). The autistic continuum. In L. Wing (Ed.), *Aspects of autism: Biological research.* London: Gaskell/Royal College of Psychiatrists.

Wing, L., Gould, J., Yeates, S. R., & Brierley, L. M. (1977). Symbolic play in severely mentally retarded and in autistic children. *Journal of Child Psychology and Psychiatry, 18,* 167–178.

Witelson, S. (1976). Sex and the single hemisphere: Specialization of the right hemisphere for spatial processing. *Science, 193,* 425–427.

Witelson, S. (1989). Hand and sex differences in the isthmus and genu of the human corpus callosum. *Brain, 112,* 799–835.

Witelson, S. (1991). Neural sexual mosaicism: Sexual differentiation of the human temporo-parietal region for function asymmetry. *Psychoneuroendocrinology, 16,* 131–153.

Witkin, H., Oltman, P., Raskin, E., & Karp, S. (1971). *A manual for the embedded figures test.* Palo Alto, CA: Consulting Psychologists Press.

Zelinski, C., Taylor, M., & Juzwin, K. (1991). Neuropsychological deficits in obsessive-compulsive disorder. *Neuropsychiatry, Neuropsychology and Behavioral Neurology, 4,* 110–126.

18 Autism: A Genetic Perspective

Susan L. Santangelo and Susan E. Folstein

HISTORICAL PERSPECTIVE

In 1943, Leo Kanner, the director of the first academic program in child psychiatry in the United States, published a series of 11 cases of a heretofore unrecognized syndrome. He called it *infantile autism: infantile* because it started very early in life and *autism* because the lack of social contact exhibited by these children resembled the Bleulerian symptom of schizophrenia of the same name.

Both these words became embroiled in controversies about the etiology of autism. Kanner (1943) surmised that because it began in infancy, autism must be "constitutional" in nature. Yet, in the 1950s and early 1960s, Kanner and his student, Leo Eisenberg (1957), both under the very powerful influence of the psychoanalytical movement that claimed that autism was caused by parental neglect, questioned this formulation. However, their initial view proved correct, and the etiology of idiopathic autism now is considered to be largely genetic. The term *autism* encouraged the view that the disorder is a very early form of schizophrenia, but no evidence corroborates that the two are etiologically related. The epidemiology, signs and symptoms, and course of illness are very different, and the two conditions, though both strongly genetically influenced, generally do not occur in the same families.

In the decades after Kanner's original description, interest in this new syndrome increased rapidly. Population surveys (Victor, 1966) and case series (Eisenberg, 1957; Rutter et al., 1967; Rutter & Lockyer, 1967) were carried out to establish the frequency of the syndrome and to determine the rates and distribution of various clinical features and course of illness.

We now know that autism manifests by age $2\frac{1}{2}$ and is defined by the failure to develop normal social interaction, by inflexible use of language or the failure to develop language at all, and by restricted and repetitive activities and interests. The manifestations may improve or change with age, but few individuals who meet full criteria in childhood ever become normal. Although low intelligence has never been a defining feature, some three-quarters of individuals with autism have IQs in the retarded range (Smalley et al., 1988). Even those with normal intelligence have a poor prognosis for social adjustment and the ability to function in the workplace. Although autism is not the most common of the childhood-onset neuropsychiatric disorders (with a prevalence of perhaps 2 to 4 per 10,000 school-aged children; Piven & Folstein, 1994), it is very costly in terms of both economics and human suffering. Most autistic individuals require one-to-one education, basic caretaking, and close supervision throughout their lives.

Though clearly the behaviors that define autism are neurobiological in origin and usually have a genetic cause, not all cases likely will have the same cause. In the study of autism, we are at the stage wherein we have a clear definition of the clinical syndrome but no clear biological markers. At this point in our investigations, autism is analogous to heart failure or pneumonia. Each of these disorders is clearly identifiable by clinical examination but has several different etiologies. The specific virus or bacterium relevant to the individual case of pneumonia needs to be identified to prescribe the most effective treatment. Thus, we feel confident that autism is mainly genetic in etiology, but the identity, number, and nature of the specific genes that cause autism—and the way in which these genes cause the neuropathology and consequent behavior—for the most part are unknown. In samples chosen for meeting criteria for autism, perhaps 2% have a mutation on the X chromosome known as *fragile* X (reviewed by Piven et al., 1991), and fewer than 1% are caused by other genetic disorders, such as tuberous sclerosis (Piven & Folstein, 1994).

We also know very little about how these genes act on the brain to cause the symptoms of autism. Brain-imaging studies have demonstrated slightly larger head size and occasional focal heterotopias (Berthier et al., 1990; Piven et al., 1990, 1992). Autopsy reveals consistent abnormalities of neuronal size, number, and organization in some limbic and cerebellar areas, regardless of the IQ of the subjects (Bauman & Kemper, 1994). Cerebellar hypoplasia has been reported by one group (Courchesne et al., 1988, 1994) but has not been confirmed by others (Garber & Ritvo, 1992; Holttum et al., 1992; Piven & Arndt, 1995).

In each of the early published case series, some 2% to 3% of the families contained more than one autistic child. It was pointed out by Rutter (1968) that this was 50 to 100 times greater than was expected by chance, given the population prevalence. At the same time, case reports of concordant twin pairs began to appear in the literature (reviewed in Folstein & Rutter, 1977). These two findings suggested the need to explore more formally the possibility of a genetic etiology.

RECURRENCE RISK FOR AUTISM

To explore possible genetic mechanisms of a disorder and estimate its heritability, geneticists use an estimate of the frequency with which a condition recurs in subsequently born children, after the parents have had one child with the condition. This estimate is called the *recurrence risk*. For many conditions, this can be approximated by the prevalence in siblings. However, when a condition is severely handicapping from an early age, it changes parents' reproductive behavior; they are likely to have no subsequent children or to have just one subsequent child (Jones & Szatmari, 1988). When these "stoppage rules" operate, prevalence in siblings underestimates the risk that the disease will recur in subsequently born offspring. This is true in autism; most nonautistic siblings are older than the proband. Counting only those siblings who are born after the autistic proband, the rate of recurrence for autism is approximately 6% to 8%, more than twice the prevalence in all siblings (Ritvo et al., 1989).

Twin Studies

Distinguishing between familiality and genetic heritability is important. The observation that a trait is familial is genetically uninterpretable. Traits or diseases that run in families may be due also to cultural or infectious transmission. Always possible is that conditions defined only by behavior for which we have no independent biological markers or tests aggregate in families because of some aspect of shared environment. To determine whether a trait is heritable in humans and to control for shared environment, genetic epidemiologists have used twin and adoption studies. Although no adoption studies of autism exist, three twin studies using geographically defined samples have been carried out.

The twin method is based on the assumption that the influence of the shared environment is the same for both identical, or monozygotic (MZ), and fraternal, or dizygotic (DZ), pairs. Genetically, however, the two types of twins are different. MZ pairs are genetically identical, whereas DZ pairs are genetically like siblings who share, on average, 50% of their genes in common. Therefore, differences in the concordance rates for the two kinds of twins are attributed to differences in their degree of genetic similarity.

In the three epidemiologically based twin studies of autism (Folstein & Rutter, 1977; Steffenberg et al., 1989; Bailey et al., 1995), all twins (one or both of whom were affected) who lived in a geographically defined population were sought out; twin studies necessitate attempts to find all the affected twins who live in a geographical area. When twin pairs are found through advertisements for volunteers, families with MZ and concordant twins (both twins affected) are more likely to come forward than are families with twins who are DZ or discordant (only one twin affected). So, studies that are based on advertising for volunteers will overestimate the concordance rate.

Autism twin studies have used only same-gender pairs. As autism is so much more common in boys (the male-female ratio is nearly 3:1), opposite-gender pairs would be more likely to be discordant. The combined number of pairs studied in the three autism twin studies was 66: 36 MZ and 30 DZ. The average MZ concordance rate is 70%, compared with a DZ rate of 0%.

These rates were obtained after excluding three of the original twin pairs from the Folstein and Rutter (1977) study: one pair, because the twins had fragile X and two pairs because the pair had atypical autism and did not meet current International Classification of Diseases ICD-10 criteria (Bailey et al., 1995). One additional DZ pair, concordant for autism, was found by Bailey et al. after ascertainment had closed. If this pair were included, the combined DZ concordance rate for the three studies would be 3%. The concordance of autism in the MZ pairs could not be explained by shared prenatal or perinatal difficulties.

Given the prevalence in siblings, the expected DZ concordance rate is at least 3%. The observed rate of 0% is undoubtedly a chance finding resulting from the small sample size (n = 30) of DZ pairs. Even assuming that the true DZ rate is 3% to 6%, this is a very large MZ/DZ difference, suggesting that autism is highly heritable. The heritability, calculated from the recurrence risk and the MZ/DZ concordance ratio, is more than 90%. This means that 90% of this population's variation in phenotype (the observable manifestation of an individual's genotype in interaction with the environment) can be attributed to variation in genotype, whereas 10% is due to environmental variation.

Perfect heritability (100%) would mean that all the phenotypic variance (differences between individuals) observed in a given population would be due to the genotypic variance and that none would be due to environmental variance. However, that would not necessarily imply that the environment had no influence on phenotypic differences between individuals. It might simply mean that very little environmental variation existed in the particular population studied. Equally possible, for example, is that in countries with a high rate of encephalitis (which may sometimes cause autism), the heritability would be lower.

The MZ concordance rate of 70% suggests other causative factors; if the etiology were purely genetic, the MZ concordance rate would be 100%. However, when concordance is examined for a phenotype consisting of *either* autism *or* milder cognitive and social deficits, 82% of MZ twins, compared with perhaps 10% of DZ pairs, are concordant (Folstein & Rutter, 1977). Most of the nonautistic MZ cotwins had language-based learning disabilities, and several were socially reticent. The social reticence was even more striking when the twins were reexamined in adulthood (Bailey et al., 1995).

Early Studies of Nonautistic Family Members: The Broader Autism Phenotype

The finding that many of the nonautistic cotwins had similar cognitive and social deficits was not anticipated, although perhaps it should have been. As early as 1957 (Eisenberg, 1957) Eisenberg reported that, compared to the fathers of other patients that they had seen, many of the fathers of autistic children had unusual personality traits, such as rigidity and a lack of interest in social interaction. All these men were married, and most were successful professionals who clearly were able to socialize adequately for those purposes; however, in their free time, they preferred solitary activities and tended to follow set routines. The article actually was published in response to the outpouring of psychoanalytical speculation that autism was caused by "refrigerator mothers" (Bettelheim, 1967). Eisenberg wanted to point out that if either parent fit that model, it was more likely to be the father. Eventually, published studies demonstrated that the parents of autistic children were normally affectionate with their children (Cantwell et al., 1979), and considerable other empirical evidence was put forward to refute the refrigerator mother theory (Rimland, 1964). Nevertheless, this gross and unjust disservice to the conscientious and long-suffering parents cast a pall over the study of the family members of autistic children for many years. Following the Folstein and Rutter twin study (1977), several groups resumed the study of families, this time with a genetic hypothesis and with the goal of using the information to establish the genetic mechanism by which autism might be inherited and to find specific genes.

Several of these studies suggested cognitive abnormalities in the non-autistic first-degree relatives of autistic probands. A study comparing autistic children and children with developmental language disorder noted a family history of speech delay in members of 25% of the autism families (Cox et al., 1975). The study used unsystematic family history methods to elicit this information: That is, information on relatives was gathered by interviewing (without the aid of a structured interview) one key informant about all the other relatives, as opposed to interviewing all relatives directly. Family history studies are known to underestimate the true rates of several psychiatric disorders (Thompson et al., 1982).

Another group tested IQ and reading ability in the siblings of autistic and Down syndrome (DS) probands (August et al., 1981). More of the autism siblings scored poorly on reading (but probably not lower than expected for their IQs). Many of the autistic probands were severely retarded, and several of their siblings had low-normal to borderline IQs.

Social abnormalities also were documented in the relatives of individuals with autism. Wolff et al. (1988) compared the parents of autistic children with those of mentally retarded children. The interviewers, who were blind to family membership, conversed with the parents and rated them on a number of traits. More often, the autism parents were rated as being ungregarious, lacking in emotional responsiveness and empathy, oversensitive to criticism, and both over- and undercommunicative. This subset of the autism parents tended to pursue special interests with single-mindedness and had little rapport with the examiner.

The Hopkins autism research group carried out telephone interviews with the parents of 37 autistic adults to get information about the 67 nonautistic siblings of the probands, whose mean age was 33 years (Piven et al., 1990).

Eighteen of the probands had been diagnosed by Kanner. Ten percent of the siblings were reported by their parents to have a history of learning problems in childhood (which mostly had been overcome by adulthood), and 10% had been treated for mood disorders. Three (4.4%) of the adult brothers met criteria for Asperger syndrome.

Asperger syndrome is similar to autism, except that intelligence is usually normal or superior and language development is superficially normal (Asperger, 1944): That is, speech onset is not delayed, nor are obvious semantic or phonemic abnormalities seen. Use of pragmatic language, however, is abnormal. Similarly, the social deficits are less severe, with usually normal attachments to parents but lifelong difficulty in forming peer friendships. Motor stereotypies usually are lacking, but their rigid, stereotyped behavior patterns and circumscribed interests often are striking. Considerable discussion has centered on the relationship between autism and Asperger syndrome. Though the clinical definitions of the two are a little different, the quality and type of abnormalities are very similar, and many individuals who meet criteria for autism early in life, "recover" with development to resemble Asperger syndrome. Very likely, the disorders are genetically related, as one finds individuals with Asperger syndrome in autism families and vice versa.

The siblings of the cases diagnosed by Kanner had a much higher rate of social, cognitive, and mood disorders than did the other cases, and all the Asperger cases were from Kanner's families. Kanner's cases did not have higher IQs, but they did have a rich array of autistic features, including the insistence on sameness, which was a key autistic feature for Kanner.

Taken together, these studies—Eisenberg's descriptions of fathers, the twin studies, and the four studies of family members just described—provided clear evidence that idiopathic autism was not only highly familial but that its etiology had a strong genetic component. However, the mode of inheritance of autism was (and still is) unknown. The difficulty in discerning the mechanism of inheritance is partly due to the fact that families generally are small because of the stoppage rules previously mentioned, wherein parents decide not to have more children after the birth of an autistic child. Small families provide limited opportunity to observe patterns of genetic transmission. In addition, autistic individuals rarely have children, thereby affording little opportunity to observe vertical transmission of the classic disorder.

These studies also suggested that limiting the phenotype to classic autism and dichotomizing it (present-absent) may not be the most powerful or accurate approach to investigating possible genetic mechanisms operating in autism or in finding genes. In fact, evidence from the studies described suggested the hypothesis that some parents and siblings of autistic children had features that bore a striking resemblance to the core features of autism, although much milder than either autism or Asperger syndrome. These features, which include cognitive difficulties, social awkwardness, language abnormalities, and certain personality characteristics (in addition to Asperger syndrome), have come to be called the *broader autism phenotype*. We hypothe-sized that these features might be manifestations of the genetic liability.

Comprehensive Studies of Parents and Siblings

The hypothesis that the features comprising the broader autism phenotype were more common in autism parents than in parents of controls was tested in two family studies, parallel in design and carried out simultaneously in London by Rutter et al. (Pickles et al., 1995; Bolton et al., 1994) and in Baltimore by Folstein et al., (Piven et al., 1990; Piven et al., 1994; Santangelo & Folstein, 1995; Landa et al., 1992). Results of these studies still are being analyzed, but the work completed to date on the Baltimore study clearly indicates that perhaps a third of parents and siblings of autistic children have one or more traits qualitatively similar to the features of autism, although much less severe, rarely coming to clinical attention and, in some cases, hav-ing important adaptive value.

The two parallel studies used a case-control design, comparing families of autistic and DS probands. The main purpose of the DS comparison group was to control for the effect of having a handicapped child but one with a diagnosis that did not confer any genetic liability for similar difficulties on any of the other family members. The Baltimore group obtained all their cases and controls from local family support groups and area schools, asking for volunteers for a study of the causes of autism but without any reference to our genetic hypothesis. In this, we hoped to avoid attracting an excess of families who thought that other family members also were affected.

The initial challenge for these studies was to design or adapt methods for the reliable documentation of the various deficits that, though often easy to discern during conversation with the relatives of autistic children, lacked specific methods for documentation. We set out to develop methods to doc-ument family member characteristics that resembled the three diagnostic features of autism: social deficits, language deficits, and rigid and repetitive behavior and interests. We also included cognitive testing and a psychiatric interview, based on our pilot data suggesting problems in these areas. Several of our approaches were unsuccessful, but most showed differences between autism and DS family members.

Social Deficits   Social deficits were documented by an interview designed to measure personality traits that were extreme enough to cause difficulties variously in work, domestic, or social circumstances. The personality assess-ment schedule (PAS), originally developed by Tyrer (1988), was modified to include more traits that we thought were common in family members of autistic children. The autism parents and adult siblings more often described themselves as aloof, untactful, and undemonstrative of emotion (Piven et al., 1994). Twenty-five percent of the parents scored significantly higher than did the controls on at least one of these traits; 16% scored high on two or more. The main disadvantage of this method was the impossibility of remaining blind to family membership. However, we took great pains to establish reliability and coded an abnormality only when subjects or their spouses gave examples of difficulties that it caused; we did not code difficulties that were noticed only by the research staff.

As a second approach to documenting social difficulties, we developed a friendship interview and rating scale. We asked parents and adult siblings to give the names of three friends outside their family members, and we then asked about the nature of these friendships: whether they were reciprocal, supportive, and intimate. The interview consists of 13 items designed to assess an individual's social interactions outside the immediate family. Rating scale scores are best estimates of an individual's capacity for friendships, based on answers given in the interview. The scores range from 1, which is normal (i.e., the individual has two or more relationships characterized by reciprocity and intimacy), to 5 (for an individual who has never had relationships of this type). The scores for 180 parents of 90 autism probands were significantly higher (worse) than those for 80 parents of 40 DS control probands. In fact, 20% of the autism parents, representing one-third of autism families, versus 6% of the parents of DS controls (10% of DS families) scored in the deviant range on the rating scale (Santangelo & Folstein, 1995).

Language Deficits Dr. Rebecca Landa, a speech and language scientist, developed two methods for assessing language deficits on the basis of linguistic classifications. She developed a rating scale for pragmatic aspects of language (Landa et al., 1992) and used the story stem method for documenting the parents' difficulties in narrative discourse (Landa et al., 1991). Though we did not document an increased rate of delayed onset of speech and language in autism relatives, we observed that deficits in pragmatic language use and in narrative language were striking and, again, present in some 20% to 30% of the autism parents and adult siblings. These instruments were rated from audiotapes, blind to family membership. Landa's current work (Landa, 1996) extends the investigation of language development to the young siblings of autistic children.

Rigid and Repetitive Behaviors and Interests We had expected to find an increased rate of obsessive-compulsive disorder (OCD) or obsessional personality traits among the relatives of autistic probands. However, on the basis of interviews using a structured psychiatric interview—the Schizophrenia and Affective Disorder Schedule–Lifetime version (SADS-L) (Endicott & Spitzer, 1978) no parents received a diagnosis of OCD (Piven et al., 1991). Our method of inquiry about obsessional and rigid personality traits by use of the PAS probably was not designed well. In a subsequent study of the parents of two autistic probands carried out in Iowa, this part of the interview was modified and also was rated from videotapes, blind to family membership. In addition to the traits *aloof* and *untactful* identified in the Baltimore Family Study, a rigid adherence to routine emerged as significantly more common in autism family members than among controls in the subsequent study (Piven et al., 1997).

Cognitive Disorders We did not find any excess of mental retardation in either the parents or the siblings of autistic probands. In fact, they had higher-than-average IQs (though not different from the control families who were ascertained from similar support groups and schools) and were matched for education and social class. Additionally, the autism family members did not differ from controls on standard tests of reading, including reading comprehension, and spelling (Wzorek et al., 1991). Two interesting findings emerged. First, autism parents more often had large verbal performance discrepancies on the Wechsler Adult Intelligence Scale (Wechsler, 1981), with verbal scores higher than those of performance. Secondly, autism parents performed significantly worse on picture arrangement, often conceived as an estimate of "social intelligence," and on picture completion (Wzorek et al., unpublished manuscript).

Psychiatric Disorders Using the SADS-L (Endicott & Spitzer, 1978; Piven et al., 1991), we found a higher rate of anxiety disorders (in a combination of all types of anxiety disorders) and a rate of major depression in the autism relatives higher than that in the DS relatives. Minor depression was equally prevalent in the two groups. This has been reported previously in parents of handicapped children (Breslau & Davis, 1986). For most parents, the onset of the anxiety and mood disorders preceded the birth of their autistic child and, therefore, could not be explained as a response to the burden of having a handicapped child.

DEFINITION OF THE BROADER AUTISM PHENOTYPE FOR USE IN GENETIC LINKAGE STUDIES

For the purposes of defining the traits present in the family members of autistic children more often than in controls, each of our findings is important in itself. However, for the purpose of finding genes for autism in a genetic linkage study, we want to define a broader autism phenotype that provides a maximum distinction between cases and controls, is likely to be "genetically valid" (in that its pattern in families roughly conforms to the expectations of Mendelian genetic transmission), and provides documentation practical for use in a very large sample, the size necessary for a genetic linkage study.

One approach is to define as "affected" only those family members who score abnormally in at least two of the three areas—social deficits, pragmatic language abnormalities, and rigid behaviors or circumscribed interests—that define autism. This approach has been taken by the London group in the analysis of their family history data from the parallel study (Bolton et al.,

1994). Perhaps 1% of the parents and 12% of the siblings in the London sample were termed *affected* by this scheme. It includes all persons in the families who meet criteria for autism, for pervasive developmental disorder (PDD: individuals meeting two of the three basic criteria for autism), and for Asperger syndrome and family members with a similar but milder phenotype. When deficits in only one of the three areas were required, approximately 20% of siblings and 11% of parents were included. When the autistic, PDD, and Asperger cases were excluded, the rates of the milder traits were lower: 7% of siblings had two or more traits, and 9% had one. These rates, not surprisingly, are lower than those found in direct testing of similar traits reported in the Baltimore study. The family history method is always less sensitive than are direct interviews and tests.

Another approach is to use multivariate analyses to determine empirically which of the direct test measures, and in what combination, is most powerful in specifying family membership correctly. For example, using logistical regression, the model that best discriminated the cases from controls included several traits from the PAS (aloof, untactful, anxiously worrying, and undemonstrative of emotion), the friendship score, a history of early trouble with reading and language, and the performance IQ.

The friendship score, the one variable so far analyzed in this way, appears to conform to expectations of genetic transmission. When one or both parents scored abnormally, as occurred in one-third of the families, 25% of their nonautistic adult children also scored in the abnormal range. Among the two-thirds of families in which both parents scored normally, only 3% of their adult children scored abnormally. Unlike the family history measures used in the London report, which found that siblings were affected more often than were parents, siblings and parents in the Baltimore Family Study were equally likely to have abnormal friendship scores. This also was true for several other measures.

Possibly, in the friendship score, we have happened onto a measure of one of the several putative genes that converge to cause autism. Equally possible is that (as described in the next section) each of the several genes hypothesized to act in concert to cause autism has a definable phenotype [e.g., pragmatic deficits, rigidity, executive function deficits (Ozonoff et al., 1991) or social deficits].

POSSIBLE GENETIC MECHANISMS

Defined Genetic Etiologies

Autism already is known to be a genetically heterogeneous disorder (i.e., not all the cases with a genetic cause have the same gene as the cause). Several single-gene conditions are more frequently associated with autism than would be expected, and many individual case reports speak of autism with visible chromosomal (cytogenetic) abnormalities. However, these single-gene conditions, including phenylketonuria (PKU), tuberous sclerosis, and fragile X syndrome, account for only a small proportion (perhaps 3%) of the cases. Nevertheless, these conditions are important because of the clues that they might provide about idiopathic autism and because the diagnosis is important to genetic counseling.

The associations between autism and the single-gene conditions—PKU, tuberous sclerosis, and fragile X syndrome—remain controversial for two reasons. First, it has not always been clear that the cases meet diagnostic criteria for autism. This is especially true for untreated PKU (reviewed in Folstein & Rutter, 1988). The associations were reported at a time when the standard of clinical description for published cases was low, and the studies cannot be repeated using current methods because now PKU is treated. The second reason for controversy is the fact that mental retardation is a prominent feature of these syndromes. That mental retardation also is a common feature of autism (although not a defining one) has created difficulty in sorting out whether the associations have been between these syndromes and autism or between the syndromes and severe mental retardation, wherein social and language abnormalities also are very common. Recent studies of tuberous sclerosis do confirm a high prevalence of autism among the cases with mental retardation (Smalley et al., 1992; Hunt & Shepherd, 1993). The detailed studies of the fragile X phenotype suggest that the language and social characteristics, though similar to autism, often are distinguishable (reviewed in Folstein & Piven, 1991).

In addition to the single-gene disorders that have been associated with autism, many case reports have cited autistic children (usually with accompanying severe mental retardation) who have detectable cytogenetic abnormalities that are likely to involve several genes. The most intriguing are the reports of partial duplications of chromosome 15 (Baker et al., 1994). These are interesting because a fairly large number of chromosome 15 partial duplications have been reported and because, as opposed to deletions, duplications (extra chromosomal material) are uncommon and often are associated with increased gene dosage. Both deletions and duplications can be useful in pointing to genetic loci of general importance to etiology. Once a general area is identified using linkage analysis, a case with a deletion in that area sometimes can be used to pinpoint the location of the gene.

Possible Mechanisms for Idiopathic Autism

The most parsimonious genetic model for the remaining cases of idiopathic autism may be one in which three or four genes interact with one another to produce the autism phenotype. In an analysis of the Baltimore Family Study data, Van Eerdewegh (unpublished data) rejected a single-locus model and heterogeneity models and found that a model with three to six epistatic (interacting) loci was the simplest model consistent with the data. The data for this analysis, which used a graphical method (Craddock et al., 1995), included the population prevalence of classic autism, the rate of autism in siblings of autistic probands, and the rate in MZ co-twins. In an analysis of the London family history data, using a latent-class analytical approach, Pickles et al. (1995) also rejected a single-locus model and heterogeneity models in favor of a multilocus epistatic model involving anywhere from 2 to 10 loci, with 3 loci being most plausible. This analysis examined rates of autism-PDD, and both narrow and broad definitions of the broader autism phenotype, in first-, second-, and third-degree relatives of autistic probands. Though whether all idiopathic cases share the same mode of genetic transmission is not clear, presently the most compelling hypothesis for the genetic transmission of autism is a model involving three or four interacting genes. That is, children with autism are most likely to result when they inherit three or four genes from the parents, each of which contributes to causing the defining phenotype. The model cannot specify whether these are always the same three or four genes or whether several combinations of three or four genes from a larger array of predisposing genes could cause autism.

This model also provides an explanation for the variation in severity of autism in sibling pairs and for the fact that, in families ascertained through an autistic proband, other members are found with Asperger syndrome or PDD. One would expect that the milder phenotypes result when a child inherits fewer of the same genes that predispose to autism. Similarly, the traits that are found (often in isolation) in parents of autistic children could be the manifestations of just one or two of the predisposing genes.

Some have speculated that because of the preponderance of male cases, genes on the X chromosome might be involved. It seems unlikely that a single gene located on the X chromosome causes autism. Diseases and traits that are transmitted on the X chromosome never show father-to-son transmission because fathers give only their Y chromosome to their sons. Hall-mayer et al. (1996) reported on 11 families having multiple affected autistic members wherein the family structures were such that inheritance could be traced through at least two generations. Half these families were incompatible with X linkage because of father-to-son transmission. We have observed this also with transmission of the broader autism phenotype: Many fathers with some of the traits of the broader phenotype have autistic sons. However, still possible is that one of the several genes that interact to cause autism is located on the X chromosome.

One regularly sees affected cousins and occasionally sees several autistic individuals in a few collateral lines of a single family. Though such families with multiple affected members in more than one branch of the family are uncommon, they do exist; probably, in these families, autism is caused by just one or two genes, owing to the low probability that three or four genes, the number thought necessary to cause a multigenic form of autism, would co-occur in the same extended family so frequently. However, we expect that cases caused by single genes will be rare.

One sort of single-gene mutation, known as a *dynamic mutation*, is seen in families in which manifestation of the disease worsens as it is passed from one generation to another, a phenomenon known as *anticipation*. The dynamic mutations so far have been characterized by repetitive sequences of three base pairs (trimeric repeat sequences) that enlarge as the gene is transmitted from one generation to the next (Ross, 1995). Fragile X is one such mutation (see chapter 3). A parent who has the broader autism phenotype and has children with autism is an example of anticipation, but the mechanism by which it might occur to produce autism is unknown. Possibly, each parent carries one or two of the relevant genes, causing a mild phenotype in the parent and a more severe phenotype in offspring who receive a larger gene dose from the two parents.

GENETIC COUNSELING

The recurrence risk for autism is 6% to 8% for siblings born after the first affected child. Preliminary evidence demonstrates that if there are two autistic children in a family, the risk for having a third affected child may be as high as 25% (Piven, personal communication). However, this result is based on a very small sample and must be replicated.

The risk for Asperger syndrome to a family with an autistic child is also very likely to be elevated, but the evidence for this is more anecdotal and not based on systematic study. Among the adult siblings seen in the Baltimore Family Study, 4.2% (2 of 48) met criteria for Asperger syndrome (Folstein & Santangelo, unpublished manuscript). In the family history study described earlier (Piven et al., 1990) 4.4% (3 of 67) of siblings of autistic probands met criteria for Asperger syndrome.

The risk to siblings for having one or more of the features of the broader autism phenotype may be as high as 30% in adult siblings. How this might manifest in children is not yet clear.

CONCLUSIONS

Evidence from family and twin studies indicates that idiopathic autism is strongly familial and heritable. Though the prevalence of autism among the siblings of autistic individuals is some 3%, the recurrence risk is at least twice that number: 6% to 8%. The MZ/DZ twin concordance ratio is high and, in combination with the recurrence risk, yields a heritability estimate of nearly 90%. However, the MZ twin concordance rate of 70% suggests nongenetic risk factors as well. The mode of transmission of a gene or genes for autism is as yet unknown, in part because of the added difficulty of trying to discern transmission patterns in small families, with little opportunity to observe vertical transmission.

The task of identifying chromosomal locations for autism genes may become easier with the reliable identification of milder but qualitatively similar traits that appear to be present in some of the relatives of autistic probands. The possible presence of several relevant traits in parents that are markers for some of the genes that cause autism will provide a greater opportunity to observe more affected individuals per family, increasing the power of family and linkage studies. In light of the evidence that autism is unlikely to be a monogenic disorder (and rather probably involves three to four genes), adequate power is critical to the success of linkage studies of autism. In broadening the criteria for the relevant phenotype however, we must be conservative and scrupulous in our definition of what constitutes being affected, so as not to increase the number of false-positive diagnoses, which can seriously compromise the success of linkage analyses. We are in the process of defining the broader autism phenotypes so as to be as inclusive as possible while simultaneously minimizing the potential for false-positive diagnoses.

ACKNOWLEDGMENTS

This study was supported by United States Public Health Services grants MH39936 and MH01338.

REFERENCES

Asperger, H. (1944). Die autistischen psychopathen im kindesalter. *Archiv fur Psychiatrie und Nervenkrankheiten, 117,* 76–136.

August, G. J., Stewart, M. A., & Tsai, L. (1981). The incidence of cognitive disabilities in the siblings of autistic children. *British Journal of Psychiatry, 138,* 416–422.

Bailey, A., Le Couteur, A., Gottesman, I., et al. (1995). Autism as a strongly genetic disorder: Evidence from a British twin study. *Psychological Medicine, 25*(1), 63–77.

Baker, P., Piven, J., Schwartz, S., & Patil, S. (1994). Brief report: Duplication of chromosome 15q11–13 in two individuals with autistic disorder. *Journal of Autism and Developmental Disorders, 24*(4), 529–535.

Bauman, M., and Kemper, T. (1994). Neuroanatomic observations of the brain in autism. In: M. Bauman & T. Kemper (Eds.), *The neurobiology of autism* (pp. 119–145). Baltimore: Johns Hopkins University Press.

Berthier, M. L., Starkstein, S. E., and Leiguarda, R. (1990). Developmental cortical anomalies in Asperger's syndrome: Neuroradiological findings in two patients. *Journal of Neuropsychiatry and Clinical Neuroscience, 2*(2), 197–201.

Bettelheim, B. (1967). *The empty fortress: Infantile autism and the birth of the self.* New York: Free Press.

Bolton, P., Macdonald, H., Pickles, A., et al. (1994). A case-control family history study of autism. *Journal of Child Psychology and Psychiatry, 35*(5), 877–900.

Breslau, N., & Davis, G. C. (1986). Chronic stress and major depression. *Archives of General Psychiatry, 43*(4), 309–314.

Cantwell, D. P., Baker, L., & Rutter, M. (1979). Families of autistic and dysphasic children: I. Family life and interaction patterns. *Archives of General Psychiatry, 36*(6), 682–687.

Courchesne, E., Townsend, J., & Saitoh, O. (1994). The brain in infantile autism: Posterior fossa structures are abnormal. *Neurology, 44*(2), 214–223.

Courchesne, E., Yeung-Courchesne, R., Press, G. A., Hesselink, J. R., & Jernigan, T. L. (1988). Hypoplasia of cerebellar vermal lobules VI and VII in autism. *New England Journal of Medicine, 318*(21), 1349–1354.

Cox, A., Rutter, M., Newman, S., & Bartak, L. (1975). A comparative study of infantile autism and specific developmental receptive language disorder: II. Parental characteristics. *British Journal of Psychiatry, 126,* 146–159.

Craddock, N., Khodel, V., Van Eerdewegh, P., & Reich, T. (1995). Mathematical limits of multi-locus models: The genetic transmission of bipolar disorder. *American Journal of Human Genetics, 57*(3), 690–702.

Eisenberg, L. (1957). The fathers of autistic children. *American Journal of Orthopsychiatry, 127,* 715–724.

Endicott, J., & Spitzer, R. L. (1978). A diagnostic interview: The schedule for affective disorders and schizophrenia. *Archives of General Psychiatry, 35*(7), 837–844.

Folstein, S. E., & Piven, J. (1991). Etiology of autism: Genetic influences [review]. *Pediatrics, 87*(5), 767–773.

Folstein, S. E., & Rutter, M. L. (1988). Autism: Familial aggregation and genetic implications [review]. *Journal of Autism and Developmental Disorders, 18*(1), 3–30.

Folstein, S., & Rutter, M. (1977). Infantile autism: A genetic study of 21 twin pairs. *Journal of Child Psychology and Psychiatry and Allied Disciplines, 18*(4), 297–321.

Garber, H. J., & Ritvo, E. R. (1992). Magnetic resonance imaging of the posterior fossa in autistic adults. *American Journal of Psychiatry, 149*(2), 245–247.

Hallmayer, J., Spiker, D., Lotspeich, L., et al. (1996). Male-to-male transmission in extended pedigrees with multiple cases of autism. *American Journal of Medical Genetics: Neuropsychiatric Genetics, 67,* 13–18.

Holttum, J. R., Minshew, N. J., Sanders, R. S., and Phillips, N. E. (1992). Magnetic resonance imaging of the posterior fossa in autism. *Biological Psychiatry, 32*(12), 1091–1101.

Hunt, A., Shepherd, C. (1993). A prevalence study of autism in tuberous sclerosis. *Journal of Autism and Developmental Disorders, 23*(2), 323–339.

Jones, M. B., & Szatmari, P. (1988). Stoppage rules and genetic studies of autism. *Journal of Autism and Developmental Disorders, 18*(1), 31–40.

Kanner, L. (1943). Autistic disturbances of affective contact. *Nervous Child, 2,* 217–250.

Landa, R. (1996 June). *Evidence for specific impairment in siblings of autistic individuals.* In Presentation at the Symposium for Research on Child Language Disorders, Madison, WI.

Landa, R., Folstein, S. E., & Isaacs, C. (1991). Spontaneous narrative-discourse performance of parents of autistic individuals. *Journal of Speech and Hearing Research, 34*(6), 1339–1345.

Landa, R., Piven, J., Wzorek, M. M., Gayle, J. O., Chase, G. A., & Folstein, S. E. (1992). Social language use in parents of autistic individuals. *Psychological Medicine, 22*(1), 245–254.

Ozonoff, S., Pennington, B. F., & Rogers, S. J. (1991). Executive function deficits in high-functioning autistic individuals: Relationship to theory of mind. *Journal of Child Psychology and Psychiatry and Allied Disciplines, 32*(7), 1081–1105.

Pickles, A., Bolton, P., Macdonald, H., et al. (1995). Latent-class analysis of recurrence risks for complex phenotypes with selection and measurement error: A twin and family history study of autism. *American Journal of Human Genetics, 57*(3), 717–726.

Piven, J., & Arndt, S. (1995). The cerebellum and autism [letter]. *Neurology, 45*(2), 398–402.

Piven, J., Berthier, M. L., Starkstein, S. E., Nehme, E., Pearlson, G., & Folstein, S. (1990). Magnetic resonance imaging evidence for a defect of cerebral cortical development in autism. *American Journal of Psychiatry, 147*(6), 734–739.

Piven, J., Chase, G. A., Landa, R., et al. (1991). Psychiatric disorders in the parents of autistic individuals. *Journal of the American Academy of Child and Adolescent Psychiatry, 30*(3), 471–478.

Piven, J., & Folstein, S. (1994). The genetics of autism. In M. Bauman & T. Kemper (Eds.), *The neurobiology of autism* (pp. 18–44). Baltimore: Johns Hopkins University Press.

Piven, J., Gayle, J., Chase, G. A., et al. (1990). A family history study of neuropsychiatric disorders in the adult siblings of autistic individuals. *Journal of the American Academy of Child and Adolescent Psychiatry, 29*(2), 177–183.

Piven, J., Gayle, J., Landa, R., Wzorek, M., & Folstein, S. (1991). The prevalence of fragile X in a sample of autistic individuals diagnosed using a standardized interview. *Journal of the American Academy of Child and Adolescent Psychiatry, 30*(5), 825–830.

Piven, J., Nehme, E., Simon, J., Barta, P., Pearlson, G., & Folstein, S. E. (1992). Magnetic resonance imaging in autism: Measurement of the cerebellum, pons, and fourth ventricle. *Biological Psychiatry, 31*(5), 491–504.

Piven, J., Palmer, P., Jacobi, D., & Childress, D. & Arndt, S. (1997). The broader autism phenotype: Eridence from a family study of multiple-incidence autism families. *American Journral of Psychiatry, 154*, 185–190.

Piven, J., Wzorek, M., Landa, R., et al. (1994). Personality characteristics of the parents of autistic individuals. *Psychological Medicine, 24*(3), 783–795.

Rimland, B. (1964). *Infantile autism: The syndrome and its implications for a neural theory of behavior.* New York: Appleton-Century-Crofts.

Ritvo, E. R., Jorde, L. B., Mason-Brothers, A., et al. (1989). The UCLA-University of Utah epidemiologic survey of autism: Recurrence risk estimates and genetic counseling. *American Journal of Psychiatry, 146*(8), 1032–1036.

Ross, C. A. (1995). When more is less: Pathogenesis of glutamine repeat neurodegenerative diseases [review]. *Neuron, 15*(3), 493–496.

Rutter, M. (1968). Concepts of autism: A review of research [review]. *Journal of Child Psychology and Psychiatry and Allied Disciplines, 9*(1), 1–25.

Rutter, M., Greenfeld, D., & Lockyer, L. (1967). A five to fifteen year follow-up study of infantile psychosis: II. Social and behavioural outcome. *British Journal of Psychiatry, 113*, 1183–1199.

Rutter, M., & Lockyer, L. (1967). A five to fifteen year follow-up study of infantile psychosis: I. Description of sample. *British Journal of Psychiatry, 113*, 1169–1182.

Santangelo, S. L., & Folstein, S. E. (1995). Social deficits in the families of autistic probands. *American Journal of Human Genetics, 57*(4), 89.

Smalley, S. L., Asarnow, R. F., & Spence, M. A. (1988). Autism and genetics. A decade of research [review]. *Archives of General Psychiatry, 45*(10), 953–961.

Smalley, S. L., Tanguay, P. E., Smith, M., & Gutierrez, G. (1992). Autism and tuberous sclerosis. *Journal of Autism and Developmental Disorders, 22*(3), 339–355.

Steffenburg, S., Gillberg, C., Hellgren, L., et al. (1989). A twin study of autism in Denmark, Finland, Iceland, Norway and Sweden. *Journal of Child Psychology and Psychiatry and Allied Disciplines, 30*(3), 405–416.

Thompson, W. D., Orvaschel, H., Prusoff, B. A., & Kidd, K. K. (1982). An evaluation of the family history method for ascertaining psychiatric disorders. *Archives of General Psychiatry, 39*(1), 53–58.

Tyrer, P. (1988). *Personality assessment schedule. Personality disorders: Diagnosis management and course* (pp. 140–167). London: Butterworth.

Victor, L. (1966). Epidemiology of autistic conditions in young children: I. Prevalence. *Social Psychiatry, 1,* 124–147.

Weschler, D. (1981). *Wechsler Adult Intelligence Scale–Revised.* San Antonio, TX: The Psychological Corporation.

Wolff, S., Narayan, S., & Moyes, B. (1988). Personality characteristics of parents of autistic children: A controlled study. *Journal of Child Psychology and Psychiatry and Allied Disciplines, 29*(2), 143–153.

Wzorek, M., Landa, R., Piven, J., & Folstein, S. (1991 October). *Cognition in parents and sibs of autistic probands.* Presentation at the Annual Meeting of the American Psychiatric Association, New Orleans.

IV   Broader Perspectives on Neurodevelopmental Disorders

19 On Neurodevelopmental Disorders: Perspectives from Neurobehavioral Teratology

Jane Adams

Neurobehavioral teratology is the study of abnormal development of the nervous system and behavior as a consequence of prenatal environmental insult. The history of this discipline is deeply steeped in a regulatory context and, as a result, most research has focused on risk assessment issues. This context has produced an overriding emphasis on the continuum of outcomes in an effort to establish "no-effect" levels for chemically induced teratogenesis. Current neurobehavioral research exists in five major forms: (1) examinations of the prevalence of behavioral deficits in exposed individuals; (2) examinations of the relationships between dose and time of exposure and the syndromes of resulting physical and behavioral abnormalities; (3) examinations of the relationships between brain insult and the disruption of other developing systems in an effort to identify early correlates or predictors of risk status for functional or behavioral deficits; (4) integrations of information in an effort to derive governing principles of neurobehavioral teratogenesis; and (5) research directed at the understanding of mechanisms through which teratogens disrupt development. Most studies in neurobehavioral teratology are conducted using animal models. Human studies have primarily focused on the identification during infancy of syndromes of physical abnormalities after prenatal exposure, with behavioral evaluations receiving less attention. Historically, the detection and definition of human cognitive deficits has been limited to the identification of mental retardation through psychometric approaches and in conjunction with some attention to neuroanatomy. However, newer work is beginning to focus on specific strengths and weaknesses in cognitive processing abilities in lesser affected children, and a continuum of deficits within the cognitive domain has been clearly established.

Research in neuroteratology that has been directed at the understanding of mechanisms of teratogenesis has primarily examined effects at the severe end of the continuum. In vitro cellular and molecular approaches have been used to identify mechanisms responsible for pronounced neuroanatomical and craniofacial abnormalities. An integration of information provided from the five separate, sometimes divergent research avenues provides a conceptual pathway for understanding the factors relevant to the early emergence of disrupted neural development that is reflected in neurobehavioral aberration.

This chapter first presents a brief history of neurobehavioral teratology in order to provide a context for understanding the principles that have emerged and the issues that warrant further attention. A conceptual overview of fundamental principles of teratogenesis and how they may inform the study of all congenital neurobehavioral disorders is presented. The discussion highlights the continuum and syndromic nature of outcomes over which teratogenesis is expressed, individual factors that influence vulnerability to teratogenic insult and contribute to variations in outcome, the stage- and dose-specific nature of teratogenicity, and mechanisms of teratogenesis. Principles are illustrated primarily through information on the teratogenicity of retinoid compounds. Retinoids, members of the vitamin A family of compounds, are among the most thoroughly studied teratogens, owing to their potency and their use as experimental tools for studying the production of insults. The nature of retinoid teratogencity has been a major contributor to establishing principles of teratogenesis and neurobehavioral teratogenesis, as well as to determining the validity of animal models for the full spectrum of outcomes (from death to dysfunction). Throughout the discussion of principles, parallels to research on genetic mental retardation syndromes are presented when possible. Finally, common governing principles are proposed that appear to exist among neurodevelopmental disorders, whether of environmental or genetic etiology. These commonalities then are used to suggest how certain comparisons and contrasts may elucidate knowledge relevant to disorders from each etiology and might facilitate understanding of more general underpinnings of cognitive neuropsychological dysfunction. The question posed is as follows: "Given that aberrant behavior is a final common pathway for the expression of neural dysfunction resulting from multiple possible etiologies, what is the most parsimonious approach to understanding cognitive developmental disorders?" From the teratological perspective, the clearest pathway to understanding is to begin by examining the embryological context in which a disorder emerges and the syndrome and continuum of defects that characterize its manifestations.

FORCES IN THE EVOLUTION OF NEUROBEHAVIORAL TERATOLOGY

The first reports of prenatal drug effects on postnatal behavior were published in the early 1960s. However, greater activity began in the early 1970s (see reviews by Butcher, 1985; Vorhees, 1986), when behavioral effects first were suggested to represent the "subtle" end of a continuum in the expression of prenatal insult. Early studies were conducted mostly in animal species, with some precedent from human data on the effects of exposure to radiation or methyl mercury. Early research in neurobehavioral teratology emerged within the context of a science of teratology that focused rather narrowly on death and malformation as manifestations of teratogenesis. It also emerged in a budding regulatory context that sought to determine the nature and extent of screening requirements for teratogenicity that would be imposed by the US Food and Drug Administration, a major impetus having been the identification of thalidomide as a teratogen. Thalidomide, the drug identified as a teratogen in the early 1960s, was described primarily according to its most salient feature, reduction deformities of the limbs. It should be noted, however, that the syndrome includes certain major organ abnormalities, craniofacial abnormalities, ocular and ophthalmic abnormalities, and related sensory dysfunction, as well as cranial nerve abnormalities (see reviews by Newman, 1985, and Stromland & Miller, 1993). An increased incidence of mental retardation has not been reported in thalidomide-exposed individuals, though several cases of autism with mental retardation have been reported (Stromland et al., 1994). Neuropsychological characteristics apparently have never been evaluated systematically.

The most salient of the embryopathic features induced by thalidomide, radiation, and methyl mercury were grossly observable. In this context, federal regulations for screening of compounds relevant to the US Food and Drug Administration were deemed feasible for visible anatomical abnormalities; screening for behavioral dysfunction was not. Some researchers expressed the belief that, from a teratogen identification perspective, behavioral testing was unnecessary given that the identification of malformations would already classify compounds as teratogenic. Others expressed concern that behavioral data could never stand alone in the risk assessment process as a means of identifying no-effect levels of exposure: Measurements of behavior were considered not to meet "scientific" standards for validity, reliability, or methodological standardization necessary to support incorporation into regulatory screening requirements (Kimmel & Buelke-Sam, 1985). Further, some workers held that behavioral aberrations may not be governed by the same principles as were established for death and malformation end points of teratogenesis. Thus, the stage was set for the emergent discipline of neurobehavioral teratology to be largely separate from conventional teratology rather than viewed as an integral part of it. Correspondingly, several "criteria" were put forth that had to be satisfied by neurobehavioral teratology to establish its importance. The mission then was to demonstrate the validity, reliability, and sensitivity of behavioral methodologies for the assessment of risks while simultaneously demonstrating that behavioral aberration could occur in the absence of other manifestations of teratogenesis. To be successful, neurobehavioral teratogenic effects had to be demonstrated at levels of exposure lower than, or at later developmental stages than, those that produce gross structural malformations. Additionally, cognitive aberrations had to be shown to be unconfounded by other factors such as reduced weight or sensorimotor dysfunction. Prevalent in the regulatory and scientific milieu was the idea that the interpretation of behavioral data would be severely compromised by the presence of *any* form of malformation or any type of sensory or motor system anomaly. Thus, researchers in neurobehavioral teratology have always paid careful attention to possible confounders in the interpretation, particularly in performance on cognitive measures. However, it has been customary to restrict animal behavioral evaluations to dose levels or stages of exposure that do not produce physical, sensory, or motor abnormalities rather than to develop methods that tease things apart. Thus, neurobehavioral teratology has emerged with a focus on the more subtle end of the spectrum of abnormalities produced by an agent.

In human neurobehavioral teratology, where control of dosing is not possible, evaluations and discussions of cognitive functioning have been presented clearly as a continuum, alongside the general physical status of the individuals. Thus, the cognitive status of individuals with fetal alcohol syndrome who, by definition, have growth retardation and physical malformations diagnosable at birth, generally is presented separately from that of children with fetal alcohol effects who lack gross physical markers of exposure (see discussions by Streissguth, 1986; Randall et al., 1990; West & Goodlett, 1990; West et al., 1994).

HISTORICAL FORCES ON RESEARCH IN NEUROBEHAVIORAL TERATOLOGY VERSUS GENETIC MENTAL RETARDATION SYNDROMES

At this point, let us contrast the historical foci of neurobehavioral teratology with those for the study of genetic neurodevelopmental disorders. First, animal models have played a more central role in neurobehavioral teratological studies (wherein they are easily established) than in studies of genetic disorders. Second, understanding the continuum of expression of dysfunction and the variables that determine it has been of paramount importance in neurobehavioral teratology. Only recently have genetic mental retardation syndromes been examined for and determined to display a continuum of medical and cognitive severity over which they are expressed. Third, for the neurobehavioral teratologist, both addressing and avoiding the relationships between physical and behavioral characteristics have been driving forces in experimental design and data interpretation. Thus, cognitive data are reported in conjunction with a careful presentation of the malformation or anomaly status of an individual and his or her performance on sensory and motor tasks. In contrast, the physical characteristics (malformation status, general health status, sensory characteristics, motor characteristics) of the specific subjects in studies of genetic disorders rarely are reported. Fourth, neurobehavioral teratologists have had the advantage of knowing exposure characteristics (relatively precisely in animal studies, less so in humans) and, therefore, the task of addressing relationships between stage- and dose-response issues and the continuum of expression of dysfunction has been rather straightforward. The exploration and understanding of causative genetic factors and their mechanistic relationship to phenotype have been technologically limited, until recently, in studies of the genetic disorders.

RELEVANT PRINCIPLES OF NEUROBEHAVIORAL TERATOGENESIS

Given the *Zeitgeist* for the ontogeny of neurobehavioral teratology as a discipline, many of the neurobehavioral teratological studies conducted since the 1970s have aimed to establish the principles that do govern behavioral teratogenicity and the extent to which they overlap with or diverge from established principles of classical teratology. A solid empirical foundation now substantiates the common principles that govern vulnerability in all organ systems, including the brain and its behavioral controlling systems (see Vorhees, 1986; Adams, 1993a). Effects appear to be manifest in a continuum of expression from death and malformation to growth and functional abnormalities. Let us now consider the principles that are most relevant to the examination of developmental disorders from the perspectives of neurobehavioral teratology.

Teratogenic Effects Expressed Over a Continuum of Severity

A hallmark of teratology is that effects are variably expressed over a continuum of severity, from death and malformation at one end to effects on growth and function at the other. Thus, the same administered dose at the same point in embryonic development may be lethal in one case, produce a cluster of malformations in another, and produce no physical abnormalities in another case. For example, exposure to isotretinoin ([13-*cis*-retinoic acid (Accutane)] during the first 60 days of human pregnancy produces a spectrum of outcomes (Lammer et al., 1985; Adams & Lammer, 1991). Risks associated with human exposure during embryogenesis include a 40% risk for spontaneous abortion, 4% to 5% risk for perinatal mortality, 16% risk for premature birth, and 25% risk for major malformation (Lammer et al., 1985, 1988). The characteristic pattern of malformations involves craniofacial, cardiac, thymic, and central nervous system (CNS) structures. Major malformations of the CNS include cerebellar hypoplasia, agenesis of the vermis, enlargement of the fourth ventricle, malformation-induced hydrocephalus, cortical abnormalities, and microcephaly in some cases. Importantly, these CNS abnormalities have not been systematically evaluated but instead emerge from clinically motivated evaluations. Autopsy of the brains of affected fetuses or infants has revealed abnormalities in the cerebellum, pons, medulla, thalamus, and hippocampus, heterotopias in frontal cortex, and white-matter gliosis (Lammer & Armstrong, 1992). Craniofacial abnormalities include external ear abnormalities (anotia or microtia), abnormal ear canals, mild facial asymmetry, facial nerve paresis, and mild mandibular hypoplasia. This constellation of major organ, CNS, and craniofacial abnormalities is consistent with disruption of adjacent neuroectodermal and normal cranial neural crest cell migration prior to and around the time of neural tube closure (Lammer et al., 1985; Adams, 1996).

A continuum of cognitive deficits also is expressed by a number of tera-togens, although historically more attention has been paid to a dichotomous description of cognitive outcome as mentally retarded versus "normal." Thus, individuals functioning in the borderline range were deemed normal, as were significantly learning-disabled individuals with average IQ status. As a result, the sensitivity of risk assessment has been highly restricted. Attention to profiles of neuropsychological performance is now evident in research on lead (see chapter 20), ethanol (Streissguth, 1986; Streissguth et al., 1983, 1990, 1991; Don & Rourke, 1995), and isotretinoin (Adams & Lammer, 1991, 1995; Adams et al., 1991). This focus is critical to both risk assessment and understanding of underlying substrates. Human data on iso-tretinoin teratogenicity exemplifies this point.

A longitudinal follow-up of the children exposed prenatally to isotretinoin clearly reveals a continuum of cognitive deficits from profound mental retar-dation through apparent intellectual normality. At the age of 5 years, 13.6% of the children prenatally exposed to isotretinoin performed in the mentally retarded range (Stanford-Binet IV), and 29.4% performed in the borderline range of intelligence (70–84 full-scale IQ). Thus, 43% of the exposed chil-dren were performing at below-average levels of general mental ability, as compared to 9.8% of the prenatally matched control children.

However, this psychometric categorization does not identify all the affected children because additional children have learning disabilities. In nonretarded 5-year-old children prenatally exposed to isotretinoin, the areas of greatest difficulty involve visuomotor integration, visuoperceptual analysis, attention, and organizational abilities. Language-based abilities are a relative strength. When performance on information and vocabulary subtests was compared to performance on pattern analysis and bead memory (Stanford-Binet IV), sig-nificant "nonverbal" weaknesses were present in 61.5% of the children in the borderline to low-average range of general mental ability, whereas only 14.3% of the controls in this range demonstrated this profile. When adverse outcome after early embryonic isotretinoin exposure is described in psycho-metric terms, 43% of our exposed children are identified as being mentally retarded or of borderline intelligence, as compared to only 9.8% of the age- and demographically matched controls. An additional 16% of exposed cases demonstrate the significant learning disability profile, whereas only 7% of the control children met these defining criteria. Collectively, then, early embyonic isotretinoin exposure is associated with a 59% incidence of intel-lectual compromise, as compared to an incidence of 17% in matched control children. Knowledge of this profile supports specific hypothesis testing of the integrity of underlying structures demonstrated to be involved in the impaired neuropsychological processes and, ultimately, should further our understanding of the relationships between stage-specific embryonic pertur-bation, consequent abnormal substrates, and cognitive functioning.

Examples of a continuum of variation in outcome after exposures to com-parable doses and at comparable stages are well established, but one must understand also that a continuum of expression of teratogenic outcomes results from stage-specific and dose-specific effects. Indeed, individual variations in outcome after comparable administered doses often are interpreted to result from as yet misunderstood variation in individual metabolism or disposition of the agent—thus, conceivably, a dose-response effect. Let us now consider individual factors that are related to teratogenic response, then discuss stage-specific and dose-dependent factors.

Individual Factors That Contribute to Vulnerability and Variability of Expression

Whether it be the most potent modern-day neurobehavioral teratogens (the retinoids) or perhaps the most prevalent (ethanol), susceptibility to teratogenesis varies across individuals, and the manifestations of the syndromic cluster vary in extent. These differences appear to be due to the parental and fetal genotype and to nutritional, metabolic, and general health status. The role of nongenetic maternal environmental factors is illustrated in a reported case of monzygotic twins, one with the fetal alcohol syndrome and one without (Don & Rourke, 1995). Variations in the expressions of genetic disorders may also be viewed in this manner, whereby the genotype would govern the presence of redundant "backup" or, perhaps, compensatory systems relevant to the mechanism of abnormal development.

Stage Specificity and Dose Dependence of Vulnerability to Teratogenesis

All organ systems have embryonic periods of heightened vulnerability to teratogenic agents. Heightened vulnerability is characterized by both the severity of the responses to exposure and sensitivity to lower dose levels. When death and readily identifiable or life-threatening malformations are examined as end points, the period of greatest vulnerability is the period of embryogenesis (days 14 to 60) in human pregnancy. At this time, cells that compose most organ systems (heart, lungs, kidneys, major glands) are proliferating rapidly, migrating, and assembling to form the particular structure (for the embryological timetable for major organs, see Moore & Persaud, 1993).

A protracted development confined to the embryonic period characterizes the establishment of structural integrity of all major organ systems except the brain. Excellent single-chapter-level reviews of brain development can be found in Kandel et al. (1995) and Martin (1996); a detailed presentation is found in O'Rahilly and Muller (1992). At the end of the embryonic period, the brain consists of defined (though smooth) hemispheres and midbrain and hindbrain structures (see O'Rahilly & Muller, 1992). During the fetal period, certain forebrain structures and the cortex are established and initially elaborated.

The extended period of development and vulnerability of the human brain has received less research attention by anatomically focused teratologists who have invested more effort in the study of gross malformations caused by insult in early embryogenesis, prior to neural tube closure (approximately 24–28 days in human pregnancy). In contrast, neurobehavioral teratologists have focused primarily on later exposure periods or nonmalforming dose levels so that the behavioral consequences of insult could be studied without "confounding" by physical abnormalities.

Given the differences in interests and study design for research directed at understanding conventional malformation end points as opposed to postnatal functional ones, it is difficult to derive smooth stage-response and dose-response curves across end points of teratogenesis. Nevertheless, in an attempt to demonstrate that the expression of neurobehavioral malformation end points of teratogenesis are governed by similar principles, Adams (1993b) examined the literature on the teratogenicity of retinoid compounds. Table 19.1 demonstrates the stage- and dose-specific nature of the effects of exposure to all-*trans*-retinoic acid, the active agent of teratogenesis for retinoids in the rat. As shown, at earlier gestational stages, lower doses are capable of producing embryonic death (resorptions) and gross brain malformations (exencephaly, anencephaly) than can do so at later stages.

Table 19.1 Stage- and dose-response relationships derived from studies of retinoid teratogenesis in rats

Time of Treatment (days of gestation)[a]	End point	Lowest Effective Dose of All-Trans-Retinoic Acid
Days 8–10	Resorptions[b]	10 mg/kg
	Brain malformations	
	Postnatal death	> 5 mg/kg
	Postnatal weight reduction	> 5 mg/kg
	Postnatal behavioral dysfunction	5 mg/kg
Days 11–13	Resorptions	20 mg/kg[c]
	Brain malformations	
	Postnatal death	≥ 5 mg/kg
	Postnatal weight reduction	≤ 5 mg/kg
	Postnatal behavioral dysfunction	≤ 2.5 mg/kg
Days 14–16	Resorptions	(too late for these end points)
	Brain malformations	
	Postnatal death	> 6 mg/kg
	Postnatal weight reduction	≥ 6 mg/kg
	Postnatal behavioral dysfunction	≥ 2.5 mg/kg

[a] In the laboratory rat, gestational length is 21–22 days.
[b] In the rat, embryos that do not survive are resorbed, not aborted.
[c] This value is estimated on the basis of exposures on days 9–11 or 10–12; data were not available for this end point in studies that used the day 11–13 exposure period.
Source: Adapted from Adams, 1993b.

It is plausible to assume that variation in the manifestations of genetic syndromes may reflect a conceptual dose response in which the number of genes involved or the interaction between redundant systems determines the amount of the adverse compound present and available to produce disruption. Indeed, gene-dosing models have been developed to explain the relationship between genetic variations and phenotypic outcome in individuals with fragile X syndrome (see chapter 3). Conceptually similar arguments have also been made to account for relationships between mosaicism and phenotypic characteristics for both Down syndrome (see chapters 8, 9) and Turner syndrome (see chapter 11).

Syndromology in the Manifestations of Teratogenesis: An Effect of Shared Vulnerability to Common Mechanisms

Our understanding of causes (identification of teratogenic agents) and manifestations (phenotypic characteristics) is reasonably well established and catalogued, but our understanding of mechanisms (exactly how exposure translates into abnormal development) is not. Even thalidomide teratogenesis defies explanation in mechanistic terms. Nevertheless, a clear defining principle of teratogenesis is that manifestations appear in clusters (e.g., specific malformations of the heart, of craniofacial structures, of the brain or its functioning) representing a syndrome of abnormalities (Cohen, 1990). The constituents of the syndrome of detectable abnormalities appear to share a common embryological timetable, a common cellular ancestry, or common controlling mechanisms. Thus, the development of a cluster of tissues or organ systems may be disrupted by a generalized toxic event (such as hypoxia or destruction of the cell membrane) that damages or kills all cells undergoing rapid proliferation at the time [see discussions of alcohol (West et al., 1994; Don & Rourke, 1995) and methyl mercury (Burbacher et al., 1990; see also chapter 20] or by an agent with tissue-specific, receptor-mediated affinity (such as the retinoids).

We are beginning to understand mechanisms of teratogenesis for retinoid compounds. Exogenously administered retinoids appear to accomplish their potent teratogenicity through the disruption of precisely timed and complexly orchestrated receptor-mediated actions that normally would subserve responses to endogenous retinoids. During normal development, endogenous retinoic acids play an important role in the morphogenesis of the embryo, especially for limb and nervous system development (Maden et al., 1990). Disruption of this role by exogenously administered retinoids produces potent teratogenicity. All the retinoid compounds (which precludes beta-carotene) are teratogenic at some level and appear to accomplish their teratogenicity through conversion to the *trans* isomer and *trans* metabolite (Creech Kraft et al., 1987, 1989; Kochhar et al., 1988; Klug et al., 1989). Within the embryo, receptor-binding substrates for these compounds provide them with a regulatory role during embryogenesis (Wolf, 1990). At a cellular level, retinol and retinoic acid bind with cellular retinol-binding protein and cellular retinoic acid-binding protein as a potential means of gaining entry into the nucleus (Wolf, 1990, 1991). Once in the nucleus, retinoic acids interact with nuclear receptors for retinoic acid (retinoic acid receptors) and, as a result, rates of gene transcription are modified by interaction with specific sequences on the cell's DNA (for review, see Wolf, 1990). Such receptor interactions are known to play a regulatory role in DNA function in nervous system and craniofacial development in both the mouse and the rat embryo (Madden et al., 1990; Dencker et al., 1991; Morris-Kay, 1993). High levels of the cellular and nuclear binding proteins have been found in the cellular anlage for CNS structures, craniofacial structures, and branchial arches (Dencker et al., 1991; Wolf, 1991; Gustafson et al., 1993). As previously discussed, these structures are core features of isotretinoin embryopathy in animals as well as humans. Thus, the normal role of retinoids during embryogenesis is believed to be disturbed by the high levels that occur after exogenous administration, and abnormal development of relevant structures results.

Not only do certain structures of the face, head, and hindbrain and parts of the heart and thymus gland share common embryonic primordia with regulation by retinoids, but their formation also appears to be controlled by a common family of regulatory genes that coordinate the development of the bodily structures (Durston et al., 1989; Lonai & Orr-Urtreger, 1990; Holland, 1992; Thorogood & Ferretti, 1992). These genes are members of families of genes known as *homeogenes*, the expression of which controls the embryonic development of specific bodily "segments." Retinoids are one of many molecular types known to play a role in regulating the activity of certain homeogenes (Gilbert, 1994).

When homeogenetic activity is disrupted by exogenously administered retinoids such as isotretinoin, by genetic knockout experiments, or by genetic abnormalities, syndromic abnormalities of the face, brain, heart, and thymus gland have been shown to result (Gilbert, 1994). This occurrence suggests that differing etiologies may produce similar phenotypic expressions. An understanding of the fundamental regulatory actions of this family of genes is important if we are to recognize the potential role that multiple families of homeogenes may play in the embryogenesis of multiple neurodevelopmental disorders. One must assume that abnormalities in genes that produce molecular triggers for homeogene expression or that themselves are triggered to produce substances after homeogene activation would disturb the translation of assembly rules coded by these genes. Through this mechanistic path, both teratogenic agents and genetic abnormalities may produce craniofacial, brain, and certain major organ abnormalities. Thus, a teratogen may interfere with cellular or molecular activity relevant to the initiation or implementation of homeogene activity. Likewise, a genetic abnormality relevant to the production of regulatory chemicals or in the homeogenes themselves might disrupt normal genetic expression.

THE POTENTIAL FOR SIMILAR MECHANISMS UNDERLYING GENETIC MENTAL RETARDATION SYNDROMES

Shared embryological primordia, controlling substances, or regulation through similar homeogene activities may begin to explain the commonality of co-occurrence of the syndrome of abnormalities so prominent among neurobehavioral teratogenic and mental retardation syndromes: craniofacial abnormalities, hindbrain abnormalities, and certain organ malformations. With respect to mental retardation syndromes of known or suspected genetic causation, phenotypic characteristics suggest an early embryological origin owing to the prototypical co-occurrence of these common outcomes. Table 19.2 presents the characteristics of several mental retardation syndromes discussed in this book. Though focusing on overlapping "generic" features and ignoring specific attributes and differences is a superficial means of addressing a potentially shared embryology for these diverse disorders, we will entertain this approach briefly in order to address theoretical possibilities. Albeit a superficial examination, Table 19.2 clearly shows that craniofacial and hindbrain abnormalities coexist in all the disorders. Also apparent is that a continuum of cognitive dysfunction occurs in individuals with these disorders. This fact suggests that the specific mechanisms through which cause translates into effect may overlap somewhat and points to an early embryonic period of insult, be it from exposure to an exogenous agent or abnormal endogenous production of some substance due to genetic abnormality.

Let us now consider how the understanding of these mechanisms and the previously discussed principles of neurobehavioral teratogenesis may directly contribute to the study of neurodevelopmental disorder. Rodier (Rodier et al., 1996, 1997, 1998) first suggested commonalities between teratogenic and other neurodevelopmental disorders with respect to the disorder of autism, the etiology of which is unknown. Awareness of thalidomide-induced cases of autism (Stromland et al., 1994) led Rodier to undertake an evaluation of the specific features of thalidomide-exposed autistic children that might shed light on the relevant neuropathology of autism. She has presented a compelling argument that thalidomide-induced autistic cases bear neuropathological and behavioral similarities to other cases of autism.

In the case of thalidomide exposure, autism occurs at an unusually high incidence (5 of 15) after exposure between days 20 and 24 of pregnancy (Stromland et al., 1994). Rodier et al. (1997) argue that thalidomide-induced autism results from interference with pattern formation of the rhombomeres from which the brainstem nuclei arise or from interference with neuron production of cranial nerve motor nuclei. These abnormalities reflect injury to basal plate derivatives of the neural tube. It is argued that the hindbrain and cerebellar abnormalities that have been reported in autistic individuals are consistent with a severe developmental injury to these same structures. Thus, Rodier argues that early insult to the basal plate can cause

Table 19.2   Characteristics of children with specific genetic mental retardation syndromes

Disorder	Physical malformations (noncephalic)	Craniofacial features	Brain abnormalities	Other physical characteristics	Intellectual characteristics
Autism	None reported	Increased number of nonspecific anomalies; increased ear anomalies	Increased brain weight; increased neuron density in limbic structures; cerebellar abnormalities; hypoplasia of cerebellar vermis; hyperplasia of cerebellar vermis; reduced size of brainstem structures	None reported	Profound MR to low-average status
Down syndrome	Heart malformations; shortened limbs; small thymus gland	Upslanted palpebral fissures; epicanthal folds; broad, flat nasal bridge; protruding tongue; microcephaly; ear and eye abnormalities	Reduced weight and volume; reduced frontal-occipital distance; reduced size of frontal lobes, hippocampus, cerebellum, and brainstem; flattened occiput	Immunodeficiencies	Profound MR to borderline (related to karyotype)
Fragile X syndrome	Macroorchidism	Increased head circumference; long face; prominent ears; high arched palate	Enlarged lateral ventricles; hypoplasia of cerebellar vermis; enlarged hippocampus and caudate nucleus; reduced synaptic fields	Abnormal elastin fibers (flat feet; hyperextensible fingers)	Profound MR to average status (related to karyotype)
Prader-Willi syndrome	Small hands and feet; hypogonadism	Dolichocephaly; long, narrow face; narrow bifrontal diameter; almond-shaped eyes; small mouth; thin upper lip	Not reported	Altered hypothalamic functioning; obesity; hypotonia in infancy; hypopigmentation; short stature; visual disturbances	Profound MR to average status
Turner syndrome	Heart malformations; digital hypoplasia	Short, webbed neck; ptosis micronathia; high arched palate; ear abnormalities	Decreased volume in limbic structures; decreased volume in parietal-occipital areas	Ovarian dysfunction; short stature	Borderline to above-average range

Table 19.2 (continued)

Disorder	Physical malformations (noncephalic)	Craniofacial features	Brain abnormalities	Other physical characteristics	Intellectual characteristics
Williams syndrome	Heart malformations	Facial assymmetry; bitemporal narrowing; low nasal root; long philtrum; flat mala; full cheeks; periorbital fullness; wide mouth; stellate iris; prominent ear lobes	Dolichocephaly; microcephaly; hyperplasia of the cerebellar vermis	Associated hypercalcemia	Profound MR to low-average status

MR, mental retardation.

the development of the brain to deviate in a way that leads to autism. She suggests that specific disruptions in the early embryogenesis of the hindbrain and cranial motor nerve nuclei may account for the disorder of autism.

Further, Rodier argues that the existence of a *Hoxa-1* transonic knockout mouse with similar neuropathology (Chisaka et al., 1992) suggests that the failure of formation of the fifth rhombomere may be particularly relevant and that abnormalities in certain homeogenes may underly the disorder of autism. Though Rodier's arguments are compelling, whether the teratogen-induced autistic symptomatology represents the cognitive features that are shown in nonretarded autistics, or primarily reflects the symptomatology seen in mentally retarded individuals with autism remains unclear. Regardless, this work clearly exemplifies the application of a teratological and neurodevelopmental perspective to the study of a disorder that has defied etiological understanding and offers a new model for exploring the etiology of autism. Rodier (Rodier et al., 1996, 1997) has now developed a valproic acid–induced animal model of autism in which specific early embryonic exposure results in neuropathological similarities. She is also examining the genetic characteristics of families with autistic members.

Inherent in Rodier's hypothesis for autism are three major points:

1. Understanding the embryonic origin of the neuroanatomical abnormalities present in a disorder helps to clarify its etiology, be it teratogen-induced interference or genetic abnormality.

2. The etiology and manifestations may then be seen to be consistent with disruptions of the role of certain regulatory molecules or genes in development.

3. Teratological events and abnormal genetic events may be expressed through similar mechanisms of abnormal development.

These points and Rodier's approach demonstrate how guidance from principles of teratogenesis can advance the study of the etiology of a neurodevelopmental disorder along a somewhat different path from that typically pursued by researchers of genetic disorders. Whether a disorder be caused by teratogenic or genetic insult, embryonic development may proceed abnormally owing to the disruption of common mechanisms critical to normal development. Thus, shared underlying mechanisms potentially may translate genetic or teratogenic insult into similar physical *and* neuropsychological sequelae.

CONCLUSIONS

This neurobehavioral teratological perspective on neurodevelopmental disorders has emphasized mechanisms and governing principles that may be shared in the production of syndromes involving cognitive dysfunction, whether the dysfunction results from genetic or environmental causes. An implication of these direct or conceptual commonalities is that the study of each causative category should inform the understanding of the other. Given this assumption, researchers should begin to consider the benefits of designing studies using embryologically selected and matched contrast groups to examine the specificity of purported disorder-specific neuropsychological profiles. In this approach, the cause of the disorder present in the contrast group is somewhat irrelevant: What matters is the nature of the common embryology suggested by somewhat common manifestations and the relationship between structural and functional abnormality. The question becomes: When anatomical manifestations suggest a particular prenatal period in which development was disrupted, is this disruption also reflected in a similar resultant neuropsychological profile? If structure-function relationships are assumed to be relatively invariant despite developmental abnormality, one would assume that commonalities in neuropsychological characteristics should be present in individuals with overlapping neuropathology. However, compensatory mechanisms may force reorganization of brain systems and their mediational roles so that overlapping but nonidentical anatomical features may result in a spectrum of cognitive outcomes. No doubt both may be true to an extent that will begin to account for the similarities and differences present across disorders.

It appears prudent to explore the relationships between neuroanatomical and neuropsychological characteristics by comparing and contrasting the features of individuals who have phenotypic similarities despite differing etiologies and diagnoses. Within this context, perhaps it also is time to focus on the role of hindbrain structures in general intellectual ability as well as in specific neuropsychological characteristics. Recent data on the role of hindbrain and cerebellar structures in cognition (Akshoomoff and Courchesne, 1992; Daum & Ackerman, 1995) forces attention to these developing systems and challenges our established focus on forebrain and cortical systems as somewhat exclusive mediators of higher-order cognitive processes. Interestingly, with the exception of autism, all the disorders in Table 19.2 share a profile of visuospatial and organizational deficits in which relative strength in language-based processing is retained. This profile also is exhibited by children with myelomeningocele and related hindbrain and cerebellar abnormality (see chapter 22; Wills et al., 1990). Further, neurologically normal children prenatally affected by isotretinoin exposure exhibit a similar cognitive profile.

Understanding the prenatal stage-specific disruption of particular neuroanatomical systems and neuropsychological processes would greatly advance our understanding of disorders of unknown etiology and provide direction to the search for causes and controlling mechanisms. Likewise, it should inform the selection of both medical and educational therapeutic interventions.

ACKNOWLEDGMENTS

This work was partially supported through National Institute of Child Health and Human Development grant RO1-HD29510. The author wishes to thank Doug Annis, Jennifer Hamel, and Kara Stutz for assistance in producing this chapter.

REFERENCES

Adams, J. (1993a). Structure-activity and dose-response relationships in the neural and behavioral teratogenesis of retinoids. *Neurotoxicology and Teratology, 15,* 193–202.

Adams, J. (1993b). Neural and behavioral pathology following prenatal exposure to retinoids. In G. Koren (Ed.), *Retinoids, in clinical practice* (pp. 111–128). New York: Marcell-Dekker.

Adams, J. (1996). Similarities in genetic mental retardation and neuroteratogenic syndromes. *Pharmacology, Biochemistry, and Behavior, 55,* 683–690.

Adams J., & Lammer, E. J. (1991). Relationship between dysmorphology and neuropsychological function in children exposed to isotretinoin "in utero." In T. Fujii & G. J. Boer (Eds.), *Functional neuroteratology of short term exposure to drugs* (pp. 159–170). Tokyo: Tokyo University Press.

Adams, J., & Lammer, E. J. (1995). Human isotretinoin exposure: The teratogenesis of a syndrome of cognitive deficits. *Neurotoxicology and Teratology, 17,* 386.

Adams, J., Lammer, E. J., & Holmes, L. B. (1991). A syndrome of cognitive dysfunctions following human embryonic exposure to isotretinoin. *Teratology, 43,* 497.

Akshoomoff, N. A., & Courchesne, E. (1992). A new role for the cerebellum in cognitive operations. *Behavioral Neuroscience, 106,* 731–738.

Burbacher, T. M., Rodier, P. M., & Weiss, B. (1990). Methylmercury developmental neurotoxicity: A comparison of effects in humans and animals. *Neurotoxicology and Teratology, 12,* 191–201.

Butcher, R. E. (1985). A historical perspective on behavioral teratology. *Neurobehavioral Toxicology and Teratology, 7,* 537–540.

Chisaka, O., Musci, T. S., & Capecchi, M. R. (1992). Developmental defects of the ear, cranial nerves, and hindbrain resulting from targeted disruption of the mouse homeobox gene *Hox-1.6. Nature, 335,* 516–520.

Cohen, M. M., Jr. (1990). Syndromology: An updated conceptual overview. VII. Aspects of teratogenesis. *International Journal of Oral and Maxillofacial Surgery, 19,* 26–32.

Creech Kraft, J., Kochhar, D. M., Scott, W. J., & Nau, H. (1987). Low teratogenicity of 13-*cis* retinoic acid (isotretinoin) in the mouse corresponds to low embryo concentrations during organogenesis: Comparison to the all-*trans* isomer. *Toxicology and Applied Pharmacology, 87,* 474–482.

Creech Kraft, J., Lofberg, B., Chahoud, I., Bochert, G., & Nau, H. (1989). Teratogenicity and placental transfer of all-*trans*-, 13-*cis*, 4-Oxo-all-*trans*-, and 4-Oxo-13-*cis*-retinoic acid after administration of a low oral dose during organogenesis in mice. *Toxicology and Applied Pharmacology, 100,* 162–176.

Daum, I., & Ackerman, H. (1995). Cerebellar contributions to cognition. *Behavioural Brain Research, 67,* 201–210.

Dencker, L., Gustafson, A., Annerwall, E., Busch, C., & Eriksson, U. (1991). Retinoid-binding proteins in craniofacial development. *Journal of Craniofacial and Genetic Developmental Biology, 11,* 303–314.

Don, A., & Rourke, B. P. (1995). Fetal alcohol syndrome. In B. P. Rourke (Ed.), *Syndrome of nonverbal learning disabilities: Neurodevelopmental manifestations* (pp. 372–406). New York: Guilford Press.

Durston, A. J., Timmermans, J. P. M., Hage, W. J., Kendriks, H. F. J., de Vries, N. J., Heideveid, M., & Nieuwkoop, P. D. (1989). Retinoic acid causes an anteroposterior transformation in the developing central nervous system. *Nature, 340,* 140–144.

Gilbert, S. F. (1994). *Developmental biology* (4th ed.). Sunderland, MA: Sinauer Associates.

Gustafson, A., Dencker, L., & Eriksson, U. (1993). Nonoverlapping expression of CRBP I and CRABP I during pattern formation of limbs and craniofacial structures in the early mouse embryo. *Development, 117,* 451–460.

Holland, P. (1992). Homeobox genes in vertebrate evolution. *BioEssays, 14,* 267–273.

Kandel, E. R., Schwarz, J. H., & Jessel, T. M. (1995). *Essentials of neural science and behavior.* Norwalk, CT: Appleton & Lange.

Kimmel, C. A., & Buelke-Sam, J. (1985). Collaborative behavioral teratology study: Background and overview. *Neurobehavioral Toxicology and Teratology, 7,* 541–545.

Klug, S., Creech Kraft, J., Wildi, E., Merker, H. J., Persaud, T. V. N., Nau, H., & Neubert, D. (1989). Influence of 13-*cis* and all-*trans* retinoic acid on rat embryonic development in vitro: Correlation with isomerisation and drug transfer to the embryo. *Archives of Toxicology, 63,* 185–192.

Kochhar, D. M., Penner J. D., & Satre, M. A. (1988). Derivation of retinoic acid metabolites from a teratogenic dose retinol (vitamin A) in mice. *Toxicology and Applied Pharmacology, 96,* 429–441.

Lammer, E. J., & Armstrong, D. L. (1992). Malformations of hindbrain structures among humans exposed to isotretinoin (13-*cis*-retinoic acid) during early embryogenesis. In G. Morriss-Kay (Ed.), *Retinoids in normal development and teratogenesis* (pp. 281–295). London: Oxford University Press.

Lammer, E. J., Chen, D. T., Hoar, R. M., Agnish, N. D., Benke, P. J., Braun, J. T., Curry C. J., Ferhnoff, P. M., Grix, A. W., Lott, I. T., Richard, J. M., & Sun, S. C. (1985). Retinoic acid embryopathy. *New England Journal of Medicine, 313,* 837–841.

Lammer, E. J., Hayes, A. M., Schunior, A., & Holmes, L. B. (1988). Unusually high risk for adverse outcomes of pregnancy following fetal isotretinoin exposure. *American Journal of Human Genetics, 43,* A58.

IV. Broader Perspectives on Neurodevelopmental Disorders

Lonai, P., & Orr-Urtreger, A. (1990). Homeogenes in mammalian development and the evolution of the cranium and central nervous system. *Federation of the American Society for Experimental Biology, 4*, 1436–1443.

Madden, M., Ong, D. E., & Chytil, F. (1990). Retinoid-binding protein distribution in the developing mammalian nervous system. *Development, 109*, 75–80.

Martin, J. H. (1996). *Neuroanatomy: Text and atlas.* Stamford, CT: Appleton & Lange.

Moore, K. L., & Persaud, T. V. N. (1993). *The developing human: Clinically oriented teratology* (5th ed.). Philadelphia: Saunders.

Morris-Kay, G. (1993). Retinoic acid and craniofacial development: Molecules and morphogenesis. *BioEssays, 15*, 9–15.

Newman, C. G. H. (1985). Teratogen update: Clinical aspects of thalidomide embryopathy—a continuing preoccupation. *Teratology, 32*, 133–144.

O'Rahilly, R., & Muller, F. (1992). *Human embryology and teratology.* New York: Wiley-Liss.

Randall, C. L., Ekblad, U., & Anton, R. F. (1990). Perspectives on the pathophysiology of fetal alcohol syndrome. *Alcoholism: Clinical and Experimental Research, 14*, 807–812.

Rodier, P. M. & Hyman, S. (1998). Early environmental factors in autism. *Mental Retardation and Developmental Disabilities Research Reviews, 4*, 121–128.

Rodier, P. M., Ingram, J. L., Tisdale, B., & Croog, V. (1997). Linking etiologies in humans and animal models: Studies of autism. *Reproductive Toxicology, 11*, 417–422.

Rodier, P. M., Ingrain, J. L., Tisdale, B., Nelson. S., & Romano, J. (1996). An embryological origin for autism: Developmental anomalies of the cranial motor nerve nuclei. *Journal of Comparative Neurology, 370*, 247–261.

Streissguth, A. P. (1986). The behavioral teratology of alcohol: Performance, behavioral, and intellectual deficits in prenatally exposed children. In J. R. West (Ed.), *Alcohol and brain development* (pp. 3–44). New York: Oxford University Press.

Streissguth, A. P., Aase, J. M., Clarren, S. K., Randalls, S. P., LaDue, R. A., & Smith, D. W. (1991). Fetal alcohol syndrome in adolescents and adults. *Journal of the American Medical Association, 265*, 1961–1967.

Streissguth, A. P., Barr, H. M., & Martin, D. C. (1983). Maternal alcohol and neonatal habituation assessed with the Brazelton Scale. *Child Development, 54*, 1109–1118.

Streissguth, A. P., Barr, H. M., & Sampson, P. D. (1990). Moderate prenatal alcohol exposure: Effects on child IQ and learning problems at age $7\frac{1}{2}$ years. *Alcoholism: Clinical and Experimental Research, 14*, 662–669.

Stromland, K., & Miller, M. T. (1993). Thalidomide embryopathy: Revisited 27 years later. *Acta Ophthalmologica, 71*, 238–245.

Stromland, K., Nordin, V., Miller, M., Akerstrom, B., & Gillberg, C. (1994). Autism in thalidomide embryopathy: A population study. *Developmental Medicine and Child Neurology, 36*, 351–356.

Thorogood, P., & Ferretti, P. (1992). Heads and tales: Recent advances in craniofacial development. *British Dental Journal, 173*, 301–306.

Vorhees, C. V. (1986). Principles of behavioral teratology. In Riley, E. P., & Vorhees, C. V. (Eds.), *Handbook of behavioral teratology* (pp. 23–48). New York: Plenum Press.

West, J. R., Chen, W. A., & Pantazis, N. J. (1994). Fetal alcohol syndrome: The vulnerability of the developing brain and possible mechanisms of damage. *Metabolic Brain Disease, 9*, 291–322.

West, J. R., & Goodlett, C. R. (1990). Teratogenic effects of alcohol on brain development. *Annals of Medicine, 22*, 319–325.

Wills, K. E., Holmbeck, G. N., Dillon, K., and McLone, D. G. (1990). Intelligence and achievement in children with myelomeningocele. *Journal of Pediatric Psychology, 15*(2), 161–177.

Wolf G. (1990). Recent progress in vitamin A research: Nuclear retinoic acid receptors and their interaction with gene elements. *Journal of Nutritional Biochemistry, 1*, 284–289.

Wolf G. (1991). The intracellular vitamin A–binding proteins: An overview of their functions. *Nutrition Reviews, 49*, 1–12.

20 Environmental Toxicants and Child Development

Kim N. Dietrich

ENVIRONMENTAL TOXICANTS AS HUMAN TERATOGENS

Cognitive developmental deficits are the most common form of birth defect and yet, in most instances, their cause is unknown. Thus, for example, figure 20.1 shows the distribution of diagnoses for mentally retarded children in the Swedish birth registry of infants born in 1978 and followed until January 1, 1986. Among the causes of mental handicap, the category of *unknown* had the highest percentage of cases (Kallen, 1988). Some have speculated that environmental chemical exposures during prenatal or early postnatal development may play an etiological role in mental developmental deficits and delays of otherwise uncertain etiology (Kallen, 1988; Rees et al., 1990).

The exact role of environmental chemicals in the development of most cognitive deficits and learning problems remains obscure. Although hundreds of exogenous agents have been demonstrated to produce morphological and functional developmental defects in controlled experiments with laboratory animals, very few environmental chemicals are known to be teratogenic in humans (Shephard, 1994). Indeed, Shephard lists only two: (1) a class of compounds known collectively as the *polychlorinated aromatic hydrocarbons* [such as polychlorinated biphenyls (PCBs) and dioxinlike compounds (e.g., 2,3,7,8-tetrachlorodibenzo-p-dioxin)] and (2) mercury, especially organic mercurials, such as methyl mercury. Although lead at high doses prenatally is an abortifacient or gives rise to growth-retarded and constitutionally weak infants (Cantarow & Trumper, 1944), it is listed only as a *possible* teratogen in the latest edition of Shephard's authoritative catalog.

The small number of identified human teratogens in the environment could be viewed as an indication of the robustness of the species. However, probably the small number of human environmental chemical teratogens identified thus far is a reflection of our lack of knowledge. Thus, for example, though estimates hold that approximately 70,000 chemicals are now in commercial use, few of these substances have been evaluated scientifically for their developmentally toxic potential. If one excludes pharmaceutical agents, fewer than 10% of chemicals currently in commercial use have been subjected

Percent of Cases

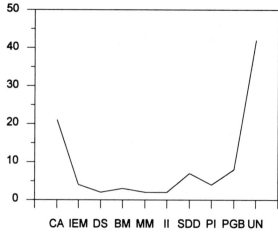

CA IEM DS BM MM II SDD PI PGB UN

Diagnoses of Infants Reported to the Swedish Registry of Mental Handicap

Figure 20.1 Diagnoses of infants reported to the Swedish Registry of Mental Handicaps. CA, chromosomal anomalies; IEM, inborn errors of metabolism; DS, defined syndromes; BM, brain malformations; MM, multiple malformations; II, intrauterine infections; SDD, suspected delivery damage; PI, postnatal infections; PGB, probable genetic background; UK, unknown. (Adapted from table 8 of Kallen, 1988.)

to neurotoxicity testing (Landrigan et al., 1994), and only a small portion of these have been examined for their developmental neurotoxic potential (Rees et al., 1990).

Determining the number of known exogenous human teratogens also depends on one's concept of what exactly constitutes an environmental agent. A strong tendency seeks to equate toxic environmental agents with humanmade substances that subsequently are introduced into the environment as products people use and dispose of or the waste by-products of production. However, certain natural substances in the environment have teratogenic potential, including plants, fungi, bacteria, and viruses (Wilson, 1977). Nutritional deficiencies during pregnancy also have the potential to increase the risk of congenital central nervous system defects (Trevathen et al., 1991).

However, this chapter is concerned primarily with studies of substances introduced into the environment through human industrial activities, thus limiting the number of agents considered in detail to three: PCBs, methyl mercury, and lead. These substances are ubiquitous in developed and developing countries and have been subjected to methodologically rigorous examination in both animal experiments and in epidemiological studies of humans (Burbacher et al., 1990; Davis et al., 1990; Tilson et al., 1990). Exposure to these substances in combination with nutritional deficiencies or exposure to teratogens in nature may enhance the adverse effects of environmental toxicants, but a full discussion of this question is beyond the scope of this chapter. However, notably, nutrition in particular plays an important role in the absorption of environmental contaminants and the expression of health effects (Mahaffey, 1985).

THE SCOPE OF MODERN NEUROTOXICOLOGY AND TERATOLOGY

Many scientists regard James G. Wilson as one of the founders of modern teratology. His *Six Principles of Teratology* published more than two decades ago still constitutes the field's scientific foundation (Wilson, 1973, 1977). Although Wilson was a classical structural pathomorphologist, he was among the first senior scientists in this field to recognize the fundamental importance of behavioral teratology (Vorhees, 1987). Of particular significance to the cognitive neurosciences is his fifth principle (Wilson, 1973): "The four manifestations of deviant development are death, malformation, growth retardation and *functional deficits*" (emphasis added). Wilson expands the definition of a teratogen to agents that are capable of producing deficits in cognitive and other measures of neurobehavioral performance in the absence of gross malformations of the central nervous system.

Many of the axioms of modern developmental neurotoxicology are embodied in Wilson's fifth principle. Thus, chemically mediated interference with the conceptus prior to or shortly after implantation is likely to result in death. Interference with early organogenesis during the first 2 to 8 weeks of postconceptual life can result in malformations that sometimes are so severe that many of these conceptuses are aborted spontaneously or are born with major neurostructural defects that are incompatible either with life or with grossly normal mental and motor functioning (e.g., anencephaly, holoprosencephalopathy, spina bifida). However, the risks for suboptimal central nervous system development do not end with the conclusion of the embryonic stage of primordial differentiation. Although the central nervous system is refractory to the induction of major malformations during the fetal period of advanced organogenesis and maturation, it remains at risk for more subtle developmental deviations throughout the fetal period (Wilson, 1977; Dobbing, 1981).

Parturition does not mark the end of neurodevelopmental vulnerability. This is because such processes as cell proliferation, growth, and (especially) cortical cellular migration, myelination, dendritic arborization, and synaptogenesis continue for a considerable period postnatally. In fact, owing to the long-term process of myelination of neural fibers postnatally, the human brain does not reach its completely mature form until approximately 21 years conceptual age (Rodier, 1994). Thus, an environmental agent that is capable of interfering with these long-term developmental processes may be associated also with subtle functional cognitive or neuromotor deficits, even when gross histological or neuroradiological examination of the brain is unrevealing.

EFFECTS OF SPECIFIC TOXICANTS ON THE CENTRAL NERVOUS SYSTEM AND BEHAVIOR

Elemental and Methyl Mercury

Much of what is understood about the neuroteratogenic properties of methyl mercury in humans comes from two episodes of mass poisoning that occurred in the 1950s and early 1970s in Japan and Iraq, respectively. Prior to these disasters, mercury poisoning of the developing central nervous system was associated predominantly with exposure to inorganic mercury contained in prescription and over-the-counter medicines. For example, calomel (mercurous chloride) often was prescribed by physicians to treat various childhood disorders ranging from teething pain to helminthism. For reasons that are still unknown, only a relatively small percentage of infants and children who were administered these preparations developed a complex of cutaneous, neurological, and psychiatric symptoms that doctors termed as *acrodynia*. This disease sometimes proved fatal. Although mercury was identified as the iatrogenic agent in these medicines as early as 1920, more than 30 years passed before mercurials were eliminated from the pharmacist's shelf (Warkany, 1966). The identification of medicinals as a cause of acrodynia in infants and children represents a fascinating chapter in human behavioral teratology. The late Josef Warkany wrote a vivid "postmortem" of this disease (Warkany, 1966).

Mercury in its organic form (e.g., methyl mercury) is extremely toxic to the developing nervous system. Ingested methyl mercury is absorbed almost completely by humans. Methyl mercury readily crosses the human placenta with newborn blood concentrations exceeding maternal levels by up to $2:1$ (Clarkson et al., 1988). In epidemiological studies, prenatal exposure to methyl mercury often is assessed indirectly by analyzing the concentration of the metal in maternal hair. Scalp hair grows at a known rate during pregnancy (1.1 cm per month), so the history of embryo-fetal exposure can be reconstructed by sectioning strands of maternal hair for elemental analyses. A high correlation between the concentration of methyl mercury in maternal hair during pregnancy and infants' brains recently was reported by a group of investigators studying a population of women whose source of dietary protein comes primarily from ocean fish (Cernchiari et al., 1995).

The first published report of methyl mercury poisoning was in male adults occupationally exposed to the metal (Hunter & Russel, 1954). The authors described a syndrome that began with paresthesia and progressed to deficits in fine-motor coordination, constriction of the peripheral visual fields, and gross ataxia.

The best-known and documented mass poisonings occurred in Minamata and Niigata, Japan, in the 1950s and 1960s and in Iraq in the early 1970s. In Minamata, an acetaldehyde and vinyl chloride manufacturer dumped massive amounts of methyl mercury into waters from which residents harvested fish for human consumption. The methyl mercury bioaccumulated in the marine food chain, beginning with protozoa and plankton, and reached its highest levels in pisciverous fish and crustaceans. As seafood was the principal source of dietary protein in this population, many were exposed to methyl mercury at relatively high levels.

Fetuses and children were the most affected, presenting with a syndrome that resembled cerebral palsy but almost always accompanied by severe sensory and cognitive deficits. In some victims, the disease progressed to extreme emotional disturbances, coma, and untimely death (Tsuchiya, 1992).

The other major methyl mercury poisoning epidemic occurred in Iraq in the winter of 1971 to 1972. Methyl mercury had been used as a fungicide for imported seed grain which, owing to a drought, was misused to make bread. More than 6000 documented poisonings and more than 600 deaths resulted. As in Japan, fetuses also were affected, as numerous cases of congenital methyl mercury–cerebral syndrome dominated by hypertonicity, blindness, deafness, and mental retardation were recorded (Clarkson, 1992; Marsh et al., 1987). Another common finding in the Japanese and Iraqi outbreaks was that this cerebral syndrome was observed in the infants of mothers who often were only mildly symptomatic (e.g., paresthesia) or clinically unaffected.

Methyl mercury has highly selective effects in the adult nervous system, attacking the visual cortex and granule layer of the cerebellum and resulting in ataxia, dysarthria, and blindness. However, in the fetal and infant brain, the damage is much more widespread, with atrophy of the cerebellum, underdevelopment of the corpus callosum and subcortex and enlarged ventricles. Microcephaly was common among newborns exposed transplacentally to methyl mercury (Takeuchi, 1968).

When environmental chemicals are found to be developmentally toxic at high doses, the usual custom is for investigators to examine more subtle deficits at so-called asymptomatic levels. Such regulatory and advisory agencies as the World Health Organization, the US Environmental Protection Agency, and the Centers for Disease Control have a keen interest in estimating the lowest observed adverse effect level for exposures of sensitive populations to environmental chemical agents. For methyl mercury, the focus has centered on populations that obtain most of their dietary protein from seafood, including sea mammals.

McKeon-Eyssen et al. (1983) studied 234 Cree Indian children from four communities in northern Quebec. All four communities subsist on freshwater fish from bodies of water known to support elevated methyl mercury concentrations in fish tissues. Dose-related deficits in the psychomotor development index of the Bayley Scales of Infant Development (Bayley, 1969) were observed, with male individuals being affected more often than female persons. Kjellstrom et al. (1989) found that, at the age of 4 years, New Zealand children with mothers that had the highest maternal-hair methyl mercury concentrations had lower scores on the Denver Developmental Screening Test (Frankenberg et al., 1981) and at 6 years had significantly lower scores on the Wechsler Intelligence Scale for Children–Revised (Wechsler, 1974) and the Test of Language Development (Hammill & Newcomer, 1988). Maternal-hair methyl mercury levels accounted for perhaps 3% of the variance in IQ after adjustment for covariates.

A methodologically rigorous study of low-level methyl mercury exposure and child development is underway in the Seychelles (Marsh et al., 1995). This multiple-island republic lies in the western Indian Ocean approximately 1500 kilometers from the eastern coast of Africa, and its inhabitants consume large amounts of fish and other seafoods. The study has been conducted in two stages. In pilot studies involving more than 780 Seychellois infants, a statistically significant relationship was observed between maternal-hair methyl mercury concentrations during pregnancy and nonoptimal scores on the Denver Developmental Screening Test–Revised; (Frankenburg et al., 1981) after adjustment for such covariates as socioeconomic and perinatal status variables (Myers et al., 1995a). The authors were able to assess 217 of these subjects at 5.5 years of age. Maternal-hair concentrations of methyl mercury were associated negatively with the McCarthy Scales of Children's Abilities (McCarthy, 1972), General Cognitive Index and Perceptual Performance subscale, and the Preschool Language Scale (Zimmerman et al., 1979), Language and Auditory Comprehension subscales (Meyers et al., 1995b).

Results forthcoming from the main prospective study appear to contradict those reported for the pilot investigations. Thus, for example, no relationship was found between gravid maternal methyl mercury concentrations on a measure of infant memory (Fagan & Shephard, 1987) or scores on the Bayley Scales of Infant Development (Bayley, 1969) at 19 and 29 months of age (Davidson et al., 1995; Myers et al., 1995c).

The negative nature of the outcomes measured in the main Seychellois prospective study must be interpreted with caution. For example, environmental epidemiological studies of lead have shown that the effects of early exposure become more pronounced as children mature and that the measures employed to assess later neurobehavioral health become more reliable, precise, and predictive of adolescent and adult academic and vocational success (Baghurst et al., 1992: Dietrich et al., 1993b; Needleman et al., 1990).

Methyl mercury appears to have very specific effects on the developing nervous system. The inhibition of cell division and maturation are two of the important mechanisms by which developmental toxicity is expressed. The molecular mechanism underlying this process is interference with microtubular assembly. A biological target of methyl mercury is the protein tubulin. Methyl mercury depolymerizes microtubules that play essential roles in neuronal and neuroglial cell duplication, migration, and nutrition. The result is fewer neurons and misalignment of the cytoarchitecture of the brain (Sager et al., 1984; Rodier et al., 1984).

Polychlorinated, Polycyclic Aromatic Compounds

Polyhalogenated and, in particular, polychlorinated polycyclic aromatic compounds are persistent in the human environment, owing to the fact that halogens deactivate the aromatic nuclei, making many such compounds resistant to chemical or metabolic decomposition. Residues of these chemicals can be detected in biological tissues (especially fat) of most residents in industrialized nations (Jensen, 1989). These compounds are found also in human breastmilk. In fact, lactation is the single physiological circumstance in which substantial quantities of PCBs are excreted over a relatively brief period of time (Masuda et al., 1978).

The PCBs are a family of 209 synthetic hydrocarbons (congeners) that once were used in a wide array of commercial products, including insulating oil and hydraulic fluids. The manufacture and use of these compounds were banned in the United States in the 1970s, but their use persists in underdeveloped nations.

As with methyl mercury, the developmental toxicity of PCBs in humans was made apparent by two disasters where the compounds found their way into the diets of pregnant women and children. PCBs and their thermodegradation by-products first were identified as a human teratogen in 1968 when, in Japan, substantial quantities of PCBs and polychlorinated dibenzofurans (PCDFs) were mixed accidentally with cooking oil during the decolorization process (Kuratsune, 1989). Another mass poisoning occurred in Taiwan in 1979 when, once again, these compounds were mixed accidentally with cooking oil during processing. The infirmities that followed these intrauterine exposures were referred to as *Yusho* and *Yucheng* (oil disease) in Japan and Taiwan, respectively.

Neonates exposed in utero in both epidemics were born with low birth weights, dark pigmentation of the skin and nails, natal teeth, swollen eyelids, and an acneiform rash. In some cases, intrauterine exposure resulted in newborn fatalities (Hsu et al., 1985). The survivors of prenatal poisoning have been described as developmentally delayed in sensorimotor and cognitive abilities in comparison to their unexposed peers (Harada, 1976; Rogan, et al., 1988).

As with methyl mercury, the results of these mass poisonings raised the question of the health effects of lower-level exposures. However, the amount of data in this area is quite meager. In fact, only two studies of substantial methodological rigor have been conducted. These two studies focused on 300 families who lived along the southeastern shores of Lake Michigan and consumed variable quantities of PCB-contaminated sportfish (Fein et al., 1984) and a random sample of approximately 1000 children in North Carolina exposed to background levels of PCBs (Rogan et al. 1986).

Neuropsychological examination of children born to women in these two birth cohorts began shortly after parturition. Neonates of Michigan mothers who consumed large quantities of PCB-contaminated fish exhibited feeble reflexes and were more likely to be unresponsive to visual and auditory stimulation (Jacobson et al., 1984). In North Carolina, weak reflexes and unresponsiveness to visual and auditory stimuli also were observed in neonates exposed to higher levels of PCBs transplacentally (Rogan et al., 1986).

Except those in infants with substantial central nervous system maldevelopment or injury at birth, measures of neonatal behavior are of little or no prognostic value. Therefore, the Michigan and North Carolina studies extended their follow-up examinations into the later infancy and preschool periods of development.

In North Carolina, prenatal exposure to PCBs was associated with lower scores on the Bayley (1969) Psychomotor Development Index at 12, 18, and 24 months (Gladen et al., 1988). However, no measures of perinatal PCB exposure were associated significantly with the Bayley Mental Development Index. Furthermore, the North Carolina study did not observe a relationship between any measure of *intrauterine* exposure and the cognitive skills and academic achievement of children after their entry into the primary grades (Gladen & Rogan, 1991).

In Michigan, no measures of perinatal PCB exposure were associated significantly with the Bayley mental or psychomotor developmental indices, although cord serum PCB concentrations were associated significantly with deficits on a cluster of Bayley items that assess fine-motor coordination (Jacobson & Jacobson, 1994). Subjects in the Michigan study also were administered the Fagan Test of Infant Development (Fagan & Shephard, 1987). This is a new instrument in the field of neurobehavioral teratology and of developmental psychology. The instrument examines the infant's mastery in the discrimination of a novel visual stimulus when it is paired with another visual stimulus that was presented previously during a "familiarization" period. Thus, if the infant gazes for a longer period at the novel stimulus, the neurocognitive inference is that the familiar stimulus has been encoded mentally, retained, and discriminated. In the Michigan study, both cord serum PCB concentrations and the quantity of maternal consumption of contaminated fish were associated significantly in a dose-dependent fashion with poorer visual recognition memory scores on the Fagan Test of Infant Development at 7 months of age (Jacobson et al., 1985).

The Michigan study stands out in comparison to other studies in the area of environmental chemical neuroteratogenesis in the specificity of the neurobehavioral effects that have been reported. Thus, for example, when these children were evaluated with the McCarthy Scales of Children's Abilities (McCarthy, 1972) at the age of 4 years, the most robust associations were between measures of perinatal PCB exposure, such as cord serum and breastmilk concentrations, and performance on the McCarthy Memory Subscales (Jacobson et al., 1990). The skills necessary to encode and retain information appeared to be affected especially by *intrauterine* exposure to PCBs.

The authors of the Michigan study also noted in their data a paradoxical relationship that speaks to the complexity of conducting investigations of this kind. Thus, the children of mothers who breast-fed for longer periods of time postnatally (and therefore received higher doses of PCBs during early postnatal development) did not, as predicted, score more poorly on measures of cognitive development. The confounding factor seemed to be that mothers that breast-feed for longer periods postnatally provided an environment that was more favorable to mental developmental advancement in their children and thus compensated for any adverse developmental effects of postnatal exposure to PCBs via breastmilk. Authors of these studies have concluded that the inverse association between the absolute concentration of PCBs in breastmilk reflected prenatal (as opposed to postnatal) exposure, as the concentration of PCBs in maternal breastmilk after birth would be highly correlated with prenatal maternal body burden of the chemical and its trans-placental transfer to the fetus. The fact that the neurocognitive effects associated with maternal-milk PCB levels paralleled those associated with cord serum PCB concentrations lends substantial support for this interpretation (Jacobson & Jacobson, 1994).

Due to the apparent specificity of the cognitive effects of transplacental PCB exposure in the Michigan data, the effect of PCBs on information-processing efficiency was assessed further in the cohort using supplementary neuropsychological measures of memory, reaction time, visual discrimination, and sustained attention (Jacobson et al., 1992). Thus, for example, as with the McCarthy scales, cord serum and breastmilk PCB concentrations were associated significantly in a dose-dependent fashion with information-processing efficiency as examined by measures of memory, stimulus discrimination, and reaction time. However, as observed previously, the duration of breast-feeding was not associated inversely with any measures of cognitive function. Therefore, maternal breastmilk PCB concentration probably reflected higher prenatal (rather than postnatal) breast-feeding exposure.

A great deal of discussion in the area of PCB developmental neurotoxicity has focused on reasons for the seemingly discrepant findings in the Michigan and North Carolina studies (United States Environmental Protection Agency, 1993). Both studies observed an association between intrauterine exposure to PCBs and measures of neonatal neuromotor and sensory functions. However, effects on central nervous system function persisted only in the Michigan study. Furthermore, the neurobehavioral deficits in the Michigan study were mostly cognitive and rather specific to mnemonic functions, whereas only psychomotor effects were observed in the North Carolina data. Dose to the conceptus appeared to overlap, but differences in the chemical analytical procedures used to assess the concentration of PCBs in sampled tissues varied and thus complicated attempts to estimate the absolute level of prenatal exposures in the two studies. Another difference between the two studies is that in Michigan, perinatal exposure to PCBs was assessed directly in cord serum whereas, owing to the overwhelming number of nondetects, the North Carolina study had to construct perinatal dose using several highly intercorrelated measures of fetal exposure, including concentrations in maternal serum and breastmilk. Nevertheless, what must be emphasized is that both of these studies were using the best analytical techniques available at the time of sampling. Many of the problems associated with PCB analysis at low dose have now been resolved (Mullin et al., 1984).

Although the possibility is open to conjecture, the neurobehavioral data collected in the Michigan study may have been somewhat more precise, owing to the fact that all assessments were administered individually by a relatively small number of highly trained psychometricians whose proficiency and reliability for the purposes of the study were established before collection of study data.

The biological mechanism responsible for the developmentally neurotoxic properties of PCB congeners has not been identified with complete certainty. A considerable body of scientific evidence holds that PCBs and related compounds express many of their toxic effects through changes in hormonal function. They do so by altering the concentrations of hormones or by affecting hormonal receptor numbers or affinity in target cells. For example, some of the developmental neurotoxicity of dioxinlike PCB congeners may be associated with the antiestrogenic characteristics of these compounds. These compounds can affect neurochemistry during development, such as dopaminergic functions (Korach et al., 1987; United States Environmental Protection Agency, 1993).

Of considerable significance is that PCBs and related compounds are structurally similar to the thyroid hormones. These hormones are essential for the normal development of the central nervous system. Thus, for example, they serve to increase the rate of neuronal proliferation and help to initiate the process of neuronal maturation and differentiation (Hambaugh et. al., 1971). PCBs and related compounds have been speculated to alter central nervous system development through their action on thyroid hormone availability during sensitive periods of development (Porterfield, 1994). Such alterations in hormonal output and cellular affinity could express themselves in subtle deficits in infant and child neuropsychological functions (Jacobson & Jacobson, 1994).

Inorganic Lead

No other environmental chemical contaminant has been studied as thoroughly as lead. Most clinicians and scientists no longer seriously debate whether chronic high-level exposure to this metal poses a mental developmental risk to the conceptus, infant, and child (Bellinger, 1995). As Cantarow and Trumper (1944 p. 85) observed more than five decades ago in their classic text describing, among other things, exposure among women working in the lead industry, "It is generally agreed that if pregnancy does occur it is frequently characterized by miscarriage, intrauterine death of the fetus, premature birth and, if living children are born, they are usually smaller, weaker, slower in development and have a higher infant mortality."

Presently, the most controversial question is whether exposures to lead at lower levels prenatally and postnatally pose a risk to normal central nervous system development.

The literature in this area is immense, rendering a comprehensive critical review of the available studies impractical in a single chapter concerned with several environmental chemical influences on child development. After a brief historical overview, the chapter focuses on findings of the most recent and methodologically rigorous studies.

Although lead has been recognized in one form or another as a poison since antiquity, the special problem of lead poisoning in children was not acknowledged generally until the 1890s, when Gibson et al. (1892; Gibson, 1904) described a series of patients with stunted physical development and other health problems due to the consumption of chalking lead-based paint in domestic residences in and around Brisbane, Australia. During the first part of the twentieth century, a common belief was that children surviving the acute stage of the disease would not be burdened with irreversible mental deficits. Then, in 1943, Byers and Lord (1943) identified 20 children who had survived the acute stages of lead encephalopathy and found that 19 of them were learning- or behaviorally disordered. Thus, these authors were the first to illustrate lead's long-lasting and perhaps irreversible developmental neurotoxicity in young children.

Fatal or life-threatening lead poisoning is now rare, although occasional cases continue to be reported (Selbst et al., 1985; Centers for Disease Control, 1991). Concern currently is focused on the mental developmental effects of low-dose "asymptomatic" exposures that are associated with blood lead concentrations in the range of 10 to 30 μg/dL.

The modern era of pediatric lead research began with an investigation of a cohort of first and second graders in Chelsea and Somerville, MA (Needleman et al., 1979). This study was the first to address some of the methodological problems noted in previous investigations. Thus, cumulative historical exposure to lead was assessed by determining the concentration of the metal in shed deciduous teeth, potential confounding factors were measured, and multivariate statistical procedures were employed.

Needleman et al. reported in full-scale IQ between "high" and "low" tooth lead groups a covariate-adjusted difference of 4.5 points. Teachers' ratings of the behaviors of study subjects also revealed significantly more behavioral problems and academic difficulties in children with higher concentrations of lead in teeth. The questions of low-level lead effects raised by this study inspired a number of later cross-sectional and prospective studies of lead and child development in the United States, Europe, and Australia (Bellinger & Dietrich, 1994). This study served as a stimulus for an increased concern that low-level or so-called subclinical lead exposure may contribute to learning disabilities in children.

Even before the landmark report of Needleman et al., most generally accepted that a prospective methodology would be necessary to resolve some of the issues raised by such cross-sectional studies as those in the Chelsea and Somerville investigation (World Health Organization, 1977). A longitudinal methodology is believed to be better suited to the task of establishing a causal link between early exposure to lead and later cognitive or other neurobehavioral deficits. For example, a common characteristic of the severely developmentally delayed or mentally retarded is that they continue to engage in hand-to-mouth or *pica* behaviors well into later childhood and adolescence. This finding raises the question as to whether lead exposure was a *cause* or *effect* of cognitive deficits. Recruiting subjects prior to birth of their children also allowed studies to evaluate the effects of lower-level prenatal exposure to lead.

In the early 1980s, birth cohort studies were initiated in Australia, Scotland, the former Yugoslavia, and the United States. In general, these studies documented developmental exposure to lead, potential confounding factors, and neurobehavioral development with greater precision and detail than that in earlier investigations (Bellinger & Dietrich, 1994; World Health Organization, 1997).

Several of these prospective studies reported a significant dose-effect relationship between various measures of low-level prenatal lead exposure (e.g., concentration of lead measured in maternal, cord, or neonatal blood) and lower scores on the Bayley Scales of Infant Development (Bellinger et al., 1987; Dietrich et al., 1987; Ernhart et al., 1987; Wigg et al., 1988). The reported effects were small, and further follow-up of these cohorts revealed that the observed deficits related to prenatal lead exposure for the most part were transient or limited to the kinds of skills assessed by global measures in infancy (i.e., principally sensorimotor abilities). Prenatal or cord blood lead concentrations in these studies generally were in the range of 1 to 25 µg/dL.

The exception to the later results of these studies of prenatal lead exposure and mental functioning came from a prospective investigation that recruited birth cohorts in the lead smelting region of Kosovo and the nonindustrial community of Pristina, Mitrovica Province, of the former Yugoslavia (Wasserman et al., 1994). A significant dose-effect relationship was observed between prenatal maternal blood lead concentrations and mental developmental status as measured by the McCarthy Scales of Children's Abilities at 3 and 4 years of age. Furthermore, the effects observed were large in comparison to other cross-sectional and prospective studies. Thus, for example, on the perceptual-performance subscale, which has a mean of 50 and standard deviation of 10, children of mothers with prenatal blood lead values greater than 20 µg/dL scored a full standard deviation below children in the lowest exposure group (< 5µg/dL prenatal blood lead). However, importantly, this cohort differed from subjects studied in the other prospective studies in that more than one-third of the 300 children examined were anemic, and maternal prenatal blood lead concentrations were relatively high (i.e., exposures to lead during pregnancy were more typical of occupational exposures in factories with poor environmental controls as opposed to gen-

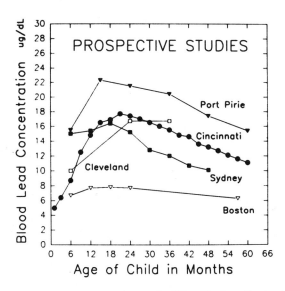

Figure 20.2 Average longitudinal blood lead profiles for the international prospective studies of lead exposure and child development.

eral community exposures). Thus, for example, 25% of the women in the study had integrated prenatal blood lead concentrations from midpregnancy to delivery of between 20 and 42 µg/dL. The study also was conducted in a country in the throes of political instability and civil war. These factors seriously undermine the generalizability of the Kosovo study's findings to the more widespread problem of lower-level exposures in most communities without a point source of heavy lead contamination.

Another interesting exception to the results of the other longitudinal investigations can be found in later results from the Cincinnati Prospective Study. A significant covariate-adjusted inverse relationship was reported between neonatal blood lead concentrations and visuomotor control, motor speed, dexterity, and fine-motor (manipulatory) skills as revealed in the administration of the Bruininks-Oseretsky Test of Motor Proficiency (Bruininks, 1978) to subjects just after school entry (Dietrich et al., 1993a).

Lower-level postnatal exposure to lead also was examined in these prospective studies. Figure 20.2 presents the average serial blood lead concentrations by age of sampling for the prospective studies conducted in the United States and Australia. These studies sampled the concentration of lead in children's blood at variable intervals, with the Cincinnati study having the most comprehensive assessment of historical exposure over the preschool and early school-age years. Also found was that exposures between cohorts were fairly variable, with the highest in studies of children near smelting operations—Kosovo (not pictured) and Port-Pirie—and to a somewhat lesser degree in children residing in old, deteriorating inner-city housing (Cincinnati, Cleveland) and the lowest in a sample of middle- to upper-class New England families (Boston).

Four of these studies have reported on the relationship between earlier postnatal lead exposure and intellectual and academic achievement in school-age children (Cooney et al., 1991; Baghurst et al., 1992; Bellinger et al., 1992; Dietrich et al., 1993b). Using global measures of intellectual attainment, all these studies except the one conducted in Sydney found a significant inverse relationship between earlier blood lead concentrations and IQ after accounting for potential confounders and covariates. Nevertheless, the effects observed at the lowest levels of lead exposure were small. Thus, for example, meta-analytical studies of these data estimated that an increase in blood lead concentration from 10 to 20 μg/dL was associated with a decrease in full-scale IQ of approximately 2 points (95% confidence interval = −0.3 to −3.6 points). (World Health Organization, 1997). However, very important is that this analysis did not address the intellectual and other neurobehavioral ramifications for blood lead concentrations in excess of 20 μg/dL. Many children in our inner cities continue to present with blood lead concentrations equal to or often in excess of this level. For example, in the study by Dietrich et al., (1993b), first-graders with average lifetime blood lead concentrations of greater than 20 μg/dL had covariate-adjusted performance IQs that were up to nine points lower than those of children whose blood lead concentrations remained below 10 μg/dL. Children with lifetime average blood lead concentrations greater than 10 μg/dL also displayed statistically and clinically significant deficits in fine-motor coordination as assessed in kindergarten (Dietrich et al., 1993a).

Attempts to describe the neuropsychological bases for lead-associated deficits in IQ and academic achievement have been difficult, owing to the reliance on global measures of cognitive development in the prospective and other studies. Limited data exist, but poorer performance on measures of motor speed, executive regulatory functions, visuospatial and visuomotor integration appear to be affected in particular (Winneke et al., 1990; Dietrich et al., 1993a; Stiles & Bellinger, 1993; Baghurst et al., 1995).

Lower-level lead exposure has been examined also in relationship to behavioral conduct disorders in older children and young adults. Byers and Lord (1943) noted that children treated for lead poisoning often were referred back to him by their families and schools for violent and aggressive behavioral tendencies (Needleman et al., 1996). Exposure to lead has been linked to hyperactive behavior and attentional deficits in some studies, but until recently no link has been made between childhood lead exposure and antisocial behaviors. Needleman et al. (1996) examined the relationship between bone lead concentrations assessed by K-shell x-ray fluorescence spectroscopy (an experimental measure of cumulative childhood lead exposure) and delinquent behavioral trends in children enrolled in the Pittsburgh Youth Study at 7 and 11 years of age. A statistically significant lead-related association with the delinquency and aggressive clusters of the Achenbach Child Behavior Checklist (Achenbach & Edelbrock, 1983) was observed in interviews with both teachers and parents. Higher concentrations of lead in bone were associated with an increased risk of exceeding the clinical score for the factors of attention, aggression, and delinquency at 11 years of age. Although these findings are intriguing, the question must be studied further in other cohorts.

Data describing the long-term effects of early lead exposure on the neurobehavioral status of older adolescents and adults are rather paltry. The only rigorous study in the peer-reviewed literature is a follow-up of the Chelsea and Somerville cohorts when they reached 17 to 18 years of age (Needleman et al., 1990). Among subjects with dentine lead concentrations greater than $20\,\mu g/gm$ as compared to those with concentrations of less than $10\,\mu g/gm$, the covariate-adjusted odds ratio for failure to graduate from high school was 7.4 (95% confindence interval = 1.4–40.8). The likelihood of a reading disability also was significantly higher in young adults with higher concentrations of lead in shed deciduous teeth. Other adverse outcomes associated with higher tooth lead concentrations were lower class rank, increased absenteeism, and poorer academic performance in the areas of grammatical reasoning and vocabulary. Subjects in the higher-tooth-lead groups also exhibited slower finger tapping, poorer eye-hand coordination, and longer reaction times in response to auditory and visual stimuli.

With the establishment of lower-level lead effects in the immature human central nervous system, animal studies now are focused on determining the possible biological mechanisms underlying lead's apparent developmental neurotoxicity. Recent investigations suggest that lead may disrupt the process whereby synaptic connections are established in the developing brain (Goldstein, 1992). Thus, for example, Marcovac and Goldstein (1988) found that lead activated phosphokinase c at very low concentrations. This finding may represent a fundamental mechanism for the neurodevelopmental toxicity of lead. A key event in the human central nervous system is the programmed death of neural cellular aggregations. Thus, the increase in neuronal responsivity promoted by an increase in phosphokinase c activity could alter the higher-order cerebral architecture of the brain.

In studies of rodents, lead has been shown to disturb desialylation of neural cell adhesion molecule, a morphoregulator that is important in neural fiber outgrowth, neural migration, and synaptogenesis (Cookman et al., 1987). Furthermore, low-level lead exposure has been shown as well to induce precocious glial cell development in rodent brains, thus disrupting their trophic, supportive, and nutritional roles in central nervous system development (Cookman et al., 1988). As a neuropharmacological agent, lead has been shown to affect calcium-dependent aspects of neurotransmission and signal transduction. Such effects could alter the process whereby connections are established in the fetal and infant brain (Pounds & Rosen, 1988).

As an environmental contaminant capable of producing central nervous systems effects in children, lead is unique in that sometimes it is treated with medicines that aid the body in excreting the toxicant. The standard of treatment at this time calls for medical intervention when a child's confirmed blood lead concentration exceeds 44 µg/dL. For many years, a diagnosis of lead poisoning has meant treatment in hospital with parenteral administration of calcium disodium ethylene diamine tetraacetic acid. At higher blood lead concentrations, this is often accompanied by the painful procedure of repeated intramuscular injections of dimercaprol. Now, medical treatment of lead toxicity at moderate levels increasingly is conducted on an outpatient basis with dimercaptosuccinic acid, or succimer (Chemet), a congener of dimercaprol. A question of critical public health importance is whether such therapies reverse cognitive developmental damage or prevent additional damage (Bellinger & Dietrich, 1994). Under the auspices of the National Institute of Environmental Health Sciences, a multicenter double-blind clinical trial is under way to determine whether treatment with an oral chelator (succimer) is developmentally beneficial to infants from 12 to 32 months of age with presenting blood lead concentrations ranging from 20 to 44 µg/dL.

CONCLUSIONS

As in many areas of epidemiological research, clinicians and investigators have reached a wide range of conclusions concerning the impact of environmental chemical exposures on child development. Some researchers have noted that these conclusions seem at times to reside in the *transcientific* domain, wherein the investigator's values may interfere with an objective appraisal of the data (Needleman, 1992). Nevertheless, most clinicians and environmental health scientists agree that limiting the exposure of fetuses, infants and children to the environmental contaminants covered in this review is an important goal. The effects of environmental chemical exposures at low levels in utero and postnatally often seem trivial in comparison to the devastating impacts of what has come to be known as the *social welfare state*, with its accompanying poverty, crime, feelings of hopelessness, and child neglect. However, the exposure to the fetus and child by neuroteratogenic agents can be eliminated through practical human engineering, and such endeavors should be encouraged and granted the financial and technical support necessary for implementation.

Finally, what should be recognized also is that not all nonpharmaceutical chemical exposures to the conceptus are involuntary, as is mostly the case for methyl mercury, PCBs, and lead. For example, some reports cite an increase of commercial solvent abuse in women of reproductive potential. Estimates posit that as many as 4% of teenagers of reproductive potential engage in this activity on a regular basis (Lowenstein, 1985). Such exposure creates a temporary "high," which can result in central nervous system, renal, and hepatic effects in the abuser. Toluene, a solvent found in commercial aerosol paints, is the chemical agent most commonly abused by women whose surviving offspring sometimes bear a striking similarity to infants and children with fetal alcohol syndrome (Pearson et al., 1994; Arnold et al., 1994).

Overall, our health and quality of life have been enhanced greatly by humanmade substances and the exploitation of minerals and other natural resources. However, we must continue to monitor the impact of the use and disposal of these materials on the reproductive and developmental health of the population. Owing to the lengthy period of maturation of the human central nervous system, developmental neurotoxicology and the cognitive neurosciences will continue to play an important role in determining the adverse consequences of perinatal exposures to environmental chemicals.

REFERENCES

Achenbach, T. M., & Edelbrock, C. (1983). *Manual for the child behavior checklist and revised child behavior profile*. Burlington, VT: University of Vermont Department of Psychiatry.

Arnold, G. L., Kirby, R. S., Langendoerfer, S., & Wilkins-Haug, L. (1994). Toluene embryopathy: Clinical delineation and developmental follow-up. *Pediatrics, 93*, 216–220.

Baghurst, P. A., McMichael, A. J., Tong, S., Wigg, N. R., Vimpani, G. V., & Robertson, E. F. (1995). Exposure to environmental lead and visual-motor integration at age 7 years: The Port Pirie Cohort Study. *Epidemiology, 6*, 104–109.

Baghurst, P. A., McMichael, A. J., Wigg, N. R., Vimpani, G. V., Robertson, E. F., & Tong, S. (1992). Environmental exposure to lead and children's intelligence at the age of seven years: The Port Pirie Cohort Study. *New England Journal of Medicine, 327*, 1279–1284.

Bayley, N. (1969). *Manual for the Bayley scales of infant development*. San Antonio, TX: The Psychological Corporation.

Bellinger, D. C. (1995). Interpreting the literature on lad and child development: The neglected role of the "experimental system." *Neurotoxicology and Teratology, 17*, 201–212.

Bellinger, D. C., & Dietrich, K. N. (1994). Low level lead exposure and cognitive function in children. *Pediatric Annals, 23*, 600–605.

Bellinger, D. C., Stiles, K. M., & Needleman, H. L. (1992). Low-level lead exposure, intelligence and academic achievement: A long-term follow-up study. *Pediatrics, 90*, 855–861.

Bellinger, D., Leviton, A., Waternaux, C., Needleman, H., & Rabinowitz, M. (1987). Longitudinal analyses of prenatal and postnatal lead exposure and early cognitive development. *New England Journal of Medicine, 316*, 1037–1043.

Bruininks, R. H. (1978). *The Bruininks-Oseretsky test of motor proficiency*. Circle Pines, MN: American Guidance Service.

Burbacher, T. M., Rodier, P. M., & Weiss, B. (1990). Methylmercury developmental neurotoxicity: A comparison of effects in humans and animals. *Neurotoxicology and Teratology, 12*, 191–202.

Byers, R. K., & Lord, E. E. (1943). Late effects of lead poisoning on mental development. *American Journal of Diseases of Children, 66*, 471–494.

Cantarow, A., & Trumper, M. (1944). *Lead poisoning*. Baltimore: Williams & Wilkins.

Centers for Disease Control (1991). Fatal pediatric poisoning from leaded paint—Wisconsin, 1990. *Journal of the American Medical Association, 265*, 2050–2051.

Cernichiari, E., Brewer, R., Myers, G. J., Marsh, D. O., Lapham, L. W., Cox, C., et al. (1995). Monitoring methylmercury during pregnancy: Maternal hair predicts fetal brain exposure. *Neurotoxicology, 16*, 705–710.

Clarkson, T. W. (1992). Mercury: Major issues in environmental health. *Environmental Health Perspectives, 100,* 31–38.

Clarkson, T. W., Hursh, J. B., Sager, P. R., & Syverson, T. L. M. (1988). Mercury. In T. W. Carkson, L. Friberg, G. F. Nordberg, & P. R. Sager (Eds.), *Biological monitoring of toxic metals* (pp. 199–246). New York: Plenum.

Cookman, G. R., Hemmens, S. E., Keane, G. J., King, W. B., & Regan, C. M. (1988). Chronic low-level lead exposure precociously induces rat glial development *in vitro* and *in vivo. Neuroscience Letters, 86,* 33–37.

Cookman, G. R., King, W. B., & Regan, C. M. (1987). Chronic low level lead exposure impairs embryonic to adult conversion of neural cell adhesion molecule. *Journal of Neurochemistry, 49,* 399–403.

Cooney, G., Bell, A., & Stanrov, C. (1991). Low level exposure to lead and neurobehavioral development: The Sydney study at seven years. In: *Proceedings of the international conference on heavy metals in the environment (Vol. 1,* pp. 16–19) Edinburgh: CEP Consultants Ltd.

Davidson, P. W., Myers, G. J., Cox, C., Shamlaye, C. F., Marsh, D. O., Tanner, M. A., et al. (1995). Longitudinal neurodevelopmental study of Seychellois children following *in utero* exposure to methylmercury from maternal fish ingestion: Outcomes at 19 to 29 months. *Neurotoxicology, 16,* 677–688.

Davis, J. M., Otto, D. A., Weil, D. E., & Grant, L. D. (1990). The comparative developmental neurotoxicity of lead in humans and animals. *Neurotoxicology and Teratology, 12,* 215–229.

Dietrich, K. N., Berger, O. G., & Succop, P. A. (1993a). Lead exposure and the motor developmental status of urban six-year-old children in the Cincinnati Prospective Study. *Pediatrics, 91,* 301–307.

Dietrich, K. N., Berger, O. G., Succop, P. A., Hammond, P. B., & Bornschein, R. L. (1993b). The developmental consequences of low to moderate prenatal and postnatal lead exposure: Intellectual attainment in the Cincinnati Lead Study cohort following school entry. *Neurotoxicology and Teratology, 15,* 37–44.

Dietrich, K. N., Krafft, K. M., Bornschein, R. L., Hammond, P. B., Berger, O., Succop, P. A., et al. (1987). Low-level fetal lead exposure effect on neurobehavioral development in early infancy. *Pediatrics, 80,* 721–730.

Dobbing, J. (1981). The later development of the brain and its vulnerability. In J. A. Davis & J. Dobbing (Eds.), *Scientific foundations of pediatrics* (pp. 744–759). London: Heinemann.

Ernhart, C., Morrow-Tlucak, M., Marler, M., & Wolf, A. (1987). Low level lead exposure in the prenatal and early postnatal periods: Early preschool development. *Neurotoxicology and Teratology, 9,* 259–270.

Fagan, J. F., & Shephard, P. A. (1987). *Fagan test of infant intelligence.* Cleveland: Infantest Corporation.

Fein, G. G., Jacobson, J. L., Jacobson, S. W., Schwartz, P. M., & Dowler, J. K. (1984). Prenatal exposure to polychlorinated biphenyls: Effects on birth size and gestational age. *Journal of Pediatrics, 105,* 315–320.

Frankenberg, W. K., Fandal, A. W., Sciarillo, W., & Burgess, D. (1981). The newly abbreviated and revised Denver Developmental Screening Test. *Pediatrics, 99,* 995–999.

Gibson, J. L. (1904). A plea for painted railings and painted walls of rooms as the source of lead poisoning amongst Queensland children. *Australian Medical Gazette, 23,* 149–153.

Gibson, J. L., Love, W., Hardine, D., Bencroft, P., & Turner, D. (1892). Note on lead poisoning as observed among children in Brisbane (pp. 76–83). In *Transactions of the third intercolonial medical congress.* Sydney.

Gladen, B. C., & Rogan, W. J. (1991). Effects of perinatal polychlorinated biphenyls and dichlorodiphenyl dichlorethene on later development. *Journal of Pediatrics, 119*, 58–63.

Gladen, B. C., Rogan, W. J., Hardy, P., Thullen, J., Tingelstad, J., & Tulley, M. (1988). Development after exposure to polychlorinated biphenyls and dichlorodiphenyl dichloroethene transplacentally and through human milk. *Journal of Pediatrics, 113*, 991–995.

Goldstein, G. (1992). Developmental neurobiology of lead toxicity. In H. L. Needleman (Ed.), *Human lead exposure* (pp. 125–135). Boca Raton, FL: CRC Press.

Hambaugh, M., Mendoza, L. A., Burkhart, J. F., & Weil, F. (1971). The thyroid as a time clock in the developing nervous system. In D. C. Pease (Ed.), *Cellular aspects of neuronal growth and differentiation* (pp. 321–328). Berkeley, CA: University of California Press.

Hammill, D., & Newcomer, P. (1988). *Test of language development–intermediate*. Austin, TX: Pro-Ed.

Harada, M. (1976). Intrauterine poisoning: Clinical and epidemiological studies of the problem. *Bulletin of the Institute of Constitutional Medicine of Kumamoto University, 25*, 1–60.

Hsu, S. T., Ma, C. I., Hsu, S. H., Wu, S. S., Hsu, N. H., Yeh, C. C., et al. (1985). Discovery and epidemiology of PCB poisoning in Taiwan: A four year follow-up. *Environmental Health Perspectives, 59*, 5–10.

Hunter, D., & Russel, D. S. (1954). Focal cerebral and cerebellar atrophy in a human subject due to organic mercury compounds. *Journal of Neurology, Neurosurgery, and Psychiatry, 17*, 235–241.

Jacobson, J. L., & Jacobson, S. W. (1994). The effects of perinatal exposure to polychlorinated biphenyls and related contaminants. In H. L. Needleman & D. C. Bellinger (Eds.), *Prenatal exposure to toxicants: developmental consequences* (pp. 130–147). Baltimore: Johns Hopkins University Press.

Jacobson, J. L., Jacobson, S. W., Fein, G. G., Schwartz, P. M., & Dowler, J. K. (1984). Prenatal exposure to an environmental toxin: A test of the multiple effects model. *Developmental Psychology, 20*, 523–532.

Jacobson, J. L., Jacobson, S. W., & Humphrey, H. E. B. (1990). Effects of *in utero* exposure to polychlorinated biphenyls on cognitive functioning in young children. *Journal of Pediatrics, 116*, 38–45.

Jacobson, J. L., Jacobson, S. W., Padgett, R. J., Brumitt, G. A., & Billings, R. L. (1992). Effects of prenatal PCB exposure on cognitive processing efficiency and sustained attention. *Developmental Psychology, 28*, 297–306.

Jacobson, S. W., Fein, G. G., Jacobson, J. L., Schwartz, P. M., & Dowler, J. K. (1985). The effect of PCB exposure on visual recognition memory. *Child Development, 56*, 853–860.

Jensen, A. A. (1989). Background levels in humans. In R. D. Kimbrough & A. A. Jensen (Eds.), *Topics in environmental health; Vol. 4. Halogenated biphenyls, napthalenes, dibenzodioxins, and related products* (pp. 385–390). Amsterdam: Elsevier.

Kallen, B. (1988). *Epidemiology of human reproduction*. Boca Raton, FL: CRC Press.

Kjellstrom, T., Kennedy, P., Wallis, S., Stewart, A., Friberg, L., Lind, B., et al. (1989). *Physical and mental development of children with prenatal exposure to mercury from fish: Stage 2. Interviews and psychological tests at age 6*. National Swedish Environmental Protection Board Report 3642, Solna, Sweden.

Korach, K. S., Sarver, P., Chae, K., McLachlan, J. A., & McKinney, J. D. (1987). Estrogen receptor-binding activity of polychlorinated hydroxybiphenyls: Conformationally restricted structural probes. *Molecular Pharmacology, 33*, 120–126.

Kuratsune, M. (1989). Yusho with reference to Yucheng. In R. D. Kimbrough & A. A. Jensen (Eds.), *Halogenated biphenyls, terphenyls, napthalenes, dibenzodioxins, and related products* (pp. 381–400). New Amsterdam: Elsevier.

Landrigan, P. J., Graham, D. G., & Thomas, R. D. (1994). Environmental neurotoxic illness: Research for prevention. *Environmental Health Perspectives, 102*(suppl.), 117–120.

Lowenstein, L. F. (1985). Recent research into glue-snifffing: Extent of the problem, its repercussions and treatment appproaches. *International Journal of Social Psychiatry, 31*, 93–104.

Mahaffey, K. R. (1985). Factors modifying susceptibility to lead toxicity. In K. R. Mahaffey (Ed.), *Dietary and environmental lead: Human health effects.* New York: Elsevier.

Markovac, J., & Goldstein, G. (1988). Picomolar concentrations of lead stimulate brain protein kinase C. *Nature, 334*, 71–73.

Marsh, D. O., Clarkson, T. W., Cox, C., Myers, G. J., Amin-Zaki, L., & Al-Tikriti, S. (1987). Fetal methylmercury poisoning. *Archives of Neurology, 44*, 1017–1022.

Marsh, D. O., Clarkson, T. W., Myers, G. J., Davidson, P. W., Cox, C., Cernchiari, E., et al. (1995). The Seychelles study of fetal methylmercury exposure and child development: Introduction. *Neurotoxicology, 16*, 583–596.

Masuda, Y, Kagawa, R., Kuroki, H., Kuratsune, M., Yoshimura, T., Taki, I., et al. (1978). Transfer of polychlorinated biphenyls from mothers to fetuses and infants. *Food and Cosmetic Toxicology, 16*, 543–546.

McCarthy, D. (1972). *McCarthy scales of children's abilities.* San Antonio, TX: The Psychological Corporation.

McKeown-Eyssen, G. E., Reudy, J., & Neims, A. (1983). Methylmercury exposure in Northern Quebec: II. Neurological findings in children. *American Journal of Epidemiology, 118*, 470–479.

Mullin, M. D., Pochini, C. M., McCrindle, S., Romkes, M., Safe, S., & Safe, L. (1984). High resolution PCB analysis: The synthesis and chromatographic properties of all 209 PCB congeners. *Environmental Science and Technology, 18*, 468–476.

Myers, G. J., Davidson, P. W., Cox, C., Shamlaye, C. F., Tanner, M. A., Choisy, O., et al. (1995b). Neurodevelopmental outcomes of Seychellois children sixty-six months after *in utero* exposure to methylmercury from a maternal fish diet: Pilot study. *Neurotoxicology, 16*, 639–652.

Myers, G. J., Marsh, D. O., Cox, C., Davidson, P. W., Shamlaye, C. F., Tanner, M. A., et al. (1995a). A pilot neurodevelopmental study of Seychellois children following *in utero* exposure to methylmercury from a maternal fish diet. *Neurotoxicology, 16*, 629–638.

Myers, G. J., Marsh, D. O., Davidson, P. W., Cox, C., Shamlaye, C. F., Tanner, M., et al. (1995c). Main neurodevelopmental study of Seychellois children following *in utero* exposure to methylmercury from a maternal fish diet: Outcome at six months. *Neurotoxicology, 16*, 653–664.

Needleman, H. L. (1992). Salem comes to the National Institutes of Health: Notes from inside the crucible of scientific integrity. *Pediatrics, 90*, 977–981.

Needleman, H. L., Gunnoe, C., Leviton, A., Reed R., Peresie, H. Maher, C., et al., (1979). Deficits in psychologic and classroom performance of children with elevated dentine lead levels. *New England Journal of Medicine, 300*, 689–695.

Needleman, H. L., Riess, J. A., Tobin, M. J., Biesecker, G. E., & Greenhouse, J. B. (1996). Bone lead levels and delinquent behavior. *Journal of the American Medical Association, 275*, 363–369.

Needleman, H. L., Schell, A., Bellinger, D. Leviton, A., & Allred, E. N. (1990). The long-term effects of low doses of lead in childhood, an 11-year follow-up report. *New England Journal of Medicine, 322*, 83–88.

Newcomer, P. & Hammill, D. (1988). *Test of language development*. Austin, TX: ProEd.

Pearson, M. A., Hoyme, E., Seaver, L. H., & Rimsza, M. A. (1994). Toluene embryopathy: Delineation of the phenotype and comparison with fetal alcohol syndrome. *Pediatrics, 93,* 211–215.

Porterfield, S. P. (1994). Vulnerability of the developing brain to thyroid abnormalities. Environmental insults to the thyroid system. *Environmental Health Perspectives, 102,* 125–130.

Pounds, J., & Rosen, J. (1988). Cellular Ca^{2+} homeostasis and Ca^{2+}-mediated cell processes as critical targets for toxicant action: Conceptual and methodological pitfalls. *Toxicology and Applied Pharmacology, 94,* 331–341.

Rees, D. C., Francis, E. Z., & Kimmel, C. A. (1990). Scientific and regulatory issues relevant to assessing risk for developmental neurotoxicity: An overview. *Neurotoxicology and Teratology, 12,* 175–181.

Rodier, P. M. (1994). Vulnerable periods and processes during central nervous system development. *Environmental Health Perspectives, 102*(suppl. 2), 121–124.

Rodier, P. M., Aschner, M., & Sager, P. R. (1984). Mitotic arrest in the developing CNS after prenatal exposure to methylmercury. *Neurobehavioral Toxicology and Teratology, 6,* 379–385.

Rogan, W. J., Gladen, B. C., Hung, K. L., Koong, S. L., Shih, L. Y., Taylor, J. S., et al. (1988). Congenital poisoning by polychlorinated biphenyls and their contaminants in Taiwan. *Science, 241,* 334–336.

Rogan, W. J., Gladen, B. C., McKinney, J. D., Carreras, N., Hardy, P., Thullen, J. et al. (1986). Neonatal effects of transplacental exposure to PCB's and DDE. *Journal of Pediatrics, 109,* 335–341.

Sager, P. R., Aschner, M., & Rodier, P. M. (1984). Persistent differential alterations in developing cerebellar cortex of male and female mice after methylmercury exposure. *Brain Research and Developmental Brain Research, 12,* 1–11.

Selbst, S. M., Henretig, F. M., & Pearce, J. (1985). Lead encephalopathy. *Clinical Pediatrics, 24,* 280–285.

Shephard, T. H. (1994). *Catalog of teratogenic agents* (8th ed.). Baltimore: Johns Hopkins University Press.

Stiles, K. M., & Bellinger, D. C. (1993). Neuropsychological correlates of low-level lead exposure in school-age children: A prospective study. *Neurotoxicology and Teratology, 15,* 27–35.

Takeuchi, T. (1968). Pathology of Minamata disease. In *Study Group of Minamata disease*. Kumamoto University, Japan: Study Group of Minamata Disease.

Tilson, H. A., Jacobson, J. L., & Rogan, W. J. (1990). Polychlorinated biphenyls and the developing nervous system: Cross-species comparisons. *Neurotoxicology and Teratology, 12,* 239–248.

Trevathen, E., Chavez, G. F., & Sever, L. W. (1991). Epidemiology of congenital malformations of the central nervous system. In D. W. Anderson (Ed.), *Neuroepidemiology: A tribute to Bruce Schoenberg* (pp. 217–238). Boca Raton, FL: CRC Press.

Tsuchiya, K. (1992). The discovery of the causal agent of Minamata disease. *American Journal of Industrial Medicine, 21,* 275–280.

United States Environmental Protection Agency (1993). *Workshop report on developmental neurotoxic effects associated with exposure to PCB's.* Lexington, MA: Eastern Research Group.

Vorhees, C. V. (1987). Origins of behavioral teratology. In E. P. Riley & C. V. Vorhees (Eds.), *Handbook of behavioral teratology* (pp. 3–22). New York: Plenum.

Warkany, J. (1966). Acrodynia-postmortem of a disease. *American Journal of Diseases of Children, 112,* 147–156.

Wasserman, G., Graziano, J. H., Factor-Litvak, P., Popovac, D., Morina, N., Musabegovic, A., et al. (1994). Consequences of lead exposure and iron supplementation on childhood development at age 4 years. *Neurotoxicology and Teratology, 16,* 233–240.

Wechsler, D. (1974). *Weschler Intelligence Scale for Children—Revised.* San Antonio, TX: Psychological Corporation.

Wigg, N. R., Vimpani, F. V., McMichael, A. J., Baghurst, P. A., Robertson, S. F., & Roberts, R. J. (1988). Port Pirie cohort study: Childhood blood lead and neuropsychological development at age two years. *Journal of Epidemiology and Community Health, 42,* 213–219.

Wilson, J. G. (1973). *Environment and birth defects.* New York: Academic.

Wilson, J. G. (1977). Current status of teratology—general principles and mechanisms derived from animal studies. In J. G. Wilson & R. C. Fraser (Eds.), *Handbook of teratology* (Vol. 1, pp. 47–74). New York: Plenum.

Winneke, G., Brockhaus, A., Ewers, U., Kramer, U., & Neuf, M. (1990). Results from the European multicenter study on lead neurotoxicity in children: Implications for risk assessment. *Neurotoxicology and Teratology, 12,* 553–559.

World Health Organization (1977). *Environmental Health Criteria 3 Lead.* Geneva: World Health Organization.

World Health Organization (1995). *Environmental health criteria for inorganic lead.* Geneva: World Health Organization International Programme on Chemical Safety.

Zimmerman, I., Steiner, V., & Pond, R. (1979). *Manual, preschool language scale* (rev. ed.). Columbus, OH: Charles E. Merrill.

21 Synesthesia: A Challenge for Developmental Cognitive Neuroscience

Simon Baron-Cohen and John Harrison

The mapping between sensory modalities and cross-modal transfer recently has begun to receive considerable attention. Often nature reveals itself through exceptions, and two relevant exceptional instances of cross-modal percepts (as a consequence of brain trauma) recently were reported by Halligan et al. (1996) and by Ramachandran and Rogers-Ramachandran (1996). In both cases, visual information appears to have been experienced as touch, suggesting that this is a form of *acquired synesthesia*. This type of synesthesia does not seem to occur naturally. In contrast, *colored-hearing* synesthesia does occur naturally. In this chapter, we explore the phenomenon of colored hearing and propose a neural mechanism that might account for the condition, a model that explains synesthesia not by means of additional brain connections but as a failure of apoptosis, leading to a breakdown in sensory modularity.

The topic of synesthesia currently enjoys a controversial reputation, with some scientists dismissing it as an illusion and others perceiving it as a genuine natural phenomenon, in need of explanation and with important implications for developmental cognitive neuroscience. First, what is synesthesia? We, along with others, (Vernon, 1930; Marks, 1975; Cytowic, 1989, 1994; Motluk, 1994) define synesthesia as the stimulation of one sensory modality that automatically triggers a perception in a second modality in the absence of any direct stimulation to this second modality. So, for example, a sound automatically and instantly might trigger the perception of vivid color, or vice versa. EP, the subject of a study by Baron-Cohen et al., (1997), provided a number of descriptions of color-word correspondences, describing the word *Moscow* as "darkish gray, with spinach green and pale blue." Those with the condition describe the percept not as part of their external visual experience nor in their "mind's eye" but somewhere else, phenomenologically.

Many combinations of synesthesia are reported to occur naturally, including sound giving rise to visual percepts (colored hearing) and smell giving rise to tactile sensation, as in Cytowic's (1993) subject MW. Our experience suggests that colored-hearing synesthesia is the most common form and that certain combinations of synesthesia almost never occur (e.g., touch to hearing). Synesthesia also is sometimes reported by those who have used hallucinogenic drugs, such as lysergic acid diethylamide (LSD) or mescaline. For the most part, this chapter will focus on the naturally occurring form of synesthesia, while acknowledging that a connection may be found with the drug-induced form.

BACKGROUND

The closing decades of the nineteenth century saw a considerable number of accounts of synesthesia, including further accounts of blind people who claimed to be able to "see" colors (Starr, 1893), perhaps the most notable being Galton's (1883) "Inquiries into Human Faculty and Its Development." Scientific interest in the condition declined with the rise of behaviorism as the dominant psychological paradigm, and very little on the topic appears in the literature since the late 1920s. Marks's (1975) review of the topic yields 74 publications in the 50-year period of 1881 to 1931, as compared with a mere 16 in the 42-year period between 1932 and 1974. This paucity probably occurred because behaviorism banished reference to mental states from scientific language. As synesthesia could be defined only by self-report and reference to mental states, it was not considered amenable to "scientific" investigation.

Within the last few years, synesthesia has had something of a renaissance, with researchers from various disciplines within cognitive neuroscience contributing both new data and theory. Such developments have led, for the first time, to wide recognition of the condition as having a neurological reality. This new acceptance of the condition is due in part to current availability of objective approaches to studying it.

TESTING FOR SYNESTHESIA

Our test for the presence of the condition involves assessing a subject's *consistency* in reporting color descriptions for words across two or more occasions: when the subject has no prior warning of the retest and irrespective of the length of interval between testing sessions (Baron-Cohen et al., 1987, 1993). Use of this method results in consistency typically as high as 90%, even when subjects are retested over years and even when stringent criteria are set for retest descriptions. In the case of EP's color correspondences for *Moscow*, for example, her original description would be compared for similarity with retest descriptions, and the two responses would be judged for similarity.

However, the advent of such neuroimaging techniques as positron emission tomography (PET) and functional magnetic resonance imaging (fMRI) now provides an opportunity to image the brains of individuals with synesthesia in vivo. Cytowic and Wood (1982) used the xenon inhalation technique to image the brain of a single subject, and our own group has used both PET (Paulesu et al., 1995) and, more recently, fMRI. Given the marked consistency of patterns of activation in synesthetes studied in the Paulesu et al. study, determining the presence of synesthesia objectively using functional brain imaging techniques ultimately might prove possible. Neuroimaging data are discussed later.

TERMINOLOGY

A standing tendency has been to use the term *synesthesia* whenever a person reports a "mixing of the senses." In this vague usage, *synesthesia* covers at least five very different situations, producing a hopeless muddle. We shall try to draw sharper distinctions by separate discussions of the following: (1) "developmental" synesthesia; (2) synesthesia caused by neurological dysfunction; (3) synesthesia as the consequence of psychoactive drug use; (4) metaphor as pseudosynesthesia; and, finally, (5) association as pseudosynesthesia.

Developmental Synesthesia

We adopt the term *developmental synesthesia* to distinguish it from acquired synesthesia (of which there are at least two forms) and pseudosynesthesia. Developmental synesthesia, in most cases, has several characteristics: (1) It appears to have a childhood onset, in all cases before 4 years of age; (2) it differs from hallucination, delusion, or other psychotic phenomena; (3) it differs from imagery arising from imagination; and (4) it is not induced by drug use. It is vivid, automatic or involuntary, and unlearned.

Synesthesia Caused by Neurological Dysfunction

A variety of neuropathological conditions apparently give rise to acquired synesthesias. According to Krohn (1893), Carnaz speculated that synesthesia of all forms was "pathological and due to some optical lesion" (Krohn, 1893, p. 33) and could therefore be seen as being due to "hyperaesthesia of the sense of colour." A rather fuller account of the variety of acquired synesthesia is given in Critchley (1994), who provided evidence that synesthesia can be acquired. Note that the resultant synesthesic percepts often are much simpler than the complex forms seen in developmental synesthesia.

Synesthesia as a Consequence of Psychoactive Drug Use

Additionally, a number of accounts cite individuals reporting synesthesia as a result of the use of psychoactive drugs (Cytowic, 1989). The mechanisms by which drug-induced synesthesia occur are not well understood, though the use of LSD, mescaline, and psilocin are reported to cause confusion between the sensory modalities, so that sounds are perceived as visions (Rang & Dale, 1987). Neurophysiological studies reported by Aghajanian (1981) have suggested different sites of action for LSD and mescaline, with LSD seeming to work by inhibiting the serotonin-containing neurons of the raphé nuclei and mescaline seeming to work by acting on the noradrenergic system. Note that drug-induced synesthesia differs from developmental synesthesia in several ways: (1) often it is accompanied by hallucinations and loss of reality monitoring; (2) it is transient; (3) it usually has an onset only in adult life (or whenever the drug was used); and (4) it can produce sensory combinations that otherwise do not occur naturally.

Metaphor as Pseudosynesthesia

Almost all writers on the topic of synesthesia have been drawn into discussion of the possibility that a number of authors, poets, painters, and musicians may have had synesthesia. A typical list of these individuals would include the composers Liszt, Rimsky-Korsakov, Messiäen, and Scriabin; the poets Basho, Rimbaud, and Baudelaire; the artists Kandinsky and Hockney; and, finally, the novelist Nabokov. We are unaware of any evidence that demonstrates that these individuals have been tested formally for synesthesia; thus, we have no data with which to make a "diagnosis." However, rather than describing instances of genuine synesthesia, much of the literature cited probably reflects a form of metaphor or analogy.

Thus, Charles Baudelaire appears to have believed in the unity of sensation (as implied by his poem "Correspondances"), but substantial doubt exists over whether Baudelaire was a developmental synesthete, especially given his account of hashish intoxication in which he suggests that "sounds are clad in colour."

In sum, we suggest that the metaphor widespread in language provides ripe conditions for confusion with developmental synesthesia. Distinguishing between the metaphor as pseudosynesthesia and developmental synesthesia is difficult and will rely on objective tests, such as those described earlier. However, the key differences are that in metaphorical pseudosynesthesia, no percept *necessarily* is triggered, the subject often will acknowledge that the description is only of an analogy, and it is voluntary.

Association as Pseudosynesthesia

Possibly, a second form of pseudosynesthesia may include individuals who have simply learned to pair words or letters with colors. Western European culture provides a number of possible means by which colors and letters may be paired. For example, in childhood many of us are given alphabet books in which letters are depicted in a variety of colors. Similarly, a traditional training in needle craft has been the production of samplers. These samplers often depict embroidered letters, each of which often is shown in different colors. The example of sampler production seems an unlikely explanation for developmental synesthesia in that most synesthetes are aware of having had color-word or color-letter associations before having learned handicrafts of this sort. The example of colored letter books seems a more plausible route in that, typically, exposure to these books occurs in infancy. Nevertheless, detailed examination of the color-letter alphabets of individuals with developmental synesthesia often yields the finding that successive letters have very similar colors. This is in marked to contrast to colored alphabet books in which successive letters have markedly different color representations. We suggest that the term *associative pseudosynesthesia* should be retained, however, to describe those individuals who can give a good learning account of their own form of synesthesia. Whether associative pseudosynesthesia has any of the features of developmental synesthesia (e.g., vivid, automatic percepts) remains unknown.

CAUSES OF SYNESTHESIA

Over the last 200 years, a number of hypotheses have been forwarded to explain the cause of synesthesia. Some of the early theories are reviewed by Marks (1975), so we shall concentrate on later theories. However, we point out Marks's dismissal of neurobiological accounts. His stance should be seen in the context of the time in which Marks was writing and, as we describe later, a number of recent findings suggest plausible neurobiological causes of the condition.

Preserved Neural Connectivity

The normal adult human brain does not contain direct neural connections between auditory and visual areas. However, the early developing brain in many species does. Probably for genetic reasons, according to this first theory, in individuals with synesthesia, pathways between auditory and visual areas in the brain continue to exist beyond neoteny, such that when words or sounds give rise to activation in auditory areas, the visual cortex also is stimulated. What is the evidence for this theory?

One method of investigation would be to look at the brains of people with synesthesia to establish whether such pathways are present. This is currently impossible to do both in living individuals or at postmortem. The potential for doing such postmortem studies does, however, exist, and two fluorescent carbocyanine tracers have been used to trace pathways in postmortem brain tissue (Honig & Hume, 1989). However, these fluorescent carbocyanine tracers are lipid-soluble and, therefore, only effective in tracing pathways in relatively unmyelinated neurons (i.e., in fetal tissue). Consequently, to establish that such pathways exist, we must await further technological developments in the field of neurophysiology.

However, evidence supports the presence of such connective pathways in other species (see Kennedy et al., 1996). Kennedy and others in a number of studies (Dehay et al., 1984; Kennedy et al., 1989) have found that connections between auditory and visual areas exist in the brain structure of species, such as the macaque monkey (*Macaca irus*) and the domestic cat (*Felis Domesticus*). These projections appear to be transient, typically disappearing approximately 3 months postpartum.

Some evidence also suggests that these transitory pathways exist in human neonates and may, as in cats and macaques, be "pruned" as part of the biological maturation of the brain. Much of this evidence is reviewed by Maurer (1993). Maurer's hypothesis was that human babies mix the input from different senses and that this gives rise to normal "synesthesia." We know from the work by Meltzoff and Borton (1979) that babies who suck on either a "nubby" or a "smooth" pacifier (dummy) will prefer to look at a picture of the pacifier they sucked on, thereby showing a match between touch and vision. The Meltzoff and Borton study usually is taken as evidence for cross-modal transfer. Maurer goes one step further in suggesting that synesthesia might be a normal stage of perceptual experience in addition to cross-modal transfer.

Maurer's evidence in support of this view comes from other studies of neonates. One such study is that reported by Lewkowicz and Turkewicz (1980). In their experiment, 1-month-old children who had seen a patch of white light for 20 trials were presented with bursts of white noise presented at different intensities. During the noise presentation, the patch of light that they had been trained on was interspersed repeatedly, and the children's heart rate was measured. Normally, heart rate increases as a function of noise intensity, but Lewkowicz and Turkewicz found that the heart rate recorded at a noise intensity of 74 dB showed the lowest heart rate change and that, for values greater or less than this value, heart rate increased. These authors' interpretation of this finding was that "infants were responding to the auditory stimuli in terms of their similarity to the previously presented visual stimulus" (p. 597) or, as Maurer put it, "the children responded least to the 'familiar' intensity" (p. 110). Maurer also cited evidence from electrophysiological studies of neonates showing that the amplitude of somatosensory evoked potentials increases when they are played white noise. Normally, these potentials only increase as a consequence of tactile stimulation. Finally, Maurer cited the work of Neville (1991) that posited that in early infancy, auditorily evoked potentials to language evoke a potential in the occipital cortex, whereas in older individuals, these stimuli yield potentials only in auditory areas, such as the temporal lobes.

The foregoing evidence is consistent with the notion that synesthesia might be due to the persistence of neural information passing from auditory to visual brain areas, beyond the neonatal stage. Taken in the context of development, it also suggests the intriguing possibility that we might *all* be colored-hearing synesthetes until we lose connections between these two areas somewhere near 3 months of age, at which point cortical maturation gives rise to sensory differentiation. This theory is consistent with Cytowic's (1989) view of synesthetes as "cognitive fossils."

Sensory Leakage Theory

Jacobs et al. (1981) proposed what we shall call the *sensory leakage theory*. This is an account of how simple photisms arise in cases of acquired synesthesia, though in principle it could be extended to account for idiopathic synesthesia. As mentioned, most cases of *acquired* synesthesia arise in individuals who suffer brain damage to anterior portions of the brain, often the optic nerve. Close examination of the nine patients reported in Jacobs et al. reveals that four of these patients (cases 1, 2, 4, & 7) also experienced photisms in the *absence* of auditory stimulation, casting doubt on whether these instances should be described as cases of auditory visual synesthesia at all. Also worth observing is that seven patients always experienced their photisms when they were "relaxed, drowsy or dozing" (Jacobs et al., 1981, p. 214), circumstances in which hypnagogic hallucinations are possible.

The essence of the Jacobs group's theory is that auditory information "leaks" into pathways and areas in the brain that ordinarily deal with visual information. These authors expanded this leakage theory by suggesting the presence of "numerous regions of the brain where visual and auditory pathways lie in close anatomic proximity" (Jacobs et al., 1981, p. 216) and that at these points, postsynaptic fibers might converge to cause the synesthesia seen in a range of pathological states, such as congenital blindness and drug intoxication.

Evidence to support leakage between areas subserving different forms of sensory information is sparse, causing some difficulties for this theory. However, recent work has suggested that rather than positing the need for leakage, at certain locations in the brain there are classes of neurons responsive to stimulation from more than one sensory modality. For example, in a study of nonhuman primates carried out by Graziano et al., (1994), recordings were made from neurons (N = 141) in the ventral portion of the premotor cortex. Of these neurons, 27% to 31% were found to be bimodally responsive, firing as a result of either (or both) visual and somasthetic stimulation.

More recent work by Sadato et al. (1996) has shown that congenitally blind subjects show increased blood flow to primary visual areas when reading braille, a finding the authors account for by suggesting that in these subjects "cortical areas normally reserved for vision may be activated by other sensory modalities" (p. 526). Such an account also might explain the case of acquired synesthesia reported by Rizzo and Eslinger (1989). Their subject, a 17-year-old who had developed retrolental fibroplasia as the consequence of perinatal difficulties, exhibited a florid form of colored hearing for musical tones. Rizzo and Eslinger failed to find evidence to suggest visual area activation as a consequence of auditory stimulation but limited themselves to the use of electroencephalography as a means of detecting such activity. These authors' finding suggests that functional neuroimaging might prove to be a useful technique for investigating cases of acquired synesthesia.

Cytowic's Theory of Synesthesia

Perhaps the most controversial theoretical account of the cause of synesthesia is that most recently advanced by Cytowic (1993) in his book, *The Man Who Tasted Shapes*. Cytowic proposes that synesthesia occurs because "parts of the brain get disconnected from one another ... causing the normal processes of the limbic system to be released, bared to consciousness, and experienced as synesthesia" (p. 163). His assertion that the limbic system is the critical brain locus can and has been tested.

In the final chapter of Cytowic's book, the author concedes that though he has no direct evidence to implicate a particular neural structure, given the "stunning shut-down of the cortex" (p. 152) observed in the ^{133}Xe studies of blood flow in MW's brain, he points to the limbic areas as being "the seat of synesthesia." Direct evidence of the involvement of the limbic system would have been provided by evidence of blood flow changes in this brain region; however, neuroimaging using ^{133}Xe inhalation does not permit imaging of such deep structures.

On the other hand, this is not a limitation shared by PET, so the importance of the limbic system in synesthesia can be evaluated using this technique. This question was one of those addressed in the study of colored-hearing synesthesia reported by Paulesu et al. (1995). This study compared brain activity in synesthetes and control while listening either to words or to pure tones. The synesthetes selected reported color percepts for words but not for nonword sounds, so comparing brain activation of synesthetes listening to words as compared with tones with control subjects should yield clues to the neural basis of colored-hearing synesthesia. From this analysis, two areas of particular interest emerged—posterior inferotemporal cortex and the parietol-occipital junction, both of which have known involvement in color perception. However, neither the between-groups nor the within-groups comparisons demonstrated any suggestion of limbic system involvement. Of course, possibly Cytowic's subject (MW) is different in *kind* from the subjects scanned by Paulesu et al. (1995). Given both MW's grossly abnormal resting blood flow levels and his polymodal synesthesia, this conjecture remains a strong possibility.

The Learned Association Theory

The theoretical proposition originally called the *learned association* was suggested as an explanation of synesthesia by Calkins (1893) and holds that in colored-hearing synesthesia, the color-word and sound correspondences reported are due entirely to learned association. The idea is that the color-letter associations are derived from colored alphabet books or from colored letters that the individual saw as a child. Though we regard this theory as a plausible account of the acquisition of pseudosynesthesia, we suspect for a number of reasons that it is an unsatisfactory account of developmental synesthesia. Several reasons substantiate our contention.

The Gender Ratio   The gender ratio in synesthesia is 6:1. Why should so many more women, as compared to men, form such associations? A socialization account that would lead to this gender ratio is not immediately obvious, though transmission from mothers to daughters via modeling may be a possibility (though tenuous).

Consecutive Letters   We have examined the "colored alphabets" of many of the subjects who have contacted us. Careful scrutiny yields the finding that often consecutive letters are closely described in color terms (e.g., M = olive green, N = emerald green, O = washed-out pale green). We have compared this finding with colored alphabet books and have found, in contrast, that publishers logically go to great lengths to ensure that consecutive letters are printed in very different colors. Learned association, therefore, cannot account for the specific colors of particular letters or phonemes.

Synesthesic Twins   A comparison of the colored alphabets of twins so far has yielded substantial variation in the color-letter correspondences made by each of the pair. The same variation is given by siblings and by mothers and daughters in the same family. Surprising is the lack of greater similarity in the color-letter correspondences of family members if colored alphabets are acquired as learned associations.

Lack of Recollection   We have yet to meet a person with synesthesia who is able to report *knowing* that their letter-color associations were learned either purposefully or incidentally via exposure to colored alphabet letters or books.

The learned association theory of synesthesia has not yet provided satisfactory explanations of these anomalies.

The Genetic Theory of Synesthesia

The possibility that synesthesia might be an inherited trait seems first to have been forwarded by Galton (1883). We share this view and suspect that genetic mechanisms might cause the preserved neural connectivity described. Earlier, we reviewed the evidence for transitory connections between auditory and visual brain areas in other mammalian species. Assuming that such connections also are to be found in our species, one explanation for synesthesia is that in individuals with the condition, these neonatal pathways persist owing to inherited mechanisms. A recent study (Baron-Cohen et al., 1995) has provided evidence to support the notion that synesthesia might be an inherited trait. In that study, the pedigrees of seven families of probands suggested that the condition is transmitted as an autosomal dominant X chromosome linked condition (figure 21.1). We are testing this theory by extending the number of pedigrees tested and by taking blood for linkage analysis.

Support of the genetic theory begs the question of the mechanism by which such a biological inheritance has its effect. A candidate mechanism would be the expression of genes that regulate the migration and maturation of neurons within the developing brain. A second candidate mechanism is "neuronal pruning" (apoptosis). On this account, synesthesia can be explained best not by positive forces creating neural pathways that in nonsynesthetes do not exist but by maturational effects that lead to neonatal pathways being left active. This theory would be consistent with Maurer's observations regarding the mergence of modality-specific responses in 3-month-old human neonates.

The Cross-Modal Matching Theory

The cross-modal matching theory is based on evidence of cross-modal matching in normal subjects, in addition to those found by Lewkowicz & Turkewicz (1980). Do the presence of such abilities in normal subjects represent a *forme fruste* of the condition? Much of the work looking at cross-modal analogs of characteristics, such as brightness-loudness and the like, has been carried out by Marks (1982a,b, 1987) . The following review of whether mild synesthesia is found in "normal" subjects draws on both his work and that of Zellner & Kautz (1990).

Marks (1982a) showed that normal subjects exhibited remarkable consistency when asked to rate a selection of auditory-visual synesthetic metaphors using scaled ratings of loudness, pitch, and brightness. For example, *sunlight* was rated as louder than *glow*, which was in turn rated as louder than *moonlight*. A second study reported by Marks (1982b) required subjects to set the loudness of a 1000-Hz tone and the brightness of white light for 15 cases of visual-auditory metaphor taken from works of poetry. Again, marked consistency characterized the performance of these subjects, leading Marks to propose that intensity might be a common sensory dimension.

The Modularity Theory

For us to "know" that a percept is visual, auditory, olfactory, and so on, we must have a method of identifying information as being of one sensory kind or another. We may achieve this via a *modular* structure to sensation (Fodor, 1983). The modularity theory holds that whereas in nonsynesthetes audition and vision are functionally discrete, in individuals with synesthesia a breakdown in modularity has occurred (Baron-Cohen et al., 1993). The consequence of this, in the case of colored-hearing synesthesia, is that sounds have visual attributes. Testing the modularity theory is a challenge for future research.

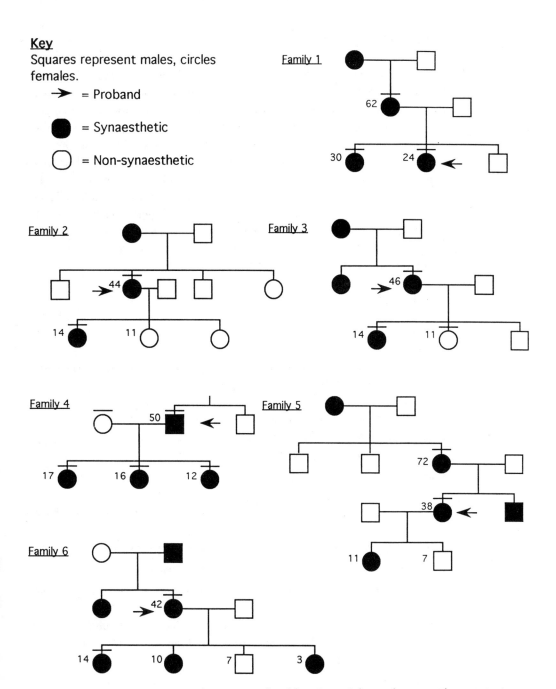

Figure 21.1   Six pedigrees. (Reproduced from Baron-Cohen et al., 1996, with permission.)

CONCLUSION

Investigations of colored-hearing synesthesia suggest that individuals with the condition are consistent in their descriptions of word-color correspondence, and these investigations report similar phenomenological accounts of the condition. Further, synesthetes appear to show different patterns of brain activation when listening to color-evoking sound stimuli. We posit the existence of unusual neural connections between auditory and visual areas to explain synesthetic experience, perhaps as the result of a failure of apoptosis. This theory seems to be a parsimonious explanation of the condition. Recent accounts of familiality of the condition suggest that genetic factors may sustain neonatal auditory-visual pathways. If this proves to be the case, studies of synesthesia may have the potential to inform us of the mechanisms of programmed cell death in the neonatal period.

REFERENCES

Aghajanian, G. K. (1981). In R. Hoffmeister & G. Stille (Eds.), *Handbook of Experimental Pharmacology, 55*(2), 89–110.

Baron-Cohen, S., Burt, L, Laittan-Smith, F., Harrison, J. E., & Bolton, P. (1995). Synaesthesia: Prevalence and familiarity. *Perception, 25*(9), 1073–1079.

Baron-Cohen, S., Harrison, J., Goldstein, L., & Wyke, M. (1993). Coloured speech perception: Is synaesthesia what happens when modularity breaks down? *Perception, 22,* 419–426.

Baron-Cohen S., Wyke M., & Binnie C. (1997). Hearing words and seeing colours: An experimental investigation of synaesthesia. *Perception, 16,* 761–767.

Calkins, M. W. (1893). A statistical study of pseudo-chromesthesia and of mental-forms. *American Journal of Psychology, 5,* 439–466.

Critchley, E. M. R. (1994). Synaesthesia. In *The neurological boundaries of reality.* London: Farrand Press.

Cytowic, R. E. (1989). *Synaesthesia: A union of the senses.* New York: Springer.

Cytowic, R. E. (1993). *The man who tasted shapes.* New York: Putnam.

Cytowic, R. E. & Wood, F. B. (1982). Synesthesia I: A review of major theories and their brain basis. *Brain and Cognition, 1,* 23–35.

Dehay, C., Bullier J., & Kennedy, H. (1984). Transient projections from the fronto-parietal and temporal cortex to areas 17, 18 and 19 in the kitten. *Experimental Brain Research, 57,* 208–212.

Fodor, J. (1984). *The modularity of mind.* MIT Press.

Galton, F. (1883). *Inquiries into human faculty and its development.* London: Dent & Sons.

Graziano, M. S. A., Yap, G. S., & Gross, C. G. (1994). Coding of visual space by premotor neurons. *Science, 266,* 1054–1057.

Halligan, P. W., Hunt, M., Marshall, J. C., & Wade, D. T. (1996). When seeing is feeling—acquired synaesthesia or phantom touch. *Neurocase, 2*(1), 21–29.

Honig, M. G., & Hume, R. I. (1989). DiI and diO—versatile fluorescent dyes for neuronal labeling and pathway tracing. *Trends in Neurosciences, 12*(9), 333.

Jacobs, L., Karpik, A., Bozian, D., & Gøthgen, S. (1981). Auditory-visual synesthesia: Sound induced photisms. *Archives of Neurology, 38,* 211–216.

Kennedy, H., Batardiere, A., Dehay, C., & Barone, P. (1996). In S. Baron-Cohen & J. Harrison (Eds.), *Synaesthesia: Classic & contemporary readings.* Oxford: Blackwell.

Kennedy, H., Bullier, J., & Dehay, C. (1989). Transient projection from the superior temporal sulcus to area 17 in the newborn macaque monkey. *Proceedings of the National Academy of Science of the United States of America, 86,* 8093–8097.

Krohn, W. O. (1893). Pseudo-chromesthesia, or the association of colors with words, letters and sounds. *American Journal of Psychology, 5,* 20–39.

Lewkowicz, D. J., & Turkewicz, G. (1980). Cross-modal equivalence in early infancy: Auditory-visual intensity matching. *Developmental Psychology, 16*(6), 597–607.

Marks, L. (1975). On colored-hearing synesthesia: Cross-modal translations of sensory dimensions. *Psychological Bulletin, 82*(3), 303–331.

Marks, L. E. (1982a). Bright sneezes and dark coughs, loud sunlight and soft moonlight. *Journal of Experimental Psychology Human Perception and Performance, 8*(2), 177–193.

Marks, L. E. (1982b). Synesthetic perception and poetic metaphor. *Journal of Experimental Psychology: Human Perception and Performance, 8*(1), 15–23.

Marks, L. E. (1987). On cross-modal similarity: Auditory-visual interactions in speeded discrimination. *Journal of Experimental Psychology, 13*(3), 384–394.

Maurer, D. (1993). Neonatal synaesthesia: Implications for the processing of speech and faces. In B. de Boysson-Bardies, S. de Schonen, P. Jusczyk, P. McNeilage & J. Morton (eds), *Developmental neurocognition: Speech and face processing in the first year of life.* Dordrecht: Kluwer.

Meltzoff, A. N., & Borton, R. W. (1979). Intermodal matching by human neonates. *Nature 282,* 403–404.

Motluk, A. (1994). The sweet smell of purple. *New Scientist, 143,* 32–37.

Neville, H. (1991). Neurobiology of cognitive and language processing: Effects of early experience. In K. Gibson & A. C. Peterson (Eds.), *Brain maturation and cognitive development: Comparative and cross-cultural perspectives* (pp. 355–380). New York: Aldine Gruyter.

Paulesu, E., Harrison, J., Baron-Cohen, S., Watson, J., Goldstein, L., Heather, J., Frackowiak, R. S. J., & Frith, C. D. (1995). The physiology of coloured hearing. *Brain, 118,* 661–676.

Ramachandran, V. S., & Rogers-Ramachandran, D. (1996). Synaesthesia in phantom limbs induced with mirrors. *Proceedings of the Royal Society of London Series B: Biological Sciences, 263,* 377–386.

Rang, H. P., & Dale, M. M. (1987). *Pharmacology.* Edinburgh: Churchill Livingstone.

Rizzo, M., & Eslinger, P. J. (1989). Colored hearing synaesthesia: An investigation of neural factors. *Neurology, 39,* 781–784.

Sadato, N., Pascual-Leone, A., Grafman, J., Ibanez, V., & Deiber M. P. (1996). Activation of the primary visual-cortex by braille reading in blind subjects. *Nature 380,* 526–528.

Starr, F. (1893). Note on color-hearing. *American Journal of Psychology, 51,* 416–418.

Vernon, P. E. (1930). Synaesthesia in music. *Psyche 10,* 22–40.

Zellner, D. A., & Kautz M. A. (1990). Color affects perceived odor intensity. *Journal of Experimental Psychology, 16*(2), 391–397

22 Congenital Hydrocephalus as a Model of Neurodevelopmental Disorder

Maureen Dennis, Marcia A. Barnes, and
C. Ross Hetherington

The relation between brain structure and cognitive function is central to understanding any neurodevelopmental disorder. To study structure-function relations in a particular disorder, however, a desirable approach is to have both a clear-cut set of structural features and a characteristic behavioral phenotype. Congenital hydrocephalus, the common factor in several neurodevelopmental disorders affecting the brain and ventricular system, offers the possibility of relating diagnostic structural anomalies to a reliable behavioral phenotype. In this chapter, we consider the unique perspective that hydrocephalus affords on the relation between congenital brain dysmorphologies and both elementary and higher-order cognitive functions in neurodevelopmental disorders.

STRUCTURE-FUNCTION RELATIONS

Hydrocephalus is a good model for understanding structure-function relations in neurodevelopmental disorders. Study of this disorder is useful because hydrocephalus meets a number of important criteria.

Definitive Brain Dysmorphologies

Congenital hydrocephalus is diagnosed on the basis of defining dysmorphologies rather than on the basis of a behavioral syndrome. The dysmorphologies primarily affect four main brain regions: the medial and lateral cerebellum, the midbrain and tectum, the corpus callosum, and the posterior cortex.

Early, Prenatal Onset

The prototypical dysmorphologies of congenital-onset (as opposed to infantile-onset) hydrocephalus occur at defined points in prenatal brain development and of themselves are not progressive. For example, spina bifida, a defect in closure of the neural tube associated with meningomyelocele and hydrocephalus, originates in gestational week 10. With conditions having precise onsets within a narrow time window during gestation, age at test effects provides information about the relation of cognitive development and dysmorphology that may be interpreted reliably.

Congruent Structure-Function Correlations

Many functional deficits of hydrocephalus are congruent with the known abnormalities of structure in this condition. This finding allows the establishment of structure-function relations based on established neuroanatomical models.

Specific Psychometric Profile

The profiles of psychometric deficits in congenital hydrocephalus show specific areas of strength and weakness.

Core Cognitive Deficits

Some cognitive deficits of hydrocephalus are robust across levels of cognitive development ranging from low to high (i.e., certain deficits are evident in both low- and high-ability children). These may be considered core cognitive deficits of hydrocephalus, and they are amenable to experimental decomposition. The cognitive processes impaired in hydrocephalus often cohere across modalities and functional domains, allowing the investigation of putative core deficits by means of standard cognitive experiments.

Functional Deficits Interpretable Through Models of Normal and Disordered Function

The application of cognitive models of normal function allows the deficits in hydrocephalus to be delineated more clearly in terms of component processes, in turn allowing the study of specific performance compromises with real-time tasks and decisions between different models of the nature of the cognitive deficit. Functional deficits in hydrocephalus can be compared with those of children who have no brain dysmorphism but show cognitive deficits parallel to those in hydrocephalus.

Taxonomic Agenda

Other neurodevelopmental disorders share both some of the behavioral deficits of hydrocephalus and some of its brain dysmorphism, similarities that ultimately should provide the basis of a taxonomy of neurodevelopmental disorders.

In this chapter, we consider the foregoing qualities in relation to the descriptive information about cognitive function in this population and also in relation to an established research program conducted with the participation of individuals with hydrocephalus. This program, based in linguistic and cognitive theory, has illuminated cognitive and linguistic issues central to the disorder and has validated theoretical constructs derived from research with normally developing individuals. The cognitive issues that have been explored include the assembly of meaning from context (a core deficit in hydrocephalus); how clinical observations about the cocktail party syndrome (CPS) relate to linguistic-pragmatic theory about textual and interpersonal rhetoric; and the development of algorithms for the study of brain dysmorphism—cognitive deficit correlations. The approach described is pertinent not only to hydrocephalus but to the emergence of a methodology for understanding other neurodevelopmental disorders.

DEFINITION

Hydrocephalus is the common feature in a set of neurodevelopmental disorders that affect early brain development through raised cerebrospinal fluid pressure and enlarged ventricles. It is a disturbance of pressure in the brain arising from an imbalance in the production and absorption of cerebrospinal fluid, causing dilated ventricles and a loss of brain volume. From a developmental perspective, hydrocephalus is important because it alters the microstructure of brain development and function in a number of ways. It impairs the maturation of neurons, it reduces the vascularization in the corpus callosum and white and periventricular gray matter, and it alters the tortuosity of the extracellular space, which in itself impairs neuronal function (Del Bigio, 1993).

DEFINITIVE BRAIN DYSMORPHOLOGIES

The taxonomy of hydrocephalus may be based on time of onset or neurological diagnostic procedures, with considerable overlap between the resulting classifications (Harwood-Nash & Fritz, 1976). Spina bifida meningomyelocele and aqueduct stenosis are congenital malformations, arising during the early months of gestation and affecting the structural formation of the brain. In contrast, intraventricular hemorrhage is a condition arising postnatally or in early infancy, sometimes leading to hydrocephalus. Hydrocephalus in the first year of life can result from congenital or postnatal (infantile) causes.

The most common cause of congenital hydrocephalus is spina bifida meningomyelocele, a neural tube defect (Chuang, 1986) leading to dysraphism of the spine that, when severe, can result in an outpouching of the meninges containing spinal cord through a gap in the vertebral column, known as a *meningomyelocele*. Hydrocephalus develops in some 90% of these severe cases (Brunt, 1984), usually resulting from a malformation of the brainstem and cerebellum termed the *Arnold-Chiari II deformation* of the hindbrain. This disorder involves significant cerebellar compromise, involving a reduction in the size of the cerebellar hemispheres, which are pushed down through the exits of the fourth ventricle, and, together with the vermis, are pushed up into the midbrain area (Menkes, 1995).

Hydrocephalus also may develop congenitally from aqueduct stenosis, a focal reduction in the cerebral aqueduct at the level of the colliculus, in the absence of the major cerebellar malformation frequently associated with hydrocephalus secondary to spina bifida (Barkovich, 1994). Aqueduct stenosis accounts for 20% of cases of congenital onset hydrocephalus (Menkes, 1995).

A less common cause of congenital hydrocephalus is the Dandy-Walker syndrome, a major malformation of the posterior fossa. The gross dysmorphology of the Dandy-Walker syndrome involves the triad of agenesis of the cerebellar vermis, associated posterior fossa cyst, and callosal agenesis.

Infantile hydrocephalus may be produced by various perinatal or postnatal events, with intraventricular hemorrhage secondary to prematurity and low birth weight being the most common cause (Fletcher & Levin, 1987). Intraventricular hemorrhage occurs in up to 50% of infants weighing less than 1500 gm at birth, with hydrocephalus developing in 50% of the survivors (Burstein et al., 1979). Enlargement of the lateral ventricles and hydrocephalus usually occurs in the more severe forms.

The main etiologies of hydrocephalus are associated with clear dysmorphologies of brain macrostructure. The defining brain dysmorphisms of hydrocephalus are obvious and consistently present, unlike the more elusive brain anomalies of conditions defined by behavioral deficits (autism, dyslexia, specific language impairment) or conditions in which the genotype is well defined but the ontogenetic consequences for brain morphology are not fully understood (e.g., Turner, Prader-Willi, Williams, and Down syndromes). To understand structure-function relations in hydrocephalus, we may begin with a focus on areas of principal dysmorphology, because these brain dysmorphologies are defining and characteristic of the various subgroups.

Early studies using postmortem material or older imaging techniques, such as air encephalograms and ventriculograms, identified cerebellar abnormalities in many forms of hydrocephalus and also in the selective thinning of the posterior cortex (Dennis et al., 1981). Newer imaging techniques applied to the brains of children with hydrocephalus have confirmed four principal dysmorphologies: the cerebellum and the corpus callosum (each of which may be agenetic or hypoplastic), the midbrain (abnormal in structure or position, and the posterior cortex (selectively thinner than the anterior cortical mantle). Of these, only the corpus callosum and posterior cortex have been studied quantitatively (Fletcher et al., 1995, 1996). Hydrocephalus thus produces a variety of dysmorphologies of the brain that are quite pronounced and that may involve primary developmental malformations or secondary hypoplasia of brain structures as a result of increased intracranial pressure.

Primary dysmorphologies occur in the corpus callosum, midbrain, and cortex as part of the basic formation of the brain. The cerebellum is also the site of primary dysmorphologies. The Dandy-Walker syndrome involves a primary hypoplasia of the cerebellar vermis associated with a variety of other malformations. Some 95% of children with spina bifida meningomyelocele develop the Arnold-Chiari malformation, which involves caudal herniation of the hindbrain and cerebellum into the upper cervical canal, thereby blocking exits to the fourth ventricle; reduced posterior fossa size; reduced cerebellar volume; effacement of the cerebellar cortex; reduction in all types of cerebellar neurons; small and gliotic cerebellar gyri; and asymmetry and dorsal flattening of the cerebellar hemispheres (Smith, 1974; Caviness, 1976; Harding, 1992; Bennett, 1993).

Secondary dysgenesis may result from abnormal pressures of adjacent structures, leading to a degree of hypoplasia. The midbrain is subject to abnormal pressures in hydrocephalus; for example, in the Arnold-Chiari condition, the tectum is pushed upward by the elevation of the cerebellar vermis, giving rise to the "beaked" tectum. Cortical thinning also is a likely secondary effect of hydrocephalus, and this thinning is selective, being particularly pronounced in the vertex and parietal regions.

For the most part, the brain dysmorphologies distinctive to hydrocephalus (e.g., cerebellar vermis dysgenesis) have been characterized qualitatively rather than quantitatively. A qualitative description of dysmorphology, though somewhat interesting, is not amenable to parametric study because the dysmorphologies have not been measured quantitatively.

Morphological differences in brains of children with neurodevelopmental disorders may involve volume, form, and geometrical topology: the spatial relation of a particular structure to the rest of the brain regardless of its volume or form. Magnetic resonance imaging—based volumetric analyses, including techniques for anatomical segmentation and cortical parcellation that permit calculations of volumes of subcortical structures and functionally defined cortical regions, recently were developed (Kennedy & Nelson, 1987; Kennedy et al., 1989; Caviness, et al., 1996). As well, recently developed morphometric techniques permit the visualization and biomathematical analysis of group morphological differences, expressed as differences between sets of unique, neuroanatomically meaningful geometrical points in magnetic resonance images (Bookstein, 1993). The dysmorphologies of hydrocephalus, then, are amenable to quantitative measure with respect to both global and regional morphometric analyses of brain volume and to measurement of the dysmorphology itself.

PRENATAL ONSET AND PROTRACTED DEVELOPMENTAL COURSE

One feature of congenital hydrocephalus that makes it a good model for neurodevelopmental disorders is that its dysmorphologies originate in prenatal brain development. For all etiologies of congenital hydrocephalus, time of onset is before birth, which allows for the evaluation of the developmental effects of other age and time variables, such as time since onset.

However, congenital hydrocephalus also allows comparisons to be made across etiologies, which is interesting in another way: Etiologies whose origins are separated by only a few gestational weeks may be associated with different patterns of brain dysmorphology through different mechanisms in neuroembryogenesis, and, thereby, likely with different long-term cognitive outcomes.

Hydrocephalus is consistent with a long life span and with a degree of stability in terms of medical conditions, leading to a relatively stable developmental course. In the absence of major treatment complications, therefore, testing neurocognitive function is possible in individuals with hydrocephalus over a protracted period, from infancy to adulthood.

The combination of a prenatal onset in development and the ability to look at neurobehavioral functions over an extended time span readers hydrocephalus a useful model for explicitly developmental questions in neurodevelopmental disorders. The study of individuals of different ages with a common history of early-onset hydrocephalus allows us to test lag versus deficit models of particular skills and allows us to test between alternate views of the developmental trajectory of a particular neurocognitive function.

CONGRUENT STRUCTURE-FUNCTION CORRELATIONS

The unique pathology of hydrocephalus is enormously interesting, and the study of structure-function relations in this condition is of recent origin. With respect to hydrocephalus, magnetic image–based structure–cognitive function relations have been reported for two brain regions. The cross-sectional area of the corpus callosum has been related to nonverbal IQ in children with hydrocephalus (Fletcher et al., 1992). With a larger sample (Fletcher et al., 1996), the corpus callosum again was found to be smaller in the hydrocephalus group, and corpus callosum volume was related to nonverbal cognitive skills and motor function. Selective posterior cortex thinning also has been studied. When hydrocephalus occurs, the ventricles expand along a posteroanterior direction, so that posterior regions of the brain may be more susceptible to damage because of this posteroanterior progression and of initial effects on cerebral white matter. Early studies that used air encephalograms found that global measures of intelligence were related to the thickness of the cortical mantle before and after treatment (Young et al., 1973). Using the same air encephalograms–ventriculogram technology, Dennis et al. (1981) examined regional patterns of cortical mantle thinning based on radiological review in a group of children with classic hydrocephalus etiologies.

Proportionately greater thinning of posterior brain regions relative to anterior brain regions was associated with lower nonverbal IQ scores; in contrast, children with proportionate anteroposterior thinning had comparable verbal and nonverbal IQ scores. Using quantitative measures from magnetic resonance images, Fletcher et al. (1996) confirmed this earlier finding:

When children with hydrocephalus were separated according to quantitative assessment of the distribution of cerebrospinal fluid percentages in anterior and posterior brain regions, those with proportionately greater amounts of cerebrospinal fluid in posterior relative to anterior brain regions had much lower nonverbal and motor skill performance.

Many dysmorphologies in hydrocephalus occur in brain regions with well-established elementary level functions in the adult brain. For example, lesions of the cerebellar hemispheres produce an ipsilateral limb ataxia. Until recently, core clinical functions of some of the brain regions that are dysmorphic in hydrocephalus have not been related to the relevant brain dysmorphology. Individuals with the Arnold-Chiari malformation of the hindbrain have significant cerebellar compromise involving a reduction in the size of the cerebellar hemispheres. Though many descriptions of clumsiness, poor handwriting, and poor motor skills are found in individuals with hydrocephalus and spina bifida, only recently have clear demonstrations shown that frank limb ataxia occurs in congenital hydrocephalus and that it is of greater magnitude in this condition than in children with hydrocephalus from infantile onset (Hetherington & Dennis, 1999). The combination of predictable dysmorphology in the principal etiologies of congenital hydrocephalus with the fact that the dysmorphic structures have fairly well-understood normal function suggests the possibility to propose structure-function relationships that are theoretically motivated and meaningful.

SPECIFIC PSYCHOMETRIC PROFILE

The effects of hydrocephalus on cognitive function long have been studied (see Wills, 1993; Dennis & Barnes, 1994; Fletcher et al., 1995), with intelligence being the most commonly studied outcome measure (see Fletcher & Levin, 1987; Donders et al., 1990; Wills, 1993 for recent reviews). Cognitive deficits in hydrocephalus tend to be relatively specific rather than cutting across all cognitive domains. Children with hydrocephalus have good grammar, vocabulary, and rote memory but a variety of deficits in nonverbal intelligence, coordinate movement, visual attention and orientation, and discourse. Patterns of preserved function in many areas with specific deficits in other domains is a useful property in the study of structure-function relations.

Intelligence

On the basis of IQ studies conducted over the last 20 years (Lonton, 1977; Jamison & Fee, 1978; Dennis et al., 1981; Shaffer et al., 1985; Donders et al., 1990; Wills et al., 1990; Fletcher et al., 1992), a pattern appears to hold over a variety of etiologies and treatments. Hydrocephalus is associated with IQ scores 1 to 2 standard deviations below the mean, with the greatest deficits occurring on the performance IQ scale (Dennis et al., 1981; Donders et al.,

1990; Wills et al., 1990; Fletcher et al., 1992; Riva et al., 1994). The disorder displays no consistent gender difference (Lonton, 1985) or handedness IQ difference.

Though hydrocephalus typically involves a compromise of intelligence, it is compatible with preserved IQ; in fact, the brain may be thinned significantly without concurrent IQ deficit (Lorber, 1980). However, specific neuropsychological deficits are common, regardless of the level of IQ.

Coordinate Movement

Motor deficits frequently are reported in children with hydrocephalus. The presence of motor impairment is not surprising in this population because hydrocephalus frequently involves brain regions implicated in motor control, such as the cerebellum and brainstem, the corpus callosum, periventricular white matter tracts (including the corticospinal tract), and the cerebral cortex. Despite the evident relation between functional outcome and structural brain dysmorphology in hydrocephalus, few studies have characterized the motor profile associated with this condition or have placed such a profile in the context of normal motor development.

Gross motor function studies in children with hydrocephalus often are restricted to the spina bifida etiology (Anderson & Plewis, 1977; Brunt, 1980, 1984; Laatsch et al., 1984). Lower-limb dysfunction is common in spina bifida because of the spinal lesion, and level of mobility has been used to relate degree of motor disability to general or specific cognitive skills, such as development of visuomotor ability or nonverbal IQ (Dennis et al., 1981; Ziviani et al., 1990). Gait abnormalities have been reported in almost all of a group of children with spina bifida and hydrocephalus (Fletcher et al., 1995), and gait abnormalities also occur, albeit less frequently, in other etiologies of hydrocephalus, both congenital and infantile. Motor strength, as a component of upper-limb motor function, is impaired in children with hydrocephalus (Tew, 1991).

Some effort has been directed toward characterizing the fine-motor skills of children with hydrocephalus, a concern arising from the requirements of handwriting, drawing, and other school-related skills. Regardless of gross motor status or strength, deficits in upper-limb and hand function, including fine-motor skills and psychomotor speed, commonly are reported. Children with spina bifida had abnormal upper-limb function (Wallace, 1973). Children with meningomyelocele with or without hydrocephalus scored lower than did normally developing children on tests of motor speed and dexterity (Grimm, 1976; Andersen & Plewis, 1977; Laatsch et al., 1984; Evans et al., 1985; Zeiner et al., 1985; Holler et al., 1995). Tests of hand function are performed poorly (Sand et al., 1973; Grimm, 1976; Shaffer et al., 1986; Mazur et al., 1988). Three-quarters of a large group of children with shunted hydrocephalus from mixed etiologies showed abnormalities in fine-motor coordination (Fletcher et al., 1995).

Motor deficits may be related to sensory and motor planning functions. Brunt (1980, 1984) has suggested an apraxic feature to the motor difficulties experienced by children with spina bifida meningomyelocele and hydrocephalus, characterized by difficulty in initiating movement to command and in executing sequential motor tasks. Praxic difficulties on sensory motor tasks were reported also in children with this condition (Land, 1977). Children with meningomyelocele approach fine-motor tasks in a deliberate or precise manner and frequently fail to develop continuous, flowing movements (Shaffer et al., 1986), which may reflect difficulty in motor automatization.

Recent research shows that core motor functions, not just complex visuomotor integration tasks, are impaired in hydrocephalus (Hetherington & Dennis, 1999). We administered age-normed motor tests (McCarron, 1976) to 42 children between the ages of 5 and 15, all of whom had conditions diagnosed as hydrocephalus, treatment with shunts during the first year of life, and no generalized intellectual impairment. Children with hydrocephalus had impairments in a broad range of motor functions: balance, coordination, and kinesthetic integration; fine-motor control and manual dexterity; persistence and smooth motor control; and motor strength. Mean performance was between 1 and 3 standard deviations below the mean for normally developing children in the standardization sample. In fact, on 9 of 10 subtests, the upper limit of 95% confidence intervals fell below 1 standard deviation of the mean for normally developing children.

Etiology and time of hydrocephalus onset are markers of a range of brain dysmorphologies and abnormal microstructure in brain regions important for motor development. Differences in motor profiles between etiological groups and in the functional role of specific brain dysmorphologies remain to be understood. Correlating motor function with magnetic resonance imaging–based morphometric analysis of the dysmorphic structures would increase understanding of the degree to which dysmorphism of relevant brain structures limits motor development.

Visuomotor Coordination

Visuomotor function involves a variety of skills, and they are impaired in children with hydrocephalus (Willoughby & Hoffman, 1979; Tew et al., 1980; Horn et al., 1985; Fletcher et al., 1995), especially those with brain infections, shunt revisions, and high lesions (Tew et al., 1980), but not low IQ (Lollar, 1990). Children with hydrocephalus have poor handwriting (Anderson, 1975; Pearson et al., 1988; Ziviani et al., 1990), with reduced writing speed and legibility (Anderson, 1975; Ziviani et al., 1990). In a group of children with spina bifida (most with hydrocephalus), freehand drawing skill was impaired (Sandler et al., 1993).

One of two factors important for spatial function has been termed *visualization*, and it is related to tasks involving the mental transformation of visual images (McGee, 1979). The second important spatial factor is *orientation*, involved in such tasks as field dependence–field independence, map reading, and sense of direction (McGee, 1979). Visualization and orientation are consistent areas of deficit for children with spina bifida and hydrocephalus (Miller & Sethi, 1971a,b; Sand et al., 1973; Land, 1977; Soare & Raimondi, 1977; Simms, 1987; Wills et al., 1990; Friedrich et al., 1991; Sandler et al., 1993). Spina bifida children with shunt infections have visuomotor problems (McLone et al., 1982) and visuospatial problems (Miller & Sethi, 1971a,b; Anderson & Spain, 1977; Willoughby & Hoffman, 1979; Culatta & Egolf, 1980; but see Shaffer et al., 1986). Drawing skill is impaired (Sandler et al., 1993). Explanations for visuospatial deficits include a primary motor deficit that compromises performance on nonverbal speeded IQ tests (Shaffer et al., 1986; Thompson et al., 1991; Wills, 1993); ocular deficits including oculomotor and acuity deficits (Dennis et al., 1981; Zeiner et al., 1985; Donders et al., 1990) that interfere with visuospatial tasks; impairments in white-matter association tracts (Wills et al., 1990), and posterior cortex thinning (Dennis et al., 1981; Fletcher et al., 1996). Children with hydrocephalus have deficits in spatial cognition even on tasks with minimized motor demands (Fletcher et al., 1995).

Visual Attention and Orientation

Visual attention and orientation are also areas of deficit for children with hydrocephalus; they have difficulty with tasks involving visual attention, visual analysis, and judgment of orientation (Willoughby & Hoffman, 1979; Tew et al., 1980; Horn et al., 1985; Fletcher et al., 1995). Performance on attentional measures varies with brain infection, shunt revisions, and high lesions (Tew et al., 1980), but not with IQ (Lollar, 1990).

Recently (1997), the authors studied the question of central attentional mechanisms using age-referenced tests of vigilance and distractibility (Gordon, 1988) in children with hydrocephalus arising from two classic etiologies associated with beaking of the tectum and midbrain eye syndromes (i.e., spina bifida and aqueduct stenosis). Children with hydrocephalus were less accurate than were age norms at visual target detection, even though their detection speed was comparable to age norms. Under conditions of distraction, both accuracy and detection speed were lower than were age norms in the hydrocephalus group. When the no-distraction and distraction conditions were compared within subjects, response latency (but not accuracy) was different. Children with hydrocephalus have poor visual attention accuracy, even under conditions barring distraction and on a task with minimal motor requirements.

Text-Level Language and Discourse

Hydrocephalus long has been associated with content-poor but fluent language. The term *cocktail party syndrome* (CPS) originally was used to describe a pattern of fluent speech and language that, while fluent, was characterized by verbal perseveration, excessive use of stereotyped social utterances, irrelevant verbosity, and overfamiliar manner (e.g., Hadenius et al., 1962). Language facilitated social contact rather than conveying meaning (Taylor, 1961).

Studies from our laboratory have shown that children with hydrocephalus have many adequately developed oral language skills (Dennis et al., 1987) and written language skills (Barnes & Dennis, 1992), including unimpaired access to the oral lexicon through visual (picture) and phonological (rhyme) routes (Dennis et al., 1987); rapid access to names for colors, pictures, and letters (Dennis et al., 1987); and good grammar (Dennis et al., 1987). Nevertheless, they have oral discourse impairments and content-poor oral language. The narratives of children with hydrocephalus are verbose, imprecise, and lacking in core semantic content (Dennis et al., 1994). These children fail to make inferences, to understand ambiguous sentences, and to comprehend idioms as well as do peers (Dennis & Barnes, 1993). Language impairment in hydrocephalus is of a specific rather than a global nature.

CORE COGNITIVE DEFICITS

Deficits Across Levels of Intellectual Function

In approaching neurodevelopmental disorders, one strategy has been to study individuals with severe forms of retardation and to search for islands of preserved function (e.g., Williams syndrome). The congenital etiologies associated with hydrocephalus, however, are consonant with a range of intelligence levels. This means that deficits that are found only at the lower end of the IQ distribution can be separated from those that are found across the condition regardless of intellectual level.

The methodology we have adopted involves examining cognitive deficits in nonretarded but diverse IQ groups of children with hydrocephalus including a subgroup of these children who have average or above-average IQs. The reasoning is that cognitive deficits found to vary with intelligence are likely to share common processing resources or mechanisms with very general cognitive skills and, hence, are poor candidates for a core deficit. In contrast, cognitive deficits that persist in a neurodevelopmental disorder into that segment of the sample with the highest levels of intelligence are likely part of the core deficits of the condition. Intact general cognitive abilities are not enough to compensate for a specific deficit.

Across a number of studies, we have shown that discourse difficulties of children with hydrocephalus cannot be explained by low levels of verbal intelligence. Further, the component skills of nonverbal IQ scales do not overlap with those that contribute to deficient discourse in these children. Discourse skills that are disrupted in hydrocephalus are only modestly related to verbal IQ, and all are unrelated to performance IQ (Dennis et al., 1987;

Barnes & Dennis, 1992; Dennis & Barnes, 1993; Dennis et al., 1994). What interested us, however, was whether the same patterns of discourse strengths and deficits found in children with hydrocephalus across a broad IQ spectrum also existed for those children at average and above-average cognitive levels.

In terms of written language in children with hydrocephalus, both groups with average or higher verbal IQs and groups unselected for IQ show poor comprehension of text despite adequate word-level skills. That is, the children with average verbal IQ are proficient at reading words and using phonological skills to decode nonsense words, such as "frip." Their written vocabulary knowledge is also as good as that of normally developing children of the same age, in contrast to children with lower IQ. For children with average or higher IQ, however, competence in all these written language skills still resulted in poorer understanding of texts in comparison to controls and in a reading comprehension level that was lower than expected on the basis of adequate word recognition and vocabulary (Barnes & Dennis, 1992).

Impaired comprehension for oral language also is evident. A higher level of general verbal function brings some advantage for understanding certain aspects of discourse but not for others. Children with hydrocephalus of average or higher IQ, for example, understand some aspects of figurative language as well as do normally developing controls (Dennis & Barnes, 1993); unlike lower-IQ children with hydrocephalus, these children demonstrate no impairment in understanding idiomatic expressions, such as "It's all water under the bridge." Like peers with lower IQ, however, they have difficulty with inferencing (Dennis & Barnes, 1993; Barnes & Dennis, 1996; Barnes & Dennis, 1998), which is an important component of oral and written language comprehension (Kintsch, 1994; Oakhill & Garnham, 1988).

Previous studies, in short, have shown that children with hydrocephalus, regardless of their cognitive level, have discourse-related deficits that include poor reading comprehension and poor inferencing skills. Deficits in vocabulary and idiom comprehension, in contrast, consistently are seen in groups that include the lower (but nonretarded) end of the IQ range but are not seen in children of average or higher verbal intelligence.

Skills that are *not* categorically impaired in hydrocephalus—those that are intact in children with average or higher IQ—appear to be those that rely relatively little (or not at all) on particular discourse contexts for their computation (Barnes & Dennis, 1998). For example, word recognition and phonological analysis skills are considered to operate independent of context (e.g., "It's all water under the bridge" has the same figurative meaning, regardless of context). Once basic decoding skills have been acquired and automatized, context does not influence word recognition processes (reviewed in Adams, 1990). The meanings of single words and idioms also can be derived without respect to context. The figurative expressions we studied use stale metaphors or idioms. How different types of idiomatic expressions are understood is a matter of some debate (Cacciari & Tabossi, 1993), although what is known is that the meaning of many idiomatic expressions sometimes may be understood at least as quickly as their literal meaning (Gibbs, 1980). This finding suggests that some idioms might be represented directly in semantic or lexical memory, so that access to their meanings is relatively independent of the discourse context in which they occur (Swinney & Cutler, 1979).

The discourse skills that *are* impaired in hydrocephalus across the IQ range studied are those that must be computed from a particular discourse context. These are skills, such as making inferences and understanding written and oral texts, and nonidiomatic figurative language, such as novel metaphors or similes (Barnes & Dennis, 1996; Barnes & Dennis, 1998). Word meanings stored in semantic memory facilitate comprehension of individual words and phrases in a text; however, the meaning of a text as a whole must be constructed both by linking propositions within the text and also by integrating general information about the world with the propositions in the text. In the former case, the various propositions must be connected meaningfully to one another to form a semantic representation referred to as a *text base* (Kintsch & van Dijk, 1978). In the latter case, the listener or reader goes beyond the propositions given by constructing a representation of the real-world situation described by the text (Johnson-Laird, 1983).

The advantage of the average-IQ children with hydrocephalus concerns the ability to retrieve meaning directly from semantic memory but not the ability to compute meaning from context, which may involve the integration of propositions within a text or the integration of general knowledge with explicit text. How children with hydrocephalus understand idioms and metaphors is particularly interesting in this context. When meaning (of words, phrases, idioms) can be accessed directly from semantic memory, children with hydrocephalus and average intelligence are not disadvantaged, compared to their age peers. They process common, idiomatic, figurative expressions in which figurative meaning, when accessed, is relatively context-free; in contrast, they have more difficulty in interpreting similes when the context establishes meaning. The "anger" meaning of "My mother saw red," for example, is true outside a discourse context or within any discourse context, whereas the precise meaning of "He was like a boxer who had lost a fight" is established through a specific story context in which, for example, reference is made to the scrapes and bruises the character sustained in falling on the ice as opposed to his feeling down-hearted, defeated, or angry. In effect, "My mother saw red" is figuratively true anywhere; "He was like a boxer who had lost a fight" is true with reference to the particular discourse context established within the story.

To summarize the studies of the higher IQ spectrum in congenital hydrocephalus, the discourse deficits that disappear or are attenuated as IQ increases involve the understanding of vocabulary, idioms, and the understanding and production of syntax (Dennis et al., 1987; Dennis & Barnes, 1993). The discourse deficits that persist in the higher-IQ spectrum in hydrocephalus involve inferencing and understanding novel figurative expressions (Barnes & Dennis, 1998).

Inability fully to compute meaning from context may be considered to be a core deficit for several reasons. The deficit is relatively independent of intelligence (i.e., it is demonstrable even in individuals with average to superior IQ). Also, it is a deficit specific to discourse contexts in that it cannot be explained by limitations in other language skills, such as a restricted vocabulary, that might in their own right produce deficits in discourse. Further, it is specific to derivation of a particular form of meaning; it is apparent when meaning must be constructed from the discourse context but is not categorically associated with the derivation of meaning because context-independent meanings are well understood by average-IQ children with hydrocephalus (Barnes & Dennis, 1996).

Experimental Decomposition

In the past, the balance of studies of hydrocephalus reported mainly psychometric data that were not related easily to brain structure. With newer linguistic and cognitive approaches to defining cognitive function, domain-specific and condition-specific deficits that have emerged may be studied with the conventional methodology of cognitive and developmental psychology in which complex tasks are decomposed into a set of component skills. The value of studying cognitive impairments in neurodevelopmental disorders experimentally is that it allows one to investigate the core cognitive deficits underlying more complex cognitive skills. In turn, these core deficits may be related more easily to brain structure than is performance on psychometric tests that tap several skills at once. Later, we discuss in hydrocephalic children an experimental decomposition of one of the deficits that holds across the IQ range.

Inferencing is an important part of discourse comprehension (Oakhill & Garnham, 1988; Kintsch, 1994), but it is not a unitary function. Different types of inferences exist, and not all might be related equally to text comprehension. In addition, the failure to integrate different sources of information within and without a text to make an inference may be due to all or one of several factors, including a lack of world knowledge (Kintsch, 1994), problems in holding the information necessary to make an inference in working memory (Oakhill, 1993), or problems in the reasoning needed to make some types of inferences (Das Gupta & Bryant, 1989). Understanding more about inferencing deficits in children with hydrocephalus necessitated analyzing more specifically some of these components of inferencing.

General world and domain-specific knowledge is important for successful inferencing. Logically, these kinds of knowledge are a precondition for some types of inferences in the sense that they form part of the information needed to make the appropriate inference. The typical advantage in inferencing for children with higher versus lower IQ can be reversed when the domain knowledge of the lower-IQ children is more comprehensive than that of the higher-IQ children. For example, lower-IQ children knowledgeable about soccer make more inferences when listening to soccer stories than do higher-IQ children with less soccer knowledge (Yekovich et al., 1990). Given the influence of the knowledge base in skilled performance (see Chi, 1978), including inferencing, a deficient or circumscribed knowledge base may contribute to poor inferencing in children with comprehension problems.

Children with hydrocephalus might lack the knowledge needed to make some inferences. For example, physical disabilities in some cases may restrict their experiences (and hence their knowledge base) of particular situations and event sequences that involve activities, such as riding on a bus or hiking. Thus, distinguishing inferencing difficulties is important in children with hydrocephalus and in other groups of poor comprehenders from limitations in a deficient knowledge base from which inferences are to be made. To do this, we devised a novel method to study inferencing within a controlled knowledge base involving a make-believe world called *Gan*, the features of which the children learned through words and pictures (e.g., "The shoes on Gan have wings"). The children were required to make inferences by listening to a story in which inferences were to be made using the newly learned knowledge base. Inferencing was conditional on knowledge base items that were recalled over the period in which inferences were to be made. Coherence inferences and elaborative inferences, each of which has a different function in text comprehension were tested (Casteel, 1993; Barnes et al., 1996).

A particular class of inference—knowledge-based inferences—link elements in a text with general or world knowledge. Within knowledge-based inferences, different types of inferences serve different discourse functions. Specifically, coherence inferences and elaborative inferences have different functions in text comprehension (Casteel, 1993; Barnes et al., 1996).

Coherence inferences (Barnes et al., 1996) maintain a coherent story line by adding unstated but important information to explicit text. They form a causal link between knowledge and text, which helps to infer *why* an event occurred, and they would be considered obligatory for comprehension. For example, on hearing that a family ate lunch at home after starting out for a picnic in their car, an inference about the car's implied condition or a sudden change in the weather is important for understanding the events in the story.

Elaborative inferences, although not necessary for narrative coherence, serve to elaborate on story content and strengthen memory for stories. By rendering concepts more concrete, elaborative inferences also may facilitate the integration of subsequent propositions within a text even though they are not central to textual cohesion (Whitney et al., 1991). Elaborative inferences specify a fuller description to help infer *what* an event is like and contribute to the building of a richer mental model of the situation (Johnson-Laird, 1983). For example, on hearing "It was a gorgeous sunny day," an inference about the color of the sky might be made, though this is not essential for comprehension.

Inferences that maintain coherence are made more frequently by both children and adults than are those that elaborate story content (Keenan et al., 1984; Duffy, 1986; Garrod et al., 1990; McKoon & Ratcliff, 1990, 1992; Casteel, 1993; Barnes et al., 1996; review in Whitney, 1987). Elaborative inferences, however, are more frequent when the comprehender has rich, highly accessible knowledge of the physical setting of the story (Morrow et al., 1990; see Singer et al., 1994 for a more general discussion of the factors guiding inference processes).

Elaborative and coherence inferencing was investigated in children who had hydrocephalus and average or higher intelligence and in two groups of children without known brain dysmorphism: One group contained normally developing average readers, the other was composed of children who were poor readers with respect to both decoding and comprehension. This latter group is interesting, because inferencing deficits are characteristic not only of children with hydrocephalus but of some proportion of children who do not have frank brain injury but are poor comprehenders (Oakhill, 1993).

The controlled knowledge base was taught to all children, and the only inferences required were those that drew on this newly acquired knowledge base. By exploring how children with hydrocephalus access information from an available knowledge base to make different types of inferences, and by contrasting this with inferencing in normally developing readers and poor readers without frank brain injury, we hoped to delineate the deficient underlying processes that cause inferencing failure in each group. Data of this kind also bear on another issue: whether the origins of inferencing deficits in children with hydrocephalus are the same as those in children without known brain anomalies (discussed later).

The inferencing decomposition study showed that the hydrocephalus group had more difficulty in learning the new knowledge base and had more difficulty in remembering that knowledge over the course of the story, meaning that (in absolute terms) they made fewer inferences because they could not retrieve necessary information from their knowledge base. However, even when inferencing was made conditional on available or recalled knowledge, the children with hydrocephalus made fewer coherence and elaborative inferences. Children with hydrocephalus also were less successful in recalling the literal aspects of the story.

All groups made more coherence inferences than elaborative inferences, suggesting some knowledge of the importance of maintaining coherence in stories. Poor readers, however, made significantly fewer coherence inferences than did average readers, and they also made fewer elaborative inferences when inferencing was conditionalized on having recalled the pertinent knowledge base information (Barnes & Dennis, 1996). Unlike children with hydrocephalus, however, these poor readers remembered the knowledge base as well as did average readers, and they were as accurate as average readers in answering questions about literal story content. The inferencing failures of both poor and average readers were due to failure to integrate recalled premise information (the proposition from the text important for making the inference) and knowledge base information; the poor readers simply made more of these errors than did the average readers (Barnes & Dennis, 1996).

In summary, both children with hydrocephalus and poor comprehenders without brain anomalies (whether good or poor at decoding) have difficulty in making inferences. These groups also differ in several important ways. For the most part, children with hydrocephalus had difficulty in making inferences because they failed to access either pertinent text-based or knowledge-based information, in agreement with their problems in retrieving literal text content. For children with hydrocephalus, then, inferencing difficulties seem related to problems in rapidly accessing information from memory during comprehension. Poor comprehenders without frank brain injury, on the other hand, quickly can access the information needed to make an inference but cannot integrate text with knowledge-based information. As Oakhill (1993) has suggested, these integration difficulties in poor comprehenders may reflect limits in working memory to the extent that such integration relies on concurrent storage and processing capabilities.

FUNCTIONAL DEFICITS INTERPRETABLE THROUGH MODELS OF NORMAL AND ABNORMAL FUNCTION

A claim that we made earlier in support of hydrocephalus as a model for neurodevelopmental disorders concerns the possibility of assembling large cohorts of individuals with normal levels of intelligence, which would render possible the performance of standard cognitive psychology experiments in this population. This methodology leads to the identification of core cognitive deficits of the condition (as discussed). Identified deficits then can be conceptualized within models of normal cognitive function. We investigated the core deficit in reading comprehension using cognitive models of the normal reading comprehension process.

Two paths lead to the meaning of discourse or text. One concerns the *construction of the semantic meaning of the text*, termed the *representation of the text-base* in propositions that carry the meaning of the text. The other is a representation of the text that the listener constructs, which goes beyond what is given in the text and represents the real-world situation described by the text (Johnson-Laird, 1983). These *situation models* are thought to represent story events in the following dimensions: time, space, protagonist, causality, and intentionality (Zwaan et al., 1995). Comprehension failure could occur because an inadequate mental model of the situation described by the text was constructed (i.e., a model that facilitates knowledge-based inferences). Comprehension problems may arise from a failure to represent text-based information or, alternatively, from a failure to create a situation model described by the text (a component of which is the type of knowledge-based inference already discussed). We investigated whether the comprehension difficulties of children with hydrocephalus involve one or both sources of comprehension failure.

On the basis of models of the reading comprehension process, we proposed that very early in the comprehension process, words that are read activate a pool of relevant information from semantic memory. Shortly after, irrelevant information is suppressed, so that only contextually-relevant information is used for comprehension. At the same time, the reader must use the context rapidly to select, enhance, or keep mnemonically active the contextually relevant information (Gernsbacher & Faust, 1991). Also, comprehension of new text sometimes requires the reader to make an inference using previously read text. Such inferences are called *text-based inferences*, because the information needed to make the inference is contained in the propositions given in the text. These activation, suppression, contextual selection, and text-based inferencing processes were tested in children with hydrocephalus and in age-matched controls. Recently, we investigated on-line reading comprehension processes that may be used to construct a text-based representation (Barnes & Dennis, unpublished data).

Children with hydrocephalus initially activated information from semantic memory during reading as well as did controls, and they were as fast as controls at suppressing irrelevant semantic information; they could also make text-based inferences as well as did controls when the two critical propositions in the text were separated by one or four sentences. However, children with hydrocephalus were less efficient than were controls in using context rapidly to select the appropriate meaning of words and sentences.

In reading, children with hydrocephalus have comprehension deficits because they have more difficulty than their peers in making rapid use of context to derive meaning, not because they fail to activate information from semantic memory, nor because they fail to suppress irrelevant information. This difficulty likely results in the formation of an inadequate semantic representation of the text. An incomplete representation of the text means that the text was not understood as well as it might have been *during* reading. Incomplete or inadequate text representations also may affect comprehension in another way. Children's understanding of what they have read often requires them to reflect on the text, and such textual comprehension after reading involves constructive processing. When the representation of the text is semantically incomplete or inadequate, constructive processing on that representation also will suffer. Some converging evidence for this hypothesis comes from our studies of story reproduction in children with hydrocephalus. They retell stories that are as long as those of their age peers but contain less of the story's core semantic content (Dennis et al., 1994).

To summarize the results, children with hydrocephalus performed as efficiently as did controls with respect to activation and suppression processes in on-line text comprehension. Contextual enhancement differences emerged between the groups: Children with hydrocephalus were generally slower than were controls to use context, and the facilitative effect of a biasing context was not as large for children with hydrocephalus as for controls. The effects are not at a single-word level (because fluency of single-word naming in these children was similar to that in controls) but rather the effect is based on the rapid use of context to specify meaning as it emerges on line.

In integrating data from the text-based comprehension studies and from the inferencing studies already discussed, apparently children with hydrocephalus are likely to have problems with rapidly assembling meaning from context, in assembling and integrating either new or old information relevant to an unfolding context. Thus, they will be unable to perform language functions requiring the use of knowledge to make inferences, the establishment of mental models, and the integrative use of context during oral and written comprehension (Barnes & Dennis, 1996; Barnes & Dennis, 1998). The broader entailment of this body of data is that children with hydrocephalus will be successful at routine operations that serve the acquisition of knowledge but somehow will lack the processing redundancy or capacity successfully to integrate partial information that unfolds over time or within a temporal structure (Jones & Boltz, 1989) or information from diverse sources.

Generally, we have been able to demonstrate that model-driven testing of the status of the components of reading comprehension can discriminate between intact and deficient processes in the neurodevelopmental condition hydrocephalus. Investigation of cognitive deficits in hydrocephalus can be well served by decomposing those deficits using models of normal cognitive function and cognitive tasks developed to test explicitly the hypothesized components of the model. Nonetheless, much remains to be found out about discourse and reading comprehension deficits in children with hydrocephalus. For example, why do these children have difficulty in bringing general knowledge to bear to make an inference? Which aspects of building a situation model of what they hear or see are deficient, and which are intact?

If models of normal function are useful for testing hypotheses about disordered function, abnormal function can inform models of normal function. A central tenet of cognitive neuropsychology is that the way in which a skill decomposes under conditions of brain damage is revealing of the normal functional architecture for that skill. If a skill, such as inferencing, decomposes differently in poor comprehenders depending on the presence or absence of a history of early brain pathology, a logical consideration is that early lesions impose changes on neural development that alter the normal relations among developing skills. In the context of development, this conclusion highlights the importance of comparing basic cognitive processes in populations who show the same defective cognitive outcome on measures of more global skills.

Data exploring the specificity of deficits of hydrocephalus are important because they test assumptions about brain-damage dissolution as a direct link to normal function. On the basis of findings from lesion studies with adults and children, hypotheses have been put forth about possible brain dysfunction in children who exhibit aberrant behavioral typologies and do not have demonstrable brain damage (Rourke et al., 1983; Barkley et al., 1992). A closer look at the cognitive processes underlying superficially similar disabilities in children with and without frank brain damage sometimes may reveal that different core deficits underlie similar behavioral outcomes. The processes that produce good decoding coupled with poor comprehension in the child with hydrocephalus, for example, do not appear to be the same as those that produce this pattern in children without demonstrable brain damage. This suggests that brain-behavior inferences need to incorporate what is known about similarities and differences in the core processing deficits of children with and without known neuropathology, in addition to data provided by brain imaging in well-defined groups of children with similar core processing deficits; for similar models in dyslexia research, see the review in Hynd & Semrud-Clikeman (1989). The quality of data about brain-behavior relations, importantly, depends on the clarity of the behavioral data.

THEORETICALLY GROUNDED ANALYSES

Neurodevelopmental conditions often have clinical symptoms associated with them. For hydrocephalus, a long-standing observed clinical deficit has been termed *cocktail party speech*. Studies that have sought to document the prevalence of CPS and understand it by relating CPS symptoms to psychometric and neuropsychological measures largely have been unsuccessful. We have taken a different approach to this problem by studying the social-pragmatic language of children with hydrocephalus by means of linguistic analyses. The results have provided not just a fuller description of the linguistic deficit but a more theoretically grounded understanding of the long-observed clinical deficit in the oral discourse of children with hydrocephalus. The following example illustrates the set of steps that has related clinical observations regarding the CPS in hydrocephalus to a linguistic distinction between textual and interpersonal rhetoric.

In the studies described, cognitive and linguistic theories were used as tools to help to derive a better understanding of cognitive function in hydrocephalus. In turn, data from these studies may be used to refine cognitive and linguistic models. The particular properties of hydrocephalus allow one to take a clinical observation, define it through psychological tests, and cast it within the framework of a theoretical issue in cognitive science. In this manner, the linguistic framework provides an interpretative heuristic for the data from individuals with hydrocephalus, which data, in turn, functionally validate the linguistic theory. An example of this may be seen in the studies of narrative discourse in children with hydrocephalus.

As hydrocephalus long has been associated with content-poor but fluent language, our recent language studies have supported one aspect of the original clinical observation of language development after early-onset hydrocephalus: Children with hydrocephalus produce fluent language that is a good vehicle for social contact but a poor means of conveying the meaning of a text (Taylor, 1961).

A distinct pattern of preserved and impaired language function has emerged. Children with hydrocephalus produce single words in isolation better than they use the same words in context, and they are slower than are age peers to produce content words appropriate to semantic contextual cues, even though they are as successful as age peers at producing the same words in referential naming tasks (Dennis et al., 1987). Children with hydrocephalus have relatively preserved interpersonal rhetoric. In narratives and conversations they take an appropriate number of turns and are avid participants in conversational dyads; however, they communicate with considerable redundancy. In narrative discourse tasks, they relate fluent, fairly well-structured stories that nevertheless fail to capture important aspects of the discourse content; their narratives are verbose and content-poor (Dennis et al., 1994). Thus, children with hydrocephalus fail to produce and understand much core semantic content, particularly when semantic content is communicated by an appreciation of contextual information.

Earlier, we argued that children with hydrocephalus are well able to understand aspects of discourse that may be interpreted free of context, such as the meaning of words, idioms, and so forth, and can be accessed directly from semantic memory. The preservation of a certain number of directly accessed meanings in a subset of higher-IQ children with hydrocephalus has important implications for discourse function, not only in this subset but in the broader sample of children with hydrocephalus. Even at lower levels of language skill, children who probably have a less complete lexicon than do controls may rely largely on direct-access mechanism for discourse.

To the extent that discourse in children with hydrocephalus is composed largely of directly accessed meanings (as opposed to constructed meanings), their conversations and narratives should sound stereotyped to the listener. In fact, an abundance of stereotyped phrases was noted as a characteristic feature of the original descriptions of CPS in this population. What has been noted, for example, is that children with hydrocephalus exchange verbal patterns instead of conversing (Taylor, 1961; Tew & Laurence, 1979). Children with hydrocephalus often are described as sociable, and this sociability contributes to the enthusiasm with which they engage in conversations or storytelling. They obey many of the social conventions of discourse; in conversations, for example, they take as many turns (Murdoch et al., 1990), or even more turns (Swisher & Pinsker, 1971) as do controls.

Elements of discourse concerned with turn taking and gaining the interest of the audience are important for discourse but are far from sufficient. A narrative or conversation is successful to the extent that it balances the old or stereotyped elements with new story or conversational content. The imbalance of the hydrocephalic children arises because they convey stereotyped elements more successfully than core semantic content.

The particular pattern of intact and deficient narrative discourse skills produced by early-onset hydrocephalus has implications for theories of discourse (Leech, 1983) that distinguish between interpersonal rhetoric (including such principles as cooperation, turn taking, politeness, and irony, that are based on social conventions) and textual rhetoric (involving clarity of discourse meaning, the economy with which discourse is delivered, and the expressivity of discourse, which includes the full elaboration of literal, figurative, and inferential meaning). Early-onset hydrocephalus appears to produce a dissociation between interpersonal rhetoric, which at least in some ways is proficient, and textual rhetoric, which in many ways is impaired (Dennis et al., 1994).

TAXONOMIC AGENDA: CONNECTIONS WITH OTHER NEURODEVELOPMENTAL DISORDERS

Other neurodevelopmental disorders share some of the behavioral deficits of hydrocephalus and some of its brain dysmorphisms. At a behavioral level, the sociability, conversational responsiveness, and affective prosody characteristic of children with hydrocephalus also has been described in other special populations (i.e., children with Williams syndrome). The functional effect of these behaviors is to engage the attention of the listener during conversations and narratives, so perhaps direct access to meanings in semantic or lexical memory is a part of the mechanism underlying this pragmatic strategy in both conditions. At the level of brain dysmorphology, the cerebellar vermis abnormalities described in some children with autism are the defining dysmorphology of the Dandy-Walker syndrome, although, because the latter condition is rare, pragmatic language has not been studied in any detail in individuals with this condition. As they become better understood, the distinctive profiles of cognitive dysfunction and brain dysmorphology in congenital hydrocephalus conditions should provide important input into a rational taxonomy of neurodevelopmental disorders.

ACKNOWLEDGMENT

This research was supported by project grants to Maureen Dennis and Marcia A. Barnes from the Ontario Mental Health Foundation and by a project grant to Ross Hetherington and Maureen Dennis from the Spina Bifida Association of Canada. We thank the Hamilton-Wentworth Roman Catholic Separate School Board for its participation in the studies involving control groups.

REFERENCES

Adams, M. J. (1990). *Beginning to read: Thinking and learning about print*. Cambridge, MA: MIT Press.

Anderson, E. (1975). Cognitive deficits in children with spina bifida and hydrocephalus: A review of the literature. *British Journal of Educational Psychology, 45,* 257–268.

Anderson, E. M., & Plewis, I. (1977). Impairment of motor skill in children with spina bifida cystica and hydrocephalus: An exploratory study. *British Journal of Psychology, 68,* 61–70.

Barkley, R. A., Grodzinsky, G., & DuPaul, G. J. (1992). Frontal lobe functions in attention deficit disorders with and without hyperactivity: A review and research report. *Journal of Abnormal Child Psychology, 20,* 163–188.

Barkovich, A. J. (1994). Congenital malformations of the brain and skull. In A. J. Barkovich (Ed.), *Pediatric neuroimaging* (2nd ed.). New York: Raven.

Barnes, M. A., & Dennis, M. (1992). Reading in children and adolescents after early onset hydrocephalus and in normally developing age peers: Phonological analysis, word recognition, word comprehension, and passage comprehension skills. *Journal of Pediatric Psychology, 17,* 445–465.

Barnes, M. A., & Dennis, M. (1996). Reading comprehension deficits arise from diverse sources: Evidence from readers with and without developmental brain pathology. In C. Cornoldi & J. Oakhill (Eds.), *Reading comprehension difficulties: Processes & interventionz* (pp. 251–278). Hillsdale, NJ: Erlbaum.

Barnes, M. A., & Dennis, M. (1998). Discourse after early-onset hydrocephalus: Core deficits in children of average intelligence. *Brain and Language, 61,* 309–334.

Barnes, M. A., Dennis, M., & Haefele-Kalvaitis, J. (1996). The effects of knowledge availability and knowledge accessibility on coherence and elaborative inferencing in children from six to fifteen years of age. *Journal of Experimental Child Psychology, 61,* 216–241.

Bennett, H. S. (1993). AC II malformations. In R. Lechtenberg (Ed.), *Handbook of cerebellar diseases.* New York: Marcel Dekker.

Bookstein, F. L. (1993) Landmarks, edges, morphometrics, and the brain atlas problem. In R. W. Thatcher, M. Hallett, T. Ceffiro, E. R. John, & M. Huerta (Eds.), *Functional neuroimaging: Technical foundation* (pp. 107–119). San Diego: Academic.

Brunt, D. (1980). Characteristics of upper limb movement in a sample of meningomyocele children. *Perceptual and Motor Skills, 51,* 43–47.

Brunt, D. (1984). Apraxic tendencies in children with myelomeningocele. *Adapted Physical Activity Quarterly, 1,* 61–67.

Burstein, J., Papile, L., & Burstein, R. (1979). Intraventricular hemorrhage and hydrocephalus in premature newborns: A prospective study with CT. *American Journal of Roentgenology, 132,* 631–635.

Cacciari, C., & Tabossi, P. (1993). Idioms processing, structure, and interpretation. Hillsdale, NJ: Erlbaum.

Casteel, M. A. (1993). Effects of inference necessity and reading goal in children's inferential generations. *Developmental Psychology, 29,* 346–357.

Caviness, V. S. (1976). The Chiari malformations of the posterior fossa and their relation to hydrocephalus. *Developmental Medicine and Child Neurology, 18,* 103–116.

Caviness, V. S., Meyer, J., Makris, N., & Kennedy, D. N. (1996) MRI-based topographic parcellation of human neocortex: An anatomically specific method with estimate of reliability. *Journal of Cognitive Neuroscience, 8,* 566–587.

Chi, M. T. H. (1978). Knowledge structures and memory development. In R. Siegler (Ed.), *Children's thinking: What develops?* (pp. 73–96). Hillsdale, NJ: Erlbaum.

Chuang, S. (1986). Perinatal and neonatal hydrocephalus: Part 1. Incidence and etiology. *Peerinatal Neonatology, 10,* 8—19.

Das Gupa, P., & Bryant, P. E. (1989). Young children's causal inferences. *Child Development, 60,* 1138—1146.

Del Bigio, M. R. (1993). Neuropathological changes caused by hydrocephalus. *Acta Neuropathologica, 85,* 573—585.

Dennis, M., & Barnes, M. A. (1993). Oral discourse after early-onset hydrocephalus: Linguistic ambiguity, figurative language, speech acts, and script-based inferences. *Journal of Pediatric Psychology, 18,* 639—652.

Dennis, M., & Barnes, M. A. (1994). Developmental aspects of neuropsychology: Childhood. In D. Zaidel (Ed.), *Handbook of perception and cognition: Neuropsychology* (pp. 219—246). New York: Academic.

Dennis, M., Barnes, M. A., & Hetherington, C. R. (1997, June). Visual attention in children with congenital hydrocephalus. Paper presented at the Canadian Psychological Association Toronto, CA.

Dennis, M., Fitz, C. R., Netley, C. T., Sugar, J., Harwood-Nash, D. C. F., Hendrick, H. B., Hoffman, H. J, & Humphreys, R. P. (1981). The intelligence of hydrocephalic children. *Archives of Neurology, 38,* 607—715.

Dennis, M., Hendrick, E. B., Hoffman, H. J., & Humphreys, R. P. (1987). Language of hydrocephalic children and adolescents. *Journal of Clinical and Experimental Neuropsychology, 9,* 593—621.

Dennis, M., Jacennik, B., & Barnes, M. A. (1994). The content of narrative discourse in children and adolescents after early onset hydrocephalus and in normally developing age peers. *Brain and Language, 46,* 129—165.

Donders, J., Canady, A. I., & Rourke, B. P. (1990). Psychometric intelligence after infantile hydrocephalus. *Child's Nervous System, 6,* 148—154.

Duffy, S. A. (1986). Role of expectations in sentence integration. *Journal of Experimental Psychology: Learning, Memory, and Cognition, 12,* 208—219.

Evans, R., Tew, B., Thomas, M., & Ford, J. (1985). Selective surgical management of neural tube malformations. *Archives of Disease in Childhood, 60,* 415—419.

Fletcher, J. M., Bohan, T. P., Brandt, M. E., Brookshire, B. L., Beaver, S. R., Francis, D. J., Thompson, N. M., & Miner, M. E. (1992). Cerebral white matter and cognition in hydrocephalic children. *Archives of Neurology, 49,* 818—824.

Fletcher, J. M., Brookshire, B. L., Bohan, T. P., Brandt, M. E., & Davidson, K. C. (1995). Early hydrocephalus. In B. P. Rourke (Ed.), *Syndrome of nonverbal learning disabilities: Neurodevelopmental manifestations* (pp. 206—238). New York: Guilford.

Fletcher, J. M. & Levin, H. S. (1987). Neurobehavioural effects of brain injury in children. In D. Routh (Ed.), *Handbook of pediatric psychology.* New York: Guilford.

Fletcher, J. M., McCauley, S. R., Brandt, M. E., Bohan, T. P., Kramer, L. A., Francis, D. J., Thorstad, K., & Brookshire, B. L. (1996). Regional brain tissue composition in children with hydrocephalus. *Archives of Neurology, 53,* 549—557.

Friedrich, W. N., Lovejoy, M. C., Shaffer, J., Shurtleff, D. B., & Beilke, R. L. (1991). Cognitive abilities and achievement status of children with myelomeningocele: A contemporary sample. *Journal of Pediatric Psychology, 16,* 423—428.

Garrod, S., O'Brien, E. J., Morris, R. D., & Rayner, K. (1990) Elaborative inferencing as an active or passive process. *Journal of Experimental Psychology: Learning, Memory, & Cognition, 16,* 250—257.

Gernsbacher, M. A., & Faust, M. E. (1991). The mechanism of suppression: A component of general comprehension skill. *Journal of Experimental Psychology: Learning, Memory and Cognition, 17,* 245–262.

Gibbs, R. W. (1980). Spilling the beans on understanding and memory for idioms in conversation. *Memory and Cognition, 8,* 449–456.

Gibbs, R. W., & Nayak, N. P. (1989). Psycholinguistic studies on the syntactic behavior of idioms. *Cognitive Psychology, 21,* 100–138.

Gordon Systems, Inc. (1988). *Instruction manual for the Gordon diagnostic system.* Dewitt, NY: Gordon Systems.

Grimm, R. A. (1976). Hand function and tactile perception in a sample of children with hydrocephalus. *American Journal of Occupational Therapy, 30,* 234–240.

Hadenius, A., Hagberg, B., Hyttnas-Bensch, K., & Sjögren, I. (1962). The natural prognosis of infantile hydrocephalus. *Acta Paediatrica, 51,* 117–118.

Harding, B. N. (1992). Malformations of the nervous system. In J. H. Adams & L. W. Duchen (Eds.), *Greenfield's neuropathology* (5th ed., pp. 521–543). New York: Oxford University Press.

Harwood-Nash, D. C. F. & Fritz, C. R. (1976). *Neuroradiology in Infants and Children, Volume 2,* St Louis, MO: C. V. Mosby.

Hetherington, C. R., & Dennis, M. (1999). Motor function profile in children with early onset hydrocephalus. *Developmental Neuropsychology, 15,* 25–51.

Holler, K. A., Fennell, E. B., Crosson, B., Boggs, S. R., & Mickle, J. P. (1995). Neuropsychological and adaptive functioning in younger versus older children shunted for hydrocephalus. *Child Neuropsychology, 1,* 63–73.

Horn, D. G., Lorch, E., Lorch, R. F., Jr., & Culatta, B. (1985). Distractibility and vocabulary deficits in children with spina bifida and hydocephalus. *Developmental Medicine and Child Neurology, 27,* 713–720.

Hynd, G. W., & Semrud-Clikeman, M. (1989). Dyslexia and brain morphology. *Psychological Bulletin, 106,* 447–482.

Jamison, E., & Fee, F. (1978). Spina bifida and the WPPSI. *Irish Journal of Psychology, 4,* 14–21.

Johnson-Laird, P. N. (1983). *Mental models: Towards a cognitive science of language, inference, and consciousness.* Cambridge: Harvard University Press.

Jones, M. R., & Boltz, M. (1989). Dynamic attending and responses to time. *Psychological Review, 96,* 459–491.

Keenan, J. M., Baillet, S. D., & Brown, P. (1984). The effects of causal cohesion on comprehension & memory. *Journal of Verbal Learning and Verbal Behavior, 23,* 115–126.

Kennedy, D. N., Filipek, P. A., Caviness, V. S. (1989). Anatomic segmentation and volumetric calculations in nuclear magnetic resonance imaging. *IEEE Transactions on Biomedical Engineering, 8,* 1–7.

Kennedy, D. N., & Nelson, A. C. (1987). Three-dimensional display from cross-sectional tomographic images: An application to magnetic resonance imaging. *IEEE Transactions on Biomedical Engineering, 6,* 134–140.

Kintsch, W. (1994). Text comprehension, memory, and learning. *American Psychologist, 49,* 294–303.

Kintsch, W., & van Dijk, T. A. (1978). Toward a model of text comprehension and production. *Psychological Review, 85,* 363–394.

Laatsch, L. K., Dorman, C., & Hurley, A. D. (1984). Neuropsychological testing and survey forms to indicate possible losses of neurological functioning. *Zeitschrift fur Kinderchirurgie, 39*(suppl 2), 125–128.

Land, L. C. (1977). A study of the sensory integration of children with meningomyelocele. In R. L. McLaurin (Ed.), *Myelomeningocele* (pp. 112–117). New York: Grune & Stratton.

Leech, G. N. (1983). *Principles of pragmatics.* New York: Longmans.

Lollar, D. J. (1990). Learning patterns among spina bifida children. *Zeitschrift fur Kinderchirurgie, 45*(suppl 1), 39.

Lonton, A. P. (1977). Location of the myelomeningocele and its relationship to subsequent physical and intellectual abilities in children with myelomeningocele associated with hydrocephalus. *Zeitschrift fur Kinderchirurgie, 22,* 510–519.

Lonton, A. P. (1985). Gender and spina bifida—some misconceptions. *Zeitschrift fur Kinderchirurgie, 40,* 34–36.

Lorber, J. (1980). Is your brain really necessary? *Science, 210,* 1232–1234.

Mazur, J., Aylward, G., Colliver, J., Stacey, J., & Menelaus, M. (1988). Impaired mental capabilities and hand function in myelomeningocele patients. *Zeitschrift fur Kinderchirurgie, 43,* 24–27.

McCarron, L. T. (1976). *Mand McCarron assessment of neuromuscular development: Fine and gross motor abilities.* Dallas: Common Market Press.

McLone, D. G. Czyzewski, D., Raimondi, A. J., & Sommers, R. C. (1982). Central nervous system infections as a limiting factor in intelligence of children with myelomeningocele. *Pediatrics, 70,* 338–342.

McGee, M. G. (1979). Human spatial abilities: Psychometric studies and environmental, genetic, hormonal, and neurological differences. *Psychological Bulletin, 86,* 889–918.

McKoon G., & Ratcliff, R. (1990). Dimensions of inference. *The Psychology of Learning and Motivation, 25,* 313–328.

McKoon, G., & Ratcliff, G. (1992). Inference during reading. *Psychological Review, 99,* 440–466.

Menkes, J. (1995). *Textbook of child neurology* (5th ed.). Philadelphia: Lea & Febiger.

Miller, E., & Sethi, L. (1971a). The effect of hydrocephalus on perception. *Developmental Medicine and Child Neurology, 13,* 77–81.

Miller, E., & Sethi, L. (1971b). Tactile matching in children with hydrocephalus. *Neuropaediatrie, 3,* 191–194.

Morrow, D. G., Bower, G. H., & Greenspan, S. L. (1990). Situation-based inferences during narrative comprehension. *The Psychology of Learning and Motivation, 25,* 123–135.

Murdoch, B. E., Ozanne, A. E., & Smyth, V. (1990). Communicative impairments in neural tube disorders. In B. E. Murdoch (Ed.), *Acquired neurological speech/language disorders in childhood* (pp. 216–244). London: Taylor & Francis.

Oakhill, J. (1993). Children's difficulties in reading comprehension. *Educational Psychology Review, 5,* 1–15.

Oakhill, J., & Garnham, A. (1988). *Becoming a skilled reader.* Oxford: Basil Blackwell.

Pearson, A., Carr, J., & Halliwell, M. (1988). The handwriting of children with spina bifida. *Zeitschrift fur Kinderchirurgie, 43,* 40–42.

Riva, D., Milani, N., Giorgi, C., Pantaleoni, C., Zorzi, C., & Devoti, M. (1994). Intelligence outcome in children with shunted hydrocephalus of different etiology. *Child's Nervous System, 19,* 70–73.

Rourke, B. P., Bakker, D. J., Fisk, J. L., & Strang, J. D. (1983). *Child neuropsychology: An introduction to theory, research, & clinical practice.* New York: Guilford.

Sand, P., Taylor, N., Hill, M., Kosky, N., & Rawlings, M. (1973). Hand function in children with myelomeningocele. *American Journal of Occupational Therapy, 28,* 87–90.

Sandler, A. D., Macias, M., & Brown, T. T. (1993). The drawings of children with spina bifida: Developmental correlations and interpretations. *European Journal of Pediatric Surgery, 3*(suppl 1), 25–27.

Shaffer, J., Friedrich, W. N., Shurtleff, D. B., & Wolf, L. (1985). Cognitive and achievement status of children with myelomeningocele. *Journal of Pediatric Psychology, 10*(3), 325–336.

Shaffer, J., Wolfe, L., Friedrich, W., Shurtleff, H., Shurtleff, D., & Fay, G. (1986). Developmental expectations: Intelligence and fine motor skills. In D. B. Shurtleff (ed). *Myelodysplasias and exstrophies: Significance, prevention, and treatment* (pp. 359–372). New York: Grune & Stratton.

Simms, B. (1987). The route learning ability of young people with spina bifida and hydrocephalus and their able-bodied peers. *Zeitschrift fur Kinderchirurgie, 42,* 53–56.

Singer, M., Graesser, A. C., & Trabasso, T. (1994). Minimal or global inference during reading. *Journal of Memory and Language, 33,* 421–441.

Smith, J. F. (1974). *Pediatric neuropathology.* New York: McGraw-Hill.

Soare, P., & Raimondi, A. (1977). Intellectual and perceptual-motor characteristics of treated myelomeningocele children. *American Journal of Diseases of Childhood, 131,* 199–204.

Swinney, D., & Cutler, A. (1979). The access and processing idiomatic expressions. *Journal of Verbal Learning and Verbal Behavior, 18,* 523–534.

Swisher, L. P., & Pinsker, E. J. (1971). The language characteristics of hyperverbal, hydrocephalic children. *Developmental Medicine and Child Neurology, 13,* 746–755.

Taylor, E. M. (1961). *Psychological appraisal of children with cerebral defects.* Cambridge, MA: Harvard University Press.

Tew, B. (1991). The effects of spina bifida and hydrocephalus upon learning and behaviour. In C. M. Bannister & B. Tew (Eds.), *Current concepts in spina bifida and hydrocephalus* (pp. 158–179). New York: Cambridge University Press.

Tew, B. J., & Laurence, K. M. (1979). The clinical and psychological characteristics of children with the "cocktail party" syndrome. *Zeitschrift fur Kinderchirurgie, 28,* 360–367.

Tew, B. I., Laurence, K. M., & Richards, A. (1980). Inattention among children with hydrocephalus and spina bifida. *Zeitschrift fur Kinderchirurgie, 31*(4), 381–385.

Thompson, N., Fletcher, J., Chapieski, L., Landry, S., Miner, M., & Bixby, J. (1991). Cognitive and motor abilities in preschool hydrocephalus. *Journal of Clinical and Experimental Neuropsychology, 13,* 245–258.

Wallace, S. (1973). The effect of upper limb function on mobility of children with myelomeningocele. *Developmental Medicine and Child Neurology, 15*(suppl 29), 84–91.

Whitney, P. (1987). Psychological theories of elaborative inferences: Implications for schema-theoretic views of comprehension. *Reading Research Quarterly, 22,* 299–310.

Whitney, P., Ritchie, B. G., & Clark, M. B. (1991). Working memory capacity and the use of elaborative inferences in text comprehension. *Discourse Processes, 14,* 133–145.

Willoughby, R., & Hoffman, R. (1979). Cognitive and perceptual impairments in children with spina bifida: A look at the evidence. *Spina Bifida Therapy, 2,* 127–134.

Wills, K. E. (1993). Neuropsychological functioning in children with spina bifida and/or hydrocephalus. *Journal of Clinical Child Psychology, 22*(2), 247–265.

Wills, K. E., Holmbeck, G. N., Dillon, K., & McLone, D. G. (1990). Intelligence and achievement in children with myelomeningocele. *Journal of Pediatric Psychology, 15*(2), 161–176.

Yekovich, F. R., Walker, C. H., Ogle, L. T., & Thompson, M. A. (1990). The influence of domain knowledge on inferencing in low-aptitude individuals. *The Psychology of Learning and Motivation, 25*, 259–278.

Young, H. F., Nulsen, F. E., Weiss, M. H., et al. (1973). The relationship of intelligence and cerebral mantle in treated infantile hydrocephalus. *Pediatrics, 52*, 54–60.

Zeiner, H., Prigatano, G., Pollay, M., Biscoe, C., & Smith, R. (1985). Ocular motility, visual acuity and dysfunction of neuropsychological impairment in children with shunted uncomplicated hydrocephalus. *Child's Nervous System, 1*, 115–122.

Ziviani, J., Hayes, A., & Chant, D. (1990). Handwriting: A perceptual-motor disturbance in children with myelomeningocele. *Occupational Therapy Journal of Research, 10*, 12–26.

Zwann, R. A., Langston, M. C., & Grasesser, A. C., (1995). The construction of situation models in narrative comprehension: An event-indexing model. *Psychological Science, 6*, 292–297.

23 Neural Mediation of Language Development: Perspectives from Lesion Studies of Infants and Children

Elizabeth Bates, Stefano Vicari, and Doris Trauner

Aphasia is defined as the breakdown or impairment of language after injury to the brain, usually due to trauma or stroke. The study of aphasia goes back to the beginning of medical history, to comments in the Edmund Smyth Papyrus (c. 3000 BC) regarding an apparent link between loss of speech and damage to the head (O'Neill, 1980). Though aphasiology is the oldest subfield in the area currently known as *cognitive neuroscience*, surprisingly we still know very little about language development in children who have focal injuries similar to those that have inspired 5000 years of research on adults. Children with strokes or surgical lesions are relatively rare, and studies of their language outcomes are few in number. However, sample size is not the only obstacle to progress in the study of brain injury in children. The biggest problem lies in the fact that lesion studies of children and adults yield what appear to be contradictory findings.

Studies of brain-injured adults suggest that the left hemisphere (LH) plays a crucial role in the mediation of both receptive and expressive language. Specifically, aphasia is associated with LH in approximately 95% to 98% of all cases with unilateral damage (Goodglass, 1993; Willmes & Poeck, 1993), including cases of sign language aphasia (Poizner et al., 1987)

Studies of children with early unilateral brain injury reveal surprisingly few differences between LH and right-hemisphere (RH) cases. In fact, when cases with serious complications are excluded from the sample (e.g., seizure conditions), most children with early LH injury go on to acquire language abilities within the normal range.

These contradictory findings present us with a paradox: An intact LH is not required for the development of language, yet it appears to be critical for normal language functions in the adult. If the LH is not essential for normal language development, how and why does the characteristic form of brain organization for language observed in adults come about in the first place? Something at the beginning of life must favor LH mediation of language under normal circumstances. If that "something" is not language itself, then what is it?

We cannot offer a definitive answer to this question, but we suggest a plausible alternative, together with some fruitful directions for future research. We begin with a brief overview of the widely contrasting positions that have been put forward in the history of this field, ranging from *equipotentiality* (i.e., the idea that the two cerebral hemispheres are equivalent in their ability to support language) to *irreversible determinism* (i.e., the belief that from birth the LH contains the mechanisms essential for normal language development, so that early damage to this hemisphere results in irreversible forms of language impairment). Then we summarize the current literature on language outcomes in children with congenital or acquired lesions to one side of the brain, focusing on the contributions of (1) etiology, (2) lesion side (left versus right), (3) lesion site within the damaged hemisphere, (4) lesion size, (5) seizure conditions, and (6) the effects of age and time, including age of lesion onset, time elapsed since lesion onset, and age and developmental status at time of testing. Several of these sections include detailed examples from our ongoing work with the focal lesion population, illustrating the wide variability that can be observed in children with similar etiologies, and the dynamic and changing nature of lesion-symptom mappings across the course of development.

We have included data for individual subjects in many of the figures in this chapter. This approach is not typical in a review chapter, but we provide this information because it permits our readers to see the extent of variability lying behind the broad conclusions about brain and language development often found in this literature. In addition to this emphasis on variability *within* studies, we underscore the immense variability often found *between* studies—leading, in some cases, to completely contradictory conclusions. Some of these contradictions may reflect relatively uninteresting methodological differences from one study to another (e.g., differences in the methods used to identify and classify children with brain injury and in the measures used to assess cognitive outcomes). Indeed, one of our goals in this chapter is to provide the reader with some guidelines for evaluating studies of language and cognition in children with focal brain injury. However, these complications are not enough to explain the undeniable fact that homologous injuries occuring in childhood have effects radically different from the familiar effects observed in brain-damaged adults.

At the end of this chapter, we hope to have shown why most investigators have abandoned the extreme positions that characterized earlier research in this field. Now seemingly clear is that the two hemispheres do make different contributions to the language-learning process from the very beginning. However, these differences are apparently not irreversible and may reflect computational biases or styles of information processing that are related only indirectly to "language proper." Hence, alternative forms of brain organization can emerge when the normal situation is disrupted in some way.

OVERVIEW

Reviews of the literature on language outcomes in children with unilateral injuries include summaries by Hecaen (1976, 1983), Lenneberg (1967), Riva and Cazzaniga (1986), St. James Roberts (1981), and Woods and Teuber (1978). (See also Teuber, 1971; Smith, 1984; Bishop, 1988; Curtiss, 1988; Satz et al., 1990; Vargha-Khadem & Polkey, 1992; Stiles & Thal, 1993; Vargha-Khadem et al., 1994; Eisele & Aram, 1995; Riva, 1995; Stiles, 1995; and Elman et al., 1996.) The contrasting positions represented in these reviews correspond to three partially overlapping periods in history, starting with a period dominated by a belief in equipotentiality, moving to a phase characterized by a belief in irreversible determinism, leading up to the current state of affairs, a period in which most investigators working with the focal lesion population are looking for an alternative somewhere between these two extremes.

Equipotentiality

Early studies in this field underscored the surprisingly good outcomes that often are observed in the early focal lesion population, leading some to conclude that the two cerebral hemispheres are equipotential at birth (i.e., equally capable of mediating language functions). This conclusion was compatible with some startling observations by Kennard (1936), who found virtually no long-term effects of unilateral lesions to motor cortex in infant monkeys. It was also compatible with a famous set of lesion studies by Lashley (1950), who noted that the effects of surgical lesions on retention and relearning of spatial knowledge in adult rats seemed to depend more on the amount of brain removed rather than on lesion location. In fact, these results were what led Lashley to propose his twin principles of *equipotentiality* (i.e., all regions of the cortex are capable of the same kinds of learning) and *mass action* (i.e., learning capacity is a function of cortical mass). The equipotentiality perspective within the animal literature paralleled the holistic approach to adult aphasia offered by such Gestalt psychologists as Goldstein (1948) and such critics of the classic localization approach as Head (1926).

Within the human developmental literature, the equipotentiality view reached its high-water mark with Lenneberg (1967), who reviewed the literature on recovery from focal brain injury in humans and concluded that the two sides of the brain are indeed equipotential for language in their initial state. The familiar asymmetries observed in the adult were (Lenneberg argued) a consequence rather than a cause of language learning. Lenneberg based his conclusions primarily on Basser (1962), who presented evidence of spared language abilities in 35 children who had undergone hemispherectomy to control intractable seizures originating in the LH or RH. In 34 of these cases, no deficit in speech and language functions was observed; only one case displayed clear-cut evidence of a language impairment. Lenneberg assumed that the capacity for both hemispheres to acquire language ends somewhere around 12 years of age, coinciding with a supposed reduction in the ability to acquire fluent, nativelike abilities in a second language (a conclusion that is also controversial; see Johnson & Newport, 1989; Marchman,

1993; Bialystok & Hakuta, 1994). He attributed this apparent loss of plasticity to the progressive specialization of the two hemispheres for language and nonlanguage functions, complemented by a monotonic decrease in equipotentiality. However, the Basser data on which Lenneberg based his conclusions do not provide clear-cut information about the shape of this developmental function. As we see in more detail later, it is not at all clear that a single, monotonic function describes the relation between age of lesion and recovery of function.

Aside from its empirical adequacy, the equipotentiality view provides no logical answer to the paradox posed at the outset: If the two hemispheres are equivalent at the outset of language learning, why does the left-dominant pattern emerge in the vast majority of cases? Some kind of bias has to be there from the beginning—which brings us to the next phase in the history of this field.

Irreversible Determinism

Across the late 1970s and early 1980s, the theoretical pendulum swung away from equipotentiality and toward a belief in innate and irreversible LH specialization for language (for reviews, see Satz et al., 1990; Vargha-Khadem et al., 1994). This shift in perspective was influenced by a parallel change in neighboring fields, including generative linguistics, with its emphasis on the innateness of grammar and its autonomy from other cognitive systems (Chomsky, 1975; see Caplan, 1987, for a review), and Sperry and Gazzaniga's surprising findings on the independent functions of the two cerebral hemispheres in split-brain patients (Gazzaniga et al., 1962). At the same time, Geschwind's seminal writings were bringing about a revival of the localizationist view in research on brain-injured adults (Geschwind, 1965). Among other things, Geschwind & Levitsky (1968) demonstrated anatomical asymmetries revolving around the length and shape of the planum temporale, asymmetries that subsequently were reported to be present very close to birth in human infants (Witelson & Pallie, 1973). Several studies also provided evidence for behavioral asymmetries in very young infants, including an LH bias for complex speechlike stimuli (Entus, 1977; Molfese & Molfese, 1980; but see Vargha-Khadem & Corballis, 1979).

Within this climate, a number of papers showed that LH injury may have a negative effect on language functions in children, including children with hemispherectomies (Zaidel 1973, 1977; Dennis & Kohn, 1975; Dennis & Whitaker, 1976; Day & Ulatowska, 1979; Dennis, 1980; Dennis et al., 1981) and children with early unilateral injuries from cerebrovascular pathologies (Reed & Reitan, 1971; Woods & Teuber, 1973, 1978; Riva & Cazzaniga, 1986). In almost all these studies, the deficits observed after LH damage were very subtle. That is, even though their scores often fall below those of normal controls, the brain-injured children described in both the hemispherectomy and the lesion literature rarely qualify for a diagnosis of developmental aphasia. Furthermore, as Bishop (1983, 1988) has stressed in some highly critical reviews, the left-right differences reported in some of the hemispherectomy studies are so small that they fail to meet standard criteria for statistical reliability. Despite these caveats, a general message about early specialization and irreversible determinism began to emerge from this work, a message that has grown in magnitude across secondary and tertiary sources (St. James Roberts, 1981). The following quotation from Curtiss (1988, pp. 101–102) illustrates this point:

Cases of left hemispherectomy (or hemidecortication) in childhood after at least early stages of language acquisition, are reported to result in severe grammatical deficits—limited comprehension and production of many morphological and syntactic structures, largely agrammatic speech, and an inability to correct syntactic errors, despite good auditory discrimination and vocabulary test scores ... Studies of unilateral cortical lesions in childhood also instantiate the possibility of grammar being selectively impaired in acquisition (consistently as a result of left-hemisphere damage) ... The data from clear-cut neurological damage in childhood thus provide additional support for the modularity of grammar view, and further, along with considerable other data, tie this module and the mechanisms for its acquisition to the left cerebral hemisphere.

Of course the authors of original works on hemispherectomy and early stroke cannot be faulted for the treatment of their work in subsequent reviews. This kind of "rounding up" is common in textbook reviews of a complex literature, a move toward coherence that writers seek in their efforts to simplify a complex story for beginners. As we see later, Curtiss's conclusion is not compatible with the current literature on language in brain-injured children. However, it was (and is) compatible with a number of trends in linguistics and neurolinguistics, summarized in the following quotation from an influential textbook dealing with neuroscience (Kandel et al., 1995, p. 639):

Chomsky postulated that the brain must have an organ of language, unique to humans, that can combine a finite set of words into an infinite number of sentences. This capability, he argued, must be innate and not learned, since children speak and understand novel combinations of words they have not previously heard. *Children must therefore have built into their brains a universal grammar, a plan shared by the grammars of all natural languages.* [Note: Italics ours.]

Presumably, irreversible damage to this grammar organ due to trauma or stroke ought to lead to a permanent language disorder. In the next few pages, we try to show that such conclusions are incorrect, at least with regard to the literature on language outcomes after early focal brain injury, because most children with early LH damage do eventually master the grammar of their language.

CONSTRAINED PLASTICITY: EVIDENCE FOR A MIDDLE VIEW

Most researchers working within this subfield now agree that the truth lies somewhere in between the two extremes of equipotentiality and irreversible determinism (Stiles & Thal, 1993; Vargha-Khadem et al., 1994; Elman et al., 1996; Bates et al., 1997; Reilly et al., 1998). The remarkable plasticity displayed by children with early focal brain injury must be acknowledged. At the same time, clear and specific constraints apparently control rate of development in the early stages and the range of outcomes ultimately observed in this population.

Etiology and Presenting Symptoms

A few words are appropriate regarding the medical conditions that lead to unilateral brain injury in children (i.e., etiology) and regarding the symptoms that bring such children to the attention of clinicians and researchers. As we see later, these factors may help to explain some of the contrasting conclusions that have been reached in this literature.

The most common cause of early unilateral injury is an ischemic cerebrovascular accident, or stroke. Other causes include trauma, surgery to correct severe epilepsy, tumors (sometimes surgically excised), and developmental anomalies (wherein the "growth plan" goes awry for some unknown reason, including environmental toxins, genetic defects, or prenatal trauma). At the present time, we simply do not know whether these different etiologies are associated with different outcomes in children, but it has been known for some time that they can have a differential effect on outcomes in adults (Jackson, 1878; Goodglass, 1993). The classic adult aphasia syndromes usually are observed with acute and well-localized injuries due to stroke or trauma with penetration (i.e., bullet or shrapnel wounds). Closed-head injuries in adults are more likely to result in diffuse forms of damage rendering localization difficult and interpretation even more difficult (but see Levin, 1991). Injuries due to tumors have some of the same problems (e.g., diffuse damage due to pressure from the expanding tumor). However, in contrast with the diffuse symptoms that tend to accompany closed-head injury, the damage created by slowly growing tumors often is associated with a surprising degree of sparing in adults, presumably due to some kind of reorganization or relearning across the course of the disease. The difference between sudden and slow onset has been demonstrated experimentally in lesion studies of animals, wherein the "same" lesion (in terms of location and extent) is created either all at once or in successive steps separated in time. These studies show that the worst behavioral outcomes are observed when the lesion is created all at once; incremental lesions tend to be accompanied by better outcomes (Stein et al., 1995).

In children, differences in etiology often are confounded with differences in the age at which an injury occurs. By definition, developmental anomalies are assumed to arise at some point during prenatal brain evelopment. Strokes and trauma may occur prenatally, perinatally (i.e., around birth), or at any point later in childhood. Perinatal strokes and perinatal trauma usually are due to difficulties that arise during birth and may be associated with oxygen deprivation and other complications. Strokes later in childhood can occur for a variety of reasons (e.g., hypertension, venous abnormalities, blood clots that arise during heart catheterization) and thus also may reflect a range of different complications (e.g., a lifetime of oxygen deprivation in some children with congenital heart defects). Lesions due to tumor excision or neurosurgery to control epilepsy are rare in young infants, occurring predominantly in the preschool and school-age years. For obvious reasons, such confounds between etiology and age of injury greatly complicate our efforts to understand the putative loss in plasticity that takes place from birth to adolescence (see under heading of Age of Lesion Onset).

Another etiological confound arises from the factors that bring cases of unilateral injury to the attention of pediatric neurologists (i.e., selection bias). Cases of unilateral damage in childhood usually are diagnosed for one of three reasons: hemiplegia or hemiparesis (i.e., motor weakness or paralysis on one side of the body), seizure conditions, or birth complications (including prematurity) that lead the attending obstetrician to suspect that intraventricular bleeding or some other form of brain injury may have occurred. Although these different etiologies often are grouped together in studies of brain injury in children, very possibly such differences in presenting symptoms are associated with different patterns of neural damage (Isaacs et al., 1996).

For example, some investigators have used hemiplegia as a guide to locating children with early injuries. In many of the older studies on this topic (before neuroradiological measures were available), diagnosis of LH versus RH injury was based exclusively on the presence of hemiplegia on the contralateral side. As a result, these studies may be biased to reflect that subset of the focal lesion population whose lesions involve cortical or subcortical motor areas. Studies that include cases with trauma or seizure history introduce biases of another kind. As we see later, very different outcomes are observed in children with and without seizure disorders. A few laboratories have avoided these problems by studying children who suffer strokes during cardiac catherization (Eisele & Aram, 1995). Although this approach has its advantages, it generally rules out the study of cases with congenital (prelinguistic) injury, and it also introduces the confounds associated with months to years of the mild hypoxia associated with cardiological symptoms.

No obvious solution can solve this problem. For present purposes, our point is that variations in etiology and presenting symptoms complicate the interpretation of research with the focal lesion population. Etiology often is confounded with age of onset, seizure conditions, motor involvement, and oxygen deprivation and with the nature and extent of the lesion itself.

Lesion Side

Most of the literature on unilateral brain injury in children has concentrated on differences due to lesion side. These studies vary widely in (among other things) the kinds of measures that are used to assess language functions. However, comparison is possible across those studies that have included verbal IQ (as a measure of language level) and performance IQ (as a measure of visual-perceptual functions). Table 23.1 (adapted from Vargha-Khadem et al., 1994) summarizes findings of LH versus RH injury on verbal versus performance IQ in a representative range of studies of congenital and acquired lesions in childhood. As should be clear from a cursory examination of this table, results to date are contradictory, even for these relatively straightforward outcome measures.

Full-Scale IQ Most studies report that, as a group, children with focal brain injury perform below the level of normal controls in full-scale IQ. However, this does *not* mean that focal brain injury in children leads to mental retardation. In fact, the group difference between brain-injured children and normal controls is relatively small across all the studies in table 23.1 (e.g., mean-performance IQs in the 90s for the focal lesion population, compared with 100+ for controls). However, the range that is observed within the focal lesion population often is very large, from substandard to well above normal.

Figure 23.1 illustrates this mean difference and the range of variation in full-scale IQ that can be observed within and across lesion groups, based on previously unpublished data from our ongoing research projects. The flat dotted lines in the figure indicate the mean IQ of 100 that we would expect if children were drawn randomly from the normal population; the flat solid lines indicate the mean IQ actually observed within each of our focal lesion samples.

Figure 23.1A plots the relationship between age at testing and full-scale IQ scores for LH and RH children, taken from a study in progress by Vicari et al. at the Ospedale Bambin Gesù in Rome. This sample includes 33 children between 3 and 14 years of age, 18 with LH injuries and 15 with lesions on the right.[1] All these cases are congenital (i.e., lesions that occurred prenatally or perinatally, before 6 months of age), and none has a history of seizure conditions or seizure medication. Most of the cases in this particular sample (71%) have lesions restricted to white matter underlying the cortex (e.g., periventricular leukomalacia). Preliminary analyses showed that the LH and RH cases did not differ in age, gender, or social class.

Figure 23.1B illustrates the relation between age at testing and full-scale IQ for 43 children between 3 and 9 years of age (28 with LH damage and 15 with RH damage), part of a larger sample of children with congenital focal brain injuries followed by Stiles et al., in San Diego (including pooled data from a collaboration with Nass in New York). The San Diego study is restricted also to cases of prenatal or perinatal injury (before 6 months of age) to one side of the brain, excluding bilateral abnormalities and other more generalized conditions that would complicate interpretation of findings associated with lesion side or site, e.g., prenatal drug exposure, metabolic

Table 23.1 Summary of results for performance and verbal IQ in children with LH versus RH damage (Adapted from Vargha-Khadem et al., 1994)

Study	Sample size	Age at lesion onset	Time post lesion	Seizure history	Nonverbal IQ	Verbal IQ
Woods, 1980	LH = 27	Early = < 1 year	LE = 17;02	LE = 27%	LE < normal	LE < normal
	RH = 23	Late = > 1 year	RE = 14;01	RE = 50%	RE < normal	RE < normal
			LL = 8;06	LL = 19%	LL < normal	LL < normal
			RL = 10;03	RL = 15%	RL < normal	RL = normal
Riva &	LH = 22	Early = < 1 year	Early = 8;05		LE < normal	LE < normal
Cazzaniga, 1986	RH = 26	Late = > 1 year	Late = 4.02		RE < normal	RE = normal
					LL = normal	LL = normal
					RL < normal	RL = normal
Riva et al., 1986	LH = 8	Not divided by	L = 6;08	L = 37.5%	L < normal	L < normal
	RH = 8	age of lesion onset	R = 4;06	R = 37.5%	R < normal	R = normal
Nass et al., 1989	LH = 15	All pre- or	L = 6;07		L < normal	L = normal
	RH = 13	perinatal	R = 8;05		R < normal	R < normal
Vargha-Khadem	LH = 42	All congenital-	L = 12;03	2 seizure	L +S < normal	L +S < normal
et al., 1992	RH = 40	perinatal	R = 11;05	groups	L −S < normal	L −S = normal
				2 nonseizure	R +S < normal	R +S = normal
				groups	R −S < normal	R −S = normal
Muter et al., 1997	LH = 23	All congenital-	L = 4;09	L = 35%	L +S < normal	L +S < normal
	RH = 15	perinatal	R = 4;09	R = 27%	L −S < normal	L −S = normal
					R +S < normal	R +S < normal
					R −S < normal	R −S = normal
Ballantyne et al.,	LH = 8	All congenital-	L = 9;0	L = 62.5%	L < normal	L < normal
1996	RH = 9	perinatal	R = 11;2	R = 55.5%	R < normal	R < normal
					L : VIQ = PIQ	L : VIQ = PIQ
					R : VIQ > PIQ	R : VIQ > PIQ
San Diego Project	LH = 28	All congenital-	L = 5;04	L = 40.7%	L < normal	L < normal
(in progress)	RH = 15	perinatal	R = 5;05	R = 46.7%	R < normal	R < normal
					L = R	L = R

LH, left hemisphere (damage); RH, right hemisphere (damage); E, early lesion onset; L, late lesion onset; +S, with seizure history; −S, without seizure history.

disorders, and progressive or slow-growing abnormalities, such as arteriovenous malformations, tumor, or Sturge-Weber syndrome. In contrast with the Rome group, 43% of the San Diego cases in figure 23.1B have some kind of seizure history (including transitory neonatal seizures). All lesions have been confirmed by at least one neuroradiological technique, either computed tomography (CT) or magnetic resonance imaging (MRI). Also in contrast with the Rome sample, all the cases in figure 23.1B have lesions involving cortical gray matter, with or without involvement of underlying white matter or subcortical structures. Preliminary analyses indicate that the LH and RH groups within this sample do not differ significantly in age or gender.

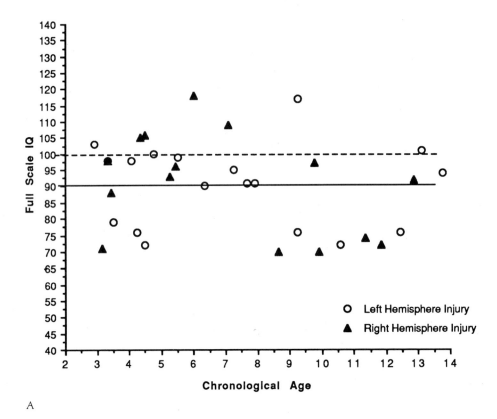

A

Figure 23.1   IQ as a function of age and side of injury in (A) Italian and (B) American children with focal brain injury. Dotted line = normal mean; solid line = focal lesion mean.

Despite differences in lesion type and incidence of seizures (see later), IQ results for the two samples are fairly similar: a mean full-scale IQ of 90.51 for the Rome group (SD, 13.98; range, 70–117), compared with a mean of 93.2 for the San Diego group (SD, 20.6; range, 44–134). Also clear from figure 23.1 is that the IQ means and ranges are fairly similar for children with LH versus RH damage: For the Rome group, mean IQ was 90.44 for LH and 90.6 for RH; for the San Diego group, mean IQ was 95.1 for LH, 90.8 for RH (all differences nonsignificant by a one-way analysis of variance and by a two-tailed *t*-test).

Of course, a group mean around 90 is lower than the mean of 100 that we would expect if these children were drawn randomly from the normal population, and a substantial number of these brain-injured children do fall below the 80–IQ cutoff for normal intelligence (including 11 cases or 33% in the Rome sample and 7 cases, or 16.3%, in the San Diego sample). In other words, some children are paying a price for their injuries and for the substantial reorganization that such injuries requires. Nevertheless, what is remarkable is that so many children are doing very well despite what are in some cases very large lesions to the LH or RH (see the heading Lesion

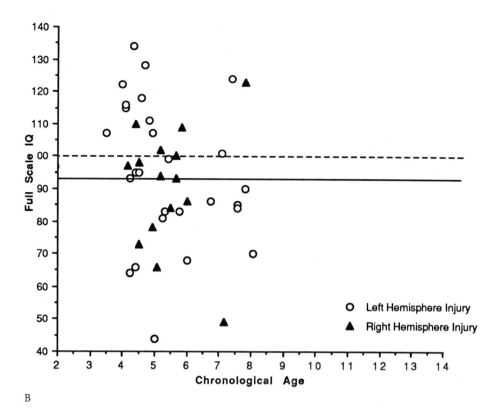

B

Figure 23.1 (continued)

Size). We are reminded here of a citation from Donald Hebb (1949), who expressed wonder and some skepticism at the degree of sparing that often is reported, even in cases of severe brain injury in adults (Hebb, 1949, pp. 18):

How is it possible that a man can have an IQ of 160 or higher after suffering an ablation (removal) of the prefrontal lobe, or that a woman can have an IQ of 115, better than 2/3 of the normal population, after having lost the entire right hemisphere of the cortex?

Performance Versus Verbal IQ In regard to results for the major IQ subscales, the studies summarized in table 23.1 do not provide evidence for a significant difference between LH and RH children in mean nonverbal or performance IQ. Instead, results for performance IQ mirror the results that we have just reported for full-scale IQ scores: Children with focal brain injury represent levels slightly but significantly below those in normal controls, with similar means and ranges in both the LH and RH groups. The one exception comes from the study by Riva et al. (1986), who found that LH children scored as did normal controls on performance IQ but only if their lesions were acquired after 1 year of age.

In contrast with the results for full-scale or performance IQ, the effects of lesion side on verbal IQ seem to vary markedly from one study to another (see table 23.1). In the studies by Woods (1980), Riva and Cazzaniga (1986), and Riva et al. (1986), children with LH lesions scored significantly below the level of normal controls on verbal IQ, a finding that was not observed in children with RH damage (at least not after age 1). Ballantyne et al. (1994) reported that verbal IQ is higher than performance IQ for RH (but not LH) children, even though both lesion groups perform significantly below levels in controls on both IQ scales. Findings in this direction are just what one would expect on the basis of the adult aphasia literature. However, the study by Nass et al. (1989) yields results in the opposite direction: Children in the LH group scored no differently from normals on verbal IQ, but children in the RH group scored significantly below controls on the same measure. In contrast to both these findings, the studies by Vargha-Khadem et al. (1992) and by Muter et al. (1997) report no significant effects of lesion side at all. Children in both groups tended to perform on levels below those in normal controls in both verbal and nonverbal IQ—a difference attributable almost entirely to children in this sample who have a seizure disorder (see heading of Seizures). Simply stated, this means that children with unilateral focal brain injury do *not* present unambiguous evidence for a dissociation between verbal and nonverbal IQ as a function of LH versus RH injury.

Note that some of the studies in table 23.1 compare each LH and RH sample with its own control group, because differences in age and other confounds preclude a direct comparison of LH and RH groups.[2] In our ongoing studies of children with congenital lesions in Rome and San Diego, we are able to escape these confounds; this means that we are able to compare the LH and RH groups directly, providing a stronger test of hypothesized group differences. As it turns out, our results to date agree with those of Vargha-Khadem et al. (1992) and Muter et al. (1997) who also were able to conduct direct LH-RH comparisons (i.e., no selective effects of side of lesion on either verbal or nonverbal IQ).

An example from the San Diego study is presented in figure 23.2, which plots the verbal IQ scores for individual children against their scores for performance IQ. The diagonal line represents the function that we would expect if verbal and nonverbal IQ were correlated perfectly. In fact, the Pearson product-moment correlation for this particular group is $+.65$ ($P < .0001$), a positive but imperfect relationship. The individual data in this figure demonstrate clearly that dissociations are distributed on both sides of the diagonal line: Performance IQ > verbal IQ in 16 cases (37% of the sample); verbal IQ > performance IQ in 27 cases (63% of the sample). Furthermore, the figure contains absolutely no evidence to support the idea that performance deficits are greater with RH damage and verbal deficits are greater with LH damage. This null result is confirmed in a multivariate analysis of variance comparing verbal and nonverbal IQ as a function of lesion side, yielding no significant main effect of side [$F(1, 41) = 0.29$, NS], no significant main effect of IQ scale [i.e., no mean difference between verbal and

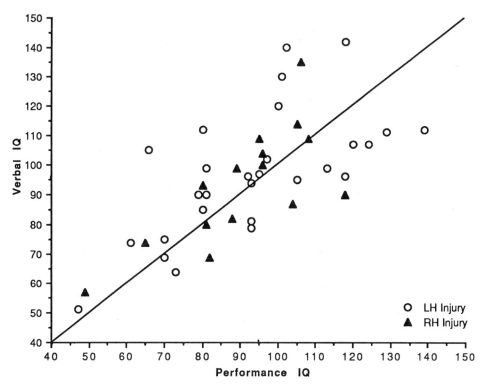

Figure 23.2 Verbal versus performance IQ from the San Diego project for children with LH versus RH injury.

performance IQ, [$F(1, 41) = 1.36$, NS], and no interaction between IQ scale and side of injury [$F(1, 41) = 0.03$, NS]. These results are identical to those reported by Vargha-Khadem et al. (1992; see table 23.1). They also are similar to a recent report by Goodman and Yude (1996), who used side of hemiparesis alone as an index to lesion side in a population-based sample of 149 hemiplegic children (i.e., no confirmation of lesion site with CT or MRI). Goodman and Yude found no effects of lesion side on either performance or verbal IQ, but they did find a large and reliable discrepancy between scales that held up independent of lesion side (with verbal IQ approximately 13 points ahead of performance IQ).

Specific Language Tests Results for lesion side are somewhat more encouraging in studies that have focused on specific language tests. However, contradictions are found in this literature as well, as indicated by the following discussion.

In an early study of older children and adults with a history of unilateral injury before age 1, McFie (1961) found patterns similar to those reported for brain injuries that occur in adulthood. That is, deficits were observed in visuospatial functions for RH patients, as were impairments in tests of language and verbal memory for LH patients.

Bates et al.: Neural Mediation of Language Development

A classic study by Alajouanine and Lhermitte (1965) reported marked interference with speech and written language after acquired lesions to the LH, although most of the children had recovered within 6 to 24 months after lesion onset (see also Hecaen, 1976). Comparable data for RH patients are not provided.

Woods (1980), Woods and Carey (1979), and Woods and Teuber (1978, 1983) reported disturbances in speech and language functions (including measures of writing and spelling) after LH damage, especially in cases of lesion acquisition after 1 year of age.

In their often-cited studies of children with left and right hemispherectomies, Dennis (1980), Dennis and Kohn (1975), Dennis and Whitaker (1976, 1977) and Dennis et al., (1981) reported that deficits in performance on some grammatical and phonological measures are more likely in individuals with a left hemispherectomy. However, the sample sizes in all these studies are very small. The cases varied widely in age at testing (e.g. from 8–28 years of age in Dennis, 1980) and in the age at which surgery was performed (from 5 months to 20 years of age in the same study). Additionally, conclusions about left and right differences are based entirely on descriptive statistics (i.e., group differences were not subjected to a significance test).

Later studies by Riva et al. (1986) reported that LH children are more impaired than are RH cases in some aspects of grammatical comprehension (i.e., complex syntax items on the token test) and on a test of sentence repetition. However, both LH and RH performed significantly lower than did their controls on receptive and expressive vocabulary (see Riva 1995 for an updated review).[2]

Vargha-Khadem et al. (1985) found that LH children performed below both RH children and controls on the token test and on a test of object naming. However, this left-right difference no longer was evident in later studies by the same research group using a larger sample and controls for presence or absence of seizures (Vargha-Khadem et al., 1994).

Reports that children with LH lesions perform below controls on some tests of grammatical comprehension and production, phonological discrimination, vocabulary, naming fluency, and lexical retrieval were cited by Aram et al. (1985, 1986, 1987, and 1990), and by Eisele & Aram (1993, 1994, 1995). On most of the same measures, RH children in the Aram et al. (1985, 1987) sample were not statistically different from their normal controls. However, further studies by Eisele (Aram et al., 1990; Eisele & Aram 1993, 1994, 1995) have qualified this initial round of findings. One study by Eisele and Aram (1994) showed that LH children performed below the level of their controls on a sentence imitation test, a pattern that was not observed in the RH group. By contrast, they observed no difference between LH and RH children on a test of syntactic comprehension, and a subset of children from both groups were at chance on this measure. Further analyses of this cohort have led these authors to conclude that most of the LH effects in the entire series of studies may be due to a subsample of children with subcortical involvement (Eisele & Aram, 1995; see heading of Lesion Site).[2]

In studies of the first stages of language development in infants with unilateral damage, Thal et al. (1991) and Bates et al. (1997) reported that both expressive vocabulary and grammar are more delayed in children with LH damage; however, this effect is due primarily to a subset of children with left temporal involvement (see heading of Lesion Site). Furthermore, delays in receptive language and communicative gesture actually were more common in children with RH damage, in direct contrast with the literature on comprehension and gesture in adults (but see Eisele & Aram, 1995).

Reilly et al. (1998) looked at lexical, grammatical, and discourse abilities in a story-telling task in a cross-sectional sample of 31 children with congenital lesions to the LH or RH. Age at testing ranged between 3 and 12 years of age. In children younger than 7 years of age, these authors reported no main effects of lesion side; however, they observed significant delays in morphology and syntax for children with left temporal involvement (in agreement with Thal et al., 1991 and Bates et al., 1997). After age 7, children with a history of early focal brain injury tended to fall behind normal controls on most of the language measures; however, none of these children would qualify for a diagnosis of aphasia, and the authors reported absolutely no specific effects of lesion location (i.e., no differences between LH and RH site and no evidence for a specific effect of lesion sites within the LH).

Kempler et al. (1996) looked at comprehension of novel sentences versus idiomatic expressions in a large group of adults with LH and RH injury, comparing the dissociations observed in adults with performance by 5- to 12-year-old children with prenatal or perinatal injuries to the LH or RH. In a replication of earlier findings, they showed that LH adults are more impaired on novel sentences, whereas RH adults are more impaired on idiomatic expressions. No such dissociation was observed in the child sample. Instead, children with LH and RH injury performed within the normal range on both subtests, although both groups scored significantly below the levels of age-matched normal controls in comprehension of novel sentences. No significant effects of lesion side were recorded in the 5- to 12-year-old children, other than a trend ($P < .06$) toward worse performance on novel sentences than on idiomatic sentences in the RH group—precisely the opposite of findings for adults.

To the extent that one can draw any generalizations at all from the foregoing list of study results, delays in language production do appear to be more likely in children with damage to the LH. Furthermore, these differences are observed more often in measures of expressive grammar. Mixed results (including worse performance by RH children) more often are observed with measures of receptive language (including some studies of sentence comprehension) or on measures of lexical ability (including vocabulary comprehension and naming). These tendencies are compatible (at least in part) with the literature on adult aphasia and hence with the idea that the LH is specialized

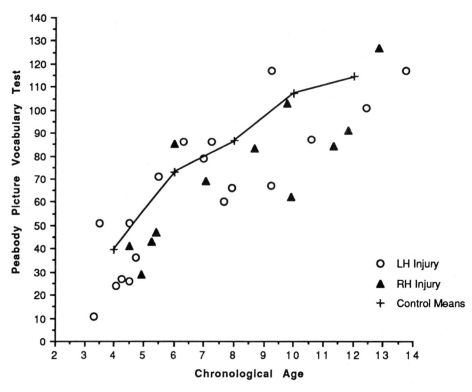

Figure 23.3 Peabody Picture Vocabulary Test for Italian children as function of side of lesion and age.

for language early in life. However, a substantial number of studies also report no effects of lesion side on specific language tasks (Feldman et al., 1992; Dall'Oglio et al., 1994; Vargha-Khadem et al., 1994; Kempler et al., 1996). Given the well-known bias in the neuropsychological literature against publication of null results, these "noneffects" must be taken seriously.

Some detailed examples from Vicari's ongoing study in Rome illustrate the latter point. The language tests administered to the sample in this study include two lexical measures: Italian translations of the Peabody Picture Vocabulary Test (PPVT), a measure of word comprehension (figure 23.3; Dunn & Dunn, 1981) and the Boston Naming Test, a measure of word production (figure 23.4; Goodglass & Kaplan, 1972). The author also used two tests of sentence comprehension: an Italian language version of the test of receptive grammar (TROG; figure 23.5; Bishop, 1979) and the Token Test (originally developed for the Italian language by DeRenzi & Faglioni, 1975; figure 23.6). In addition, children received a test of semantic category fluency in which they were required to generate in 1 minute as many examples as possible within a series of semantic categories, such as animals, fruits, and the like (Spreen & Strauss, 1991; figure 23.7). For these five measures, data for children with focal lesions are compared with those for normal controls matched for chronological age, gender, and social class.[3]

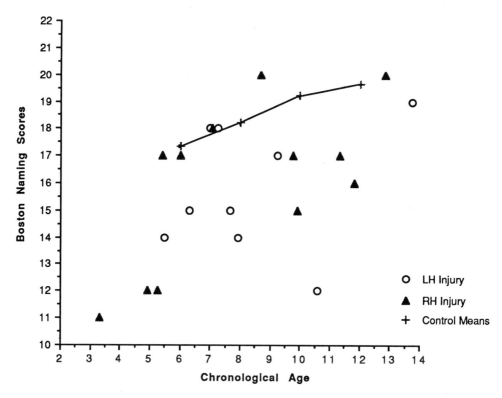

Figure 23.4 Boston Naming scores for Italian children as a function of side of lesion and age.

Vicari's results for these five language measures can be summarized briefly: *No evidence substantiates a difference between LH and RH children on any language measure*, by one-way analysis of variance or by one-tailed *t*-tests (based on the hypothesis that performance would be lower in the LH group). Because the two lesion groups do not differ significantly in age, IQ, social class, or any known neurological variables other than lesion side, this null result cannot be ascribed to other confounds. To demonstrate the range of variation and degree of overlap observed in LH children, RH children, and normal controls, we present scatterplots of individual focal lesion cases for the five measures in figures 23.3 through 23.7, compared with the mean for normal controls within age levels.

Although no evidence substantiates an effect of lesion side, the data in figures 23.3 through 23.7 indicate that children with focal brain injury do (as a group) differ from normal controls on these language measures. Simple one-way analyses of variance revealed that the brain-injured children (collapsed across side of injury) do indeed perform significantly below levels of normal controls on the Peabody Picture Vocabulary Test [$F(1, 72) = 4.57$; $P < .04$]; the Boston Naming Test [$F(1, 56) = 20.08$; $P < .0001$]; the Token Test [$F(1,47) = 4.48$; $P < .04$]; and the semantic fluency test [$F(1, 77) = 5.55$; $P < .03$] but not on the TROG [$F(1, 367) = 1.39$; NS]. However, because the

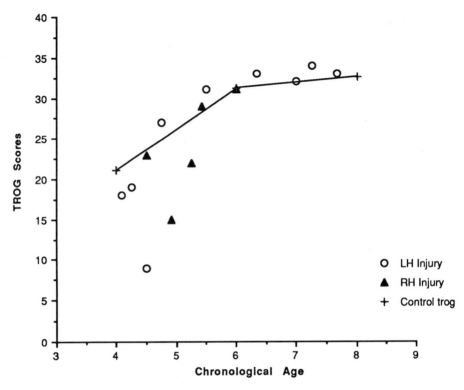

Figure 23.5 Test of receptive grammar (TROG) for Italian children as a function of side of lesion and age.

lesion population also is significantly below normal in full-scale IQ, the specificity of these effects is questionable. In fact, when the foregoing analyses of variance are repeated using mental age as a covariate, the only effect that remains significant is the difference between brain-injured children and normal controls on the Boston Naming Test [$F(1, 54) = 14.10$; $P < .0001$]. The apparent vulnerability of naming to focal brain injury is in line with previous reports by Riva et al. (1986) (based on a vocabulary subtest of Wechsler intelligence scale), as is the absence of a left-right difference on the same measure.

As Vargha-Khadem et al. (1994) noted in their review, such null effects as the foregoing are more likely in studies of children with very early injuries (i.e., congenital injuries that occur before language acquisition normally would begin). Those studies that have reported significant left-right differences on language measures tend to mix children with different lesion onset times and different etiologies (e.g., results by the Aram et al. 1985, 1986, 1987 and Riva et al. 1986 groups). Furthermore, few of the studies in the literature to date have provided information about lesion size or location in the damaged hemisphere. Reaching any conclusions about the presence or absence of LH specialization for language in children requires a consideration

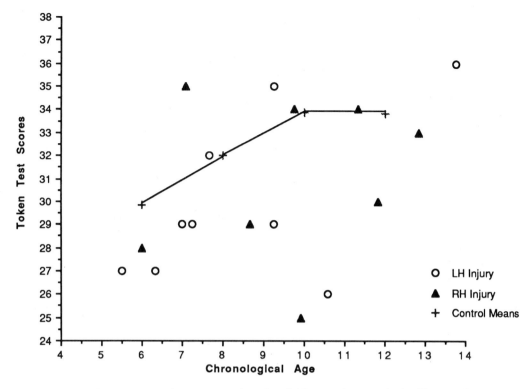

Figure 23.6 Token test scores for Italian children as a function of side of lesion and age.

of the contributions of these other variables to language outcomes in the focal lesion population.

Lesion Site

Evaluating the literature on site of lesion within the damaged hemisphere necessitates keeping in mind that good radiological measures of lesion location have been available for use with pediatric populations for only 10 to 15 years at most, and still very few centers have state-of-the-art neural imaging data available for children with focal brain injury. The relevant procedures include CT and MRI. In addition, sonography has been used as an imaging technique in some studies of infants younger than 9 months of age (prior to closing of the fontanelle). Before these tools became available, diagnosis of early unilateral injury was based entirely on secondary symptoms.

We noted earlier that early studies often relied exclusively on the presence of hemiplegia to diagnose LH versus RH injury. In the case of children whose diagnosis was based on hemiplegia, generally it was assumed that motor symptoms are associated with lesions in the contralateral hemisphere. Subsequent studies using neural imaging techniques have shown that this was a fairly safe assumption (Isaacs et al., 1996), although cases of what

Bates et al.: Neural Mediation of Language Development

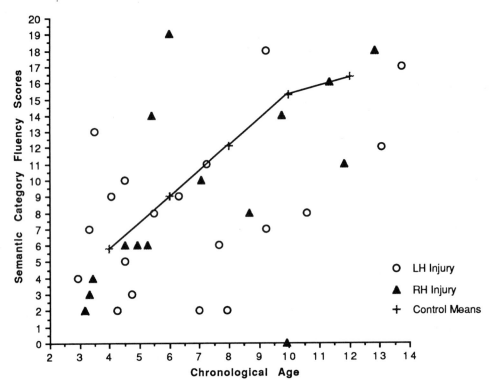

Figure 23.7 Semantic category fluency for Italian children as a function of side of lesion and age.

appears to be an ipsilateral hemiplegia have been observed (Trauner et al., 1993).

For injuries diagnosed through seizure conditions, lesion location formerly was established through electrophysiology; in current practice, neural imaging techniques with more precise spatial localization sometimes are used in conjunction with electrophysiology to locate structural damage. An important note, however, is that seizure conditions can occur in the absence of lesions visible on CT or MRI, including some cases with bilateral damage not evident with conventional neuroimaging techniques (Gadian et al., 1996; see heading of Seizures). In fact, some studies of brain-injured adults using functional brain imaging (in particular positron emission tomography) have revealed areas of hypometabolism or underactivity in regions that look quite normal on a structural scan (Metter et al., 1986, 1987, 1988; Kempler et al., 1988). In other words, structural scans may underestimate the extent and location of functional damage in patients with focal injury.

These caveats introduce a summary of the effects associated with specific intrahemispheric lesion sites in children. Using the adult aphasia literature as a guide, we might expect to find that deficits in comprehension are more common with lesions involving posterior regions of the LH, in particular the posterior region of the superior gyrus of the left temporal lobe (the presumed site of Wernicke's area). By contrast, deficits in production ought to be more common with lesions to anterior regions of the LH, in particular the third frontal convolution of the left frontal lobe (the presumed site of Broca's area).

As it turns out, surprisingly little evidence supports either of these hypotheses. Among the few studies that have looked at intrahemispheric lesion sites in brain-injured children, most have reported null results (Vargha-Khadem et al., 1994; Eisele & Aram, 1995). Aram, Eisele, and others find no specific effects of cortical sites, but they do note that the worst outcomes in their sample are observed in children whose lesions involve subcortical structures in the LH. The San Diego group has reported specific effects of lesion site, but these results are restricted to particular points in development and do not map onto findings from the adult aphasia literature in any clear or obvious way.

Note that all the cases in the San Diego studies are congenital (i.e., lesion onset before 6 months of age). Although children with a seizure history are included in the San Diego project, few cases reported seizures in the infant-toddler sample described by Bates et al. (1997), and these are restricted primarily to neonatal seizures. Based on CT or MRI data, all cases were coded to indicate whether their lesions involved the frontal, temporal, parietal, or occipital lobes in the damaged hemisphere. Comparisons were conducted not only between LH and RH but between (for example) children with left temporal injuries compared with the rest of the focal lesion sample (i.e., RH children as well as LH children whose lesions spared the temporal lobe). No specific effects were found for parietal or occipital sites, but some specific effects of temporal and frontal involvement did appear. Bates et al. (1997) reported findings for three partially overlapping samples of children between 10 and 44 months of age; except for the mean length of utterance (MLU) findings reported later, all results are based on a parent report measure: the MacArthur Communicative Development Inventories (MCDI; Fenson et al., 1993, 1994).

Between 10 and 17 months (the period in which most normal children show initial growth in vocabulary comprehension, communicative gesture, and production of first words), delays in comprehension and gesture (defined as scores in the bottom tenth percentile on the MCDI) actually were more likely in children with RH lesions. However, these effects were not associated with any particular site in the RH. Between 10 and 17 months, delays in production of first words (measured by the MCDI) were more likely in LH children but only if their lesion involved the left temporal lobe.

A similar left temporal effect was observed also for another (partially overlapping) sample of children between 19 and 31 months (the period in which most normal children show a marked acceleration in vocabulary production, accompanied by the onset of word combinations and subsequent growth of grammar). This left temporal disadvantage was equally pronounced for production of vocabulary and production of grammar, with no evidence whatsoever for a dissociation between the two.

In addition to the aforementioned left temporal effect, children between 19 and 31 months also were more delayed if their lesion involved the frontal lobe. However, in stark contrast with the adult aphasia literature (and with the left temporal effect just described), this frontal effect was statistically reliable and equivalent in size after lesions to *either* left frontal or right frontal cortex. In other words, frontal cortex does seem to be important in this dramatic phase of language development, but this frontal effect is symmetrical across the two hemispheres.

Within the same 19 to 31-month sample, children with RH lesions were reported to produce an abnormally high proportion of grammatical function words for their vocabulary size. This measure is related to a stylistic difference in early language development sometimes termed *pronominal style* (Bloom et al., 1975) or *rote-holistic style* (Bates et al., 1988; Bates et al., 1995; Shore, 1995). Bates et al. (1997) interpreted this finding to mean that the rote, unanalyzed use of grammatical function words sometimes observed in normal children in this age range may be due to an overreliance on functions mediated by the LH (e.g., some form of auditory short-term memory) without the mitigating influence of integrative processes normally mediated by the RH.

In a third (partially overlapping) sample of children between 21 and 44 months of age, left temporal lesions were associated with slower progress in mean length of utterance in morphemes, based on free-speech samples. The bilateral frontal pattern reported earlier still was present but did not reach significance.

These findings for the first stages of language development suggest that left temporal cortex may be predisposed to play an important role in the emergence of language production, with equally large and highly correlated effects on both vocabulary and grammar. However, why should this area (which is largely sensory cortex) be so important for the development of expressive language? The authors suggest that sensory analysis may be much more important in the first stages of language production than it is later on, when speakers have already acquired efficient motor templates to match their linguistic input. In fact, the left temporal lobe is now known to play a particularly important role in the extraction of perceptual detail, in both the visual and the auditory modality (Fitch et al., 1993; Stiles & Thal, 1993; Martinez et al., 1996). This kind of detailed processing may be more important for learning than it is for fluent language use later. Later, we return to this possibility, called the *local detail hypothesis* (see heading of Conclusion).

Some related findings by Reilly et al. (1998) offer support for this interpretation. These authors looked at several aspects of narrative production in brain-injured children and normal controls between 3 and 12 years of age. They report that younger children with left temporal lesions were more delayed in grammatical measures, producing fewer complex syntactical structures and more morphological errors than did normal controls or brain-injured children whose lesions spared the left temporal lobe. However, this left temporal effect was not observed in older children (i.e., children between 7 and 12 years of age). In fact, these authors found absolutely no effects of lesion site or side among the older children, even though the younger and older samples of children had identical etiologies (i.e., lesions acquired before 6 months of age).

Although these patterns must be confirmed with a longitudinal study (wherein the sample children are followed across the period from infancy through childhood), the cross-sectional results reported by Bates et al. (1997) and Reilly et al. (1998) suggest that specific effects of lesion site may be restricted to the early years when language normally is acquired. By ages 5 to 7 years, children with congenital left temporal lesions seem to have found an alternative form of brain organization for language that is at least as good as the pattern displayed by children with other forms of brain injury (including unilateral damage to the RH) and only slightly worse than the pattern displayed by age-matched normal controls. We suggest some possible reasons for this developmental pattern later.

Lesion Size

The evidence we have reviewed so far seems to argue against innate and irreversible LH specialization for language and in favor of some constrained version of the equipotentiality view. In this regard, recall that Lashley's notorious equipotentiality principle was complemented by the principle of mass action, which predicted a monotonic and (perhaps) linear drop in performance as a function of lesion size. Obviously, at some level, this theory has to be true, with removal of the entire brain as the limiting case. However, in contrast with Lashley's conclusion for lesion studies of rats, studies of humans and other primates have yielded surprisingly little evidence for a monotonic relationship between lesion size and cognitive outcomes.

An animal model for the marginal effects of lesion size may be found in studies of nonhuman primates. A review of more than 200 lesion studies by Irle (1990) revealed a significant curvilinear relationship between lesion size and reacquisition of skills in monkeys. Specifically, the worst performance of all occurs in monkeys with midsized lesions; significantly better performance is observed with small lesions (no surprise) or with lesions involving up to 60% of the brain (a very big surprise). Irle explained this unexpected finding by proposing the "fresh-start hypothesis." Put in the simplest possible terms, the author suggested that animals with midsized lesions persist in trying to solve familiar problems with familiar but damaged tissue (i.e., with broken parts), whereas animals with larger lesions are forced to find new solutions, using undamaged areas of the brain that would not ordinarily participate in those tasks.

Although human and monkey studies do agree that lesion size effects are surprisingly small, at least in unilateral cases (Goodglass, 1993; Naeser et al., 1984), the human developmental literature provides limited support for Irle's predicted curvilinear effect. Most studies that have looked at lesion size as a variable have found no relationship with language or cognitive measures. Banich et al., (1990) and Levine et al., (1987) do report a negative effect of lesion size, but this result was restricted to cases with acquired lesions (i.e., no effect of lesion size in the congenital sample). Because these studies have used linear statistics to examine the relationship between lesion size and outcome, detecting nonlinear effects of the sort proposed by Irle would be difficult for them. One study by the San Diego group does report a significant curvilinear relationship between language outcome and lesion size, with the greatest language delays observed in infants with midsized lesions (Thal et al., 1991). However, this effect no longer was significant (although it was in the same direction) in a subsequent study by the same group with a larger sample of infants (Bates et al., 1997).

Until better volumetric measures are available to assess lesion size in and across areas, detecting the predicted nonlinear effect with any reliability probably will prove fairly difficult; what, after all, is the correct definition of *middle-sized*? However, a recent study by Isaacs et al. (1996) provided indirect support for some version of the fresh-start hypothesis. These authors examined the relationship between hand preference and ear preference in a dichotic listening task in a large sample of children and adolescents with a history of early focal brain injury. Results indicated that children who are markedly impaired in use of the right hand are more likely to show a left-ear advantage in the dichotic listening task. The authors interpreted this finding to support the idea that larger lesions in the LH (associated with greater right-hand weakness) encourage a switch to RH mediation of language.

Their conclusion is compatible also with a classic report by Rasmussen and Milner (1977), based on sodium amytal tests of adults with a history of congenital LH damage. Note that all these subjects are candidates for neurosurgery to correct intractable seizures, typically due to abnormalities in the left temporal lobe. Hence, possibly their results would not generalize to the majority of individuals with congenital damage (including the cases that we have reviewed here). Nevertheless, their findings are fairly interesting and important for the issues we have raised in this chapter.

The sodium amytal test (also called the *Wada test*) involves temporary paralysis of one hemisphere while the patient performs one or more language tasks (e.g., naming pictures or repeating words). If subjects are unable to perform a task while one hemisphere is paralyzed, one may conclude that the task usually is mediated by that hemisphere. Only 40% of the individuals in this study demonstrated clear evidence for RH mediation of language (i.e., only 40% had switched to the right). Another 40% still were left-dominant for language. The remaining 20% actually showed a split in hemispheric specialization, suggesting that one language task is mediated by the LH and another is mediated by the RH.

For a subsample of these cases, lesion size and location were established with some precision during subsequent neurosurgery. Results suggested that RH mediation of language in the Wada test was more likely in individuals with larger LH lesions involving the perisylvian areas (including the parietal, temporal, and frontal lobes). This result is compatible with the idea that larger lesions force a switch in mediation and, of course, with the traditional belief that perisylvian areas are especially important for language. Interestingly, however, a switch in mediation of language from LH to RH did not necessarily entail a change in linguistic performance, at least not at the level at which language can be assessed in a Wada test.

Seizures

Seizure conditions come in different varieties. Infantile seizures are relatively common (especially febrile seizures) and can disappear after a few episodes. More persistent seizure conditions can be controlled by drugs, but these drugs may have side effects that complicate interpretation of language and cognitive delays. Although severe seizure conditions undoubtedly are associated with a structural abnormality at some level, often no evidence supports a localized lesion (i.e., areas of the brain may be "epileptogenic" or seizure-prone even though no radiological evidence can demonstrate frank structural damage). Some seizure conditions are so severe that they cannot be controlled pharmacologically; in many of these cases, children undergo surgery to remove all or part of the damaged hemisphere. Of course, the site of the surgical lesion is known in cases of this kind, but some of the confounds associated with a seizure history remain (including the possibility of bilateral damage; Gadian et al., 1996).

In the samples studied by the San Diego group, few effects of seizure condition have been reported. However, seizure cases constitute a relatively small subset of this sample, and because the San Diego group recruits most of their subjects in the first months of life, many of the seizure cases included in their studies may be transient in nature. Bates et al. (1997) looked for seizure effects in their study of early language development and found no seizure effects of any kind. We also have compared children with and without a mild seizure history in the IQ sample described earlier and found no significant differences. Children without a seizure history obtained mean scores of 96.8 on full-scale IQ, 98.6 on verbal IQ, and 95.7 on performance IQ; children with a seizure history obtained mean scores of 90.8 for full-scale IQ, 94.1 for verbal IQ, and 89.6 for performance IQ. Although all are in the predicted direction, none of these differences even approach significance by a one-tailed t-test ($P > .33$ in all three comparisons).

However, other studies show that persistent seizure conditions can make a very large contribution to language and cognitive outcomes in children with unilateral brain injury. In fact, seizure effects appear to be larger and more consistent than are effects of lesion side, site, or size. The studies cited earlier by Vargha-Khadem et al. (1992) and Muter et al. (1997) suggested that performance IQ is somewhat lower for children with focal brain injury as compared with normal controls, including children who are seizure-free; however, verbal IQ is below normal only for the children with seizures, independent of lesion side. This picture has been confirmed and extended in a more recent study by Vargha-Khadem et al. using a sample of more than 300 hemiplegic children (Vargha-Khadem, personal communication, July 1996).

At present, we cannot say whether the negative effects of seizures are due to the seizure condition itself (i.e., the problem of learning before and after a neural firestorm) or to negative effects of the drugs that are used to control seizures in many of these children with unilateral brain injury. Focal seizure conditions often are associated with temporal lobe pathology, including (in some cases) bilateral damage only evident with advanced forms of functional brain imagery (see Gadian et al., 1996). Hence, the effect of seizures could be an indirect effect of lesion site, including bilateral damage in some cases. We hasten to add that the converse is not necessarily true. Bates et al. (1997) conducted analyses to determine whether their left temporal effect on expressive language in children with congenital injuries was related to presence or absence of a seizure history and found no relationship. Once again, however, we underscore that the small group of children with seizure disorders in their infant sample may be atypical of the seizure cases included in other studies. This clearly is a matter that deserves further study.

Finally, although clearly seizure conditions or anticonvulsant medication exacerbate the effects of early focal brain injury (and are the only clear culprit in some studies), we must stress again that residual effects of unilateral injury still are observed in some children without a seizure history. The data presented here for the Rome and San Diego groups testify to the wide range of outcomes observed in children who are seizure-free—outcomes that appear to be largely independent of lesion side or site in children older than 5 to 7 years of age. This brings us to our last and perhaps most important issue for a developmental audience.

Effects of Age and Timing

Developmental studies can be distinguished from the rest of neuropsychology and neurolinguistics by their focus on timing and change over time (Bates & Elman, 1993; Elman et al., 1996). Hence this review appropriately ends with a consideration of the effects of age and timing on language outcomes in children with unilateral injuries. The review of these developmental effects contains three parts: time of lesion onset, time elapsed since lesion onset, and age at time of testing.

Time of Lesion Onset The question of lesion timing is central to arguments about equipotentiality. As noted earlier, Lenneberg's proposals regarding equipotentiality and the critical period for language rested on the assumption that plasticity decreases with progressive cortical specialization. Although Lenneberg himself took no stand on the actual shape of this function, some proponents of the critical-period view have argued—by analogy to claims in the literature on critical periods for bird song—for a sharp nonlinear drop in the capacity for language learning at some key point in development (for discussions, see Elman et al., 1996; Oyama, 1993). Further, the same nonlinear function is assumed (implicitly or explicitly) to govern recovery of a first language in children with unilateral injuries and to govern success in second-language learning in children who are neurologically intact. In fact, recent evidence on second-language learning does not provide support for this kind of "learning catastrophe," but it does suggest the possible presence of a constant, monotonic drop with age in the ability to acquire the fine morphophonological details of a second language (Johnson & Newport, 1993). Therefore, we might ask whether a similar monotonic function would hold for recovery from unilateral brain injury.

Two points along this putative recovery function are beyond dispute. First, infants with congenital LH lesions go on to acquire language abilities far in advance of the abilities displayed by adults with equivalent injuries. What is the shape of the developmental function that connects these two points? Is it monotonic (i.e., a constant decrease in long-term outcomes with age of lesion onset)? Further, if it is monotonic, is it linear or nonlinear? If it is nonlinear, what is the "point of no return" (i.e., the point after which it becomes much more difficult to recover language)? Very few empirical tests measure this important question, and the few that have been conducted yield complex and potentially contradictory results.

Woods (1980), Woods and Carey (1979), and Woods and Teuber (1973, 1978) reported some disturbance in speech functions after LH damage. In addition, Woods (1980) noted that the interacting effects of lesion side were different for verbal and performance IQ and varied with age of onset. Lesions to the LH resulted in significant lowering of *both* verbal and performance IQ, regardless of onset age. RH children whose lesions were acquired before 1 year of age showed a similar across-the-board delay. However, RH children whose injuries occurred after 1 of age were delayed significantly only on performance IQ, leaving verbal IQ at normal levels.

A somewhat different pattern of interactions is reported by Riva et al. (1986). Their RH children scored selectively lower on performance IQ measures but spared on verbal IQ measures regardless of lesion onset time. In other words, these authors failed to replicate the age-specific effects of RH damage reported by Woods. Riva et al. did observe across-the-board delays in both performance and verbal IQ tests in LH children whose lesions occurred before 1 year of age (in line with Woods' results), but children whose LH lesions occurred after 1 year of age were indistinguishable from normal controls (in contrast with Woods' results). Note that the latter finding also runs directly contrary to the monotonic drop in plasticity proposed by Lenneberg (1967).

As noted earlier, this literature is plagued by unavoidable confounds between etiology and age of lesion onset. It is limited also by the small sample sizes that have been adopted in most studies of the focal lesion population. Uncovering the "true" function connecting recovery of function with age of lesion onset will require very large and homogeneous samples of children with early focal brain injury. The largest sample that has been studied to date from this point of view comes from an ongoing project by Vargha-Khadem et al. involving more than 300 children and adolescents with congenital or acquired lesions (with or without seizure conditions) and more than 100 normal controls. Figure 23.8 presents verbal and performance IQ scores for a subset of cases from this project (Vargha-Khadem, unpublished data, July 1996): 161 children with and without a seizure history, with lesion onsets between birth and adolescence. In each figure, the group is divided into congenital cases (lesion onset in the pre- or perinatal period); early onset (between 6 months and 4 years of age); and late onset (between 4 and 10 years of age). Data are plotted separately for children with and without a

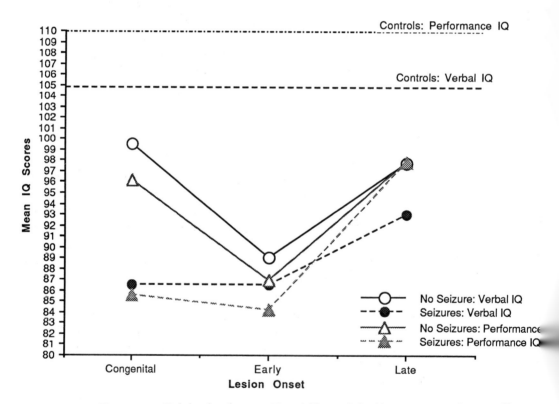

Figure 23.8 Verbal and performance IQ in children with focal brain injury, as a function of lesion onset and seizure status.

seizure history. The flat lines in the figure represent performance by normal controls on verbal and performance IQ measures, respectively.

Results are fairly surprising, providing no evidence whatsoever for the monotonic drop in plasticity predicted by Lenneberg (1967). First, figure 23.8 shows that mean verbal IQ scores for children without seizures are lowest with lesion onsets in the midrange (mean, 89), a statistically reliable U-shaped function that does not jibe with any version of the critical period hypothesis. In fact, this seizure-free subgroup is the only one that differs significantly from normal controls in post hoc tests. By contrast, verbal IQ scores are significantly lower than are scores for normal controls in all the age groups with seizures; post hoc tests for these children revealed no significant difference among any of the three lesion-onset subgroups, although figure 23.8 clearly demonstrates that verbal IQs are somewhat higher for the late-onset cases, against the critical period hypothesis.

A similar story emerges for performance IQ. For children without seizures, figure 23.8 shows that the lowest scores (mean, 87) again are observed in children whose lesion onsets occur in the middle childhood range. In fact, post hoc tests reveal that these children fall significantly below all the other seizure-free groups (i.e., below congenital cases, late-onset cases, and normal controls). For children who do have seizures, performance IQ scores are reliably below normal controls in all subgroups. However, the worst scores are associated with lesion onset before four years of age (i.e., the congenital and middle groups), providing no evidence for the expected monotonic drop in plasticity.

Although these results are fairly surprising in view of the assumption that plasticity drops monotonically with age, they are compatible with an equally puzzling finding reported by Goodman and Yude (1996). In a population-based survey of IQ scores in children with hemiplegia, they reported a mean full-scale IQ of 87 in 221 congenital cases (lesion onset before 1 month of age), compared with a mean IQ of 68 in 37 children whose lesions were acquired between 1 and 60 months of age, and a mean of 92 in the 7 cases in their sample with lesions acquired after 60 months. This inverted U-shaped function was statistically significant despite the huge variations in sample size in the three lesion-onset groups. No easy explanations account for these unexpected findings, and a good possibility is that unavoidable confounds between etiology and age of lesion onset play some role. At the very least, however, we are forced to conclude that Lenneberg's progressive-specialization hypothesis is much too simple.

Further problems for the progressive-specialization hypothesis have been raised by a recent case study of a boy who had Sturge-Weber syndrome and underwent left hemidecortication at 8.5 years of age (Vargha-Khadem et al., 1996). This child (Alex) failed to develop any expressive language prior to his surgery, beyond one correctly articulated word (*"mumma"*), a handful of sounds used consistently to refer to objects (e.g., *"oof"* for *shoe*), and vowel-like approximations for the numbers between 2 and 5. Testing Alex was difficult on most formal language measures, but results from the British Picture Vocabulary Scales suggested that he had a receptive vocabulary equivalent to a child of between 3 and 4 years of age and was able to follow simple commands. On nonverbal intelligence scales, he also achieved mental age scores between 2 and 4 years, depending on the test used. Alex showed little progress for the first few months after surgery, but shortly after the termination of anticonvulsant medication, he made a series of dramatic breakthroughs. Within a few months, he was speaking in full sentences.

Alex's language, motor, and cognitive developments were followed on a regular basis between 9 and 15 years of age, with evidence for consistent progress throughout this period. By the end of the study, he still scored in the retarded range on both verbal IQ (score, 59; mental age, 7 years, 4 months) and performance IQ (score, 50; mental age, $6\frac{1}{2}$ years). His motor abilities returned to their presurgical level soon after the surgery, with little additional improvement. Specifically, his right arm and leg are markedly weaker and smaller than the left, but he does have considerable control over the limbs on both sides (e.g., he is able to run and to kick a ball with his right leg); various neurological indices suggest that the left and right sides are controlled by separate neural pathways, suggesting a significant degree of plastic reorganization of motor control during the first years of life.

However, Alex still has marked difficulty with complex movements of the mouth and tongue, a factor that places an upper limit on the development of fluent speech. Despite this limitation, his language abilities on standardized language tests at the end of the study were equivalent to those of a normal child between 8 and 9 years of age. Alex still makes some errors in articulation, although his speech is fairly intelligible, clear, and fluent. His weakest areas within language include performance on tests of phonological awareness (which are highly correlated with reading ability, a skill that Alex had not yet mastered) and comprehension of complex syntax. Vargha-Khadem et al. note that Alex's level of performance on phonological awareness and complex syntax is compatible with his mental age and memory limitations. In fact, it is interesting that Alex actually scores much better on measures of language and auditory memory than he does on many visuospatial tasks.

What are the implications of this case for the critical period hypothesis? The authors note that some receptive language abilities were in place during the first years of life, even though Alex was virtually mute before age 9. Hence, we cannot conclude from this case that language acquisition can begin (in its entirety) after age 9. However, Alex's remarkable recovery does prove that the RH provides an adequate substrate for the development of expressive language, a potential that still is in place as late as age 9 years. An open question is whether this potential for expressive language can be maintained past puberty (e.g., the period in which famous "wild child" cases, such as Genie and Chelsea, were discovered; Curtiss, 1977, 1989).

Integrating these results for Alex with the nonmonotonic effects of lesion onset in figure 23.8, we must conclude that the function governing loss of plasticity for language still is unknown. Indeed, we may be faced with a situation in which plasticity for language waxes and wanes more than once across the course of development, in patterns incompatible with any theory that posits a single cause or a single developmental window.

Years Since Lesion Onset   In cross-sectional studies, time of lesion onset often is confounded with the amount of time that has elapsed since the lesion occurred. Garden-variety processes of learning and development undoubtedly play a role in the recovery process, so that (ceteris paribus) more time since lesion onset ought to translate into greater recovery relative to age-matched normal controls.

Interestingly, the literature to date suggests that the opposite may be true (i.e., that children with early focal brain injury actually may fall further behind age-matched controls as they grow older. Banich et al. (1990) and Levine et al. (1987) have provided some evidence for a decline in both verbal and performance IQ in a cross-sectional study of children with congenital injuries. Specifically, children younger than age 6 remained close to age-appropriate norms, but children older than age 6 were significantly more impaired. The authors suggested that the effects of focal brain injury may become more evident in later childhood and adolescence because the tasks that are used to measure normal language and cognition in this age range are more demanding.

Examination of this issue in more detail is possible using the San Diego and Rome samples of children with congenital lesions described earlier. (For our purposes here, data from the two groups are combined). Figure 23.9 presents a scatterplot illustrating the relationship between full-scale IQ and age at testing for all 76 children. The negatively accelerating line in the figure represents the linear relationship between chronological age and IQ in this cross-sectional sample. Although this line follows the direction predicted by Banich et al. (1990) and Levine et al. (1987)—lower scores with age—it represents a nonsignificant correlation of $-.18$ ($P < .06$). The low correlation is due, of course, to the broad band of variation observed throughout the age range from 3 to 14 years. A quick examination of figure 23.9 would suggest that this variance decreases with time, but this impression is an artifact of sample size (i.e., more children in the sample are between 3 and 7 years). To determine whether the absence of a linear effect masked some kind of systematic nonlinear effect, we tried fitting the data in the figure to a variety of different curvilinear functions, but this did little to improve the amount of variance for which one could account. In short, no compelling evidence in this data set demonstrates an age-related decrease in IQ among children with congenital brain injury, although trends in that direction are seen.

We do not have a complete explanation for the difference between our observations and those of Banich et al. (1990). One possibility might be the hidden effect of selection bias. In our experience, families with children who

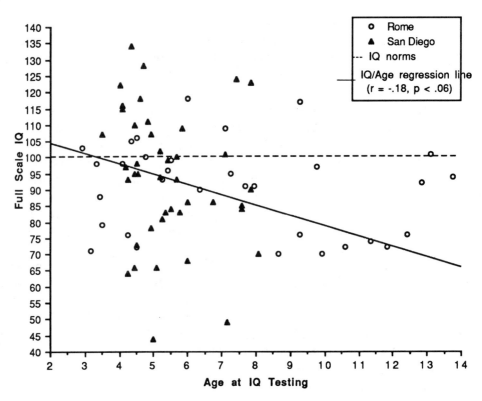

Figure 23.9 Relation between IQ and age at testing for children with congenital focal brain injury.

have suffered from early focal brain injury tend to lose interest in neuro-psychological studies if their children are doing very well. This disinterest is more likely to occur later in childhood, after parents have an opportunity to observe their child's performance in an academic setting. For this reason, older children with persistent learning problems may be overrepresented in some cross-sectional studies of the focal lesion population, an artifact that can vary in intensity from one study to another. We agree, however, that the trend proceeds consistently in the direction of a drop in scores, consistent with the argument by Levine et al. that the compensatory strategies adopted by children with focal brain injury may reach a ceiling as testing demands increase with age. Finally, another possibility is that some of this drop in performance reflects the cumulative effect of ongoing seizures in a subset of these cases.

Age at Testing Studies of time before and after onset are confounded with each other and with a third variable: the age and developmental level of the child at the time when testing occurs. In fact, investigators have made heavy use of standardized measures, such as verbal and performance IQ, precisely because these factors are among the only currently available measures offering a single score for children from age 3 through adolescence. However, this single score may be a comforting illusion, because the content and meaning of any IQ test change markedly across this age range (McCall et al., 1977).

The best way around this problem is to assess children with measures appropriate for their developmental level and to compare performance in the same sample of children longitudinally, across the age range of interest. This approach is the only sure way to determine whether individual children are catching up or falling behind relative to normal controls in any particular domain. Given the rarity of children with early focal brain injury and the difficulties involved in long-term longitudinal designs, attaining this ideal has proved very difficult.

At present, longitudinal evidence is restricted almost entirely to short-term studies across a restricted developmental period, involving single cases or very small groups. The one exception is the study by Muter et al. (1997), who found no evidence for a longitudinal change in mean IQ across a 2-year period in 20 cases of congenital brain injury. However, because these children were all between ages 3 and 7 at the first time point, their conclusions do not necessarily contradict the later drop in IQ suggested by the cross-sectional studies of Banich et al. (1990) and Levine et al. (1987).

In the handful of longitudinal studies that have been reported to date, some children do make spectacular recoveries, some maintain a constant distance from their age mates, and still others continue to lag further behind—at least across the short developmental distance that is represented in any single study. We illustrate this point with three short-term longitudinal studies of language development from 1 to 4 years. Because this is the age range in which the fundamentals of language are laid down, we have some chance of capturing important developmental events even within a short-term longitudinal study.

Marchman et al. (1991) looked at the development of babbling up to 22 months of age in 5 children with focal brain injury, compared with 10 younger normal controls matched on a free-speech measure of expressive vocabulary size. The focal lesion children included four LH cases (two with purely frontal lesions, two with posterior lesions) and one RH case (with frontal damage only). Figure 23.10 illustrates the different developmental trajectories displayed by the brain-injured children.

All five children were delayed in production of consonants prior to the appearance of meaningful speech. Two of the frontal cases (one LH and one RH) showed marked recovery just before the point at which meaningful speech finally appears and performed well within the normal range after that point. A third case with left frontal damage showed a similar pattern after a somewhat longer delay. Hence, these three frontal cases appear to represent the kind of recovery often assumed to occur in the focal lesion population at some point in development. However, the two cases with left posterior damage remained far below normal in consonant production throughout the

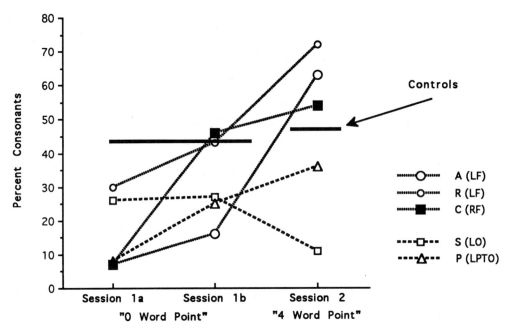

Figure 23.10 Proportions of vocalizations containing "true" consonants. (Adapted from figure 3 in the study by Marchman et al. 1991.)

study, even though they had finally (after a significant delay) begun to produce words.

A particularly optimistic example comes from a longitudinal study of free-speech development from 15 to 48 months (Feldman et al., 1992). All nine children in this study had congenital lesions, five LH (four parietal and one frontal) and four RH (one parietooccipital, one frontoparietal, one temporoparietal, and one parietal only). Most of these cases showed initial lags in expressive vocabulary, followed by normal or near-normal progress in the emergence of grammar from age 20 to 30 months. Figure 23.11 illustrates progress in grammar, indexed by mean length of utterance in morphemes (MLU). The white zone in this figure represents performance one standard deviation to either side of the mean for normal controls, the gray zone indicates performance between 1 and 2 standard deviations from the mean, and the dark zones indicate performance outside this range. Seven of the nine cases spent most of their time safely ensconced within or above the normal (white) zone throughout the course of the study. Performance well below normal (the lower dark zone) was observed in only two cases, one LH and one RH. Despite their initial lags, these two children did make significant progress over time, and both had inched into the gray zone by the conclusion of the study.

A final example comes from Dall 'Oglio et al. (1994), who carried out a longitudinal study of early language and cognitive development in six Italian

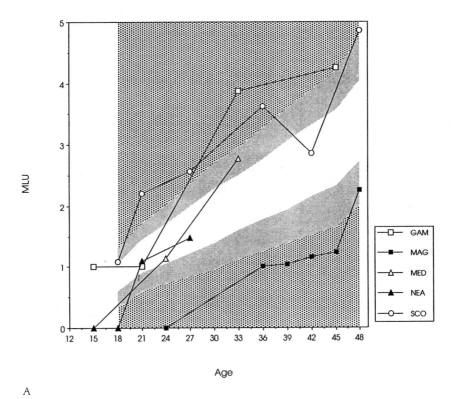

A

Figure 23.11 Mean length of utterance (MLU) as a function of age in children with (A) LH damage or (B) RH damage. (Adapted from figures 1 and 2 in the study by Feldman et al. 1992.)

infants with unilateral injuries. Although the period covered by the study and the number of sessions varied from child to child, at least two data points were available for each case. Four of the children had LH injuries (one frontal only, one frontoparietal, one parietal only, and one temporoparietal) and two had RH injuries (both frontal only). Four of the children suffered from seizure conditions, two were seizure-free (although one of these cases, EF, did display electroencephalographic abnormalities). Figure 23.12 illustrates progress in expressive vocabulary for these six children, based on an Italian version of the MCDI (Fenson et al., 1993; Caselli & Casadio, 1995). (Solid lines refer to children who are seizure-free, dotted lines to children with seizures; the open symbols are used for RH cases and filled symbols for LH cases.) Note that these are percentile scores, so that data for children whose vocabulary grew consistently over time would be reflected in a flat line, indicating that their standing relative to normal controls does not change with development; by the same token, a sharp shift upward would indicate improvement in the children's relative performance, and a sharp shift downward would indicate that the children were beginning to lag further and further behind. A quick glance at Figure 23.12 shows that every logically possible pattern can be observed in children with congenital brain injuries.

Bates et al.: Neural Mediation of Language Development

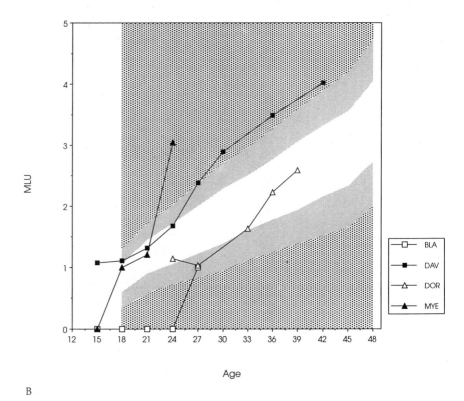

B

Figure 23.11 (continued)

Case CD had a large left frontoparietal lesion, but she was seizure-free. She started out well above normal at 19 months in expressive vocabulary and performed near the top of the normal scale by 26 months (a profile, incidentally, very close to the profile displayed by her twin sister). Excellent performance (albeit with a negative slope over time) was also displayed by AB, who had a right frontal lesion and an accompanying seizure condition.

By contrast, case MN has a large LH lesion involving the temporal and parietal lobes and had a persistent seizure condition. MN made very little progress across the course of the study, with scores at the percentile floor throughout the period from 15 to 34 months. An equally pessimistic profile was displayed by EF, who had a lesion restricted to the parietal lobe (sparing the frontal and temporal lobes, presumed sites of the "language areas") and had no seizure condition (despite electroencephalographic abnormalities).

The two most interesting profiles from a developmental perspective are displayed by cases GL and QR. GL has a lesion restricted to the left frontal lobe, with occasional resistant partial seizures. He started off making very slow progress in word production, with a decline in status from the twentieth to below the tenth percentile between 14 and 27 months. However, in only 2 months' time (27–29 months), he displayed a remarkable burst in total vocabulary, with a change in status (relative to normal controls) from

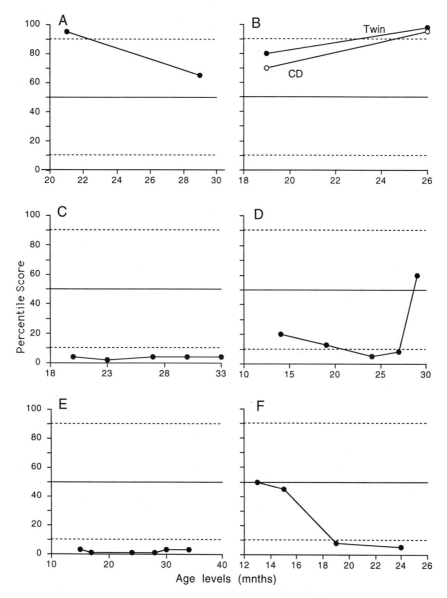

Figure 23.12 Centile scores for word production: (A) AB, (B) CD, (C) EF, (D) GL, (E) MN, and (F) QR. (Adapted from figure 1 in the study by Dall'Oglio et al. 1994.)

below the tenth percentile to well above the median. This kind of sharp acceleration is compatible with the idea that a new form of brain organization for language has emerged, permitting GL to get around obstacles to speech production that seemed to plague him for the first 2 years.

By contrast, QR was a right frontal case with partial seizures that proved resistant to drug therapy. Despite these problems (which had been with her from age 5 months), QR started off at 13 months with word production scores that placed her right at the median for normal controls. Her scores had dropped slightly by 15 months, plunged below the tenth percentile by 19 months, and stayed there until the conclusion of the study (when QR was 24 months old). QR's sharply decelerating profile provided an unhappy complement to the spectacular recovery displayed by GL.

Dall'Oglio et al. (1994) also reported on progress in nonverbal cognition for the same six children. For the most part, their data indicated that language and cognitive development travel together in these children. This was particularly clear for QR, whose cognitive and language scores dropped precipitously together. The one exception was GL, who displayed rather mediocre performance on several scales of infant intelligence despite his (eventual) burst in expressive language.

Longitudinal studies using age-appropriate measures provide a much closer and more veridical view of change in the focal-lesion population, but they also prove that the wide variability displayed by this population is an inescapable fact that must be handled in any theory of the neural mechanisms that mediate language learning. Seizure conditions clearly are a negative indicator, but their presence does not guarantee a negative outcome, nor are children who are seizure-free guaranteed a normal course of development. Lesion side and lesion site play no clear-cut role in the diverse profiles observed in figures 23.10 through 23.12. Interestingly, in light of results reported by Bates et al. (1997), the worst cases tend to have left temporal involvement (case P in Marchman et al. (1991); see figure 23.10; case MN in Dall'Oglio et al. 1994; see figure 23.12); none of the cases studied by Feldman et al. (1994) had lesions involving the left temporal cortex. However, exceptions are found to this generalization as well (e.g., case S with a left occipital lesion in Marchman et al.; see figure 23.10; case EF with a left parietal lesion in Dall'Oglio et al.; see figure 23.12). The contribution of neurological factors to language outcomes appears to be probabilistic in nature, evident only when sample sizes are large enough to detect a probabilistic effect.

CONCLUSION

We began this chapter by reviewing the two theoretical extremes that have characterized the literature on language outcomes in children with unilateral brain injuries: equipotentiality and irreversible determinism. Most of the evidence that we have described seems to favor the equipotentiality view. And yet, as noted at the outset, the overwhelming evidence for LH mediation of key language functions in adults cannot be explained unless we assume that the two hemispheres differ in some way starting from the beginning of life. Furthermore, some of the evidence that we have reviewed does show that expressive language grows more slowly in some children with LH lesions. This is particularly likely to occur if the lesions are acquired later in childhood. It also occurs in some children with congenital lesions involving the left temporal lobe, although this pattern is most evident during the early stages of language learning, before 5 to 7 years of age. On the basis of these findings, we tentatively suggest that the LH bias involves "soft" constraints that (1) are restricted primarily to the left temporal lobe, (2) are probabilistic in nature (i.e., they are not deterministic), and (3) can be overcome (i.e., they are not irreversible).

What kind of "soft" constraint could explain this peculiar set of facts? As Elman et al. (1996) discussed in some detail, that the left hemisphere comes into the world with "hard-wired" linguistic knowledge is fairly unlikely. This kind of "representational nativism" is incompatible with 15 years of evidence in developmental neurobiology regarding neural plasticity and the role of experience in determining cortical specialization and incompatible with the fact that children with severe LH injuries usually go on to acquire language abilities in the normal range. Elman et al. (1996) proposed instead that genetic constraints on cognitive outcomes are much less direct, including gross constraints on cortical architecture (i.e., from where does the information to a particular region come?) and local constraints on the kinds of computations that can be carried out in a particular zone (e.g., variations in speed, packing density, types of neural transmitters, degree of "fan in" and "fan out").

In other words, the different regions of the brain are not equipotential at birth, but they are "pluripotential." No innate knowledge exists at the cortical level, but innate limitations govern the kinds of knowledge that could be learned in a given region and govern the computations that the region can handle best. Research on brain development in other species has taught us that the process of cortical specialization involves an initial overproduction of elements (neurons and connections), with the winners and losers determined through processes of competition and recruitment (Changeux & Danchin, 1976; Huttenlocher, 1979, 1990; Edelman, 1987; Huttenlocher & de Courten, 1987; Rakic, 1988; Bates et al., 1992; Smith & Thelen, 1993; Quartz & Sejnowsky, 1995). Under normal circumstances, areas that have a slight edge in carrying out a particular kind of computation usually win the rights to processing in that domain (similar to the processes of competition and recruitment that lead tall children into basketball). However, if those areas are damaged in some way, other regions with access to the relevant inputs can take over the task (O'Leary & Stanfield, 1985, 1989; Killackey, 1990; O'Leary, 1993; Webster et al., 1995; Courchesne et al., 1995), often performing at (or only slightly below) normal levels, depending on the measure.

If this proposal is correct, we should ask what kinds of computational biases might explain the LH effects that some investigators have observed in the focal lesion population. As we noted earlier, Bates et al. (1997) did not find evidence in support of the idea that left frontal cortex plays a special role in language learning (i.e., Broca's area). Instead, unilateral damage to either the left or the right frontal region results in a greater delay in expressive language, an effect that appears to be restricted to the period between 19 and 31 months, when most normal children show a dramatic acceleration in vocabulary growth coupled with the onset of grammar. By contrast, Bates et al. (1997) did find systematic evidence for an asymmetrical effect of damage to the temporal region. This bias is evident across a variety of expressive language measures (both vocabulary and grammar), from 10 months to approximately 5 to 7 years of age. After that point, the left temporal effect no longer is evident, at least within the cross-sectional samples that these investigators have studied so far. Although possibly a residual effect of left temporal damage would show up in older children with further testing using a different set of measures, it would have to be very subtle to elude detection across a broad range of lexical and grammatical measures used by Reilly et al. (1998) and Kempler et al. (1996).

To explain the left temporal effect, Bates et al. (1997) pointed out that left temporal lesions also are implicated in particular forms of spatial cognition, causing marked deficits in children and adults in the ability to analyze the more detailed aspects of a visual display (Stiles & Thal, 1993; Stiles, 1995; Martinez et al., 1996). In nonhuman primates, lesion studies have shown that specific areas within the temporal lobe are important for object memory (the so-called what-is-it system; Mishkin et al., 1983; Webster et al., 1995). Possibly humans have evolved between the temporal lobes of the two hemispheres in these aspects of perception and cognition asymmetries greater than those usually observed in other primates, with left temporal regions predisposed to handle perceptual detail. If this "local detail" hypothesis is correct and applies to both auditory and visual processing, possibly the specific effects of left temporal damage for language may not be specific to language at all.

However, if this is the case, why does the left temporal effect disappear after 5 to 7 years of age? Perhaps it disappears because it was neither large nor irreversible, so that gradually it is eliminated with the passage of time and the increased specializations achieved by alternative cortical areas. However, another possibility exists. We know that the medial structures of the temporal lobe play a very important role in learning and memory (including the hippocampus, the amygdala, and perhaps some of the surrounding tissue in entorhinal cortex), although the general assumption is that these are not the regions in which learned information is stored in its final form. If the left temporal lesions that lead to initial delays in language learning include these medial temporal zones, we would expect a significant and selective delay in learning itself, which may not be evident after a function finally (slowly and painfully) is acquired.

What is the neurological basis of this claim? Case studies of children with bilateral medial hippocampal injuries provide evidence for massive and irreversible forms of anterograde amnesia [i.e., an inability to form new memories despite preservation of memories that were formed before the injury occurred (Vargha-Khadem et al., 1996)]. In contrast with bilateral lesions to lateral areas of temporal cortex, which show remarkable plasticity in infant primates (Webster et al., 1995), bilateral lesions to the medial temporal areas in infant monkeys lead to forms of amnesia just as serious and just as irreversible in infants as they are in adults (Bachevalier & Mishkin, 1993).

In other words, variations in the amount of plasticity can be observed from one brain region to another. Bachevalier (1996) suggested that these differences may be due to the way in which those areas are wired from the very beginning. For example, the plastic zones on the lateral surface of the temporal lobe include the final receiving stations for auditory and visual information and presumably can be replaced if the relevant information is rerouted to another resting place. By contrast, the irreplaceable zones on the medial surface of the temporal lobe are wired uniquely to receive and forward information from many different parts of the brain, a kind of wiring not available in other parts of the cortex.

In this regard, a recent study (Wood et al., 1996) used quantified MRI techniques to verify more diffuse forms of left temporal lobe pathology (including the hippocampus) in children with epilepsy. Their results suggest that this kind of unilateral temporal lobe damage is associated with deficits in verbal memory. These unilateral deficits are relatively subtle (i.e., they are not as debilitating as bilateral lesions to the hippocampal formation), but they continue to create difficulties in verbal learning and recall. Importantly, their findings also demonstrate a significant degree of dissociation between verbal memory and verbal IQ, suggesting that language learning and language use may be disrupted by different forms of temporal lobe pathology. This perspective suggests that possibly the left temporal effects observed by Bates et al. (1997) are due to cases in which the lesion has invaded these irreplaceable medial temporal structures, creating difficulties for children in learning new verbal material. However, once the material finally is learned (at a considerable delay), these memory structures no longer are as important as once they were. If this hypothesis is correct, we should not be surprised to find that left temporal effects on language are restricted to the first years of life, while language learning is still under way, and no longer are evident after that point.

Although this hypothesis is compatible with the behavioral facts and with animal models of temporal damage, it runs into difficulty when we consider the etiologies that usually lead to temporal damage in children. In particular, the middle cerebral artery strokes responsible for most temporal lesions usually spare the medial temporal structures. This fact is not a problem for the local detail hypothesis, which involves structures on the lateral surface of the temporal lobe that commonly are involved in middle cerebral artery infarctions. Ultimately, questions such as this can be settled by much more detailed specification of the lesions suffered by children with early unilateral brain injury. The variability that we have observed across all ages and measures also suggests that we are going to have to pool data from many different laboratories to achieve the statistical power necessary to control for all the factors that influence language outcomes in this population.

Our final point is that if Lashley and Lenneberg were right about equipotentiality, carrying out fine-grained neural imaging studies of brain-injured infants and children would be pointless. After all, it shouldn't matter where the lesion occurred. Conversely, if the irreversible-determinism view were correct, one could assume safely that brain organization for language is identical in children and adults. Under these circumstances, neural imaging studies of small, rare, and uncooperative children would be a waste of time and resources. We could learn all we needed to know by working with adult patients who are more numerous and render testing easier.

The results that we have reviewed in this chapter demonstrate that equipotentiality and irreversible determinism are both wrong—or, more conservatively, that they are correct about different aspects of the data. Although a great deal of evidence supports neural plasticity and a certain degree of plurifunctionality across cortical regions, areas of the brain do differ from the beginning of life in their basic wiring and in the kinds of computations that they are equipped to carry out. These patterns of specialization are related causally to the patterns that ultimately emerge in adults, but they are not the same. To understand how the initial state and the final state are related, we must take advantage of the available sophisticated tools for structural and functional brain imaging for use in human cognitive neuroscience and apply those tools to study how the neural mediation of language changes over time.

ACKNOWLEDGMENTS

The results described in this manuscript were obtained with support from the National Institutes of Health, National Institute of Neurological and Diseases and Stroke grant P50 NS22343 and National Institute on Deafness and Other Communication Disorders P50 DC01289-1351 to Elizabeth Bates, and by the Ospedale e Centro di Ricerca Bambin Gesù, Rome, Italy. Elizabeth Bates received support during manuscript preparation from NIDCD grant 2-R01-DC00216 and from the Institute of Psychology, National Council of Research, Via Nomentana 56, Rome, Italy.

We are especially grateful to Faraneh Vargha-Khadem for providing the unpublished data described herein and for her detailed comments on an earlier version of this chapter. Of course, any errors of fact or interpretation that may remain are entirely our responsibility.

NOTES

1. Language data were available for an additional three subjects for whom we do not have IQ scores; these three children will be included in the language analyses described later.

2. In the Aram studies (Aram et al., 1985, 1986, 1987) and in most of the studies by Riva et al. (Riva & Cazzaniga, 1986; Riva et al., 1986) different control groups always were used for the respective LH and RH groups, owing to marked differences between the two lesion groups in

age, gender, and social class. Although this is a defensible decision, the fact that LH and RH groups never were compared directly greatly complicates the interpretation of results.

3. Individual children within the Rome sample received only a subset of these five measures, depending on their age and developmental level, so that sample sizes vary across these five comparisons.

REFERENCES

Alajouanine, T., & Lhermitte, F. (1965). Acquired aphasia in children. *Brain, 88,* 653–662.

Aram, D., Ekelman, B., Rose, D., & Whitaker, H. (1985). Verbal and cognitive sequelae following unilateral lesions acquired in early childhood. *Journal of Clinical and Experimental Neuropsychology, 7,* 55–78.

Aram. D., Ekelman, B., & Whitaker, H. (1986). Spoken syntax in children with acquired unilateral hemisphere lesions. *Brain and Language, 27,* 75–100.

Aram, D., Ekelman, B., & Whitaker, H. (1987). Lexical retrieval in left- and right-brain-lesioned children. *Brain and Language, 28,* 61–87.

Aram, D. M., Meyers, S. C., & Ekelman, B. L. (1990). Fluency of conversational speech in children with unilateral brain lesions. *Brain and Language, 38*(1), 105–121.

Bachevalier, J. (1996, November). *The development of medial temporal lobe memory functions in monkeys.* A program in human development workshop: Brain and Cognitive Development. San Diego: University of California.

Bachevalier, J., & Mishkin, M. (1993). An early and a late developing system for learning and retention in infant monkeys. In M. Johnson *(Ed.,) Brain development and cognition: A reader* (pp. 195–207). Oxford: Blackwell.

Ballantyne, A. O., Scarvie, K. M., & Trauner, D. A. (1994). Verbal and performance IQ patterns in children after perinatal stroke. *Developmental Psychology, 10*(1), 39–50.

Banich, M., Levine, S., Kim, H., & Huttenlocher, P. (1990). The effects of developmental factors on IQ in hemiplegic children. *Neuropsychologia, 28*(1), 35–47.

Basser, L. (1962). Hemiplegia of early onset and the facutly of speech with special reference to the effects of hemispherectomy. *Brain, 85,* 427–460.

Bates, E., Bretherton, I., & Snyder, L. (1988). *From first words to grammar: Individual differences and dissociable mechanisms.* New York: Cambridge University Press.

Bates, E., Dale, P. S., & Thal, D. (1995). Individual differences and their implications for theories of language development. In P. Fletcher & B. MacWhinney (Eds.), *Handbook of child language* (pp. 96–151). Oxford: Blackwell.

Bates, E., & Elman, J. (1993). Connectionism and the study of change. In M. Johnson (Ed.), *Brain development and cognition: A reader* (pp. 623–642). Oxford: Blackwell.

Bates, E., Thal, D., Aram, D., Eisele, J., Nass, R., & Trauner, D. (1997). From first words to grammar in children with focal brain injury. *Developmental Neuropsychology* [special issue]. *13,* 275–343.

Bates, E., Thal, D., & Janowsky, J. (1992). Early language development and its neural correlates. In I. Rapin and S. Segalowitz (Eds.), *Handbook of neuropsychology: Vol. 7. Child neuropsychology* (pp. 69–110). Amsterdam: Elsevier.

Bialystok, E., & Hakuta, K. (1994). *In other words: The science and psychology of second-language acquisition.* New York: Basic Books.

Bishop, D. V. M. (1979). Comprehension in developmental disorders. *Developmental Medicine and Child Neurology, 21,* 225–238.

Bishop, D. V. M. (1983). Linguistic impairment after left hemidecortication for infantile hemiplegia? A reappraisal. *Quarterly Journal of Experimental Psychology, 35A,* 199–207.

Bishop, D. V. M. (1988). Can the right hemisphere mediate language as well as the left? A critical review of recent research. *Cognitive Neuropsychology, 5,* 353–367.

Bloom, L., Lightbown, L., & Hood, L. (1975). Structure and variation in child language. *Monographs of the Society for Research in Child Development, 40* (160).

Caplan, D. (1987). *Neurolinguistics and linguistic aphasiology: An introduction.* Cambridge: Cambridge University Press.

Caselli, M. C., & Casadio, P. (1995). *Il primo vocabolario del bambino: Guida all'uso del questionario MacArthur per la valutazione della comunicazione e del linguaggio nei primi anni di vita* [The child's first words: Guide to the use of the MacArthur questionnaire for the assessment of communication and language in the first years of life] (pp. 94–100). Milan: FrancoAngeli.

Changeux, J., & Danchin, A. (1976). Selective stabilization of developing synapses as a mechanism for the specification of neuronal networks. *Nature, 264,* 705–712.

Chomsky, N. (1975). *Reflections on language.* New York: Parthenon Press.

Courchesne, A., Townsend, J., & Chase, C. (1995). Neurodevelopmental principles guide research on developmental psychopathologies. In D. Cicchetti & D. Cohen (Eds.), *Developmental Psychopathologies* (pp. 195–226). New York: J. Wiley.

Curtiss, S. (1977). *Genie: A psycholinguistic study of a modern-day "Wild Child."* New York: Academic Press.

Curtiss, S. (1988). Abnormal language acquisition and the modularity of language. In F. Newmeyer (Ed.), *Linguistics: the Cambridge Survey II. Linguistic theory: Extensions and implications* (pp. 96–116). Cambridge: Cambridge University Press.

Curtiss, S. (1989). The independence and task specificity of language. In A. Bornstein & J. Bruner (Eds.), *Interaction in human development* (pp. 105–137). Hillsdale, NJ: Erlbaum.

Dall'Oglio, A., Bates, E., Volterra, V., DiCapua, M., & Pezzini, G. (1994). Early cognition, communication and language in children with focal brain injury. *Developmental Medicine and Child Neurology, 36,* 1076–1098.

Day, P. S., & Ulatowska, H. K. (1979). Perceptual, cognitive, and linguistic development after early hemispherectomy: Two case studies. *Brain and Language, 7,* 17–33.

Dennis, M. (1980). Capacity and strategy for syntactic comprehension after left or right hemidecortication. *Brain and Language, 10,* 287–317.

Dennis, M., & Kohn, B. (1975). Comprehension of syntax in infantile hemiplegics after cerebral hemidecortication. *Brain and Language, 2,* 472–482.

Dennis, M., Lovett, M., & Wiegel-Crump, C. (1981). Written language acquisition after left or right hemidecortication in infancy. *Brain and Language, 12,* 54–91.

Dennis, M., & Whitaker, H. A. (1976). Language acquisition following hemidecortication: Linguistic superiority of the left over the right hemisphere. *Brain and Language, 3,* 404–433.

Dennis, M., & Whitaker, H. (1977). Hemispheric equipotentiality and language acquisition. In S. J. Segalowitz & F. A. Gruber (Eds.), *Language development and neurological theory* (pp. 93–106). New York: Academic Press.

DeRenzi, F., & Faglioni, P. (1975). L'esame dei disturbi afasici di comprensione orale, mediante una versione abbreviata del test dei gettoni [The study of oral comprehension deficits in aphasia with a short form of the Token Test]. *Rivista di Patologia Nervosa Mentale, 96,* 252–269.

Dunn, L. M., & Dunn, L. M. (1981). *Peabody Picture Vocabulary Test–Revised.* Circle Pines, MN: American Guidance Service.

Edelman, G. M. (1987). *Neural Darwinism: The theory of neuronal group selection.* New York: Basic Books.

Eisele, J., & Aram, D. (1993). Differential effects of early hemisphere damage on lexical comprehension and production. *Aphasiology, 7*(5), 513–523.

Eisele, J., & Aram, D. (1994). Comprehension and imitation of syntax following early hemisphere damage. *Brain and Language, 46,* 212–231.

Eisele, J., & Aram, D. (1995). Lexical and grammatical development in children with early hemisphere damage: A cross-sectional view from birth to adolescence. In P. Fletcher & B. MacWhinney (Eds.), *The handbook of child language* (pp. 664–689). Oxford: Blackwell.

Elman, J., Bates, E., Johnson, M., Karmiloff-Smith, A., Parisi, D., & Plunkett, K. (1996). *Rethinking innateness: A connectionist perspective on development.* Cambridge, MA: MIT Press/Bradford Books.

Entus, A. (1977). Hemispheric asymmetry in processing of dichotically presented speech and nonspeech stimuli by infants. In S. Segalowitz & F. Gruber (Eds.), *Language development and neurological theory* (pp. 63–73). New York: Academic Press.

Feldman, H., Holland, A., Kemp, S., & Janosky, J. (1992). Language development after unilateral brain injury. *Brain and Language, 42,* 89–102.

Fenson, L., Dale, P., Reznick, J. S., Thal, D., Bates, E., Hartung, J., Pethick, S., & Reilly, J. (1993). *The MacArthur Communicative Development Inventories: User's guide and technical manual.* San Diego: Singular Publishing Group.

Fenson, L., Dale, P., Reznick, J. S., Bates, E., Thal, D., & Pethick, S. J. (1994). Variability in early communicative development. *Monographs of the Society for Research in Child Development, 59* (5, serial no. 242).

Fitch, R. H., Brown, C. P., O'Connor, K., & Tallal, P. (1993). Functional lateralization for auditory temporal processing in male and female rats. *Behavioral Neuroscience, 107*(5), 844–850.

Gadian, D., Isaacs, E., Cross, M., Connelly, G., Jackson, M., King, M., Neville, B., & Vargha-Khadem, F. (1996). Lateralization of brain function in childhood revealed by magnetic resonance spectroscopy. *Neurology, 46,* 974–977.

Gazzaniga, M. S., Bogen, J. E., & Sperry, R. W. (1962). Some functional effects of sectioning the cerebral commissures in man. *Proceedings of the National Academy of Sciences of the United States of America, 48,* 1765–1769.

Geschwind, N. (1965). Disconnexion syndromes in animals and man. *Brain, 88,* 585–644.

Geschwind, N., & Levitsky, W. (1968). Human brain: Left-right asymmetries in temporal speech region. *Science, 161,* 186–187.

Goldstein, K. (1948). *Language and language disturbances: Aphasic symptom complexes and their significance for medicine and theory of language.* New York: Grune & Stratton.

Goodglass, H. (1993). *Understanding aphasia.* San Diego: Academic Press.

Goodglass, H., & Kaplan, E. (1972). *The assessment of aphasia and related disorders.* Philadelpha: Lea & Febiger.

Goodman, R., & Yude, C. (1996). IQ and its predictors in childhood hemiplegia. *Developmental Medicine and Child Neurology, 38,* 881–890.

Head, H. (1926). *Aphasia and kindred disorders of speech.* Cambridge, UK: Cambridge University Press.

Hebb, D. O. (1949). *The organization of behavior: A neuropsychological theory.* New York: Wiley.

Hecaen, H. (1976). Acquired aphasia in children and the ontogenesis of hemispheric specialization. *Brain and Language, 3,* 113–134.

Hecaen, H. (1983). Acquired aphasia in children: Revisited. *Neuropsychologia, 21,* 587.

Huttenlocher, P. R. (1979). Synaptic density in human frontal cortex: Developmental changes and effects of aging. *Brain Research, 163,* 195–205.

Huttenlocher, P. R. (1990). Morphometric study of human cerebral cortex development. *Neuropsychologia, 28*(6), 517–527.

Huttenlocher, P. R., & de Courten, C. (1987). The development of synapses in striate cortex of man. *Human Neurobiology, 6,* 1–9.

Irle, E. (1990). An analysis of the correlation of lesion size, localization and behavioral effects in 283 published studies of cortical and subcortical lesions in old-world monkeys. *Brain Research Review, 15,* 181–213.

Isaacs, E., Christie, D., Vargha-Khadem, F., & Mishkin, M. (1996). Effects of hemispheric side of injury, age at injury, and presence of seizure disorder on funcitonal ear and hand asymmetries in hemiplegic children. *Neuropsychologia, 34,* 127–137.

Jackson, H. J. (1878). On affections of speech from disease of the brain. *Brain, 1,* 305–330.

Johnson, J. S., & Newport, M. (1989). Critical period effects in second language learning: The influence of maturational state on the acquisition of English as second language. *Cognitive Psychology, 21,* 60–99.

Kandel, E., Schwartz, J., & Jessell, T. (1995). *Essentials of neural science and behavior.* Norwalk, CT: Appleton & Lange.

Kempler, D., Metter, E. J., Jackson, C. A., Hanson, W. R., Riege, W., Mazziotta, J., & Phelps, M. (1988). Disconnection in cerebral metabolism: The case of conduction aphasia. *Archives of Neurology, 45,* 275–279.

Kempler, D., Van Lancker, D., Marchman, V., & Bates, E. (1996). The effects of childhood vs. adult brain damage on literal and idiomatic language comprehension. *Brain and Language, 55*(1), 167–169.

Kennard, M. (1936). Age and other factors in motor recovery from precentral lesions in monkeys. *American Journal of Physiology, 115,* 138–146.

Killackey, H. P. (1990). Neocortical expansion: An attempt toward relating phylogeny and ontogeny. *Journal of Cognitive Neuroscience, 2,* 1–17.

Lashley, K. S. (1950). In search of the engram. In *Symposia of the Society for Experimental Biology, No. 4, Physiological mechanisms and animal behaviour.* New York: Academic Press.

Lenneberg, E. (1967). *The biological foundations of language* (pp. 125–187). New York: Wiley.

Levin, H. (1991). Neuropsychological outcome of head injury in children. In A. Benton, H. Levin, G. Moretti, & D. Riva, (Eds.), *Neuropsicologia dell'età evolutiva* [Developmental neuropsychology] (pp. 171–184). Milan: FrancoAngeli.

Levine, S., Huttenlocher, P., Banich, M., & Duda, A. (1987). Factors affecting cognitive functioning in hemiplegic children. *Developmental Medicine and Child Neurology, 29,* 27–35.

Marchman, V. (1993). Constraints on plasticity in a connectionist model of the English past tense. *Journal of Cognitive Neuroscience, 5*(2), 215–234.

Marchman, V., Miller, R., & Bates, E. (1991). Babble and first words in children with focal brain injury. *Applied Psycholinguistics, 12,* 1–22.

Martinez, A., Moses, P., Frank, L., Blaettler, D., Stiles, J., Wong, E., & Buxton, R. (1996). Lateralized differences in spatial processing: Evidence from RT and fMRI. *Abstracts of the Second International Conference on Functional Mapping of the Human Brain, 3*(3), S233. San Diego: Academic Press.

McCall, R., Eichorn, D., & Hogarty, P. (1977). Transitions in early mental development. *Monographs of the Society for Research in Child Development* (serial no. 171).

McFie, J. (1961). Intellectual impairment in children with localised post-infantile cerebral lesions. *Journal of Neurology, Neurosurgery and Psychiatry, 24 ,* 361–365.

Metter, E. J., Jackson, C. A., Kempler, D., Riege, W. R., Hanson, W., Mazziotta, J., & Phelps, M. E. (1986). Left hemisphere intracerebral hemorrhages studied by (F-18)-fluoro-deoxyglucose PET. *Neurology, 36*(9), 1155–1162.

Metter, E. J., Kempler, D., Jackson, C. A., Hanson, W., Riege, W. R., Camras, L., Mazziotta, J., & Phelps, M. E. (1987). Cerebellar glucose metabolism in chronic aphasia. *Neurology, 47,* 1599–1606.

Metter, E. J., Riege, W. R., Hanson, W., Jackson, C. A., Kempler, D., & Van Lancker, D. (1988). Subcortical structures in aphasia, An analysis based on (F-18)-fluoro-deoxyglucose, positron emission tomography, and computed tomography. *Archives of Neurology, 45,* 1229–1234.

Mishkin, M., Ungerleider, L. G., & Macko, K. A. (1983). Object vision and spatial vision: Two cortical pathways. *Trends in Neurosciences, 6,* 414–417.

Molfese, D., & Molfese, J. (1980). Cortical responses of preterm infants to phonetic and nonphonetic speech stimuli. *Developmental Psychology, 16,* 574–581.

Muter, V., Taylor, S., & Vargha-Khadem, F. (1997). A longitudinal study of early intellectual development in hemiplegic children. *Neuropsychologia, 35*(3), 289–298.

Naeser, M., Helm-Estabrooks, N., Haas, G., Auerbach, S., & Levine, H. (1984). Relationship between lesion extent in "Wernicke's area" on computed tomographic scan and predicting recovery of comprehension in Wernicke's aphasia. *Archives of Neurology, 44*(1), 73–82.

Nass, R., Peterson, H., & Koch, D. (1989). Differential effects of congenital left and right brain injury on intelligence. *Brain and Cognition, 9,* 258–266.

O'Leary, D. D. (1993). Do cortical areas emerge from a protocortex? In M. Johnson (Ed.), *Brain development and cognition: A reader* (pp. 323–337). Oxford: Blackwell.

O'Leary, D. D., & Stanfield, B. B. (1985). Occipital cortical neurons with transient pyramidal tract axons extend and maintain collaterals to subcortical but not intracortical targets. *Brain Research, 336*(2), 326–333.

O'Leary, D. D., & Stanfield, B. B. (1989). Selective elimination of developing cortical neurons is dependent on regional locale: Experiments utilizing fetal cortical transplants. *Journal of Neuroscience, 9*(7), 2230–2246.

O'Neill , Y. V. (1980). *Speech and speech disorders in Western thought before 1600.* Westport, CT: Greenwood Press.

Oyama, S. (1993). The problem of change. In M. Johnson (Ed.), *Brain development and cognition: A reader* (pp. 19–30). Oxford: Blackwell.

Poizner, H., Klima, E., & Bellugi, U. (1987). *What the hands reveal about the brain*. Cambridge, MA: MIT/Bradford Books.

Quartz, S. R., & Sejnowski, T. J. (1997). The neural basis of cognitive development: A constructivist manifesto. *Behavioral and Brain Sciences, 20*, 537–596.

Rakic, P. (1988). Specification of cerebral cortical areas. *Science, 241*, 170–176.

Rasmussen, T., & Milner, B. (1977). The role of early left-brain injury in determining lateralisation of cerebral speech functions. *Annals of the New York Academy of Sciences, 299*, 355–369.

Reed, J. C., & Reitan, R. M. (1971). Verbal and performance differences among brain-injured children with lateralized motor deficits. *Neuropsychologia, 9*, 401–407.

Reilly, J., Bates, E., & Marchman, V. (1998). Narrative discourse in children with early focal brain injury. *Brain and Language, 61*, 335–375.

Riva, D. (1995). Le lesioni cerebrali focali [Cerebral focal lesions]. In G. Sabbadini (Ed.), *Manuale di neuropsicologia dell' età evolutiva* [Handbook of developmental neuropsychology] (pp. 484–504). Bologna: Zanichelli.

Riva, D., & Cazzaniga, L. (1986). Late effects of unilateral brain lesions sustained before and after age one. *Neuropsychologia, 24*, 423–428.

Riva, D., Cazzaniga, L., Pantaleoni, C., Milani, N., & Fedrizzi, E. (1986). Acute hemiplegia in childhood: The neuropsychological prognosis. *Journal of Paediatric Neurosciences, 2*, 239–250.

Satz, P., Strauss, E., & Whitaker, H. (1990). The ontogeny of hemispheric specialization: Some old hypotheses revisited. *Brain and Language, 38*(4), 596–614.

Shore, C. M. (1995). *Individual differences in language development*. Thousand Oaks, CA: Sage Publications.

Smith, A. (1984). Early and long-term recovery from brain-damage in children and adults: Evolution of concepts of localization, plasticity, and recovery. In C. R. Almli & S. Finger (Eds.), *Early brain damage* (pp. 299–324). New York: Academic Press.

Smith, L. B., & Thelen, E. (Eds.). (1993). *A dynamic systems approach to development: Applications*. Cambridge, MA: MIT Press.

Spreen, O., & Strauss, E. (1991). *A compendium of neuropsychological tests. Administration, norms, and commentary* (pp. 221–229). Oxford: Oxford University Press.

Stein, D., Brailowsky, S., & Will, B. (1995). *Brain repair*. New York: Oxford University Press.

Stiles, J. (1995). Plasticity and development: Evidence from children with early focal brain injury. In B. Julesz & I. Kovacs (Eds.), *Maturational windows and adult cortical plasticity in human development: Is there reason for an optimistic view* (pp. 217–237). Reading, MA: Addison-Wesley Publishing.

Stiles, J., & Thal, D. (1993). Linguistic and spatial cognitive development following early focal brain injury: Patterns of deficit and recovery. In M. Johnson (Ed.), *Brain development and cognition: A reader* (pp. 643–664). Oxford: Blackwell.

St. James Roberts, I. (1981). A reinterpretation of hemispherectomy data without functional plasticity of the brain. *Brain and Language, 14*, 292–306.

Teuber, H. (1971). Is it really better to have your brain damage early? A revision of the "Kennard Principle." *Neuropsychologia, 17*, 557–583.

Thal, D. J., Marchman, V. A., Stiles, J., Aram, D., Trauner, D., Nass, R., & Bates, E. (1991). Early lexical development in children with focal brain injury. *Brain and Language, 40*(4), 491–527.

Trauner D., Chase, C., Walker, P., & Wulfeck, B. (1993). Neurologic profiles of infants and children after perinatal stroke. *Pediatric Neurology, 9*(5), 383–386.

Vargha-Khadem, F., Carr, L. J., Isaacs, E., Brett, E., Adams, C., & Mishkin, M. (1996). Onset of speech after left hemispherectomy in a nine-year-old boy. *Brain, 119,* 318–326.

Vargha-Khadem, F., & Corballis, M. (1979). Cerebral asymmetry in infants. *Brain and Language, 8,* 1–9.

.Vargha-Khadem, F., Isaacs, E., & Muter, V. (1994). A review of cognitive outcome after unilateral lesions sustained during childhood. *Journal of Child Neurology, 9*(suppl.), 2S67–2S73.

Vargha-Khadem, F., Isaacs, E., Van der Werf, S., Robb, S., & Wilson, J. (1992). Development of intelligence and memory in children with hemiplegic cerebral palsy: The deleterious consequences of early seizures. *Brain, 115,* 315–329.

Vargha-Khadem, F., O'Gorman, A., & Watters, G. (1985). Aphasia and handedness in relation to hemispheric side, age at injury and severity of cerebral lesion during childhood. *Brain, 108,* 677–696.

Vargha-Khadem, F., & Polkey, C. E. (1992). A review of cognitive outcome after hemidecortication in humans. In F. D. Rose & D. A. Johnson (Eds.), *Recovery from brain damage: Advances in experimental medicine and biology: Vol. 325. Reflections and directions* (pp. 137–151). New York: Plenum Press.

Webster, M. J., Bachevalier, J., & Ungerleider, L. G. (1995). Development and plasticity of visual memory circuits. In B. Julesz & I. Kovacs (Eds.), *Maturational windows and adult cortical plasticity in human development: Is there reason for an optimistic view?* (pp. 186–201) Reading, MA: Addison-Wesley Publishing.

Witelson, S., & Pallie, W. (1973). Left-hemisphere specialisation for language in the new-born: neuroanatomical evidence of asymmetry. *Brain, 88,* 653–662.

Wood, S., Gadian, D., Isaacs, J., Cross, C., Johnson, A., Connelly, A., & Vargha-Khadem, F. (1996). The relationship between memory function and temporal lobe pathology in children. *Society for Neuroscience Abstracts, 22*(2), 575.

Woods, B. (1980). The restricted effects of right-hemisphere lesions after age one: Wechsler test data. *Neuropsychologia, 18*(1), 65–70.

Woods, B., & Carey, S. (1979). Language deficits after apparent clinical recovery from childhood aphasia. *Annals of Neurology, 6,* 405–409.

Woods, B., & Teuber, H. (1973). Early onset of complementary specialisation of the cerebral hemispheres in man. *Transactions of the American Neurological Associations, 98,* 113–117.

Woods, B., & Teuber, H. (1978). Changing patterns of childhood aphasia. *Annals of Neurology, 3,* 273–280.

Zaidel, E. (1973). *Linguistic competence and related functions in the right cerebral hemisphere of man following commissurotomy and hemispherectomy.* Unpublished doctoral dissertation, California Institute of Technology Pasadena, CA.

Zaidel, E. (1977). Unilateral auditory language comprehension on the Token Test following cerebral commissurotomy and hemispherectomy. *Neuropsychologia, 15,* 1–18.

24 Advances in the Cognitive Neuroscience of Neurodevelopmental Disorders: Views from Child Psychiatry and Medical Genetics

William M. McMahon

RELATION BETWEEN COGNITIVE NEUROSCIENCE AND NEURODEVELOPMENTAL DISORDERS

Common Interest

Neurodevelopmental disorders hold great interest for two medical subspecialties concerned with the care of children: child psychiatry and medical genetics. Both subspecialties are involved in the diagnosis, treatment, and prevention of the diverse disorders addressed in this book, and both depend on an understanding of normal and pathological development. This chapter addresses the recent advances in the study of cognition in specific neurodevelopmental disorders from the perspectives of child psychiatry and medical genetics. Historical contributions by advances in cognitive neuroscience to both subspecialties are reviewed first, followed by an examination of a model neurodevelopmental disorder under intense study by child psychiatrists: Tourette syndrome (TS). Next, concepts and vocabulary from medical genetics are reviewed and applied to examples from other chapters. Special attention is paid to the definition of the term *behavioral phenotype*. Finally, future directions are discussed.

Common History

The measurement and classification of mental retardation syndromes have been critical to progress in both child psychiatry and clinical genetics. In a review of the emergence of concepts of child and adolescent psychopathology, Lewis and Volkmar (1990) stated that the application of the methods of Binet and Simon to the classification of the kinds and degrees of mental retardation represents an important theme in the history of the conceptualization and subsequent scientific study of childhood psychopathology, and the first perspective on measurement. More recently, the measurement of intelligence in families affected by fragile X was critical to the recognition that severity increased as it was passed down through successive generations, a genetic phenomenon known as *anticipation* (see chapters 2 and 3).

The integration of cognitive measurement with new technology in molecular genetics led to the discovery of the molecular basis of anticipation in fragile X (Fu et al., 1991). Thus, an iterative process of application of advances in one discipline has facilitated advances in another discipline and has further advanced the former. This theme of progress synergized by multidisciplinary cross-fertilization, further illustrated by other chapters, lends a sense of optimistic excitement to researchers and clinicians both in child and adolescent psychiatry and in clinical genetics.

CURRENT VALUES AND CONCERNS IN CHILD PSYCHIATRY: LESSONS FROM TOURETTE SYNDROME

Tourette Syndrome as a Model Neuropsychiatric Disorder

TS and obsessive-compulsive disorder (OCD) are neurodevelopmental disorders that provide an informative comparison with disorders featured in this book. Unlike most of the disorders featured in other chapters, TS usually is not associated with mental retardation, and linkage of this phenotype to a chromosomal location has not yet occurred. Twin, adoption, and segregation analysis studies of TS support a genetic etiology, although nongenetic factors also are likely (Pauls & Leckman, 1986; Comings & Comings, 1990; Curtis et al., 1992; Allen et al., 1995; Hasstedt et al., 1995). A number of DNA linkage studies have been undertaken across the world, based on data suggesting an autosomal dominant mode of inheritance, along with the optimism that the phenotype definition would be straightforward. More than 5000 DNA markers later, linkage has not been discovered, and numerous explanations for this failure are being put forward (Comings & Comings, 1990; van de Wetering & Heutink, 1993; Hasstedt et al., 1995; McMahon et al., 1996).

TS is a complex disease currently receiving intense scrutiny from neuropsychologists, neuroimagers, psychopharmacologists, neuroimmunologists, cognitive behavior therapists, and developmental theorists. Cohen and Leckman (1994) and Leckman have et al. (1992) proposed a four-factor interactive model of the developmental psychopathology and neuropathology of TS to provide a framework for ongoing research and treatment. This model aims at an integrated view of the whole child by recognizing complex interactions between genetic susceptibility, environmental factors, the neurobiological substrate, and the clinical phenotype.

The Tourette Phenotype

The word *phenotype* derives from the Greek terms *phainen* ("to show") and *typus* ("type" or "character"). Thus, a phenotype is that character or type that shows. Human phenotypes may be studied either by beginning with a known genotype and examining the observable characteristics in a person or by beginning with a homogenous sample of people with common observable characteristics and then looking for evidence of an underlying common genotype. No genotype has yet been found for TS, but an operational definition of the phenotype has been put forth for genetic studies in the form of diagnostic criteria.

The diagnosis of TS as defined by the Tourette Syndrome Association (TSA) Study Group requires a combination of multiple motor and vocal tics that follow a characteristic waxing and waning course, beginning in childhood with a duration of at least 1 year, in the absence of other potential etiologies (The Tourette Syndrome Classification Study Group, 1993). An additional requirement to this long-standing set of criteria was added by *Diagnostic and Statistical Manual of Mental Disorders* (fourth edition) (DSM-IV) in 1994: "The disturbance causes marked distress or significant impairment in social, occupational, or other important areas of functioning" (American Psychiatric Association, 1994). This addition reflects new information about the genetics and course of TS. For example, a Utah study of 191 individuals in a single extended family showed that 38% of those with TSA criteria for TS did not experience sufficient distress or dysfunction to meet DSM-IV criteria (McMahon et al., 1996). In other words, the phenotype of tics may represent a trait with a wide spectrum of expression, from nonpathological to severely handicapping.

OCD is included in the phenotype for a number of reasons. OCD may be a heterogenous disorder with multiple familial and nonfamilial etiologies. Multiple studies of TS clinic samples report comorbid OCD at rates between 30% and 80%. Family studies of index cases with TS have shown the rate of OCD among first-degree relatives of TS cases to be 9 to 13 times higher than the population rate. Segregation analyses of families affected with TS suggest that OCD is an alternative manifestation (seen more frequently in female members of a TS family) of a probable autosomal dominant gene for TS (Pauls, 1993). OCD as defined by DSM-IV can be summarized as a disorder characterized by recurrent and persistent thoughts, impulses, images, behaviors, or mental acts that are experienced as unreasonable, difficult to suppress and causing distress, and not attributable to real-life worries or other psychiatric conditions (American Psychiatric Association, 1994). Similar to tics, obsessions and compulsions may be considered to lie on a continuum of severity, from severely handicapping to so mild as to be called *mental play*. The Utah study cited (McMahon et al., 1996) found that nonhandicapping obsessive-compulsive behaviors, such as repetitive counting or spelling, were more common among family members than was clinically significant OCD. Thus, repetitive behaviors and cognitions form the core phenomena for the TS/OCD phenotype, and such phenomena may vary in severity from a crippling impairment to what might be described as a normal trait. A potential lesson from TS applicable to studies of other neurodevelopmental disorders may be that mild versions of some neurodevelopmental disorders share fuzzy boundaries with the normal population and may not appear in more severely impaired clinical samples.

Cognitive deficits also may be associated with TS, although results across studies are inconsistent and comparison is difficult. TS symptoms may include a perceptual component, such as a sense of tension preceding a tic, or the need to have sensory stimuli manifest qualities, such as a specific texture, tightness, sound, or symmetry, that have been described as "just right." Several authors have hypothesized that tics reflect a failure of an inhibitory system mediated by executive and prefrontal dysfunction (Gedye, 1991; Pennington, 1991; Stoetter et al., 1992). As compared to siblings and to children with arithmetic disabilities, 31 TS children in a recent study demonstrated performance deficits in visuomotor and expressive language tasks and in measures of complex cognition, suggesting an "output" type of learning disability. (Brookshire et al., 1994).

Because comorbid attention deficit hyperactivity disorder and OCD may influence performance on various measures of executive function, Ozonoff et al. (1994) have studied a group of TS children free of these conditions. In their first study, information-processing paradigms testing inhibition and global-local processing were used to provide a detailed examination of executive function abilities in three groups of children: TS, high-functioning autism, and normal controls. No significant differences were found between TS and control children. In a second study, TS children were compared to normal children on a measure of inhibitory capacity, negative priming (Ozonoff et al., unpublished data). No significant differences were found between the total TS group and the control group, but when the TS group was stratified by severity or by comorbidity, significant differences in inhibitory function were found, with severe or comorbid TS children deficient as compared to controls and to mild or less comorbid TS subjects. Though further work is needed to verify this finding, a preliminary interpretation is that inhibitory deficits in TS are nonspecific and secondary symptoms in the pathogenesis and emerge only when a severity threshold is passed. Possibly, cognitive deficits found in studies of other neurodevelopmental disorders will show a similar theme, with some deficits appearing only when a certain severity is reached.

TS may affect profoundly the development of a child's sense of self, that quality "of being a whole person with desires, intentions, and feelings that are integrated and understandable to themselves and to others" (Cohen & Leckman, 1994 p. 3). The involuntary and intrusive nature of movements and noises may interrupt intentional activities. Involuntary imitative behaviors—echolalia, palilalia, and echopraxia (imitation of sounds by others, sounds by self, movements by others, respectively)—may erode the interpersonal boundaries between the TS child and family members that are normally established in the course of separation-individuation.

Social feedback may amplify the child's sense of being "possessed" by the TS demon, especially when tics take on a forbidden quality, as with self-injurious tics or coprolalia (involuntary utterance of obscene language). Yet, individuals with TS sometimes describe desirable or adaptive features of the disorder. Sensory stimuli may seem more exciting to an individual with tics triggered by such stimuli. "Just right" phenomena may be highly adaptive in perfecting valued and marketable skills and conferring the pleasure of accomplishment. Forbidden words or statements may be woven into the texture of comedy, and imitative tics may enhance a comedic or dramatic repertoire. The chaotic spontaneity provided by the apparent inhibitory deficit of TS actually may be preferred by an individual facing the alternative pharmacological inhibition provided by haloperidol or pimozide.

Sacks (1987) describes such a choice faced by Witty Ticcy Ray, a jazz drummer, for whom TS provided an exciting impetus for creative improvisation. Haloperidol suppressed both tics and musical creativity and led to Ray's refusal of full-time pharmacological treatment. As other neurodevelopmental disorders are better understood and treatments become more available, will affected individuals resist some treatments because they erode some positive aspect of the condition or undermine a sense of personal identity?

Consideration of the whole person also raises a methodological issue: How is a behavioral phenotype recognized, verified, and subjected to study? Though this topic is addressed in greater detail later, one component is illustrated by the history of TS. In 1885, the neurologist Georges Gilles de la Tourette described the core symptoms of this syndrome in nine cases, compared those cases to others reported in the literature, differentiated TS from Sydenham chorea and other overlapping conditions, and outlined the natural history (Goetz & Klawans, 1982).

As a student of Charcot, de la Tourette had the advantage of a broad medical perspective that encompassed mind and body and supported original, detailed description of the whole person in the context of a particular disease. Though modern medicine has brought advances in the diagnosis, treatment, and understanding of many diseases, the specialized knowledge necessary for such advances often obscures a view of the whole person.

For example, standardized questionnaires and structured interviews in child psychiatry have led to numerous advances in diagnosis and outcome studies but may displace efforts to recognize the personal, unique, and contextual symptoms that allow a gifted clinician to define a new syndrome. To be facetious, Georges Gilles de la Tourette could not have described his namesake syndrome from a child behavior checklist. Understanding of TS has been advanced by eloquent personal description, as in the self-report of Bliss (1980), an adult who had TS and articulated the inner experience of premonitory urges and other sensory phenomena.

This method, and others using family members, have informed TS research and clinical care. Similarly, personal descriptions by gifted individuals may be helpful for understanding the neurodevelopmental disorders in this book. Cognitive psychologists studying other conditions may further inform their studies by using self-reports by unusually eloquent subjects. Such subjective information may point to dimensions that subsequently can be quantified with existing or newly developed instruments. The relationship of cognitive functions to social, affective, or psychiatric function then may be studied.

Ross and Zinn (see chapter 11 regarding Turner syndrome) illustrated this approach. Their preliminary results suggest beneficial effects of estrogen therapy in adolescent girls with Turner syndrome on measures of self-image and behavior.

Children born to families with TS are at increased risk, as compared to population risk, for developing the disorder themselves (Carter et al., 1994). Such children offer an opportunity to study the unfolding of the TS phenotype over time. Risk and protective factors may be uncovered by comparing children within and across such families. Comorbidity and the effect of Berkson's bias can be addressed systematically (Berkson, 1946). The relationships of developmental strengths and weaknesses can be compared across motor, cognitive, behavioral, linguistic, and affective domains. The relationship of the child's features to those of the family, peer group, school, or community can be studied. This capability is critical for children with TS; as overprotection, rejection, stigmatization, or tolerance by those in the environment may influence overall outcome.

Carter et al. (1994) have presented interesting results from a preliminary prospective longitudinal study of 21 preschool children all at genetic risk for TS by virtue of having a parent or sibling with TS. Increased rates were found in these preschoolers for tic, obsessional, and anxiety symptoms and attentional and speech difficulties. Perhaps most interesting, measures of family function independent of parental psychopathology were associated with attention deficit and anxiety disorders, decreased adaptive and increased maladaptive behaviors, and lower self-esteem, but not tic or learning disorders. Thus, comorbidity in this sample of preschoolers at risk for TS depended largely on family function. Because comorbidity contributes to the total burden carried by any child with TS, these results, along with the cognitive studies of "pure" TS by Ozonoff et al. (1994), raise an important question regarding the impact of any neurodevelopmental disorder: Can any neurodevelopmental disorder be assessed or understood without understanding the other biopsychosocial variables impacting the affected child?

Future discovery of TS genes will render prospective at-risk studies even more valuable, as the presence of a TS gene coding for a specific protein will render a mechanism of pathogenesis more specific and better understood than is currently possible. If ethical considerations allow it, presymptomatic DNA testing may identify another sample of children for longitudinal, at-risk studies. The at-risk paradigm offers similar advantages for other developmental disorders. Cognitive studies of children at risk for neurodevelopmental disorders, as with female carriers of fragile X, may further define the relationship between genotype, functional protein, cognitive profile, social function, environmental stressors, or protectors and global outcome.

CONCEPTS FROM MEDICAL GENETICS

Recent History

Advances in molecular genetics have brought an explosion of discoveries in clinical genetics over the last three decades. Though disorders of cognition and neurodevelopment, most notably fragile X, have been illuminated by such advances, most new findings relate to organs other than the brain and to functions other than cognition. Many factors can be listed to account for this inequality. First, the brain is relatively inaccessibile for study, compared to such other organs as bone, blood, muscle, and skin. Neuroimaging may allow for greater access to the brain, but expense and obtaining conscious cooperation still are obstacles. Second, the diagnosis of disorders successfully linked to specific genes or chromosomal locations often has been straightforward, based on characteristics of gross anatomy, histology, or marked loss of function that are easily defined and recognized. In comparison, the diagnosis of such complex diseases as autism or TS has required much attention to more subtle aspects of diagnostic validity and reliability, particularly to those aspects that may be episodic. Third, genetic influence on a complex disease is likely to be multifactorial, involving multiple genes expressed at different times and in different places and interacting with each other and with the environment.

The technology for dissecting complex diseases is not as developed as that for single-gene disorders. The term *complex disease* is defined broadly as any disease that cannot be defined or explained accurately (Terwilliger & Ott, 1994). This term is applied to diseases in which the mode of genetic transmission is unknown or appears polygenic, further complicated by probable genetic heterogeneity and phenocopies (see following discussion). Other differences between successfully linked single-gene diseases and those diseases of cognitive development can be discussed, but the three aforementioned factors suffice to make the point that the difficulty of the challenge is greater for multiple reasons.

With such differences in mind, we still may profit from lessons learned by discoveries in single-gene disorders. The principle that rare developmental disorders provide important information for understanding normal development is supported strongly by the recent history of investigative success in single-gene disorders. Important concepts, including pleiotropy, phenocopies, penetrance, variable expression, and two types of genetic heterogeneity, are well described for a number of single-gene disorders. These will first be reviewed before turning to disorders involving multiple genes.

Pleiotropy: Lessons from Marfan Syndrome

Pleiotropy, defined as "multiple phenotypic effects of a single genetic mutation," recently was reviewed in the context of Marfan syndrome by Pyeritz

(1989). Marfan syndrome, now known to be caused by mutations in the fibrillin-1 gene, first was described 100 years ago as a skeletal disorder causing long, thin limbs. In 1914, Boerger added dislocation of the lens of the eye as a clinical feature. The autosomal dominant transmission pattern and cardiovascular features subsequently were described in the 1950s (McKusick, 1955). Current clinical diagnostic criteria vary with family history: If no first-degree relative is unequivocally affected, involvement of the skeleton and at least two of five other organ systems is required. If a first-degree relative is affected, only manifestations in two organ systems is required. Pyeritz pointed out that clinical advances have both lengthened the list of pleiotropic manifestations and provided more sensitive and specific diagnostic measures. Echocardiograms now disclose aortic dilatation in more than 90%, whereas auscultation and autopsy reports previously had recognized aortic pathology in only 40%. Computed tomography now discloses a widening of the spinal canal, known as *dural ectasia*, in 65% of Marfan cases. Dural ectasia is a rare finding in any other disorder besides von Recklinghausen neurofibromatosis. Linkage to chromosome 15, first reported in 1990, has been followed by replication in multiple samples and characterization of a number of different mutations within the fibrillin-1 gene.

Though pleiotropy may be applied to the diverse manifestations of all the neurodevelopmental disorders described in this book, fragile X may serve best to illustrate this concept. Individuals (especially male) with the expansion-mutation of fragile X may manifest any number of a long list of clinical characteristics, including long, prominent ears; high-arched palate; prominent jaw; long face; pectus excavatum (a chest deformity in which the sternum curves inward); hyperextensible joints; flat feet; large testicles; strabismus (lazy eye); and scoliosis, along with mental retardation, poor eye contact, perseverative speech, and hyperactivity (Hagerman, 1996).

Phenocopies

A disorder (phenotype) caused by a specific genotype (mutation) may be indistinguishable from a disorder caused by a different mutation or an environmental agent. An ironic example is provided once again by Marfan syndrome. Marfan's original cases may not have had what is now called *Marfan syndrome* and caused by a fibrillin-1 mutation, but rather congenital contractural arachnodactyly, a condition recently linked to the fibrillin-2 gene on chromosome 5, with phenotypic features overlapping those of Marfan. Homocystinuria, a mental retardation disorder associated with a long thin body, dislocated lens, and cardiovascular problems, also was confused with Marfan syndrome until the early 1960s. Urine chromotography allowed the identification of this disorder, now recognized to have multiple causes (among them mutations of the gene coding for the enzyme cystathionine beta-synthase, on the long arm of chromosome 21). Thus, discriminating one genetically caused disorder from another has taken 100 years because the overlap of phenotypes could be resolved only by applying biochemical and molecular techniques as they became available.

Similar struggles with phenocopies are likely to occur for the neurodevelopmental disorders. Autism, for example, may represent the final common pathway for a number of pathogenic mechanisms (Rapin, 1987).

Penetrance

Inheritance of a genotype does not always result in the occurrence of the trait or disease associated with that genotype. The relative frequency of a trait or disease (given the presence of a genotype known to cause that trait) is defined as the *penetrance* of that genotype. Penetrance may vary with age, gender, environmental factors, and the influence of other genes. Huntington's disease, a neurodegenerative disorder, offered a nearly 100% penetrance in both genders as an advantage to researchers in that it allowed successful linkage. At the same time, Huntington's disease presented a challenge for linkage, as average age at onset is near 40 years, and death may occur within 15 years of onset. Thus, pedigree size and number of cases were limited by age-related penetrance because gene carriers were not detectable until onset in middle age and were available for study only until their early death.

Penetrance also varies with mode of genetic transmission. In diseases with Mendelian inheritance, dominant transmission implies that penetrance is the same for individuals with one copy of the disease gene and one copy of the normal gene (heterozygotes) and for individuals with two copies of the disease gene (homozygotes). Recessive inheritance implies that the disease does not occur in heterozygotes. A less common mode of inheritance, known as *codominant* or *intermediate*, implies that some heterozygotes have a lower penetrance and that homozygotes have a higher penetrance. Marfan and Huntington's syndromes are examples of single-gene diseases with dominant transmission patterns. Phenylketonuria (PKU) is a recessive disease. TS has been proposed as both dominant and codominant, based on different samples. Both penetrance and mode of transmission can be estimated by studying the prevalence of a disease in affected pedigrees, but discovery of a mutation provides direct evidence for both. Penetrance of Huntington's disease initially was thought to be 100%, but DNA analysis in at-risk individuals has disclosed that some individuals asymptomatic in old age nevertheless carry the disease gene. Penetrance is likely to be an issue for neurodevelopmental disorders, most easily observed in single-gene disorders in which the mode of transmission is autosomal dominant. Prior to the discovery of the gene for such a disorder, the evidence likely to be available is the recognition that an unaffected parent of an affected child has a parent, aunt, or uncle who also is affected. Such a parent then would be designated as an *obligate carrier* of the suspected mutation.

Variable Expression

Variable expression of a mutation refers to the degree to which any of the pleitropic effects may be found in an individual. Age, gender, environmental factors, and other genes may influence the phenotypic expression of any single gene. Variable expression is distinguished from pleitropy in that pleitropy refers to a total list of pathological effects of a single mutation in all individuals with that mutation, whereas variable expression refers to the profile of differences among individuals. In contrast to penetrance, which refers to the global presence or absence of a genetic disease or trait, the variability in expression of the individual signs and symptoms of a mutation may range from absent or subtle to extremely obvious or severe.

Owing to the wide range of expression possible for each of the possible pleitropic effects, any individual with a given mutation may present a profile of symptoms that differs markedly from another individual with the same mutation. Using the Marfan syndrome example, some individuals with a fibrillin-1 mutation have severe aortic dilatation leading to death by dissection and massive hemorrhage at an early age, whereas others may live into old age without more than mild dilatation. Similarly, some individuals may manifest lens dislocation, whereas others do not. If just these two dimensions of expression are combined, a group of individuals with Marfan syndrome may include some with little aortic dilation and no lens dislocation, some individuals with one problem and some individuals with both problems. As the list of pleiotropic effects seen in any mutation syndrome becomes longer, the possible differences between any two individuals with the mutation become greater due to the variable expression of each of these pleiotropic effects.

Variable expression may account for much of the difficulty encountered to this point in linkage studies of schizophrenia, bipolar disorder, TS, and other psychiatric diseases. PKU provides an example of variable expression, particularly with respect to IQ.

Allelic and Locus Heterogeneity

Penetrance, pleiotropy, and variable expression all contribute to the remarkable variation that can be observed between individuals with the same mutation at a single locus. A given genotype may result in phenotypes that are quite different to observation. Conversely, different genotypes may result in the same apparent phenotype (as mentioned in the discussion of phenocopies). Two types of heterogeneity exist at the level of the genotype: allelic and locus.

Allelic heterogeneity refers to different mutations within the same gene. Fragile X repeat length is an example of allelic heterogeneity, in that different sizes of the CGG repeat are possible.

Locus heterogeneity refers to the existence of different major genes at different chromosomal locations that may produce the same disease phenotype. Linkage to four different loci—chromosomes 1, 14, 19, and 21—has been reported for Alzheimer disease (Online Mendelian Inheritance in Man, 1996).

Contiguous Genes, Aneuploidies, and Polygenic Disorders

Single-gene mutations produce considerable complexity. Even greater complexity results when deletions or duplications affect multiple genes or whole chromosomes. The disorders addressed in other chapters illustrate the range in the order of magnitude of disruption of DNA, from the single-gene disorders of PKU and fragile X, to the contiguous gene syndrome of Williams syndrome, to the addition or deletion of a whole chromosome in Down and Turner syndrome. As the technology for dissecting polygenic disorders advances and the influences of genes with modifying or minor effects can be studied, such complex phenotypes as autism may be better understood, and other neurodevelopmental disorders may be added to the current list. In the interim, work on contiguous gene syndromes to identify the number and identity of genes deleted by microdeletions is proceding (see chapters 4 and 5). Also, the larger task of correlating specific regions on chromosome 21 with specific Down syndrome phenotypic abnormalities is ongoing. Similar progress is being made with X chromosome critical regions and Turner syndrome features.

DEFINITION OF A BEHAVIORAL PHENOTYPE

The definition of the term *behavioral phenotype* deserves further consideration. A discrepancy exists between the meaning of the term in the medical genetics literature and its use in child psychiatry. Consistent with the meaning of the term *phenotype* in other genetic disorders, the genetics literature reflects the assumption that a phenotype is an observable expression of a genotype. It assumes that a phenotype resulting from a specific genotype may not be distinguishable from a phenocopy associated with a different genotype, because the observable trait is nonspecific and because measurement may be imperfect. Marfan and homocysteinuria (discussed earlier) were phenocopies of one another until the development of technology that allowed for their clinical discrimination.

In 1971, Nyhan introduced the term *behavioral phenotype* to describe behavior observed in the syndromes of Cornelia de Lange and Lesch-Nyhan (Nyhan, 1972). In the psychiatric literature, Flint and Yule (1994) suggested a much more limited definition for a behavioral phenotype. In their view, such a phenotype should be distinctive, occuring in almost every case with a given genetic defect but rarely in other conditions. They admitted that this definition may be overly restrictive and listed only three conditions with behaviors that fit this definition: self-mutilation in Lesch-Nyhan syndrome, food seeking in Prader-Willi syndrome, and midline hand-wringing stereotypies in Rett's syndrome. The authors went on to describe other less restrictive criteria for establishing the existence of a behavioral phenotype in a specific syndrome, using other syndromes as examples.

Though the value of finding a specific behavior pathognomonic for a given genetic defect would be great, the use of such a definition for behavioral phenotype is overly restrictive and runs against the current of established usage for the term in medical genetics. Nyhan (1995) recently pointed out that dysmorphic syndromes, such as that caused by fetal alcohol exposure, can be both acquired and genetic. He saw no reason why the term that he first defined should be limited to only those behavioral phenotypes with a genetic etiology. Furthermore, the expectation of a one-to-one correspondence between a gene defect and a phenotype appears unrealistic, given the influence of other genes, environment, and randomness. Gene knock-out experiments in mice provide ample evidence that a point mutation may result in a range of phenotypic expression rather than in an invariant phenotype. For example, targeted disruption of a known structural gene, *int-2*, in a mouse model results in dramatic phenotypic differences between individual mice with uniform genetic backgrounds (Mansour et al., 1993). One remarkable finding from this work is that development of inner-ear anomalies caused by the *int-2* knock-out more often are asymmetrical (43%, occurring in either the right or left ear of the mouse) than symmetrical (36%, occurring on both sides). Thus, the knock-out of a single gene thought to control morphogenesis of inner-ear structures results in variable inner-ear anatomy both between litter mates and within an individual mouse.

This example of variable expressivity may represent the influence of both local events in the biochemical environment and genetic redundancy in signalling pathways for inner-ear development. If such pathways exist for structural development of the inner ear, such redundancy in systems that signal the development of brain structure and function also are likely. Similarly, we should expect that no brain-related gene mutation will result in an absolute, universal, and pathognomonic phenotype, but rather that other genes and environmental effects will contribute to the expression of virtually any mutation and will result in a range of phenotypes. In practical terms, this suggests that behavioral phenotype be defined and developed by building on current usage in medical genetics with the addition of healthy skepticism and empirical methodology from the behavioral sciences.

Dykens (1995) recently proposed the following definition for *behavioral phenotype*: "[a] phenotype may best be described as the heightened *probability* or *likelihood* that people with a given syndrome will exhibit certain behavioral and developmental sequelae relative to those without the syndrome." This emphasis on probability or likelihood allows application of empirical data to quantify the relative uniqueness of any cognitive or behavioral trait. Use of this definition as a first step allows any syndrome to be assessed for the existence of a behavioral phenotype by subjecting the traits observed in a particular syndrome to a set of measurable criteria. Turk and Hill (1995) suggested that criteria be developed to measure five domains: intellectual functioning, speech and language, attentional deficits, social impairments, and other behavioral disturbances, such as self-injurious behavior. O'Brien and Yule (1995) proposed a definition that integrates a number of these elements:

The behavioural phenotype is a characteristic pattern of motor, cognitive, linguistic and social abnormalities which is consistently associated with a biological disorder. In some cases, the behavioural phenotype may constitute a psychiatric disorder; in others, behaviours which are not usually regarded as symptoms of psychiatric disorders may occur.

This definition may overly emphasize the deficits of a behavioral phenotype to the exclusion of important strengths. Dykens has emphasized that specific competencies and strengths should also be included in the definition of a behavioral phenotype and illustrates with a case vignette of Prader-Willi syndrome (see chapter 6). Other criteria for describing and measuring behavioral phenotypes have been proposed. Harris (1987) emphasized the fact that behavioral phenotypes are behaviors that are "unlearned behavior disorders." This may be expanded further to include the concept that such behavior resists extinction using operant conditioning. Neuroanatomical, neurophysiological, or molecular findings that provide a biological basis for phenotypic traits will offer further evidence for validation. An emerging example from this volume occurs in Turner syndrome. Rovet and Buchanan used behavioral, neuropsychological, and neuroimaging findings to hypothesize that the visuospatial pathway processing spatial location would be affected selectively in Turner subjects. Their subsequent studies both confirmed this hypothesis and modified it to include the likely influence of working memory (see chapter 10). Suggestions for criteria in the assessment of the validity and reliability of behavioral phenotypes for specific syndromes are summarized in table 24.1.

METHODS FOR STUDYING BEHAVIORAL PHENOTYPES

At this point in history, studies of behavioral phenotype can be divided into two main categories on the basis of what is chosen as the independent

Table 24.1 Criteria for defining behavioral phenotypes

Characteristic pattern of traits
Frequently present in index cases
Infrequently present in control or comparison groups
Similar across developmentally diverse groups
Similar across ethnic or cultural groups
Unlearned, resistant to extinction
Related to physiology or anatomy

variable: genotype or phenotype. In a study using genotype as the independent variable, index cases are included for study because of the presence of some known chromosomal or genetic abnormality. Examples are trisomy 21, Turner syndrome, Klinefelter syndrome, and (especially) fragile X, now that FMR1 mutations are known. With the genetic abnormality as the independent variable, efforts then are directed toward correlating behavioral, cognitive, linguistic, or other measures with the genetic abnormality. For example, Mazzocco and Reiss (see chapter 3) have presented their findings that the FMR1 activation ratio (proportion of cells with active normal X chromosomes versus cells with active mutated X chromosomes) in female subjects with a mutation is correlated with intellectual dysfunction and that visual-spatial and arithmetic deficits are found even among nonretarded fragile X female persons with low activation ratios.

The choice of the appropriate comparison group for studies attempting to define a behavioral phenotype is a complex topic and beyond the scope of this chapter (see review by O'Brien and Yule, 1995, and Dykens, 1995). In brief, the rare occurrence of many of these disorders, the impact of variable medical complications, and the usual distribution of IQ in the retarded range are challenges for designing a study and recruiting appropriate control subjects. Dykens (1995) recommended a multimethod approach that combines psychiatric, psychometric, and syndrome-specific observation methods to study behavioral phenotypes.

The second category of study uses the behavioral phenotype as the independent variable and tests genotypes in a sample of cases defined by clinical characteristics (e.g., dyslexia). Grigorenko et al. (1997) recently used measures of five theoretically derived dyslexia phenotypes in 94 individuals from six large families to replicate linkage previously reported for DNA markers on chromosomes 6 and 15. Measures of phonological awareness were significantly linked ($P < 10^{-6}$) to DNA markers on chromosome 6, whereas measures of single-word reading were linked to markers on chromosome 15. These genotype findings build on an impressive body of cognitive research that over the last two decades have progressively defined the parameters of the dyslexia phenotype (Pennington, 1997). The tools of cognitive analysis have propelled genetic studies of dyslexia and serve as a model for the dissection of a complex disorder. Recent efforts establishing linkage for such complex diseases as TS have failed, perhaps because of the lack of such analytical tools.

FUTURE DIRECTIONS

The reciprocal cross-fertilization of cognitive neuroscience, child psychiatry, and medical genetics is producing ever greater yield for understanding neurodevelopmental disorders. The results presented in this volume justify a sense of excitement over current and future findings. As developments in each field occur, opportunities multiply across fields of study. This section highlights some areas that hold promise for advances in the near future.

From the perspective of the whole child, between-syndrome studies of cognitive-linguistic development in children with neurodevelpmental disorders should allow for a better understanding of the cognitive and noncognitive underpinnings of social competence. Through control for cognitive skills, the contributions of other variables can be examined. How do affective variables, such as social anxiety, create an impact on children with fragile X where social anxiety is high, as compared to children with other conditions and matched IQ but less gaze aversion or other measures of social anxiety? How do psychiatric disorders in specific syndromes, such as OCD in Prader-Willi, compare to psychiatric disorders in other syndromes with different cognitive profiles, with and without controlling for IQ? How does pharmacological treatment of OCD differ in outcome across groups? How do family and other social variables affect global outcome or comorbidity?

Also from the perspective of the whole child, within-syndrome cognitive studies of children with specific neurodevelopmental disorders are likely to contribute to the knowledge of individual variability and developmental trajectories. What other genetic or environmental factors, at what point in development, contribute to the wide range of outcome in female individuals with fragile X? The chapters dealing with fragile X (see chapters 2 and 3) point to further studies that combine knowledge of specific mutations, assays of the FMR1 protein, neuroimaging, and cognitive measures in gene-brain-behavior studies. Particularly helpful in understanding individual differences, twin studies may help to define the impact of shared genetic and environmental components and nonshared environment. Those pairs of homozygous (identical) or dizygous (fraternal) twins who share a neurodevelopmental disorder are potentially valuable teachers for the investigator who is alert to their presence.

For behavioral phenotypes with evidence of susceptibility due to single or a few genes, such as TS, autism, or schizoprenia, use of newer methods of genetic study, such as sibling-pair or quantitative trait locus methods may result in successful genetic linkage. Such success would be accelerated by identifying a cognitive deficit specific to a disorder and detectable even in nonpenetrant family members—those who carry the genetic defect but who do not meet diagnostic criteria for the disorder.

The era of the study of genotype-phenotype corelations has begun. Initial success in understanding neurodevelopmental disorders both at the molecular and at the cognitive level now is evident with fragile X. Parents of children with neurodevelopmental disorders now share the hope that progress in the neuroscience will improve the lives of their children.

ACKNOWLEDGMENTS

Work on this chapter was supported by National Institute of Mental Health grant KO7 MH00980 to the author. Thanks are given to James F. Leckman, Sally Ozonoff, and John Opitz for helpful comments made in reviewing early drafts of this manuscript.

REFERENCES

Allen, A. J., Leonard, H. L., & Swedo, S. E. (1995). Case study: A new infection-triggered, auto-immune subtype of pediatric OCD and Tourette's syndrome. *Journal of the American Academy of Child and Adolescent Psychiatry, 34,* 307–311.

American Psychiatric Association. (1994). *Diagnostic and statistical manual of mental disorders* (4th ed.). Washington, DC: American Psychiatric Association.

Berkson, J. (1946). Limitations of the application of fourfold table analysis to hospital data. *Biometrics, 2,* 47–51.

Bliss, J. (1980). Sensory experiences of Gilles de la Tourette syndrome. *Archives of General Psychiatry, 37,* 1343–1347.

Brookshire, B. L., Butler, I. J., Ewing-Cobbs, L., & Fletcher, J. M. (1994). Neuropsychological characteristics of children with Tourette syndrome: Evidence for a nonverbal learning disability? *Journal of Clinical and Experimental Neuropsychology, 16*(2), 289–302.

Carter, A. S., Pauls, D. L., Leckman, J. F., & Cohen, D. J. (1994). A prospective longitudinal study of Gilles de la Tourette's syndrome. *Journal of the American Academy of Child and Adolescent Psychiatry, 33*(3), 377–385.

Cohen, D. J., & Leckman, J. L. (1994). Developmental psychopathology and neurobiology of Tourette's syndrome. *Journal of the American Academy of Child and Adolescent Psychiatry, 33,* 2–15.

Comings, D. E., & Comings, B. G. (1990). Alternative hypotheses on the inheritance of Tourette syndrome. *Advances in Neurology, 58,* 189–199.

Curtis, D., Robertson, M. M., & Gurling, H. M. D. (1992). Autosomal dominant gene transmission in a large kindred with Gilles de la Tourette syndrome. *British Journal of Psychiatry, 160,* 845–849.

Dykens, E. M. (1995). Measuring behavioral phenotypes: Provocations from the "new genetics." *American Journal of Mental Retardation, 99,* 522–532.

Flint, J., & Yule, W. (1994). Behavioral phenotypes. In M. Rutter, E. Taylor, & L. Hersov (Eds.), *Child and adolescent psychiatry: Modern approaches* (3rd ed., pp. 666–687). Oxford: Blackwell Scientific Publications.

Fu, Y. H., Kuhl, D. P., Pizzuti, A., Sutcliffe, J. S., Richards, S., Verkerk, A. J., Holden, J. A., Fenwick, R. G., Warren, S. T., Oostra, B. A., Nelson, D. L., & Caskey, C. T. (1991). Variation of the CGG repeat at the fragile site results in genetic instability: Resolution of the Sherman paradox. *Cell, 67,* 1047–1058.

Gedye, A. (1991). Tourette syndrome attributed to frontal lobe dysfunction: Numerous etiologies involved. *Journal of Clinical Psychology, 47,* 233–252.

Goetz, C. G., & Klawans, H. L. (1982). Gilles de la Tourette on Tourette syndrome. *Advances in Neurology, 35,* 1–16.

Grigorenko E. L., Wood, F. B., Meyer, M. S., Hart, L. A., Speed, W. C., Shuster, A., & Pauls, D. L. (1997). Susceptibility loci for distinct components of developmental dyslexia on chromosomes 6 and 15. *American Journal of Human Genetics, 60,* 27–39.

Hagerman, R. J. (1996). Physical and behavioral phenotype. In R. J. Hagerman & A. Chronister (Eds.), *Fragile X syndrome: Diagnosis, treatment and research* (2nd ed., pp. 3–87) Baltimore: Johns Hopkins University Press.

Hasstedt, J. S., Leppert, M., Filloux, F., van de Wetering, B. J. M., & McMahon, W. M. (1995). Intermediate inheritance of Tourette syndrome, assuming assortative mating. *American Journal of Human Genetics, 57,* 682–689.

Leckman, J. F., Pauls, D. L., Peterson, B. S., Riddle, M. A., Anderson, G. M., & Cohen, D. J. (1992). Pathogenesis of Tourette syndrome: Clues from the clinical phenotype and natural history. *Advances in Neurology, 58,* 15–24.

Lewis, M., & Volkmar, F. (1990). Historic perspective on views of child and adolescent psychopathology. In *Clinical aspects of child and adolescent development* (3rd ed.). Philadelphia: Lea & Febiger.

Mansour, S. L., Goddard, J. M., & Capecchi, M. R. (1993). Mice homozygous for a targeted disruption of the proto-oncogene *int-2* have developmental defects in the tail and inner ear. *Development, 117,* 13–28.

McKusick, V. (1955). *Heritable disorders of connectivetissue.* St Louis, MO: C. V. Mosby.

McMahon, W. M., van de Wetering, B. J. M., Filloux, F., Betit, K., Coon, H., & Leppert, M. (1996). Bilineal transmission and phenotypic variation of Tourette's disorder in a large pedigree. *Journal of the American Academy of Child and Adolescent Psychiatry, 35*(5), 672–680.

Nyhan, W. L. (1972). Behavioral phenotype in organic genetic disease (Presidential address to the Society for Pediatric Research, May 1, 1971). *Pediatric Research, 6,* 1–9.

Nyhan, W. L. (1995). Foreword. In G. O'Brien & W. Yule (Eds.), *Behavioural phenotypes* (pp. ix–x). London: Mac Keith Press.

O'Brien, G., & Yule, W. (1995). Why behavioural phenotypes? In G. O'Brien & W. Yule (Eds.), *Behavioural phenotypes* (pp. 1–23). London: Mac Keith Press.

Online Mendelian Inheritance in Man OMIM. (1996). Center for Medical Genetics, Johns Hopkins University (Baltimore, MD), and National Center for Biotechnology Informaation, National Library of Medicine (Bethesda, MD), World Wide Web URL: http://www3.ncbi.nlm.nih.gov/omim/.

Ozonoff, S., Strayer, D. L., McMahon, W. M., & Filloux, F. (1994). Executive function abilities in autism and Tourette syndrome: An information processing approach. *Journal of Child Psychology and Psychiatry, 35*(6), 1015–1032.

Pauls, D. L., & Leckman, J. F. (1986). The inheritance of Gilles de la Tourette's syndrome and associated behaviors. *New England Journal of Medicine, 16,* 993–997.

Pennington, B. F. (1991). *Diagnosing learning disorders: A neuropsychological framework.* New York: Guilford Press.

Pennington, B. F. (1997). Using genetics to dissect cognition. *American Journal of Human Genetics, 60,* 13–16.

Pyeritz, R. E. (1989). Pleiotropy revisited: Molecular explanations of a classic concept. *American Journal of Medical Genetics, 34,* 124–134.

Rapin, I. (1987). Searching for the cause of autism: A neurologic perspective. In D. J. Cohen & A. M. Donnelan (Eds.), *Handbook of autism and pervasive developmental disorders* (pp. 710–718). New York: Wiley.

Sacks, O. (1987). *The Man Who Mistook His Wife for a Hat.* New York: Harper & Row.

Stoetter, B., Braun, A. R., Randolph, C., Gernert, J., Carson, R. E., Herscovitch, P., & Chase, T. N. (1992). Functional neuroanatomy of Tourette syndrome: Limbic-motor interactions studied with FDG PET. *Advances in Neurology, 58,* 213–226.

Terwilliger, J. D., & Ott, J. (1994) *Handbook of human genetic linkage*. Baltimore: Johns Hopkins Press.

The Tourette Syndrome Classification Study Group. (1993). Definitions and classification of tic disorders. *Archives of Neurology, 50,* 1013–1016.

Turk, J., & Hill, P. (1995). Behavioural phenotypes in dysmorphic syndromes. *Clinical Dysmorphology, 4,* 105–115.

van de Wetering, B. J. M., & Heutink, P. (1993). The genetics of the Gilles de la Tourette syndrome: A review. *Journal of Laboratory and Clinical Medicine, 121,* 638–645.

Contributors

Jane Adams
Department of Psychology
University of Massachusetts
Boston, MA

Marcia A. Barnes
Department of Psychology
The Hospital for Sick Children
Toronto, ON, Canada

Simon Baron-Cohen
Department of Experimental
Psychology
University of Cambridge
Cambridge, United Kingdom

Elizabeth Bates
Center for Research in Language
University of California, San Diego
La Jolla, CA

Margaret L. Bauman
Department of Neurology
Massachusetts General Hospital
Boston, MA

Ursula Bellugi
Laboratory for Cognitive
Neuroscience
The Salk Institute for Biological
Studies
La Jolla, CA

Jacquelyn Bertrand
Division of Birth Defects and
Developmental Disabilities
Centers for Disease Control
Atlanta, GA

Lori Buchanan
Department of Psychology
The Hospital for Sick Children
Toronto, ON, Canada

Merlin G. Butler
Section on Medical Genetics and
Molecular Medicine
Children's Mercy Hospital
Kansas City, MO

Dawn Delaney
Kennedy Center
Vanderbilt University
Nashville, TN

Maureen Dennis
Department of Psychology
The Hospital for Sick Children
Toronto, ON, Canada

Kim N. Dietrich
Department of Environmental
Health
University of Cincinnati Medical
Center
Cincinnati, OH

Elisabeth M. Dykens
Department of Psychiatry
UCLA Neuropsychiatric Institute
and Hospital
Los Angeles, CA

Jack M. Fletcher
Department of Pediatrics
University of Texas—Houston
Health Science Center
Houston, TX

Susan E. Folstein
Department of Psychiatry
Tufts New England Medical Center
Boston, MA

Barbara R. Foorman
Center for Academic and Reading
Skills
University of Texas—Houston
Health Science Center
Houston, TX

Albert Galaburda
Department of Neurology
Beth Israel Deaconess Medical
Center and Harvard University
Medical School
Boston, MA

Randi Jenssen Hagerman
Child Development Unit
The Children's Hospital
Denver, CO

John Harrison
CeNes Ltd
Cambridge, United Kingdom

Ross Hetherington
Department of Psychology
The Hospital for Sick Children
Toronto, ON, Canada

Greg Hickok
Department of Cognitive Science
University of California, Irvine
Irvine CA

Terry Jernigan
Department of Veterans Affairs
University of California San Diego
School of Medicine
San Diego, CA

Beth Joseph
Kennedy Center
Vanderbilt University
Nashville, TN

William E. MacLean, Jr.
Department of Psychology
University of Wyoming
Laramie, WY

Michele M. Mazzocco
Behavioral Neurogenetics
The Kennedy Krieger Institute
Baltimore, MD

William M. McMahon
Department of Psychiatry
University of Utah Medical School
Salt Lake City, UT

Carolyn B. Mervis
Department of Psychology
University of Louisville
Lousiville, KY

Debra Mills
Center for Research in Language
University of California San Diego
La Jolla, CA

Colleen A. Morris
Departments of Pediatrics,
Pathology, and Laboratory Medicine
University of Nevada School of
Medicine
Las Vegas, NV

Lynn Nadel
Department of Psychology
University of Arizona
Tucson, AZ

Bruce F. Pennington
Department of Psychology
University of Denver
Denver, CO

Allan L. Reiss
Department of Psychiatry
Stanford University
Stanford, CA

Mabel L. Rice
Department of Speech, Language
and Hearing Sciences
University of Kansas
Lawrence, KS

Byron F. Robinson
Department of Psychology
University of Louisville
Louisville, KY

Judith L. Ross
Department of Pediatrics
Jefferson Medical College of Thomas
Jefferson University
Philadelphia, PA

Joanne Rovet
Department of Psychology
The Hospital for Sick Children
Toronto, ON, Canada

Susan L. Santangelo
Department of Psychiatry
Tufts New England Medical Center
Boston, MA

Bennett A. Shaywitz
Department of Pediatrics and
Neurology
Yale University School of Medicine
New Haven, CT

Sally E. Shaywitz
Department of Pediatrics
Yale University School of Medicine
New Haven, CT

Marian Sigman
Department of Psychology
University of California Los Angeles
Los Angeles, CA

Helen Tager-Flusberg
Department of Psychology
University of Massachusetts
Boston, MA

Travis Thompson
Department of Psychology and
Human Development
Vanderbilt University
Nashville, TN

J. Bruce Tomblin
Department of Speech Pathology
and Audiology
University of Iowa
Iowa City, IA

Doris Trauner
Department of Neurosciences
University of California, San Diego
La Jolla, CA

Stefano Vicari
Peditric Neurology
Bambin' Gesu' Hospital and
Research Center
Rome, Italy

Xuyang Zhang
Department of Speech Pathology
and Audiology
University of Iowa
Iowa City, IA

Andrew Zinn
McDermott Center for Human
Growth and Development
University of Texas Southwestern
Medical School
Dallas, TX

Index